Conceptual Foundations:
The Bridge to Professional Nursing Practice

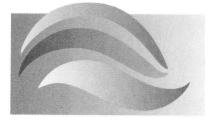

THIRD EDITION

Conceptual Foundations:
The Bridge to Professional Nursing Practice

Joan L. Creasia, PhD, RN

Professor and Dean
College of Nursing
University of Tennessee
Knoxville, Tennessee

Barbara Parker, PhD, RN, FAAN

Professor and Director
Center for Nursing Research and Doctoral Program
School of Nursing
University of Virginia
Charlottesville, Virginia

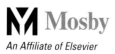
Mosby
An Affiliate of Elsevier

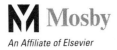
Mosby

An Affiliate of Elsevier

Vice President, Publishing Director, Nursing: Sally Schrefer
Senior Acquisitions Editor: Michael S. Ledbetter
Developmental Editor: Fran Murphy
Production Manager: Donna L. Morrissey

Library of Congress Cataloging-in-Publication Data

Conceptual foundations: the bridge to professional nursing practice/[edited by] Joan L. Creasia, Barbara Parker.—3rd ed.

   p. ; cm.

  Includes bibliographical references and index.

  ISBN-13: 978-0-323-01227-0 ISBN-10: 0-323-01227-2

   1. Nursing—Practice.   2. Nursing.   I. Creasia, Joan L.   II. Parker, Barbara, RN.   III.

Conceptual foundations of professional nursing practice.

  [DNLM: 1. Nursing.   2. Nursing Care. WY 16 C744 2001]

  RT86.7.C66 2001

  610.73—dc21   2001030284

ISBN-13: 978-0-323-01227-0
ISBN-10: 0-323-01227-2

Permissions may be sought directly from Elsevier's Health Sciences Rights Department in Philadelphia, USA: phone: (+1)215-238-7869, fax: (+1)215-238-2239, email: healthpermissions@elsevier.com. You may also complete your request on-line via the Elsevier Science homepage (http://www.elsevier.com), by selecting 'Customer Support' and then 'Obtaining Permissions'.

Mosby, Inc.
An Affiliate of Elsevier
11830 Westline Industrial Drive
St. Louis, Missouri 63146

Printed in the United States of America

Last digit is the print number: 9   8   7   6   5

Contributors

Kathleen M. Boyden, MSN, RN
Doctoral Student
University of Virginia
Charlottesville, Virginia

Barbara Brodie, PhD, RN, FAAN
Professor
School of Nursing
University of Virginia
Charlottesville, Virginia

Bonnie Jerome D'Emilia, PhD, MPH, RN
Assistant Professor
School of Nursing
University of Virginia
Charlottesville, Virginia

Sarah Farrell, PhD, RN
Assistant Professor
School of Nursing
University of Virginia
Charlottesville, Virginia

Sara T. Fry, PhD, RN, FAAN
Henry R. Luce Professor of Nursing Ethics
School of Nursing
Boston College
Chestnut Hill, Massachusetts

Audrey G. Gift, PhD, RN, FAAN
Professor
Michigan State University
East Lansing, Michigan

Mattia J. Gilmartin, PhD, RN
Research Associate
Post-Doctoral Fellow
The University of Cambridge
Judge Institute of Management
Cambridge, United Kingdom

Mary Gunther, PhD, RN
Instructor
College of Nursing
University of Tennessee
Knoxville, Tennessee

Susan K. Jacobs, MLS, RN
Health Sciences Librarian
Elmer Holmes Bobst Library
New York University
New York, New York

Kathryn Hopkins Kavanagh, PhD, RN
Professor
Northern Arizona University
Ganado, Arizona

Arlene W. Keeling, PhD, RN
Associate Professor
School of Nursing
University of Virginia
Charlottesville, Virginia

Mary L. Killeen, PhD, RN
Associate Dean for Undergraduate Programs and
    Continuing and Extended Education
College of Nursing
Arizona State University
Tempe, Arizona

Pamela A. Kulbok, DNSc, RN
Associate Professor
School of Nursing
University of Virginia
Charlottesville, Virginia

Gail O. Mazzocco, EdD, RN
Assistant Professor
School of Nursing
University of Maryland
Baltimore, Maryland

Patricia McMullen, JD, MS, RN
Associate Professor
Uniform Services University of the Health Sciences
Graduate School of Nursing
Bethesda, Maryland

Victoria Menzies, EdM, MS, RN
Doctoral Student
School of Nursing
University of Virginia
Charlottesville, Virginia

Teresa L. Panniers, PhD, RN
Associate Professor
Division of Nursing
School of Education
New York University
New York, New York

Anne Griswold Peirce, PhD, RN
Professor and Dean
School of Nursing
University of Mississippi Medical Center
Jackson, Mississippi

Nathaniel W. Peirce, EdM, EdD
Principal
St. Andrews Middle School
Ridgeland, Mississippi

C. Fay Raines, PhD, RN
Professor and Dean
College of Nursing
The University of Alabama-Huntsville
Huntsville, Alabama

Ann Gill Taylor, EdD, RN, FAAN
Betty Norman Norris Professor of Nursing
School of Nursing
University of Virginia
Charlottesville, Virginia

Sandra P. Thomas, PhD, RN, FAAN
Professor and Director, PhD Program
College of Nursing
University of Tennessee
Knoxville, Tennessee

Sharon W. Utz, PhD, RN
Associate Professor
School of Nursing
University of Virginia
Charlottesville, Virginia

Debra C. Wallace, PhD, RN
Associate Professor
College of Nursing
University of Tennessee
Knoxville, Tennessee

Janet B. Younger, PhD, NP, RN
Associate Dean, Undergraduate Nursing
School of Nursing
Virginia Commonwealth University
Richmond, Virginia

Preface

Nursing has undergone significant changes and faced many challenges during the past few decades in its quest for professionalism in practice. One influential force has been the American Nurses' Association's (ANA) 1965 recommendation that the minimum educational preparation for professional nurses be at the baccalaureate level. In more recent years, recommendations from the Pew Health Professions Commission and other esteemed groups described the need for nurses prepared at the baccalaureate level or higher. Although these recommendations have not been fully embraced by the nursing community, they have served to heighten awareness of the need for additional education. This prompted many nurses who received their basic education in an associate degree or a diploma program to return to school for a baccalaureate degree in nursing. Targeting RN-BSN students, the first edition of *Conceptual Foundations of Professional Nursing Practice* included concepts related to the nursing practice environment and concepts related to patient care, such as stress, pain, coping, crisis, and social support. The second edition omitted the patient care concepts, since they were covered in depth in other texts, and focused on the context, themes, and dimensions of nursing practice. Taking an approach similar to that used for the second edition, this edition reviews the influential forces that shaped the context of current nursing practice and analyzes dimensions and themes that have an impact on contemporary nursing practice.

Since the publication of the first edition, we became increasingly aware that our book was being used not only in RN-BSN completion programs but also in the foundational course in basic baccalaureate programs and in core courses in graduate nursing programs. This information, along with knowledge about the nurse's role in a changing and complex health care environment, influenced the selection of content for the third edition. Now titled *Conceptual Foundations: The Bridge to Professional Nursing Practice,* the book is relevant for use in both undergraduate and graduate nursing programs.

Approach

Changes in the health care delivery system have a major impact on nursing education and practice. Advanced technological developments, health policy issues, and reimbursement mechanisms play a major role in the planning and delivery of comprehensive nursing care. The focus on health promotion for individuals, families, and communities and efforts to control health care costs have given rise to alternative forms of health care delivery. In addition, the increased acuity of hospitalized patients and limited hospital stays have resulted in a greater demand for home and community health services. These changes have political, legal, and economic implications that must be incorporated into the educational foundation and professional practice of nurses. Chapters from the second edition that are included in the current edition were revised and updated to reflect these changes, with particular attention given to the ongoing evolution of nursing as a profession.

With the trend toward advanced education in nursing, a highly diverse student body is emerging. Second career men and women with valuable life experiences and students returning for renewed nursing careers are now commonplace in many nursing education programs. Nonnurses, often with degrees in other fields, are seeking entry into basic nursing programs or accelerated graduate programs. As a result, the student population as a whole tends to be more heterogeneous than traditional college students, both in terms of age and experience. These students, often described as adult learners, have an increased capacity for critical thinking and self-directed learning. Thus it is meaningful to develop a conceptual approach to nursing practice that encourages critical thinking and is applicable to diverse client groups and clinical settings. This book offers such an approach and can be used effectively to expand nursing knowledge.

Organization

Conceptual Foundations: The Bridge to Professional Nursing Practice comprehensively explores issues and concepts that influence professional practice and the delivery of nursing care. The book is divided into three parts. Part I, The Context of Professional Nursing Practice, begins with an exploration of historical events that shaped nursing practice and education. This is followed by an examination of issues related to professional socialization and role taking in nursing. Subsequently, an overview of client systems as the recipients of nursing care and frameworks and theories that provide structure for the discipline of nursing are presented. Two new chapters examining leadership and management in nursing and the case manager role are included in this section. Part I concludes with a description of the health care environment in which nurses practice and highlights current issues in health care delivery, such as cost, quality, and access.

Part II, Dimensions of Professional Nursing Practice, focuses on political, economic, legal, and ethical issues that have an impact on current practice. An overview of the legislative process and a review of health policies are followed by chapters on the economics of health care and legal aspects of nursing practice. Ethical principles and moral beliefs that are integral to nursing practice decisions are analyzed, and culturally sensitive approaches to effectively manage and treat our diverse client populations are discussed.

Part III, Themes in Professional Nursing Practice, includes client care concepts that are applicable to a variety of diverse populations and clinical practice settings as well as selected tools and strategies for effective nursing practice. An examination of the concepts of caring, health and health promotion, and teaching and learning is followed by a new chapter that examines alternative practices as a basis of holistic health care. Chapters on critical thinking and the process of change offer theories and frameworks for making decisions and effecting change in a dynamic health care environment. Chapters on nursing research and health care informatics describe the state of the discipline and highlight issues for further consideration.

Special Features

To help direct the reader's attention, each chapter begins with learning objectives. The Profile in Practice features a nurse whose practice reflects the focus of the chapter. Each chapter is developed in a similar format. An overview of the concept is followed by definitions of key terms, an in-depth discussion of the concept, and application of the concept to nursing practice. Research findings and material from current literature are integrated throughout the chapter. Significant facts and issues are highlighted at the end of the chapter as Key Points. Critical Thinking Exercises provide opportunities for the student to examine the content and apply it to nursing. A comprehensive and current reference list offers the opportunity to pursue further reading on the subject.

As each concept unfolds, the reader is challenged to discover new knowledge or reframe prior learning on a more conceptual and univer-

sally applicable level. Using this knowledge to enhance current and future nursing practice remains the final challenge.

Joan L. Creasia
Barbara Parker

Acknowledgments

We are deeply grateful to the many persons who have helped us bring this work to completion. Our special thanks go to the talented contributors who shared their knowledge, experience, and expertise in a form that is of immeasurable value to professional nurses, nursing students, and nurse educators.

The working relationship we shared as coauthors during the development of the first edition continued from afar through the development of the second and third editions. Once again, writing this book was a valuable and rewarding experience. Our working relationship, in addition to the support and encouragement of our families, enabled us to achieve our goal. We gratefully acknowledge the support of our husbands, Don Creasia and Dale Schumacher, and our children and their partners: Paul and Karen Creasia Yarrish, John and Tracey Creasia Hohenschutz, Andrea Schumacher and Bill LeConte, Meg Schumacher and John Boyd, and Peter Schumacher and Carol Brueggemeier.

We dedicate the third edition of *Conceptual Foundations: The Bridge to Professional Nursing Practice* to our grandchildren: Christina Marie Yarrish, Michael Anthony Yarrish, John Cameron Hohenschutz, Collette Schumacher LeConte, and Mollie Marie Boyd.

Joan L. Creasia
Barbara Parker

Contents

PART I

The Context of Professional Nursing Practice

The history, circumstances, frameworks, conditions, and settings of nursing practice collectively reflect its context. In this section the reader is invited to explore the evolution of nursing as a practice discipline, obtain a new awareness of the extent of the nurse's role, identify issues that cut across all areas of nursing practice, and gain an appreciation of the milieu within which nursing care is delivered.

The context of professional nursing practice constitutes those elements, both internal and external to the nurse, that are integral to the delivery of nursing care. This section begins with an overview of nursing practice and education. These chapters are presented along a historical time line, not only to illustrate the development of the profession, but also to provide an understanding of how nursing practice and education evolved to their present forms. A critical analysis of professional socialization further promotes an understanding of the evolution of nursing as a

practice discipline. A discussion of the array of roles nurses commonly assume, such as caregiver and teacher, and advanced practice roles, such as nurse practitioner and clinical specialist, provides an appreciation of the scope of nursing practice and the complexity of the nursing practice environment. A relatively new nursing role, that of case manager, is analyzed in greater depth. The chapter on nursing theories and frameworks describes an infrastructure within which nursing care may be designed, implemented, and evaluated; and an analysis of individual, family, and community client systems as the recipients of nursing care is presented. The symbiotic concepts of leadership and management and strategies for effective nursing leadership within a dynamic health care system are explored. Finally, a discussion of issues in health care delivery highlights the nursing practice environment and illustrates the movement of nursing beyond traditional boundaries to new frontiers.

Historical Highlights: The Foundations of Professional Nursing in the United States

BARBARA BRODIE, PhD, RN, FAAN, AND ARLENE W. KEELING, PhD, RN

OBJECTIVES

At the completion of this chapter, the reader will be able to:

- Describe the social, political, and governmental influences on the development of professional nursing in America from the late 19th to the 20th century.
- Describe the evolution of nurses' training from hospital-based programs to collegiate programs.
- Discuss the impact of war on the profession.
- Discuss the movement toward nursing licensure.
- Describe the history of discrimination against men and African Americans in nursing.
- Discuss the rise of advanced practice nursing, 1960–1990.
- Identify the challenges facing nursing at the turn of the 21st century.

PROFILE IN PRACTICE

Katharine C. Cook, MS, RN
Associate Professor
College of Notre Dame of Maryland
Baltimore, Maryland

I was born at the beginning of the baby-boom era in Bon Secours Hospital, Baltimore. Hospitals in America were certainly in vogue then for all matters of ailments (even natural events), and continued to be so for almost 50 years. As hospital length of stay shortens and care becomes more home and community focused, I have become fascinated by the history of nursing in cities like Baltimore before hospitals were the norm. What can we learn from the past to guide the current health care system?

Baltimore was experiencing tremendous growth in 1880 when the Sisters of Bon Secours were invited to establish a foundation. Most religious groups coming to America in the 19th century came to establish hospitals or to teach. The sisters of Bon Secours were among the earliest denominational groups to nurse the sick in their homes and minister holistically to physical, social, and spiritual needs. The sisters stayed in their patients' homes for up to 3 months at a time, nursing both rich and poor, regardless of color, creed, or religious beliefs. Nursing sisters were also assigned to home visit the poorest, especially the immigrants who settled in the slums of South and East Baltimore.

As the sisters cared for the sick through the great epidemics that plagued cities at the turn of the 19th century, they relied on guidelines conceived in the early 19th century and carried by the Bon Secours from France to America. What impressed me as I read these nursing guidelines was the similarity in content to Florence Nightingale's *Notes on Nursing,* which was not published until 17 years later.

It is evident that religious order nursing in America started as an innovative, autonomous practice and that the sisters worked collaboratively with other health professionals of the time. It gives me great pride in my profession and confidence that we, as nurses, can continue to have an impact on society's health by forging partnerships with others in public service and rendering care in community settings. It reinforces my decision to become a nurse and my desire to make a larger impact on health care. We need to communicate and celebrate this with one another and to the next generation of nurses.

"No occupation can be intelligently followed or understood unless it is, at least to some extent, illumined by the light of history. . . .

● *Dock & Stewart, 1931, p. 3*

The development of clinical nursing research is a recent phenomenon in the history of the profession. For over a century, the foundation of clinical nursing was built on a rich empirical basis of practice. To understand what led the profession to subject its clinical practice to scientific and philosophical scrutiny requires a historical examination of the development of the profession.

Today's nursing profession is a composite and distillation of over 100 years of development. Its practitioners (and the clinical and ethical dimensions of its practice), its relationship with patients, and its place in society have been forged by powerful social forces that created the American health care system. More specifically, contemporary nursing was shaped by society's views on women and nursing care, advances in medical science, the growth of hospitals and public health, changes in the philosophy of science, philanthropic and government initiatives, and the actions of nurse leaders who struggled to transform a domestic vocation into a professional discipline.

Origins

In the last quarter of the 19th century, the United States was changing from a homogeneous population in an agrarian, rural culture to a highly heterogeneous population in an industrialized, urban culture. Millions of immigrants flowed into the country, seeking new lives and economic opportunities. Joining forces with American-born citizens, they built new cities, fueled the growth of industry, and expanded the nation. With each development came new challenges and opportunities for women and men to create new roles and institutions. Caring for the ill and protecting the health of society offered the nursing profession a major role in the creation of the 20th century's health care enterprise.

WOMEN'S ROLE IN CARING

The health of the American family has always been viewed by society as a responsibility of women, usually as a function of their role as mothers. Birth, illness, and dying took place in the home under the watchful ministration of women because it was believed that women possessed a maternal instinct that directed them to care for the sick. To care for the ill without family support, colonial American communities established almshouses that served as refuges for the needy poor and infirmaries for the sick. The nursing and medical care provided to their residents, however, reflected both the low social status of the indigent and society's dismal ignorance about diseases. Physicians avoided almshouses, preferring to practice in the homes of their private patients. The scant nursing care provided almshouse residents was given by other residents or by female prisoners sentenced to serve their prison time in the infirmary ward. Although a few religious women's groups cared for the indigent sick, it was not considered proper for a "decent" woman to enter an almshouse.

THE BIRTH OF THE NURSING PROFESSION IN AMERICA

The Civil War (1861–1865) provided a strong catalyst for women to move out of their homes and into nursing. The war created a great demand for nurses to care for the sick and wounded soldiers in both the North and the South. Following Florence Nightingale's example in the Crimean War (1851–1855), women volunteered to serve in hospitals, infirmaries, and on the battlefields, caring for the injured and dying. Their experience confirmed that intelligent nursing care was essential in the treatment of hospitalized patients and that women were particularly suited for this occupation. Several prominent women and men who served in hospitals during the war drew from their experiences to create hospital nursing schools. In 1873, America's first three Nightingale-modeled schools—Bellevue Training School for Nurses, in New York City, Connecticut Training School for Nurses, in New Haven, Connecticut, and the Boston Training School for Nurses at Massachusetts General Hospital—were established (Dock, 1907).

Loosely following the Nightingale form of apprenticeship training, these nursing schools attracted single women seeking an occupation that promised higher wages and status than were generally available to females. The training programs stressed on-the-job learning, and although the work was physically daunting and the hospitals demanded loyalty, obedience, and duty from pupils, the training promised young women an opportunity to become self-supporting, independent private-duty nurses employed in patients' homes.

Hospital administrators (many of whom were physicians) of these early hospital programs recognized that, with only a modest financial investment, the quality of their patient services was dramatically improved by using "pupil nurses" (as they were known in that era). Soon, across the United States, hospitals developed nursing schools to acquire a labor force of intelligent, skillful, and obedient pupil nurses. So rapidly did schools grow that by 1900 there were 432 schools in the country (Roberts, 1954).

The birth of professional nursing coincided with dramatic advances in the medical sciences, including the discovery of anesthesia, Pasteur and Koch's work in bacteriology, and Lister's innovations in surgical antisepsis. These advances laid the foundation for modern surgery and medicine and, combined with the services of nurses, transformed almshouses from refuges for the destitute to therapeutic hospitals that provided relief from diseases and care for the ill. Although hospitals were used primarily by the poor, by the 1890s they were proving their importance in the practice and education of physicians. Physicians discovered that hospitals with nursing programs helped attract paying patients, and because student nurses dutifully followed medical orders, doctors were able to develop new treatments (Rosenberg, 1987).

The two purposes of hospital schools—to provide patient services and to train nurses—often conflicted. Although nursing superintendents, responsible for the quality of patient nursing services, believed that caring for patients was essential in the preparation of a nurse, they worried that too much of the students' time was devoted to staffing the hospital. In addition to providing clinical patient care, students were responsible for the hospital's cleanliness and organization and for preparing patients' meals. Student educational needs were often either ignored or only partially met. The demands of patient services required that nursing lectures be scheduled in the evenings after students had worked a 12-hour day (Fig. 1–1). Superintendents struggled to balance the conflicting demands of nursing service and educa-

tion but were often powerless to remedy the conflict. Furthermore, to ensure that the hospital had an adequate supply of student workers, admission and training standards were kept low. Superintendents who attempted to increase the educational content of the program or who sought auxiliary help to relieve students of housekeeping activities faced being reprimanded or discharged.

In 1893, Isabel Hampton, superintendent of the Johns Hopkins Hospital School of Nursing, brought together at the Chicago Columbian Exposition many of the superintendents of America's largest schools to discuss nursing education problems. Adopting many of the strategies used by the American Medical Association to upgrade their profession, the superintendents initiated a plan to gain control of nursing education and to raise its standards (Dock & Stewart, 1931).

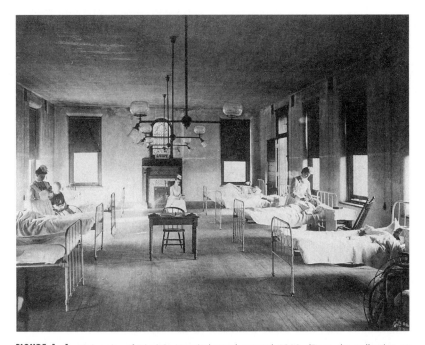

FIGURE 1–1 University of Virginia Hospital ward around 1910. (From the collection at the Center for Nursing Historical Inquiry, University of Virginia, School of Nursing, Charlottesville.)

Steps to Professionalization

The first step in the long struggle to transform nursing from a vocation to a profession was the establishment of the American Society of Superintendents of Training Schools for Nurses of the United States and Canada, in 1894. (In 1912 the organization was renamed the National League of Nursing Education, or NLNE.) This organization would serve as the focal point for ideas and strategies used by nurses across the nation to gain professional status for nursing. The early nursing leaders also recognized that graduate nurses faced serious problems in establishing their role in society, especially one that couldn't differentiate between a trained and an untrained nurse. The public's growing perception that many of their physical ills could be relieved by modern medicine created a growing demand for the services of nurses. Women who merely claimed to be nurses, however, competed with trained nurses for employment. Vexed by national census data revealing that there were almost 109,000 "untrained nurses and midwives competing with 12,000 graduate nurses," nurse leaders initiated activities to rectify this threatening situation (U.S. Bureau of Census, 1900, p. xxiii). In 1896, a small group of nurses founded the Nurses' Associated Alumnae of the United States and Canada (renamed the American Nurses Association [ANA] in 1912) (Nutting, 1926).

NURSE REGISTRATION

The first initiative of the Nurses' Associated Alumnae (and heartily endorsed by the superintendents group) was the acquisition of legal registration for nurses. Registration was first discussed by British nurses. Opposition from Florence Nightingale, who feared that legal certification would weaken the moral training of nurses, slowed the British nurses' registration movement. American nurses, however, believed that the moral underpinnings of nurses' training would not be weakened by state regulations. They understood that the legal power of the state could be utilized to upgrade the educational and clinical standards of nursing.

The swift passage of new medical practice acts at the turn of the 20th century served as an example of how medical educators and state medical societies gained legal monopolies over the provision of certain services and strengthened their powers of self-regulation over practice and medical education (Friedman, 1965). By making nursing licensure dependent on the graduates' educational credentials and performance on a qualifying examination, nursing pioneers believed that the individual state licensure boards would force nursing schools to adopt higher educational standards. Licensure would therefore protect the public from inadequately prepared nurses and, in doing so, enhance the economic and social standing of the registered nurse and the profession.

In a salient article in the first issue of the *American Journal of Nursing,* Lavinia Dock outlined a rationale for state licensure and methods that nurses could use to activate the political process. Dock, one of nursing's most analytical leaders and foremost historians, cautioned the politically neophyte nurses that in order to succeed, they would need to form medical and social coalitions. Furthermore, she noted that once legal power was attained, "continuous efforts for the rest of time" would be required to ensure nursing a professional status in the health care arena (Dock, 1900).

The Nurses' Associated Alumnae quickly moved to establish associated state organizations so that nurses could conduct the necessary political lobbying for the enactment of state registration laws. The quest for licensure encouraged cohesiveness among nurses and provided them with a structure that allowed private-duty nurses and educators to address common nursing problems. The quest also taught them ways to align themselves temporarily with special-interest groups that benefited from the closing of small hospitals whose training programs could not meet licensing standards (Tomes, 1983).

In March 1903, the North Carolina State Nurses Association was the first to acquire a registration act. Other registration acts were enacted in New Jersey, New York, and Virginia later in the same year. Although lacking in universal educational standards and in a definition of nursing practice, the first registration acts defined for the public that a "registered nurse" had attended an acceptable nursing program and passed a board evaluation examination. The licensure acts also created state nursing boards, which were empowered to employ some force to remedy educational deficits in schools of nursing.

By 1910, in spite of the fact that women lacked the right to vote, 27 states had enacted nurse registration laws. By 1923 all of the states in the nation plus Hawaii and the District of Columbia had nurse registration laws (Bullough, 1975). Over the years, nursing has used state registration and certification laws to update and expand the practice of professional nursing.

COMMUNITY HEALTH NURSING

The rapid urbanization and industrialization of the United States at the turn of the 20th century was fueled by a massive influx of immigrants. Between 1890 and 1910 almost 19 million immigrants sought new lives in America, especially in the cities. As a result, the population in cities with over 100,000 inhabitants rose by 12 million (Taylor, 1971).

Crowded into squalid tenements in ethnic ghettos, immigrants straggled to survive and raise their families. In the 1870s, groups of American women, concerned about the health conditions of the immigrants, employed graduate nurses to visit the ghetto poor. Under the auspices of private philanthropy, the Boston and Philadelphia Visiting Nurse Societies were founded in the 1880s. The role of the community health nurse, however, was firmly established by the actions of Lillian Wald, a graduate nurse (Buhler-Wilkerson, 1989).

In 1893 New York City not only served as the country's major port of entry, it was also home to the largest number of immigrants. Wald, a recent graduate of the New York Hospital Training School, was teaching a home nursing class to immigrants on the city's Lower East Side when she was asked to visit an ill woman in the tenements. The shock of finding a desperately ill, bedridden woman lying in the residue of 2-day-old hemorrhage profoundly influenced Wald's life. From this point on she devoted her life to the care of the country's forgotten poor and immigrant families (Wald, 1938).

Securing financial support from wealthy benefactors, Wald and fellow nurse Mary Brewster lived in an East Side apartment and began offering nursing services to their neighbors. The community's need for nursing care soon necessitated more nurses and a move to larger quarters. In 1895 the famed Henry Street Settlement House and Henry Street Visiting Nurse Services came into existence.

Under Wald's innovative leadership, many creative roles for community nurses were launched. In 1902, Wald offered the services of one of her nurses to the New York City school board in an experimental program. Wald believed that children's absenteeism from school because of illness could be reduced. In 1 month, the high absenteeism rates were reduced so significantly that the city hired the nurse. The following year the city employed 27 additional nurses to work within the school system. Within 2 years, in cities across the country, school nurses were being hired to provide essential health services to children (Struthers, 1917).

In 1909, community services were further expanded by Wald in a joint project with the

Metropolitan Life Insurance Company. The project sent nurses into the homes of the company's customers when they were ill. The money this project saved the company encouraged Metropolitan Life to contract for similar nursing services with over 400 visiting nurse agencies in the United States and Canada by 1912. Other major insurance companies followed suit, employing nurses to provide health services to their industrial policy owners. This business relationship subsidized the growth of individual nursing agencies and taught nurses the importance of patient record keeping and health statistics. It also taught nurses to understand how patient costs affected the outcome of their services (Hamilton, 1989). Metropolitan Life Insurance Company, through pioneer health surveys done with nurses, became the authoritative source of data on the nation's health status (Hamilton, 1992).

Additional community services, such as industrial nursing in 1895, tuberculosis nursing in 1903, and infant welfare nursing, arising from the clean milk movement of the 1900s, expanded the domain of nurses. Mary Gardner, an early public health leader and author, estimated that the 200 public health nurses existing in 1900 had grown to approximately 3,000 by 1912 (Gardner, 1936). The development of public health nursing was important to the nation and the profession because it brought essential health services to the public and provided nurses opportunities to integrate sanitation and epidemiology knowledge into the care and education of patients. Just as important, community nurses expanded the domain of nursing practice to include individuals, families, and communities. Their pioneer activities in health promotion and disease prevention and their stand on welfare reforms were vital in shaping America's public health system and the discipline of nursing (Bullough, 1978).

In 1912 the National Organization for Public Heath Nursing (NOPHN) became nursing's first clinical specialty national organization. Lillian Wald named the specialty public health nursing in the hope that the newly emerging fields of health nursing and preventive medicine could be linked to better meet the health needs of the public (Brainard, 1922).

The NOPHN worked closely with the federal government's Children's Bureau to implement studies on the nation's high infant/maternal mortality and morbidity rates. These studies, and the publicity they received, emphasized families' need for infant and obstetrical care services, especially low-income rural families. As a result, in 1921 Congress enacted the Sheppard-Towner Maternal and Infant Act. Forty-five states quickly passed legislation to qualify for the government's matching funds. With these funds the states developed new maternal and infant programs for at-risk mothers and children. Nurses were critical to the states' success in bringing, for the first time, health services to families in remote regions of the country (Brodie, 1993) (Fig. 1–2).

In 1925, 561 permanent child health and prenatal centers were opened, and a total of 21,935 health-related conferences were given by nurses and physicians. Public health nurses also provided 299,100 instructional home visits and contacted thousands of local physicians to ensure that infants and mothers in need of medical care received help (Meckel, 1990). Opposition, primarily from the American Medical Association, terminated this program in 1929, but the precedent had been set for the federal government's involvement in the provision of health care to citizens through its states.

PRIVATE-DUTY NURSING

Hospital administrators' belief that student nursing services were adequate for patient needs left little opportunity for registered nurses to find employment in hospitals. The majority of graduates therefore, continued to work as private-duty nurses in the homes of families. Working as independent practitioners and committed to individual patient care, graduate nurses enjoyed being professionally indepen-

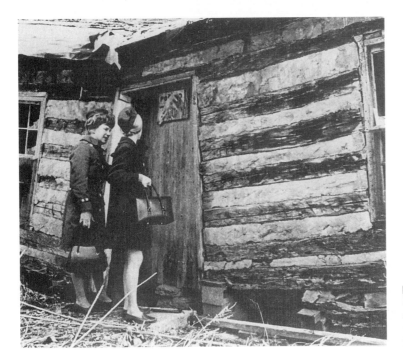

FIGURE 1-2 Home visit by a public health nurse in the 1960s. (From the collection at the Center for Nursing Historical Inquiry, University of Virginia, School of Nursing, Charlottesville.)

dent. By the 1920s, however, employment opportunities for graduates grew scarce. Improvements in public health reduced communicable diseases in the community, thus leaving fewer patients needing nurses. Those patients available were now referred to nurses by physicians or through nurse registries. To assure themselves of employment, nurses had to please physicians and be available within hours to be dispatched to patients' homes. Once assigned to a patient, the nurse worked in periods of 12 to 24 hours for as many days as necessary. The work, often involving domestic chores, was exhausting and socially isolating. In addition, the pay was poor. The annual earnings of a nurse in the late 1910s averaged about $950, a sum that sustained her but left little savings for future needs (Reverby, 1987).

By 1920 the plight of the private-duty nurse had become grimmer. Families that had been able to afford nurses in their homes when illness occurred now used hospitals. Although families might still engage a private-duty nurse for a hospitalized family member, once the medical crisis had passed they relied on the hospital's student nurse staff for the patient's recovery. Physicians and hospital administrators supported this decision because not having to pay for the services of private-duty nurses left families better able to pay the physicians' and hospitals' bills (Reverby, 1983).

Advances in medicine during this decade encouraged more people to use hospitals. Instead of adding graduate nurses to their staffs to meet the increased patient census, hospital directors increased the numbers of their student nurses. Concerned about the economic plight of graduate nurses, the NLNE, ANA, and NOPHN authorized a study of the economic status of nursing in 1926. May Ayers Burgess, the statistician who directed the study, documented both widespread underemployment of graduates and the harshness of their working conditions (Burgess, 1928).

A survey of New York State nurses by Janet Geister, a strong advocate of private-duty nurses, also confirmed registered nurses' economic difficulties. She reported that even when they found work, 80% of nurses were able to obtain patient cases that lasted only one day. This level of employment provided them with a weekly salary of $31.26. The nurses' hourly rate had sunk so low it now averaged 49 cents, less than the 50 cents an hour that scrubwomen earned (Geister, 1926).

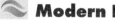 ## Modern Hospitals

By the 1920s, America's appreciation of the benefits of scientific medicine was reflected in the proliferation of hospitals and in the increased social status of physicians who used them. Between 1925 and 1929, $890 million was spent on the construction of hospitals.

Modern obstetrics, with its promise of "twilight sleep" to reduce the pain of childbirth, brought women into hospitals to deliver their babies. Furthermore, the addition of pediatric, psychiatric, and physical therapy services and private patient rooms enhanced the hospital's image in the eyes of the consumer (Roren, 1930) (Fig. 1–3).

While hospital medical care had become increasingly sophisticated, the inexpensive and unsophisticated labor provided by student nurses was still acceptable to most hospital administrators and physicians. They feared that employing registered nurses would increase hospital costs and would allow graduates unnecessary involvement in medical and hospital decisions. As one physician-administrator noted, nursing was "only a differentiation of domestic duty" and the graduate nurse a "half-baked social product thrust into the fulfillment of an uncertain social need" (Howard, 1912).

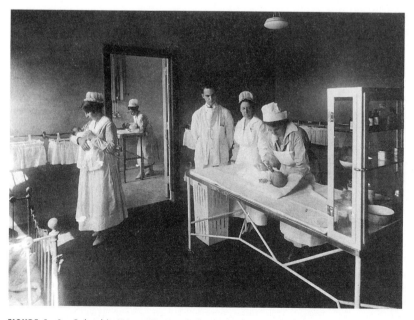

FIGURE 1–3 Columbia Women's Hospital, Washington, D.C., in the 1920s. (From the collection at the Center for Nursing Historical Inquiry, University of Virginia, School of Nursing, Charlottesville.)

Nursing educators, through the NLNE and state boards of nursing, continued in their struggle to convince hospitals that graduate nurses should provide more patient services so that students might be better educated in the science of nursing. Even after the publication of the shocking landmark Goldmark Report, a study of nursing education that uncovered glaring educational deficiencies in the country's best programs, few hospital directors were persuaded that their programs required any upgrading of their educational standards (Goldmark, 1923).

THE DEPRESSION YEARS

The economic depression that gripped the country in the 1930s drastically altered American life. The sharp decline in the world's economy caused financial, social, and health problems for the nation. Business failures and unemployment spread throughout the country, and by 1932, one out of four working Americans was without a job (Blum, 1981).

Hospital administrators, faced with a drastic reduction in the number of paying patients, were forced to examine the costs of providing care. This examination included the costs of nursing services. Many small hospitals closed or terminated their schools of nursing in an effort to reduce costs. At the same time, large hospitals, especially municipal ones, experienced a large influx of patients seeking charitable care. To rectify this situation, Blue Cross, a revolutionary prepaid health insurance plan, was developed by groups of hospitals (Numbers, 1978). Selling health plans to workers able to pay for future hospitalizations proved to be an engaging idea, and it helped ensure the financial stability of these hospitals.

The American Medical Association, however, rejected the new health plan, characterizing it as being "economically unsound, unethical and inimical to the public interests" (Kimball, 1934). In spite of the AMA's opposition, Blue Cross proved to be attractive to hospitals and patients, and because it kept community hospitals open,

it was formally endorsed by the American Hospital Association in 1937. As one hospital official noted, "Blue Cross was sired by the Depression and mothered by hospitals out of desperate economic necessity" (Sommers & Sommers, 1961, p. 21). Over 1 million people participated as members of Blue Cross in 1937, providing hospitals with enough income not only to remain open but also to grow.

STAFF NURSING

Nurses' training programs, however, continued to be seen as a financial drain by many hospitals. The cost of maintaining nursing schools proved so expensive that 570 training programs were closed in the 1930s. At first, hospitals replaced student nurses with untrained attendants. In time, however, it became evident that graduate nurses were essential to the provision of safe patient care. This recognition on the part of hospital administrators, coupled with the availability of unemployed graduate nurses willing to work for minimum wages and with the new income from health insurance and government programs, led to an increase in the employment of graduate nurses (Fitzpatrick, 1975).

The addition of graduate nurses to hospital staffs, from 4,000 positions in 1929 to 28,000 in 1937 and to over 100,000 by 1941, immensely improved the quality of patient services. It also introduced a new professional tension within the hospital system (Cannings & Lazonick, 1975). Many hospital administrators were accustomed to student nurses providing patient care. They considered paying for graduate nursing services unreasonable. In addition, registered nurses were viewed as a potential threat to administrators and physicians because they were far less compliant than students and their clinical decisions were based on their professional judgments rather than hospital routine.

Graduate nurses, although welcoming the steady hospital employment and the opportunity to develop new clinical and management skills, also experienced new professional conflicts. As independent, private-duty practitioners, they possessed the power to establish the quality care they provided their patients. Staff nursing, however, required that they function in a bureaucracy that demanded loyalty to the institution and the physician rather than to the patients. The hospital's employment of lower-paid, subsidiary nursing and housekeeping staff also added managerial responsibilities to the role of staff nurses. For many nurses, these new responsibilities were not nursing tasks, and the strict institutional control of their clinical practice reminded them of the harsh discipline, regimentation, and exploitation of their former student days (Flood, 1981).

Given the economic realities of the Great Depression, however, graduate nurses and administrators began an uneasy working alliance. Learning how to interact with professional graduates rather than a student staff challenged hospital directors for decades. Well into the 1950s and later, hospitals failed to establish personnel policies that befitted professional nurses. Instead, as historian Susan Reverby notes, hospitals offered registered nurses "low pay, long hours, split shifts, authoritarian supervision, and rigid rules" (Reverby, 1987, p. 192).

Collegiate Nursing Education: The Early Years

In 1899, with the offering of a post-diploma hospital economics program at Teachers College, Columbia University, nursing marked its first venture into an academic institution. The original program, conceived by Isabel Hampton Robb, was designed, partially taught, and voluntarily funded by NLNE members. The program prepared nurses to manage nursing services and educate pupil nurses. A generous endowment of $200,000 in 1910 by Helen Hartley Jenkins, a trustee of Teachers College, financially established the department in the

college and allowed for its expansion. Directed for 40 years by two excellent educators, Mary Adelaide Nutting and Isabel Stewart, the department offered innovative programs in administration, education, and public health nursing to thousands of nurses from the United States and abroad (Christy, 1969).

Several short-lived basic collegiate programs also opened in the 1890s, but it was the University of Minnesota in 1909 that established the first permanent university-related nursing program in the United States. The inability of hospital training programs to improve the educational experiences for students convinced nurse leaders to establish university programs, and by 1923 there were 17 schools offering 5-year degree programs. Because of time and financial costs, enrollment in these institutions remained low compared to diploma programs. While nursing had made some progress toward undergraduate collegiate status, it lacked the major financial support given to the profession of medicine by philanthropic organizations.

Large financial endowments, primarily from the Rockefeller, Carnegie, and Commonwealth foundations, moved medical education into the mainstream of university education and allowed it to expand. The famous 1910 Flexner Report, reporting on the inadequacies of medical education, acted as a catalyst for this action. The Rockefeller General Education Board alone funneled over $91 million into medical schools (Starr, 1982, p. 121). Nursing leaders, impressed with the ability of medicine to enter universities and develop into a scientific discipline, sought similar assistance for nursing education. Only the Rockefeller Foundation, however, could be persuaded to endow the establishment of two schools—Yale in 1924 and Vanderbilt in 1930 (Abram, 1993).

Annie Goodrich, noted nursing educator and director of the Army School of Nursing in 1918, was selected to direct the first independent collegiate school at Yale University. The baccalaureate program was based on the premise that nursing concepts pertinent to acute illness, the psychosocial dimensions of illness, and public health were foundational to professional nursing practice. Using a "case method" approach to patient care rather than teaching nursing techniques, and assigning nursing students to various clinical agencies for educational experiences, Yale faculty demonstrated what collegiate nursing would become (Sheahan, 1979).

In 1923, Frances Payne Bolton endowed the Department of Nursing Education at Western Reserve University, in Cleveland. Soon Western Reserve University and Yale University would offer baccalaureate and master's degrees in nursing education (Faddis, 1973). Catholic University of America began offering graduate courses in 1932, and the University of Chicago developed a graduate program in 1934 (Baer, 1992). By 1935 there was a sufficient number of collegiate programs to organize the Association of Collegiate Schools of Nursing. This organization's major mission was to establish collegiate nursing programs in America's universities. Its members strongly maintained that nursing could not become a profession until it could generate scientifically sound nursing knowledge and teach it to students (Stewart, 1943).

GOVERNMENT INITIATIVES

A characteristic of 20th century America has been the federal government's involvement in matters pertaining to the health and welfare of its citizens. Since nurses were consistently involved in this arena, the affairs of nursing have been significantly influenced by the actions of the government. The government's first involvement with nursing came as a result of wartime emergencies. Beginning with the Civil War, both the Union and Confederate armies sought the services of women to care for their ill and wounded troops. During the Spanish-American War in 1898, nurses volunteered to serve in the army to care for thousands of soldiers suffering from yellow fever. This experience persuaded Congress that nurses should be permanent members of the nation's defense forces. As a result, the Army Nurse Corps was created in 1901, and the Navy Nurse Corps in 1908.

State governments were also involved with nursing in the early years. At the turn of the century, when professional nurses sought to protect the public from untrained practitioners and to upgrade nursing educational standards, state governments supported nursing's claim to special knowledge and expertise and passed nurse registration legislation.

During World War I (1917–1919), nursing leaders cooperated with the federal government to mobilize nurses to serve in the war effort. Innovative programs designed to increase the supply of nurses, such as Vassar College's nursing program and the Army School of Nursing, were devised by nurses and supported by the government (Clappison, 1964; Koch, 1951).

The economic depression of the 1930s created a profound national emergency. The severity and length of the depression threatened the political stability of the country and the health of its people. During President Franklin D. Roosevelt's first term (1932–1936), Congress enacted emergency legislation that created jobs to improve the nation's health and welfare. The Federal Emergency Relief Act and the Works Progress Administration provided health and medical care for needy indigent citizens and also provided employment for thousands of nurses in hospitals and public health agencies. In addition, passage of the Social Security Act in 1935, with its financial aid for the elderly and Title V health care benefits, extended the government's mandate for the well-being of its citizens (Stevens, 1971).

WORLD WAR II

As war spread throughout Europe and the Eastern Hemisphere in 1939, the United States prepared for the possibility of military involvement. When Congress declared war on December 8, 1941, however, an inadequate supply of nurses for military and civilian needs created a dangerous situation. To deal with this crisis, the federal government created two programs to ease the nursing shortage: the American Red Cross volunteer nurse's aides program (1941), and the Cadet Nurse Corps (1943) (Johnston, 1966) (Fig. 1–4).

The American Red Cross nurse's aides program grew out of the country's need for nursing personnel. The loss of professional and non-professional staff to the military and defense industry left hospitals and public health agencies in need of auxiliary help to care for citizens on the home front. Through a joint venture with the Office of Civilian Defense and the American Red Cross, over 200,000 women volunteered to become certified nurse's aides and work under nursing supervision to provide nursing services. This successful venture proved to be an

important step in the stratification of nursing functions into registered, practical, and aide levels (Bullough & Bullough, 1978). This nursing stratification not only would continue after the war, it would also lead to new educational programs and licensure.

The Cadet Nurse Corps was the most significant program sponsored by the federal government to increase the supply of professional nurses. In 1943, Congresswoman Frances Payne Bolton from Ohio, long a friend of nursing, sponsored a bill that authorized the U.S. Public Health Service to establish the Cadet Nurse Corps. The Cadet Nurse Corps subsidized the education of nursing students who agreed, upon graduation, to serve in military or civilian agencies for the duration of the war. The program provided students with tuition, fees, and

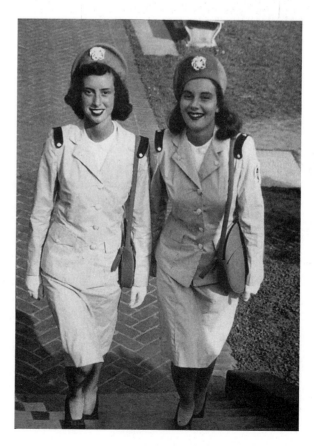

FIGURE 1–4 Cadet nurses in the 1940s. (From the collection at the Center for Nursing Historical Inquiry, University of Virginia, School of Nursing, Charlottesville.)

books, and a monthly stipend throughout their training. Nursing schools that participated in the program also received funds for instructional facilities and postgraduate education for their nursing faculty.

Although the cadet corps accepted students for only 2 years (July 1943 to October 1945), almost 170,000 cadets entered 1,125 participating schools, and two-thirds of these students graduated. The Cadet Nurse Corps not only recruited a large number of students into the profession, it also led to major changes in nursing education. The government requirements of a 30-month (versus a 36-month) program, a 48-hour (versus a 56-hour) student workweek of classes and clinical work, and the removal of school policies that discriminated on the basis of race and marital status allowed faculty an opportunity to redesign nursing education. In addition, because the federal money had to be administered by the schools' nursing directors, the costs of the educational programs and of

the services the students provided to hospitals became known. Armed with this new information, school directors were better equipped to negotiate with hospitals for the funds necessary to upgrade their programs (Brueggemann, 1992).

NURSING AND MINORITIES

As another method of increasing the availability of graduate nurses for the war, the profession turned to two groups that had long been excluded from mainstream nursing: African Americans and men (Fig. 1–5). The race and gender biases of the era led to harsh discriminatory and restrictive policies regarding admission into most nursing schools and employment opportunities for African-American and male graduate nurses. Because of their race, Negro women wishing to become nurses were restricted to attending the available Negro hospitals' schools of nursing in the country. Even after graduating

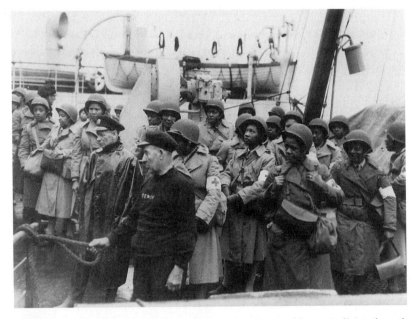

FIGURE 1–5 African-American U.S. Army nurses during World War II. (From the collection at the Center for Nursing Historical Inquiry, University of Virginia, School of Nursing, Charlottesville.)

and becoming registered nurses, many hospitals and community health agencies refused to employ Negro nurses, citing objections from white patients to being cared for by Negro nurses. The racial discrimination faced by Negro nurses extended to denying them membership in some of the state associations of the ANA. To overcome the multiple forms of discrimination experienced by these nurses, the National Association of Colored Graduate Nurses (NACGN) was formed in 1908. This group fought valiantly against the social, economical, and professional injuries inflicted on Negro graduate nurses (Staupers, 1951).

The bias against male nurses was predicated on society's belief that nursing was a feminine characteristic, and therefore men should not be nurses. Although a few nursing schools of the era were coeducational, most male nurses had attended all-male programs sponsored by religious groups or affiliated with psychiatric hospitals. Many hospitals were willing to hire male graduate nurses but often treated them as orderlies rather than as professional nurses. In 1940, male nurses formed the Men Nurses' Section of the ANA to improve the educational and employment opportunities for men and to persuade the government to allow male nurses to serve in the Army or Navy Nurse Corps (Craig, 1940).

Although Negro and male nurses numbered less than 10,000 of the 280,000 registered nurses in the United States in 1940, they represented a valuable resource to the nation. In addition, many young Negro women wished to serve their country by becoming nurses. Through the joint efforts of professional nursing groups, especially the NACGN, ANA, and NLNE, the Cadet Nurse Corps was opened to Negro schools. In addition, to meet the student quota required for Cadet Nurse Corps funding, some traditionally "white-only" programs accepted Negro students. By 1945, Negro enrollment in the nation's nursing schools reached a record high of almost 2,600 students,

a 135% increase from the 1939 figure (Hines, 1989).

Racial barriers against Negro nurses were also lifted when restrictive employment practices in hospitals and public health agencies changed. Because many civilian health facilities lost many of their graduates to the Army and Navy Nurse Corps, they were more willing to add Negro nurses to their staffs (Osborne, 1949).

For Negro nurses, however, the task of gaining admission to the Army and Navy Nurse Corps proved more difficult than gaining employment in civilian hospitals. The Army Nurse Corps maintained restrictive racial quotas, and the Navy Nurse Corps excluded all Negroes. These restrictions, combined with the willingness of Congress to consider drafting needed nurses in 1944, turned public opinion against the armed services' discriminatory policies. As a result, in January 1945, both nurse corps lifted their racial restrictions and accepted Negro female nurses.

Male nurses, however, faced a more rigid form of military discrimination than Negro female nurses. Tradition and sentiment had long dictated that nursing was a woman's field, and Congress, in establishing the nurse corps, ruled that only women could be appointed as military nurses. Thus, male students and graduates were subject to the Selective Service Act draft, and many volunteered rather than wait to be drafted into the armed forces. Although their military assignments varied, they were denied nursing status, and most served as enlisted personnel in non-health-related positions (Rose, 1947).

The ANA and other nursing groups appealed to the War Department throughout the war to secure rank and official nurse's designation for male nurses. Unfortunately, the army and navy medical departments were opposed to male nurses in the nurse corps. They shared the public's sentiment that during times of war, men served on the battlefields, and female nurses tended to the sick and wounded. It was not until 1955, after the Korean conflict, that Congress finally passed legislation that allowed the appointment of male nurses as reserve officers in the Army, Navy, and Air Force Nurse Corps (Sarnecky, 1999).

In a spirit of cooperation and change brought about by the war, a steady increase in the integration of Negro and male nurses into the country's nursing schools took place from 1945 to 1952. The substantial increase in Negro graduates encouraged many state nurses associations to remove their racial barriers to membership. General integration into the ANA was hastened in 1948, when its House of Delegates granted individual membership to Negro nurses barred from their state associations. The ANA adopted a resolution calling for the establishment of biracial integration at district and state levels. By 1950 only two state associations retained racial restrictions, and the NACGN announced its dissolution. Mabel Staupers, president of the NACGN, declared that with the acceptance of Negro nurses into the ANA, "its program of activities is no longer necessary" (Staupers, 1951).

The end of overt professional discrimination against both African-American and male nurses did not eradicate the more subtle and sophisticated forms of prejudice. It did, however, allow the profession and the health care system to benefit from the contributions of an increased number of minority graduate nurses.

THE POST-WORLD WAR II ERA

After World War II, the federal government's role in health affairs expanded to include not only funding initiatives, but also the creation of health policies and priorities for the nation. Although funding for nursing education remained modest until 1960, additional allocations were made for nursing research. Under Jessie Scott, director of the U.S. Public Health Division of Nursing and Assistant Surgeon General, the restructured Division of Nursing assisted Congress in enacting the Nurse Training Act of 1964. This act was in response to the nation's demand for more health services. The needs of

the country's baby-boom population (78 million Americans), the special needs of the growing population of the elderly, and the availability of private health insurance created widespread shortages of nurses. Congress, acknowledging that well-educated nurses were essential to meet the public's demand, awarded $242.6 million for student scholarships, loans, recruitment, school construction and maintenance, and special educational projects (Kalisch & Kalisch, 1995).

The public's growing belief in the power of modern medicine was sustained by new knowledge in pharmacology and surgery. Penicillin, the first of the so-called "miracle drugs," not only successfully treated serious infections, but, in preventing postoperative infections, it promoted new surgical advances. The creation of new drugs and technology made health professionals and patients optimistic about the conquest of disease. The public, sustained by this optimism, encouraged the government to fund medical research and to subsidize the care of the elderly and the indigent through such programs as Medicare and Medicaid in 1965 (Stevens, 1971).

Nursing, a key player in the modern health care system, received federal support to expand its role in the provision of care. To fully expand its role, however, the profession needed more than funding. It needed to sever the ties that bound nursing education to hospitals.

Nursing in Higher Education

After World War II, Congress passed the GI Bill of Rights, which enabled veterans to acquire training or a college education (Kiester, 1994). Nurse veterans took this opportunity to enroll in collegiate programs to acquire degrees in nursing education and administration. The increased enrollment gave new life to collegiate schools, and by the 1950s many colleges had developed basic baccalaureate nursing programs.

By 1962 there were 178 colleges offering undergraduate degrees in nursing, and the pool of college-educated nurses dramatically expanded (Brown, 1978) (Fig. 1–6).

COMMUNITY COLLEGE NURSING

The severity of the nursing shortage in the late 1940s also encouraged the development of experimental programs to educate new and different levels of nurses. In 1951, Mildred Montag, a nurse educator, proposed an educational study to prepare nurse technicians in 2-year associate degree (AD) community college programs. After completing a 5-year study of the graduates from seven participating colleges, the AD program was deemed successful. Success was based on the study's findings: associate graduates passed state nursing licensure examinations and demonstrated adequate clinical nursing compe-

tency, and all quickly found employment as graduate nurses (Haase, 1990).

Encouraged by these results, the W. K. Kellogg Foundation funded similar school projects in four states in 1959. The success of these schools launched the AD nursing education movement across the country. Acquiring funding from the Nurse Training Act of 1964, community colleges opened AD programs at a phenomenal rate. From 1952 to 1974, the number of associated programs in the country doubled every 4 years. During one period, new programs opened at the rate of one per week (Rines, 1977).

Several important goals were attained by the AD programs' success. A new pool of students including older individuals than the typical undergraduate men, and married women with children, were now selecting nursing careers. The AD graduates helped reduce the serious

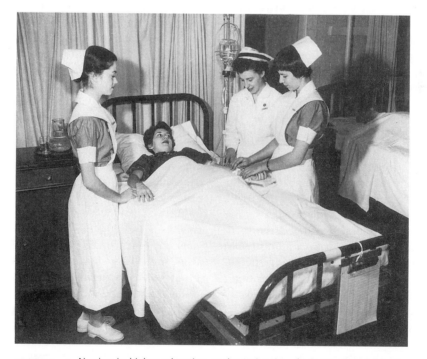

FIGURE 1–6 Nursing in higher education at the University of Virginia Hospital in the 1950s. (From the collection at the Center for Nursing Historical Inquiry, University of Virginia, School of Nursing, Charlottesville.)

nursing shortages of the 1970s and 1980s. The program's success also helped move nursing education from the hospital's diploma programs and place it in community colleges. Although this move enlarged the availability of nursing education to a wider number of people, the existence of three different educational programs—diploma, associate, and baccalaureate degree—all leading to registered nurse licensure and entry level positions, confused the public and the profession.

MASTER'S EDUCATION IN NURSING

The technological and scientific advances in medicine that started in the 1940s intensified in the 1960s. As a result, medical and surgical care became more complex, and to cope with this complexity, clinical subspecialties and intensive patient care units were developed throughout the nation. This explosion in medical knowledge and technology, coupled with advances in the social sciences, required nurses to function at a more advanced level of clinical competency. The dramatic growth in the nation's population and the public's quest for the benefits of modern medicine propelled the profession into developing advanced clinical practice graduate programs and undertaking research studies focused on the impact of nursing care on patients. To prepare nurses to understand the place of nursing research in their daily practice, research courses were incorporated into baccalaureate and graduate program curricula in the 1970s.

The expansion of professional nursing's clinical and social responsibilities changed the focus of its graduate education from administration and teaching to advance clinical nursing specialization. Adding to this expansion, the nation's lack of an adequate number of physicians to provide primary care led the federal government to fund the education of nurse practitioners. During the late 1970s and 1980s, nurses sought master's preparation to become nurse practitioners and clinical nurse specialists (Jolly & Hart, 1987). In so doing, the profession

moved another step toward defining its clinical knowledge, expertise, and identity in the health care system.

The Rise of Advanced Practice Nursing

The advent of advanced practice nursing programs, which began with psychiatric mental health nursing in the early 1960s, was to develop further with the growth of medical specialization in the hospital. The widely accepted idea of progressive patient care (Abdellah, 1959) according to which critically ill patients were grouped in special nursing units, set the stage for changes in patient care in every hospital in the United States and paved the way for new roles for nurses (Fairman & Lynaugh, 1998; Lynaugh & Brush, 1996). An example of these changes was evident in the creation of coronary care units. Influenced by research on the success of cardiopulmonary resuscitation and cardiac defibrillation, and interested in utilizing electronic monitoring technology for improving the care of cardiac patients, physicians and nurses opened CCUs to care for patients with acute myocardial infarction. Supported by the federal appropriations for medical research under Lyndon B. Johnson's Great Society program, CCUs proliferated and paved the way for the growth of other subspecialty nursing units, including those for burn, renal dialysis, and oncology patients.

Central to the advanced practice movement in nursing was the clinicians' move toward independent practice and nurse-derived standards of care and the collegial relationship they developed with physicians in the CCU. In these units, nurses and physicians shared the emerging clinical knowledge for managing cardiac patients. Together they mastered the new technology of electronic monitoring, cardiac defibrillation, and electronic pacemakers, and wrote standard "order sets" so that nurses could identify cardiac arrhythmias and treat the patients without waiting for physicians' orders. Throughout this process, CCU nurses stretched the boundaries of their practice and assumed new roles, including the conduct of nursing research and such tasks as inserting intravenous lines and defibrillating patients. Gaining acceptance as significant members of the health care team, CCU nurses helped lay the foundation for a more autonomous practice for nurses. In addition, the need for advanced practice nurses to communicate with each other about practice issues and have a forum for continuing education led to the development of national specialty organizations, including the American Association of Cardiovascular Nurses (AACN), in 1969, which was renamed the American Association of Critical Care Nurses in 1972. These specialty organizations took on the tasks of setting practice standards and developing certification for the emerging clinical specialties. Both were significant steps in the advancement of the discipline.

Throughout the process of expanding their clinical roles, nurses debated, at both the national and local levels, the place of technology in nursing. Speaking at conferences and in articles, nurse leaders challenged staff nurses to care for the "total patient" rather than machines, and to provide "patient care, not monitor care" (Pinneo, 1965). Interestingly, this debate on nursing and technology had its roots in the early 20th century, when nurses incorporated the use of such objects as the thermometer, stethoscope, and sphygmomanometer into their practice (Sandelowski, 1997). It intensified in the mid-20th century with the advent of monitors, dialysis machines, and ventilators, and continues to be of concern today as nurses move into the world of computers.

At the same time that the clinical specialist role was emerging in hospitals, the primary care nurse practitioner movement was occurring in the community setting. The idea of an advanced practice role for nurses, the rise of medical specialization, the concurrent shortage of primary care physicians, especially in rural areas,

and the public's demand for improved access to health care fostered this movement. In 1965, Loretta Ford, RN, PhD, and Henry Silver, MD, opened the first pediatric nurse practitioner program at the University of Colorado. This collaborative project, designed to prepare professional nurses to provide well child care and manage the care of children with common childhood illnesses, was extremely successful and led to federal funding for the nurse practitioner role. Like clinical nurse specialists, nurse practitioners developed organizations that created certification requirements and clinical standards. However, unlike the CNS, nurse practitioners gained prescriptive authority that was jointly regulated by state boards of medicine and nursing.

By the late 1970s, nurse practitioners were widely employed in a variety of primary care settings, including physicians' offices, clinics, and schools. In addition, some practiced in hospitals in subspecialty areas such as nephrology, oncology and neurosurgery. By the early 1990s, in response to both the growing shortage of medical residents in subspecialty areas and the need to manage patients with increasingly complex medical needs (i.e., after heart and lung transplant), numerous openings for acute care nurse practitioners (ACNPs) emerged in tertiary care centers. Today, in both primary and acute care settings, advanced practice nurses continue to expand the scope and autonomy of their practice. Part of this role expansion includes the conduct of nursing research, a movement that had its roots in the mid-20th century and grew with the development of doctoral nursing programs.

DOCTORAL EDUCATION IN NURSING

In the 1960s nursing doctoral programs began to appear. The programs, a logical step in nursing's struggle to attain disciplinary status and independence as a profession, drew upon the expanding pool of master's-prepared nurses. Understanding the nation's need for research-based nursing care, the U.S. Public Health Service in 1955 funded doctoral education for nurses through predoctoral research fellowships. The government also created Nurse Scientist Training Program grants that were awarded directly to schools of nursing to finance the formation of doctoral programs (Grace, 1978).

Doctoral education offered the profession an opportunity to attain a long-awaited goal, the chance to develop a scientific basis for its caring activities. It also provided nurse researchers and scholars opportunities to develop disciplinary knowledge beyond the confines of the medical model of practice. Strongly influenced by the prevalent views of philosophy of science, particularly the empirical method and Kuhn's ideas about the nature of science (Kuhn, 1962), early nurse scholars began to identify theories that might unify nursing's unique body of knowledge. By the 1980s, again influenced by changes in the prevailing views in the philosophy of science, the realization of the limitations of empirical science guided nurse scholars to expand their phenomena of inquiry to include the subjective nature of human experience. In so doing, they utilized qualitative research methods that emphasized a holistic nursing perspective. In addition, they focused their work on the development of theories that originated in clinical practice. The increased numbers of nurse researchers and the availability of research funding generated not only studies that addressed clinical nursing questions but also multidisciplinary studies that reflected nursing's significant role in the health care system.

Managed Care and an Aging Population: Challenges for Nursing

In an attempt to control rapidly rising costs, managed care became the focus of health care in the 1980s and 1990s, and nursing was caught in a whirlwind of cost-cutting changes sweeping through the system. Mindful of the need to be proactive in health care reform, in 1992 the ANA released its Agenda for Health Care Reform, a comprehensive plan to reduce costs and promote access to care. Today the major challenges that face the profession are (1) how to provide quality patient care that is cost-effective, (2) how to obtain adequate payment for "nursing care" in a culture that does not value "caring" (Reverby, 1987), and (3) how to provide care to an expanding aging population with a shrinking workforce of professional nurses.

Conclusion

Throughout its history, nursing has sought to fulfill its social mandate to provide nursing care to those in need. To fulfill its responsibility as a major health care provider, it first had to gain professional expertise and autonomy. The development of clinical practice domains and skills and the movement of nursing education into institutions of higher learning were essential steps in nursing's movement toward professional independence and authority.

Nurses of the 21st century must continue to be sensitive to the social and medical changes that influence clinical practice and the development of nursing knowledge. As the American health care system continues to change, it is reasonable to assume that the future system will demand new models of nursing care that are efficient, cost-effective, and responsive to human needs. These changes will require that nurses continue to search for new knowledge, skills, and health strategies. It is very important to society, however, for the profession to remember that much of what has proved to be necessary in the care of the ill, compassionate and intelligent nursing, is still essential in this century (Keeling & Ramos, 1995). Understanding the history of the profession offers an insightful analysis of the social, medical, political, and economic forces that shaped nursing's development and the decisions that nurse leaders made in response to these forces. Nursing history aids the profession in unraveling the complexity of today's health system and offers guidance as to which paths may be taken in the future.

"The ways in which we address the crises and challenges of today have much to do with our understanding and ownership of the past" (Church, 1993, p. 1).

KEY POINTS

● The nursing profession is a distillation of over 150 years of development.

● Women have traditionally been expected to care for the ill.

● In 1873 America's first three Nightingale-modeled schools of nursing were established.

● In 1893, superintendents of America's largest nursing schools met to plan ways that nurses could gain control of nursing education and raise its standards.

● By 1900 there were 432 schools of nursing in the United States.

● In 1903, North Carolina was the first state to require an acceptable program of nursing education, as well as passing an examination, before a person could use the term registered nurse.

● By 1923, all states had nurse registration laws.

● For over 100 years, nurses have played a major role in providing public health services to the community.

● During World War II, the USPHS Cadet Nurse Corps attracted thousands of needed students to the profession and provided essential nursing services in civilian hospitals throughout the war.

● African-American nurses were first accepted into the military nursing corps in 1945.

● Between 1952 and 1974 the number of associate degree nursing programs doubled every 4 years.

● Advanced practice in the clinical setting in the 1960s and 1970s coincided with an increase in

the number of master's programs to prepare clinical nurse specialists and nurse practitioners.

● Doctoral nursing programs began in the 1960s and dramatically increased the number of nurses prepared to provide leadership and conduct nursing research.

CRITICAL THINKING EXERCISES

1. What do you think might have occurred in the nursing profession if the apprenticeship model of training had not been used to prepare nurses?

2. Discuss the influence of the modern hospital on the profession. How has it changed over the years, and how does this influence affect the current role of nurses? How have nurses influenced the development of the hospital?

3. What did public health nursing add to the nursing profession?

4. How did the federal government influence the nursing profession and its educational preparation? What are some of the positive and negative implications of this influence?

5. In examining the past, how has the nursing profession shaped the current health care system?

6. How has the history of discrimination against male nurses and African-American nurses influenced current nursing practice?

7. How did the growth of medical subspecialties influence nursing in the post-World War II era?

REFERENCES

Abdellah, F. (1959, May). Progressive patient care. *American Journal of Nursing, 59,* 649–655.

Abram, S. (1993). Brilliance and bureaucracy: Nursing and changes in the Rockefeller Foundation. 1915–1930. *Nursing History Review, 1,* 119–138.

Baer, E. (1992). Aspirations unattained: The story of the Illinois Training School's search for university status. *Nursing Research, 41,* 43–48.

Blum, J. (1981). The end of an era. In J. Blum (Ed.), *The national experience* (pp. 652–669). New York: Harcourt Brace Jovanovich.

Brainard, A. (1922). *The evolution of public health nursing.* Philadelphia: Saunders.

Brodie, B. (1993). Children's Bureau: Guardian of American children. *Nursing Research, 17,* 190–191.

Brown, J. (1978). Master's education in nursing, 1945–1969. In M. Louise Fitzpatrick (Ed.), *Historical studies in nursing* (pp. 104–130). New York: Teachers College Press.

Brueggemann, D. (1992). *The United States Cadet Nurse Corps 1943–1948: The Nebraska experience.* Unpublished master's thesis, University of Nebraska at Omaha.

Buhler-Wilkerson, K. (1989). *False dawn: The rise and fall of public health nursing.* New York: Garland.

Bullough, B. (1975). The first two phases in nursing licensure. In B. Bullough (Ed.), *The law and the expanding nurse's role* (pp. 7–21). New York: Appleton-Century-Crofts.

Bullough, V., & Bullough, B. (1978). *The care of the sick: The emergence of modern nursing.* New York: Prodist.

Burgess, M. (1928). *Nurses, patients and pocketbooks.* New York: Committee on the Grading of Nursing Schools.

Cannings, K., & Lazonick, W. (1975). The development of the nursing labor force in the United States: A brief analysis. *International Journal of Health Services, 5,* 185–217.

Christy, T. (1969). *Cornerstone for nursing education.* New York: Teachers College Press.

Church, O. M. (1993, September). *In search of nursing's history: A communication service to nursing school deans, administrators, and faculty* (pp. 1–3). New York: National League for Nursing Education.

Clappison, G. B. (1964). *Vassar's Rainbow Division 1918.* Lake Mills, IA: Graphic Publishing. (Reprint of 1918 book)

Craig, L. (1940). Opportunities for men nurses. *American Journal of Nursing, 40,* 667–670.

Dock, L. (1900, October). What we might expect from the law. *American Journal of Nursing, 1,* 8–12.

Dock, L. (1907). *A history of nursing* (Vol. 2). New York: G. P. Putnam's Sons.

Dock, L., & Stewart, I. (1931). *A short history of nursing.* New York: G. P. Putnam's Sons.

Faddis, M. (1973). *A school of nursing comes of age: A history of the Frances Payne Bolton School of Nursing.* Cleveland: Alumnae of Frances P. Bolton School of Nursing.

Fairman, J., & Lynaugh, J. (1998). *Critical care nursing: A history.* Philadelphia: University of Pennsylvania Press.

Fitzpatrick, M. L. (1975). Nurses in American history: Nursing and the Great Depression. *American Journal of Nursing, 75,* 2188–2190.

Flood, M. (1981). *The troubling expedient: General staff nursing in United States hospitals in the 1930s: A means to institutional, educational, and personal ends.* Unpublished doctoral dissertation, University of California, Berkeley.

Friedman, L. (1965, March–May). Freedom of contract and licensing, 1890–1910. *California Law Review, 53,* 487–534.

Gardner, M. (1936). *Public health nursing* (3rd ed.). New York: Macmillan.

Geister, J. (1926). Hearsay and fact in private duty. *American Journal of Nursing, 26,* 515–528.

Goldmark, J., and the Committee for the Study of Nursing Education. (1923). *Nursing and nursing education in the United States.* New York: Macmillan.

Grace, H. C. (1978). The development of doctoral education in nursing: A historical education perspective. *Journal of Nursing Education, 17,* 17–27.

Haase, P. (1990). *The origins and rise of associate degree nursing education* (pp. 10–35). Durham: Duke University Press.

Hamilton, D. (1989). The cost of caring: The Metropolitan Life Insurance Company's Visiting Nurse Service, 1909–1953. *Bulletin of the History of Medicine, 63,* 414–434.

Hamilton, D. (1992). Research and reform: Community nursing and the Framingham tuberculosis project, 1914–1923. *Nursing Research, 41,* 8–13.

Hines, D. (1989). *Black nurses in white.* Bloomington: Indiana University Press.

Howard, H. B. (1912). The medical superintendent (Section on hospitals). *American Medical Association Transactions, 76.*

Johnston, D. F. (1966). *History and trends of practical nursing.* St. Louis: Mosby.

Jolly, M., & Hart, S. (1987). Master's prepared nurses: Societal needs and educational realities. In S. E. Hart (Ed.), *Issues in graduate nursing education* (NLN Publication No. 18-2196, pp. 25–31). New York: National League for Nursing.

Kalisch, P., & Kalisch, B. (1995). *The advance of American nursing* (3rd ed.). Philadelphia: Lippincott.

Keeling, A., & Ramos, M. (1995, January–February). The role of nursing history in preparing nursing for the future. *Nursing and Health Care, 16,* 30–34.

Kiester, E. (1994). The GI Bill may be the best deal ever made by Uncle Sam. *Smithsonian, 25*(8), 128–139.

Kimball, J. F. (1934). Prepayment plan of hospital care. *American Hospital Association Bulletin, 8,* 45.

Koch, H. (1951). *Militant angel: Annie W. Goodrich.* New York: Macmillan.

Kuhn, T. S. (1962). *The structure of scientific revolutions.* Chicago: University of Chicago Press.

Lynaugh, J., & Brush, B. (1996). *American nursing: From hospitals to health systems.* Cambridge, MA: Blackwell.

Meckel, R. (1990). *Save the babies* (pp. 175–180). Baltimore: Johns Hopkins University Press.

Numbers, R. (1978). The third party: Health insurance in America. In J. Leavitt & R. Numbers (Eds.), *Sickness and health in America* (pp. 142–145). Madison: University of Wisconsin Press.

Nutting, A. (1926). A sound economic basis for schools of nursing. New York: G. P. Putnam's Sons.

Osborne, E. (1949). Status and contributions of the Negro nurse. *Journal of Negro Education, 18,* 364–369.

Pinneo, R. (1965). Machines in perspective: Nursing in a coronary care unit. *American Journal of Nursing, 65*(2). Reprint, 1–4.

Reverby, S. (1983). Something besides waiting: The politics of private duty nursing reform in the depression. In E. Lagemann (Ed.), *Nursing history: New perspectives, new possibilities* (pp. 133–156). New York: Teachers College Press.

Reverby, S. (1987). *Ordered to care.* New York: Cambridge University Press.

Rines, A. (1977). Associate degree nursing education: History, development and rationale. *Nursing Outlook, 25,* 496–501.

Roberts, M. (1954). *American nursing: History and interpretation.* New York: Macmillan.

Roren, R. (1930). *The public's investment in hospitals* (Committee on the Costs of Medical Care, Publication No. 7). Chicago: University of Chicago Press.

Rose, J. (1947). Men nurses in military service. *American Journal of Nursing, 47,* 147–148.

Rosenberg, C. (1987). *The care of strangers.* New York: Basic Books.

Sandelowski, M. (1997). Making the best of things: Technology in American nursing, 1870–1940. *Nursing History Review, 5,* 3–22.

Sarnecky, M. (1999). *History of the Army Nurse Corps.* Philadelphia: University of Pennsylvania Press.

Sheahan, D. (1979). *The social origins of American nursing and its movement into the university.* Unpublished doctoral dissertation, New York University, New York.

Sommers, H., & Sommers, A. (1961). *Patients and health insurance.* Washington, DC: Brookings Institution.

Starr, P. (1982). *The social transformation of American medicine.* New York: Basic Books.

Staupers, M. (1951). Story of the NACGN. *American Journal of Nursing, 51,* 221–222.

Stevens, R. (1971). *American medicine and the public interest.* New Haven, CT: Yale University Press.

Stewart, I. (1943). *The education of nurses.* New York: Macmillan.

Struthers, L. (1917). *The school nurse.* New York: G. P. Putnam's Sons.

Taylor, P. (1971). *The distant magnet* (pp. 188–191). London: Eyre & Spottiswoode.

Tomes, N. (1983). The silent battle: Nurse registration in New York State, 1903–1920. In E. Lagemann (Ed.), *Nursing history: New perspectives, new possibilities* (pp. 107–132). New York: Teachers College Press.

U.S. Bureau of Census. (1900). *Special reports: Occupation roles, and gender.* Washington, DC: U.S. Government Printing Office.

Wald, L. (1938). *The house on Henry Street.* New York: Henry Holt.

2

Pathways of Nursing Education

JOAN L. CREASIA, PhD, RN

OBJECTIVES

At the completion of this chapter, the reader will be able to:

- Trace nursing education's history from its inception to the present.
- Compare and contrast nursing education programs for similarities and differences.
- Classify nursing education programs with respect to role preparation, scope of practice, eligibility for licensure, and eligibility for specialty certification.
- Identify and analyze trends in nursing program development, including eligibility for admission, career mobility and advancement opportunities, program accessibility, and modes of program delivery.
- Evaluate the effectiveness of available mechanisms to ensure program quality.
- Discuss and analyze the merits of the current nursing education system.
- Identify effective methodologies for addressing program models needing attention.

PROFILE IN PRACTICE

Mary Gunther, MSN, RN
College of Nursing, University of Tennessee
Knoxville, Tennessee

I was never one of those little girls who wanted to be a nurse. In fact, if early favorite toys and afterschool activities had been a predictor, I now would be a truck driver or a librarian. The high school I attended did not provide academic counseling to educate families about tuition assistance or scholarships. My grandmother, who was raising me, made it clear that a college education was beyond our financial means. It was her fervent wish that I always be able to take care of myself (that is, be able to get a well-paying job)

without relying on anyone else. She gave me two choices: become a nun or study nursing. I chose the latter.

I completed a 2-year nursing diploma program at a community hospital in Chicago. It was the type of program common at the time: students staffed the hospital round-the-clock 5 days a week and worked weekends for pay. The opportunity for hands-on clinical experience was unsurpassed. When it came time to look for a job, I chose to specialize in pediatrics, as children were less intimidating to me than adults. Furthermore, they were easier to physically move! Over the first 10 years of my career, I became a "good" nurse, developing both my intuitive and technical skills. I could recognize *what* needed to be done and *when*. What I did not know was *why*. I decided to take advantage of working at a university hospital and returned to school. It took me 15 years of on-again, off-again study to get my BSN. (Obviously, I was not exactly driven—it's more like I meandered through the undergraduate program.) By that time, I was a head nurse and had a whole new set of skills to learn.

Flushed with the success of being the first one in my family ever to graduate from college, I went back for a master's degree in nursing administration. What a difference! Almost everyone in my class had worked as a nurse for several years. Everyone had a story to tell about where they had been and where they wanted to go. The classes were not necessarily harder than those in the undergraduate program—just more interesting, because they were directly applicable to our various jobs. I fell in love with nursing all over again. I finished my MSN degree in 18

months, just in time to become the director of a large pediatric nursing department. Within a few years, I was the budget director for the entire division of nursing. Suddenly I was explaining to administrators just what it is that nurses do that makes them irreplaceable and invaluable. It was a very challenging and stressful (although not necessarily intellectually stimulating) job. I was homesick for the College of Nursing. There were so many more things I wanted to know. So back I went.

My days as a doctoral student have been among the happiest in my life. It is both the hardest and the most rewarding program I have undertaken. I also found out that I enjoy teaching, mainly because I like to talk about nursing and its place in the "real world." Over the past 4 years, I have become increasingly interested in nursing conceptual models/theories and their role in guiding nursing research, practice, and education. Studying the various models has given me an appreciation of the values and philosophies of nursing while enabling me to answer clearly the question, "What is it that nurses do, and why do they do it?" I hope the fascination never wanes.

The proliferation of nursing education programs at all levels provides multiple pathways to the attainment of one or more nursing credentials. For the individual who is planning a career in nursing, entry options into a basic or advanced nursing education program are often confusing. Chapter 1 described the social, political, and economic forces that influenced the evolution of nursing as a profession and the system of nursing education. This chapter analyzes the various educational opportunities with some considerations for selecting among the options. The programs are presented along a historical time line rather than by length or level of program. This method of presentation provides a chronology of events that influenced the development of multiple tracks of nursing

education and helps to explain how our current system of nursing education came about.

History of Nursing Education in the United States

DIPLOMA PROGRAMS

The first formal nursing education program in the United States was a 4-month hospital-based diploma program at the Boston Training School for Nurses at Massachusetts General Hospital. That program was established in 1873 and was originally intended to emulate the model put forward by Florence Nightingale when she established collegiate nursing in London, England, in 1860. Anticollegiate forces prevailed, however, and the hospital-based diploma program became the predominant model for nursing education in the United States. The model, in fact, flourished for nearly a century and still exists today.

At their peak, in 1958, diploma programs numbered 944. At that time and during the decade that followed, diploma graduates constituted nearly the entire registered nurse (RN) workforce. In 1963 the Surgeon General's Report indicated that 86% of the nursing workforce were diploma graduates. The decline in the number of programs began in earnest in the 1960s and 1970s and continues even today. By 1993 there were 126 diploma programs in 26 states, with over one-half of the programs in three states—Ohio, New Jersey, and Pennsylvania. In 2000, there were 86 diploma programs in 20 states, with one-half of them in the same three states (National League for Nursing Accrediting Commission [NLNAC], 2000a).

Diploma programs are typically 2 to 3 years in length and graduates are eligible to take the RN licensure examination (NCLEX-RN). As the length of diploma programs increased over the years from 4 months to 3 years, nursing students increasingly were used to meet hospital staffing needs rather than to function in the student role. The exploitation of nursing students was addressed in several landmark studies of nursing and nursing education, and in good time, student life became more compatible with sound educational practices. Many of these same studies also encouraged the profession to move its programs into collegiate settings (e.g., Brown, 1948; Goldmark, 1923) and to abandon the apprenticeship model. Ultimately it was the high cost of these programs, both to students and to the hospitals that offered them, coupled with an increasing number of collegiate options that brought about the closure of many diploma programs.

Some of the programs, rather than closing outright, began to align themselves with academic institutions. Others joined forces with academic institutions and began to offer joint degrees. Some became freestanding degree-granting institutions in their own right and now grant associate or baccalaureate degrees in nursing. At least 30 diploma programs have made successful transitions to college status, and many of those programs have not only been accredited by the regional accrediting body, they have also achieved professional nursing accreditation from one of the specialized accrediting agencies.

BACCALAUREATE PROGRAMS

The first baccalaureate nursing program was established in the United States at the University of Minnesota in 1909. The baccalaureate phenomenon caught on slowly and did not gain much momentum until after World War II. Until the mid-1950s many baccalaureate programs were 5 years in length and consisted of 2 years of general education followed by 3 years of nursing. The main difference between the 3 years of nursing in baccalaureate and diploma programs was the inclusion of public health nursing as part of the baccalaureate curriculum. Eventually the nursing content in baccalaureate programs was strengthened and expanded.

The proliferation of baccalaureate programs was slowed by the paucity of faculty members qualified to teach in these programs. While this was an understandable phenomenon, given the relative youth of nursing in academic centers, it created a reluctance on the part of college and university administrators to establish baccalaureate nursing programs. Those that were established were often forced to hire nursing faculty who would not otherwise qualify for university faculty appointments. It has taken several decades for this deficit to correct itself. It is to the lasting credit of the nursing profession and its members that nursing faculty teaching in baccalaureate programs today are for the most part bona fide members of their respective academic communities.

Most baccalaureate programs are now 4 academic years in length and the nursing major is concentrated at the upper-division level. Graduates are prepared as generalists, to practice nursing in beginning leadership positions in a variety of settings. To prepare nurses for this multifaceted role, several components are essential for all baccalaureate programs. These components are liberal education, professional values, core competencies, core knowledge, and role development (American Association of Colleges of Nursing [AACN], 1998a, p. 6). There are nearly 700 baccalaureate programs in existence today, and graduates are eligible to take the NCLEX-RN for licensure.

The majority of baccalaureate programs admit both prelicensure students and RNs who are graduates of diploma and associate degree nursing programs, but some programs admit only RNs. The general education requirements are the same for all students. Although some content in the RN track may be configured differently, both RN and prelicensure students meet the same program objectives. Licensed practical nurses (LPNs) also are frequently given credit for prior learning when they enroll in baccalaureate programs. The baccalaureate in nursing degree is the most common requirement for admission to graduate nursing programs (*Peterson's Guide,* 2000).

The RN track or option in the baccalaureate program is designed to recognize and reward prior learning and to capitalize on the characteristics of the adult learner. There are several models of awarding academic credit to RNs for prior education and experience to facilitate educational mobility. These include direct transfer of credits, credits awarded by examination, variable credits awarded following portfolio review of educational and professional experiences, holding lower-division nursing credits in "escrow" until completion of the program, and a number of other innovative models. "Educa-tional mobility options should respect previous learning that students bring to the educational environment . . . and build on knowledge and skills attained by learners prior to their matriculation" (AACN, 1998b, p. 1).

In 1965, the baccalaureate degree was designated by the American Nurses Association (ANA) as the entry point into professional nursing practice (ANA, 1965). Now, nearly 40 years later, there are still three educational pathways for RN licensure—baccalaureate, associate degree, and diploma programs. "The demands placed on nursing in the emerging health care system are likely to require a greater proportion of RNs who are prepared beyond the associate degree or diploma level" (Pew Health Professions Commission, 1998, p. 64).

VOCATIONAL EDUCATION

Practical/vocational nurse programs were begun in 1942 in response to the acute shortage of licensed nurses in the United States created by World War II. Because of the dramatic influx of RNs into the various military branches, U.S. hospitals were largely staffed by nurse's aides, volunteers, and other unlicensed personnel. Practical/vocational nurse programs were established to provide some formal training for those who were entering the nursing workforce with little or no knowledge about nursing and few, if any, nursing skills. The programs eventually led to a new kind of licensure for nurses, namely, licensed practical nurse/licensed vocational nurse (LPN/LVN). The license is awarded by the state board of nursing, and the examination is now known as the NCLEX-PN.

LPN/LVN programs are typically located in technical or vocational education settings. Programs are 9 to 15 months long and require proof of high school graduation for admission. Programs are designed to prepare graduates to work with RNs and to be supervised by them. Programs lead to a certificate of completion and to eligibility to take the NCLEX-PN. Currently there are about 1,100 such programs in the United States (NLNAC, 2000b). Since most courses taken by practical nurse students do not carry academic credit, these programs do not always articulate well with collegiate nursing programs. Associate degree programs, however, often have procedures for accommodation of practical nurses into their programs by way of advanced placement.

ASSOCIATE DEGREE PROGRAMS

In 1952 the associate degree in nursing (ADN) became another program option for those desiring to become RNs. Designed by Mildred Montag, these programs were intended to be a collegiate alternative for the preparation of technical nurses and a reaction to the vocational model for practical nurses.

Usually found in community or junior colleges, these 2-year programs consist of a balance between general education and clinical nursing courses, all of which carry academic credit. "Technical nurses function primarily as direct care givers within organized nursing services and use a problem-solving approach to the care of individuals and their families in institutional settings" (Williams, 1998, p. 16). ADN programs are designed to prepare technical bedside nurses for secondary care settings, such as community hospitals and long-term health care facilities. It was the founder's intent that nurses with associate degrees would work under the direction of registered professional nurses who were prepared at the baccalaureate level. Some confusion arose about roles and relationships, so that by the time the first groups of students had graduated from ADN programs, they were declared eligible for the RN licensure examination, an eligibility that graduates of these programs retain today.

The growth of associate degree programs in the United States has been nothing short of phenomenal. Not only did these programs multiply in community colleges, they also began to

appear at 4-year colleges and universities. In all cases, university-based associate degree programs are administered by a nursing unit that also offers baccalaureate and sometimes graduate nursing programs. By 1973 there were about 600 associate degree programs in the United States. By 2000 there were nearly 900 programs, which graduated nearly two-thirds of all entry-level RNs (NLNAC, 2000b).

The degree most often awarded on completion of the associate degree program is the ADN. A few institutions award the associate of arts in nursing (AAN) degree.

MASTER'S DEGREE EDUCATION

It is not surprising to note that while the establishment of associate and baccalaureate degree nursing programs was proceeding, a master's program was beginning to emerge on university campuses. The need for nursing faculty to teach in all of the new and developing nursing education programs was apparent. There was also a surge of interest in master's-prepared nurses in the service sector as the roles of clinical nurse specialists, nurse practitioners, and nurse administrators became more clearly defined.

Master's education in nursing traces its origins to 1899, when Teachers College in New York began to offer graduate courses in nursing management and nursing education. It was not until the late 1950s and early 1960s, however, that master's programs began to escalate and become nationally visible. The first programs were strong on role preparation and light on advanced nursing content. This was not surprising, since the nurses teaching in these programs did not themselves hold graduate degrees in nursing. As advanced nursing content became more clearly defined, and as increasing numbers of nursing faculty became proficient at teaching it, strong advanced nursing content became the prevailing characteristic of master's programs in nursing. Role preparation received somewhat less attention as clinical emphasis escalated, and by the 1990s advanced practice had become the predominant focus for most master's programs.

> "[T]he expanding authority of APN's [advanced practice nurses] to serve as autonomous providers of care requires that the education of the clinicians be sound and that the consumers of APN care be able to have confidence in the quality of the educational experience" (Booth & Bednash, 1994, p. 2).

Master's programs in nursing are typically 1½ to 2 years in length (full-time study) and are built on the baccalaureate nursing major. The program content includes a set of graduate-level foundational (core) courses, including a research component and a clinical component in a nursing specialty. Other recommended core content areas include theoretical foundations of nursing practice, health care financing, human diversity and social issues, ethics, health promotion, health care delivery systems, health policy, and professional role development. For specialty tracks that prepare advanced practice nurses, there is also a clinical core consisting of advanced pathophysiology, pharmacology, and assessment (AACN, 1996). While the bachelor of science in nursing (BSN) degree or its equivalent is usually a requirement for admission to a master's program in nursing, several other interesting models that accommodate other types of students have emerged. Some master's programs admit RNs without a baccalaureate degree or with a baccalaureate degree in another field into a streamlined track that includes both baccalaureate and master's level courses (Creasia, 1994). Other programs admit students who are in fact not nurses at all, and there are 15 of these programs in the United States at present (AACN, 2000).

The impetus for opening admissions to other types of students came from noting the kinds of students who were applying in significant numbers to associate degree and baccalaureate nursing programs. Frequently non-nurses with bac-

calaureate or sometimes graduate degrees in other fields were seeking admission to basic nursing programs. RNs from associate degree and diploma programs who had completed baccalaureate degrees in fields other than nursing were applying for admission to baccalaureate nursing programs so that they could present the appropriate credential for admission to a master's program in nursing. These students brought a rich and diversified background to their educational programs and were highly motivated, self-directed adult learners with a strong and clearly defined career orientation. While some of these students were well-served by a "fast track" second baccalaureate degree offered by several institutions, it became clear that master's programs could accommodate them and take them to the master's level in educationally sound and cost-effective ways.

Master's programs in nursing that admit non-nurse college graduates and RNs without a baccalaureate degree in nursing take the necessary steps to ensure that both groups complete whatever undergraduate or graduate prerequisite courses are needed to acquire the equivalent of a baccalaureate nursing major. They then pursue the same graduate-level foundational, specialty, and cognate courses required of master's students; thus, they exit the program having met the same program objectives that all graduates of both programs must meet. Non-nurses are eligible to take the NCLEX-RN examination on completion of the generalist or baccalaureate equivalent component of the program or at program completion. There are a number of master's programs in nursing across the United States that have multiple entry options such as those described here, and more are being developed as adult learners from diverse backgrounds migrate toward nursing.

One other option with respect to master's programs in nursing is worthy of note: the joint program leading to two master's degrees awarded simultaneously. These programs are especially relevant for nurses seeking administrative positions that require both advanced nursing knowledge and business/management skills. Several joint program models now exist across the country, not only reflecting nursing's responsiveness to documented student need and interest but also demonstrating nursing's ability to collaborate with other academic disciplines. Available programs in conjunction with the master's degree in nursing include the master's degree in business administration (MSN/MBA), master's degree in public administration (MSN/MPA), and master's degree in hospital administration (MSN/MHA). Degree candidates must be admitted to both programs and must fulfill requirements for both programs. However, requirements common to both programs may be consolidated. There are at least 76 such programs currently in existence, with several more under development (*Peterson's Guide,* 2000).

Master's degree programs in nursing have enjoyed phenomenal growth in the past several decades. In 1973 there were 86 such programs. By 1983 the number had increased to 154, and in 2000 there were 358 (NLNAC, 2000a). During the late 1980s and early 1990s, enrollment in master's degree programs increased rapidly as the demand for advanced practice nurses escalated, but a slight decline (1.9%) was evident in 1999 (AACN, 2000). Despite this growth, it is projected that by 2005 the shortage of nurses with advanced nursing degrees will approach 200,000 (U.S. DHHS, 1990). Master's degree programs currently are offered in all states and territories of the United States.

The degree most often awarded on completion of a master's degree program is the master of science in nursing degree (MSN). At least 90% of nursing master's degrees are MSN degrees. Other degree designations include the master's degree in nursing (MN), master of science degree with a major in nursing (MS), and master of arts degree with a major in nursing (MA). The degree designation is more a matter of institutional policy than a reflection of program type or content. There is in fact no sub-

stantive distinction among these various degree designations for master's-level nursing programs.

DOCTORAL PROGRAMS IN NURSING

As might be expected, given nursing's relative youth in academe, the profession has only recently carved out a major doctoral presence in the academic community. Until 1970 there were fewer than a dozen doctoral programs with a major in nursing across the country. Most nurses who earned doctoral degrees did so in related disciplines such as sociology, anthropology, education, and physiology. By 1983 there were 27 doctoral programs in nursing. By 1990, only 7 years later, their number had nearly doubled. In 2000, there were 75 doctoral programs in nursing in 35 states, and several more were in the planning stages (AACN, 2000; NLNAC, 2000b).

The degree most commonly awarded for the doctorate in nursing is the doctor of philosophy (PhD) with a major in nursing. Other degrees awarded include the doctor of nursing science (DNS or DNSc), doctor of science in nursing (DSN), and doctor of education (EdD). These varying degree designations do not necessarily distinguish one program from another with respect to content, rigor, or research emphasis, but some programs may have a heavier clinical emphasis than others. In most instances, the degree designation is that specified for the discipline by the institution that awards the degree. And, while some are still questioning nursing's readiness for the doctoral community of scholars, the profession is quietly preparing an array of scholars and researchers whose contributions to the health and nursing literature are qualitatively and quantitatively impressive.

Doctoral programs range in length from 3 to 5 years of full-time study or that equivalent in part-time work. Doctoral programs include advanced content in concept and theoretical formulations and testing, theoretical analyses, advanced nursing, supporting cognates, and in-depth research. The culminating degree requirement is the completion and defense of the doctoral dissertation.

NURSING DOCTORATE PROGRAMS

First conceptualized by Rozella Schlotfeldt in the 1970s (Schlotfeldt, 1978), the first nursing doctorate (ND) program was established at the Frances Payne Bolton School of Nursing, Case Western Reserve University, in 1979. The ND program, analogous to medical, dental, and legal models of education, is designed to prepare graduates for licensure and professional practice in their field. "An ND is a clinically focused degree that emphasizes research utilization (not generation) in patient care and health care policy. The goal for ND programs is to produce highly specialized practitioners for practice, teaching, consultation, and management" (Jones & Lutz, 1999, p. 246).

Students admitted to the ND program must hold at least a baccalaureate degree in another field and be capable of post-baccalaureate work. The 4-year program prepares a generalist for professional nursing practice who, as part of the program, also acquires an advanced practice specialty. Students are eligible to take the NCLEX-RN on completion of the generalist component of the ND program. Programs are designed to emulate the professional educational model followed by several other distinguished professions without sacrificing the identity of nursing as an academic discipline in its own right. The ND program is usually not listed with the doctoral programs available in nursing because the focus is on clinical practice rather than research. This program model has not enjoyed much growth since its inception, but it may become more attractive as a direct route to advanced practice now that advanced practice nurses are in such great demand. Currently there are just four programs in four states (Colorado, Illinois, Ohio, and South Carolina), but more may come.

To put the various educational programs in perspective, a comparison of their characteristics is presented in Table 2–1. The changes in the educational preparation of the nursing workforce from 1980 to 1996 are presented in Figure 2–1.

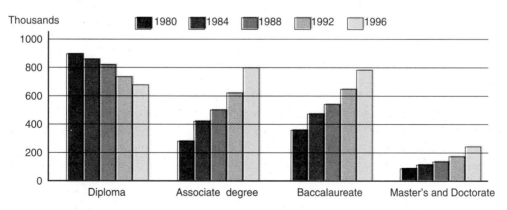

FIGURE 2–1 Highest nursing educational preparation of registered nurse population, 1980–1996. (From U.S. Department of Health and Human Services. (1996). *The registered nurse population: Findings from the national sample survey of registered nurses* (p. 7). Bethesda, MD: Author.)

TABLE 2–1 Comparison of Nursing Education Programs

	Diploma Programs	Baccalaureate Programs	Practical/Vocational Nurse Programs	Associate Degree Programs	Master's Programs	Doctoral Programs in Nursing	Nurse Doctorate Programs
Year established	1873	1909	1942	1952	Late 1950s	1960s	1979
Location	Hospitals	4-year colleges and universities	Vocational/technical schools	Community, junior, or 4-year colleges and universities	Universities and colleges	Universities and colleges	Universities and colleges
Accessibility	Limited to 86 programs in 20 states with nearly half of the programs in 3 states—New Jersey, Ohio, and Pennsylvania	Universal; all states, most cities, 695 programs; some are RN-BSN only	Universal; all states, most cities; more than 1,100 programs	Universal; all states, almost all cities, 885 programs	Very good; 358 programs with at least 1 in every state; also available through distance learning	Limited to 75 programs in 35 states	Very limited; 4 programs in 4 states
Length	2–3 years	4 years	9–15 months	2 years	1½–2 years for full-time post-baccalaureate BSN-prepared nurses; additional work for other types of students	3–5 years post master's	4 years post baccalaureate
Cost	A few hundred dollars per term	Highly variable; a few thousand to several thousand dollars per year	Minimal; mostly books and cost of living	Reasonable in state or other public colleges; a few hundred to a few thousand dollars per year	Variable; several hundred to several thousand dollars per term	Several thousand dollars per term	Several thousand dollars per term

	Prepare clinically competent bedside nurses	Prepare professional nurse generalists for acute care settings, community-based practice, and beginning leadership/management positions	Prepare assistive licensed nurse workers	Prepare competent technical bedside nurses for secondary care settings	Prepare advanced practice nurses in a clinical specialty	Prepare leaders for education, administration, clinical practice, and research	Prepare clinically adept advanced practice nurses for leadership positions in clinical settings
Purpose							
Advanced placement or acceleration opportunities	For LPNs or LVNs	For LPNs/LVNs or RNs from diploma and associated degree nursing programs	None	For LPNs or LVNs	For non-nurse college graduates, RNs with degrees in other fields, some RNs without degrees	For BSNs (limited number of programs)	Not applicable; all students are non-nurse college graduates
Degree/certificate	Diploma	BSN	Certificate of completion	ADN (usually) or AAN	MSN (most common) or MN, MS, MA	PhD (most common), or DNS, DNSc, EdD	ND
License eligibility	RN	RN (if not already licensed)	LPN/LVN	RN	RN if unlicensed at entry	Not applicable	RN
Certificate eligibility	None	Limited	None	None	Multiple	None	Multiple
Program growth pattern	Significant decline; 944 programs in 1958, 126 in 1993, and 86 in 2000.	Increasing; 420 programs in 1983, 507 in 1993, and 695 in 2000.	Slight decline; 1,200 programs in 1994 and 1,100 in 2000.	Sharp increase, then plateau; 600 programs in 1973, 900 in 1993, and 885 in 2000	Increasing; 150 programs in 1983, 300 in 1993, and 358 in 2000	Upward; 27 programs in 1983, 56 in 1993, and 75 in 2000	Very slow; 4 programs in 21 years

~ Considerations in Selecting a Nursing Education Program

A number of considerations influence an individual's choice in selecting either a basic or a graduate-level nursing program. Perhaps among the most important are cost to the student, quality of the program, and accessibility.

COST

Colleges, national summary documents, and public libraries provide relevant cost information on public and private institutions that offer nursing education programs. From this information some generalizations can be made. First, state-supported community or junior colleges tend to be less expensive than state-supported 4-year colleges and universities. Second, state-supported institutions of higher education usually give a substantial tuition reduction to instate students. Third, state- or government-supported higher education is almost always significantly less expensive than private education, but this fact should not deter investigation of private institutions because of the availability of financial aid.

Financial Assistance. Financial aid packages at most institutions are somewhat commensurate with actual costs. Assistance can take the form of scholarships, loans, work-study appointments, employment opportunities within the institution, assistantships, tutoring assignments, or some combination of these or other options. It should also be noted that many of these options are no longer limited to full-time students. Financial assistance awards may be based on scholarship alone, need alone, competitive performance alone, or a combination of two or more of these. Financial support may be, and in most cases should be, sought from more than one source. While most financial assistance awards are administered and awarded by the in-

stitution, there are a variety of packages available from community- or government-based agencies and organizations. Examples of such agencies include, but are not limited to, state and local governments, the military, chambers of commerce, minority organizations, churches, community clubs, and local or state chapters of health-related organizations (e.g., March of Dimes, American Red Cross, American Heart Association). Local banks frequently have attractive student loan packages. Local hospitals and other health care agencies often sponsor or support nursing students in exchange for a commitment from the student to work for the sponsoring agency for a specified period of time after graduation. It is clear, therefore, that some form of nursing education is fiscally and geographically within reach of all interested and qualified individuals.

QUALITY

Issues of program quality relate to the quality of the educational program itself, as well as the eligibility of its graduates to become licensed or certified. With regard to program quality, how are prospective students protected from program mediocrity or less? And how is the public protected from low-quality nursing practice, which can frequently be traced to low-quality programs?

The public is protected by licensure and certification procedures that ensure a standardized level of competence. The student is protected from marginal programs by institutional accreditation through regional accrediting bodies, by specialized accreditation of the nursing program(s) by the National League for Nursing Accrediting Commission (NLNAC) or the Commission on Collegiate Nursing Education (CCNE), and by approval of the legal regulatory body for programs preparing for licensure, specifically the respective state boards of nursing.

Appropriate questions to ask about the quality of nursing programs include the following:

• Is the parent institution accredited by the appropriate regional accrediting body?
• Is the nursing program unconditionally approved by the state board of nursing and fully accredited by a professional accrediting agency (if eligible)?
• What is the usual pass rate for first-time writers of the licensure examination from the school or program of interest?
• Are the faculty appropriately credentialed for their area of responsibility?
• Are faculty certified in their clinical specialty, if appropriate?
• Are graduates of the program eligible for the appropriate certification examination for the program being pursued?
• Does the program have a troubled history with respect to licensure examination performance, accreditation, or state approval?

Specialized Accreditation. *Accreditation* is a voluntary peer evaluation process whereby a private, nongovernmental agency grants public recognition to an institution or specialized program that meets or exceeds nationally established standards. Some new developments are occurring with respect to specialized accreditation of nursing programs that need to be factored into the assessment of program quality, especially at the master's level. Until 1999, the National League for Nursing (and subsequently the NLNAC) was the specialized accrediting body for nursing programs, LPN/LVN through master's degree. In 2000, the CCNE was approved by the Department of Education as an official accrediting agency for baccalaureate and graduate nursing education programs, thus offering a choice of accrediting agencies for those programs. Since accreditation is a voluntary process, programs are not required to seek professional accreditation to continue to operate (although all must be approved by their respective state board of nursing). It is important for students to recognize that attending a nonaccredited program may limit access to federal loans and scholarships. In addition, most graduate schools will accept only students who have earned degrees from accredited schools (*Peterson's Guide,* 2000).

In times past, when a master's program was accredited by a specialized accrediting body, the accreditation covered all specialties that were offered within the master's program. However, when a nurse-midwifery program was one of the options in the master's program, even though it was covered by master's program accreditation, separate specialized accreditation for the nurse-midwifery program was sought from the American College of Nurse Midwives. This was done so that graduates of that program could take the midwifery license/certification examination and therefore practice as nurse midwives. Now nurse anesthesia programs have been upgraded from diploma or certificate programs (which most of them were) to master's-level programs. Although several of these nurse anesthesia programs at the master's level are now accredited as one of the offerings within the master's program, these programs are continuing to seek and receive specialized accreditation from their specialty organization, the American Association of Nurse Anesthetists. This practice will continue so that nurse anesthetists are eligible for the credentials that enable them to practice their specialty. It is entirely possible that some other nursing specialties may seek programmatic accreditation that goes beyond the broader accreditation that the NLNAC or CCNE makes available. This movement is closely tied to the increasing emphasis on specialty certification and the organizations in the best position to provide it. It is an issue that persons pursuing advanced specialty preparation need to monitor with vigilance.

Certification. The certification of individual nurses is a growing quality control activity being implemented by a variety of nursing and nursing-related organizations. This effort is directed toward attesting to or endorsing the demonstrated knowledge base and clinical practice behaviors associated with high-quality performance in an area of specialization. This movement is a very important one for the profession. Initiatives are now in place to make eligibility and certification requirements more uniform, to reduce duplicate or similar certification requirements across organizations, and to match certification programs with the specialties being practiced.

> Board certification signifies those nurses who have met requirements for clinical or functional practice in a specialized field, pursued education beyond basic nursing preparation, and received the endorsement of their peers. After meeting these criteria, nurses take certification examinations based on nationally recognized standards of nursing practice to demonstrate their knowledge, skills, and abilities within the defined specialty (American Nurses' Credentialing Center, [ANCC], 2000a, p. 2).

Currently, the American Nurses' Credentialing Center, an arm of the American Nurses Association, offers 29 certification examinations, among which are 12 for generalist areas of practice, six for nurse practitioner specialties, six for clinical specialists, two for nurse administrators and one for each of the following: nursing case management, ambulatory care nursing, and informatics nurse (ANCC, 2000a; ANCC, 2000b).

Other certification examinations are offered by a variety of nursing specialty organizations. Some certifications are rather highly specialized in such areas as addiction, neuroscience, nephrology, ophthalmology, perioperative nursing, oncology, critical care, and occupational health. Many nursing specialty organizations that offer certification examinations are members of the American Board of Nursing Specialties. This board has a national peer review program that sets standards for certification and approves certification programs. All certification efforts are designed to recognize competence of nurses in specific areas and to protect the public from unsafe or uninformed nursing practice.

ACCESSIBILITY: DISTANCE EDUCATION

To improve accessibility in terms of geographic location and scheduling of classes, some nursing programs are offering all or part of their curriculum via distance education technologies. *Distance* or *distributive education* is a method of teaching and learning that takes place outside of the traditional classroom setting. Often, students are in locations that are remote from the site where the course is taught. A variety of technologies are employed to deliver education at a distance, including interactive television, e-mail and facsimile transmissions, and web-based courses with real-time interactive chat rooms. Less sophisticated and readily available technologies include audiocassettes, videotapes, and CD-ROM media. "Careful use of technology in education may well enhance the profession's ability to educate nurses for practice, prepare future nurse educators, and advance nursing science in an era when the number of professional nurses, qualified nurse faculty, and nurse researchers is well below national need" (AACN, 1999, p. 3).

As this movement gains momentum in nursing education, there are a number of issues to be addressed:

- What is the effect of distance education on the cost and quality of the program?
- What equipment is needed by both the teacher and learner to maximize distance learning?
- What impact does distance education have on the process of professional socialization?
- How can teaching strategies best match learner needs?
- What policies exist to clarify intellectual property rights and the use of copyrighted material in distance education courses?
- What effect, if any, will distance education have on student financial aid support?

It is likely that the answers to these questions will challenge traditional assumptions about the effectiveness of various teaching-learning strategies and their relationship to program quality.

⌇ Observations and Analysis

One may argue, and many have, that regardless of the reasons, the system of nursing education that has been created is chaotic, confusing, and redundant. There are those who are holding out for the day when there will be only one way to become a nurse, only one degree to be obtained, only one license to be acquired, and only one way to be approved and recognized as a specialist. That, after all, is the way medicine, dentistry, and law do it. Can there possibly be any more likely professions to which nursing might look for modeling and emulation? Probably not.

But consider for a moment how different medicine's evolution has been. Consider the venerable age of the profession. Consider how readily and completely the European model for medical education was transplanted unchanged to the United States. Consider the unquestioned dominance of the medical profession in the United States from the time the health care "system" was first defined until it began to crumble. And now that it is crumbling, consider the serious criticism being leveled at the medical profession—criticism about education, practice, costs, and societal insensitivities. Medical reform is being demanded by the federal and state governments, by consumers, and by the profession itself. And this reform must be conducted and completed by those who entered that profession in good faith and with a set of information-based expectations that they thought would last a lifetime. This state of affairs is by no means an indictment of the medical profession or the vast majority of its members. It is, instead, an example of what can happen when the status quo is unquestioned, when a service profession loses touch with its constituencies, and when hard questions are not answered because they are not asked.

Wherever the nursing education system is right now, it is clearly in a better place than many of its other health profession counterparts. Nursing does not necessarily need to look to other health professions to take the right cues or develop the right models. Rather, it needs to look within itself to examine what has been created; to retain, build on, and reconfigure as needed that which is good; to abandon or revamp that which is no longer germane; to clarify ambiguities; to underline uniqueness; to stay in touch with its consumers; and to continue the marvelous and now undeniable trend of the profession to embrace and participate fully in the higher education academic community, enjoying and benefiting from all of the collegial and professional relationships that accrue from that participation. Those, after all, are relationships that can only get better.

With those observations as a backdrop, an analysis of strengths, weaknesses, and areas needing attention is presented. The information is organized around program types and follows the historical evolution presented earlier.

DIPLOMA PROGRAMS

Strength. Programs prepare competent bedside nurses who are eligible to take the NCLEX-RN.

Weaknesses. Programs, for the most part, are not collegiate based and nursing courses are not readily transferable for career advancement purposes. In addition, they are expensive to operate.

Recommendation. Continue admirable and effective efforts to align with degree-granting institutions or become degree-granting as newly established academic institutions.

BACCALAUREATE PROGRAMS

Strengths. Programs provide a solid liberal education and a substantive upper-division nursing major. Both components are combined in ways that prepare a nurse generalist who is able to provide professional nursing services in beginning leadership positions in a variety of settings and who is eligible to take the NCLEX-RN. Programs are accessible and accommodate RNs who are graduates of associate degree and diploma programs. Baccalaureate programs in nursing have been designated by the ANA as the entry point for professional practice (ANA, 1965).

Weaknesses. The legal scope of practice for associate degree- and baccalaureate-prepared nurses is undifferentiated because both groups are awarded the same license. This limits differentiated roles in work settings and hinders the reward system for leadership responsibilities.

Recommendations. Develop a different or additional license for baccalaureate-prepared nurses. Expand community focus and give additional emphasis to managed care in the curriculum.

PRACTICAL/VOCATIONAL NURSE PROGRAMS

Strengths. Programs are short, economical, and accessible. Programs prepare assistive nurse workers who are eligible to take the NCLEX-PN.

Weaknesses. Programs are not collegiate based. Graduates are not prepared to do what they are called on to do in the workplace. Practical nurses are exploited and are frequently called on to perform functions beyond their legally defined scope of practice.

Recommendations. Elevate these programs to the community college level and award the ADN. Adjust enrollments downward to reflect market demands.

ASSOCIATE DEGREE PROGRAMS

Strengths. Programs are offered in academic/collegiate settings and are affordable, accessible,

and reasonably brief. Programs prepare competent technical bedside nurses who are eligible to take the NCLEX-RN.

Weaknesses. Programs and their graduates go beyond the purposes and scope of the practice envisioned by the program founder. When combined with practical nurses, the total number of technical nurse types being produced is excessive, given current and future market demands.

Recommendations. Collaborate with the LPN/LVN leadership to develop one program type that prepares the technical nurse, using that which is most effective from both programs to bring about this outcome. Once the two programs have become one, assess the marketplace and consumer needs for this type of nurse and adjust the program output accordingly. Seek guidance from North Dakota, where successful program unification (LPN/ADN) has already occurred.

MASTER'S PROGRAMS

Strengths. Programs are accessible. Programs prepare graduates for advanced practice in a nursing specialty. Some of the programs admit non-nurse college graduates, RNs with baccalaureate degrees in other fields, and some RNs without baccalaureate degrees. Graduates of these programs are prepared to engage in advanced practice nursing as nurse practitioners, clinical nurse specialists, nurse anesthetists, or nurse midwives, and in other specialty practices.

Weaknesses. Non-nurses take the same licensure examination as associate degree graduates (NCLEX-RN). Certificate programs for master's-prepared nurses are not uniformly consistent in terms of eligibility requirements and examination rigor.

Recommendations. Collaborate with baccalaureate nurse educators and other interested professionals in bringing to fruition the second or different examination for professional nurses. Bring greater uniformity and meaning to certification programs.

DOCTORAL PROGRAMS IN NURSING

Strengths. Programs prepare leaders for responsible advanced positions in nursing education, nursing administration, nursing research, nursing practice, or some combination of these roles. Programs are fairly accessible, as doctoral programs go.

Weakness. Program proliferation has resulted in the use of some unqualified faculty members for program delivery.

Recommendation. Stabilize program growth at the current level so that faculty can fine-tune their qualifications and participate more fully in the life of scholarship (Anderson, 2000).

NURSING DOCTORATE PROGRAM

Strength. Programs prepare clinically adroit and theoretically strong advanced practice nurses.

Weaknesses. Programs are not widely accessible (only four programs in four states) and are expensive.

Recommendation. Market the program as an effective alternative route to preparation for advanced practice nursing.

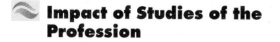 **Impact of Studies of the Profession**

Throughout this chapter the history of nursing education has been traced from professional, organizational, regulatory, and institutional perspectives. The system has been described, analyzed, compared and contrasted within itself, and presented for what it is and what it is becoming. One frame of reference that has not

been formally considered from the standpoint of impact or programmatic direction is that provided by the multiple studies that have been published about nursing and nurses. Many such studies have been conducted—some by nurses, some by the federal government, and some by human behavior experts from other disciplines (e.g., sociology, anthropology). The findings and recommendations from these studies were not ignored by the profession. The best of them were used to bring about improvements and needed change.

To analyze these studies and their impact on the developments that have occurred would constitute a book in its own right. The analysis of nursing education that completes this chapter is presented without direct reference to these studies, while recognizing fully that the studies are quite directly related to what is and what will be in nursing education. The studies that are recommended to the reader for serious review are:

- The Goldmark report, *Nursing and Nursing Education in the United States* (1923)
- The Brown report, *Nursing for the Future* (1948)
- The Lysaught report, *An Abstract for Action* (1970)
- The Institute of Medicine report, *Nursing and Nursing Education: Public Policy and Private Actions* (1983)
- The Pew Health Professions Commission reports, *Healthy America: Practitioners for 2005* (Sugars, O'Neal, & Bader, 1991) and *Recreating Health Professional Practice for a New Century* (Pew, 1998).

Looking Toward the Future

However nursing education programs are configured for the future, we must retain those facets of the system that ensure continued and growing representation of the gender and cultural diversity that exists in the society that the profession serves. This means that we must intensify efforts to attract ethnic and racial minorities and men into nursing. Ethnic and racial minority enrollment in baccalaureate and graduate programs is showing a slight increase, but it does not adequately reflect the diversity of the population. African Americans represent the largest minority group in all levels of nursing education (AACN, 1999). Male nurses are still a minority, but their ranks, too, are increasing. In 1999, 10.2% of baccalaureate students, 8.6% of master's students, and 5.4% of doctoral students were male (AACN, 2000).

Historically, transformations in nursing and nursing education have been driven by major socioeconomic factors, developments in health care, and professional issues unique to nursing. Trends to watch in terms of their potential impact on nursing education for the future are the following (Heller, Oros, & Durney-Crowley, 2000):

- The changing demographics and increasing diversity of society
- The technological explosion
- The globalization of the world's economy and society
- The era of the educated consumer, alternative therapies, genomics, and palliative care.
- The shift to population-based care and the increasing complexity of patient care
- The cost of health care and the challenge of managed care
- The impact of health policy and regulation
- The growing need for interdisciplinary education for collaborative practice
- The current nursing shortage and opportunities for lifelong learning and workforce development
- Advances in nursing science and research.

We must retain a system of nursing education that is responsive to society and that maximizes career development of nurses and ad-

vancement of the profession. We must bring greater clarity and meaning to our licensure and certification programs. And we must monitor and control the kinds and numbers of nurses we educate to meet societal and professional needs (Bellack & O'Neil, 2000). As we do so, we must bear in mind that to the extent to which the profession attracts and uses the people who earn the most respected advanced degrees and then gives them the opportunity to be role models and spokespersons for nursing, to that extent the profession will grow in viability, usefulness, and esteem.

If this chapter conveys a message of endorsement of and enthusiasm for the nursing profession and most components of its educational enterprise, a major outcome has been realized. There is every reason to believe that our successes will continue and that our problems can be solved. Nursing is a profession where exciting things are happening and where the best is yet to come.

KEY POINTS

- Health care needs in our society, along with certain historical events, influenced the development of multiple tracks of nursing education.
- Hospital-based diploma programs became the predominant model of nursing education in the United States for nearly 100 years.
- Although the first baccalaureate program in nursing was established in 1909, the development of significant numbers of these programs progressed slowly.
- Practical/vocational nursing programs were established to provide formal training for unlicensed personnel who, in large numbers, staffed U.S. hospitals during World War II.
- As a reaction to the vocational model of practical nursing, associate degree programs were established to educate technical nurses in collegiate programs.

- Master's programs prepare advanced practice nurses and other nurse specialists to assume significant roles in a variety of health care settings.

- The nursing doctorate program, similar in design to medical, dental, and legal models of education, prepares graduates for licensure and professional practice.

- Doctoral programs in nursing are designed to prepare scholars and researchers to expand the body of nursing knowledge.

- Cost and quality are two major considerations in selecting educational programs in nursing.

- Indicators of academic program quality include the status of program accreditation and approval, pass rates on licensure examinations, and pass rates on certification examinations.

- While each nursing education program has unique strengths, each also has weaknesses to which attention must be given.

- The tapestry of nursing education has the potential to be affected by societal and professional trends and issues.

CRITICAL THINKING EXERCISES

1. Defend or refute the following statement: There should be a separate licensing examination for nurses with baccalaureate degrees.

2. What is your career goal in nursing? What, if any, further education will you need to fully achieve your goal?

3. How does the certification of advanced practice nurses and nurse specialists protect the public?

4. Consult your state nurse practice act to determine the scope of practice of advanced practice nurses and other nurse specialists. What are the constraints on advanced practice nursing in your state?

5. Clarify the differences between nursing doctorate programs and doctoral programs in nursing.

6. Discuss the validity of licensure exam pass rates, regional and specialized accreditation status, and pass rates on certification examinations as indicators of the quality of a nursing education program.

7. What changes must be made in nursing education to ensure a culturally diverse nursing profession, non-punitive career advancement opportunities, and credibility in the higher education community?

8. Analyze the potential impact on nursing education and nursing practice of each trend identified on page 42.

REFERENCES

American Association of Colleges of Nursing. (1996). *Essentials of master's education for advanced practice nursing.* Washington, DC: Author.

American Association of Colleges of Nursing. (1998a). *Essentials of baccalaureate education for professional nursing practice.* Washington, DC: Author.

American Association of Colleges of Nursing. (1998b). *Position statement on educational mobility.* Washington, DC: Author.

American Association of Colleges of Nursing. (1999). *Distance technology in nursing education.* Washington, DC: Author.

American Association of Colleges of Nursing. (2000). *1999–2000 enrollments and graduations.* Washington, DC: Author.

American Nurses Association. (1965). *Educational preparation for nurse practitioners and assistants to nurses: A position paper.* New York: Author.

American Nurses' Credentialing Center. (2000a). *Certification catalog.* Washington, DC: Author.

American Nurses' Credentialing Center. (2000b). *Nurse practitioner board certification examination catalog.* Washington, DC: Author.

Anderson, C. A. (2000). Current strengths and limitations of doctoral education in nursing: Are we prepared for the future? *Journal of Professional Nursing, 16,* 191–200.

Bellack, J., & O'Neil, E. H. (2000). Recreating nursing practice for a new century: Recommendations and implications of the Pew Health Professions Commission's final report. *Nursing and Health Care Perspectives, 21*(1), 14–21.

Booth, R. Z., & Bednash, G. (1994). *Syllabus: The Newsletter of the American Association of Colleges of Nursing, 20*(5), 2.

Brown, E. L. (1948). *Nursing for the future.* New York: Russell Sage Foundation.

Creasia, J. L. (1994). Issues in designing an RN-MS track. *Nurse Educator, 19,* 27–32.

Goldmark, J., & the Committee for the Study of Nursing Education. (1923). *Nursing and nursing education in the United States.* New York: Macmillan.

Heller, B. R., Oros, M. T., & Durney-Crowley, J. (2000). The future of nursing education: 10 trends to watch. *Nursing and Health Care Perspectives, 21*(1), 9–13.

Institute of Medicine. (1983). *Nursing and nursing education: Public policies and private actions.* Washington, DC: National Academy Press.

Jones, K. D., & Lutz, K. F. (1999). Selecting doctoral programs in nursing: Resources for students and faculty. *Journal of Professional Nursing, 15,* 245–252.

Lysaught, J. (1970). *An abstract for action.* New York: McGraw-Hill.

National League for Nursing Accrediting Commission. (2000a). *Directory of accredited nursing programs.* New York: Author.

National League for Nursing Accrediting Commission. (2000b, June 30). *NLNAC Homepage* [On-line]. Available: *www.accrediting-comm-nlnac.org*

Peterson's guide to nursing programs. (2000). Princeton, NJ: Author, in cooperation with the American Association of Colleges of Nursing.

Pew Health Professions Commission. (1998). *Recreating health professional practice for a new century.* San Francisco: Author.

Schlotfeldt, R. M. (1978). The professional doctorate: Rationale and characteristics. *Nursing Outlook, 26,* 302–311.

Sugars, D. A., O'Neil, E. H., & Bader, J. D. (Eds.). (1991). *Healthy America: Practitioners for 2005. An agenda for action for U.S. health professional schools. A report of the Pew Health Professions Commission.* Durham, NC: Pew Health Professions Commission, Duke University Medical Center.

U.S. Department of Health and Human Services. (1990). *Eighth report to the President and Congress on the status of health personnel in the United States.* Bethesda, MD: Author.

U.S. Department of Health and Human Services. (1996). *The registered nurse population: Findings from the national sample survey of registered nurses.* Bethesda, MD: Author.

Williams, M. B. (1998). *Changing roles and relationships in nursing and health care.* St. Louis: Warren H. Green.

3

Socialization to Professional Nursing

MARY L. KILLEEN, PhD, RN

OBJECTIVES

At the completion of this chapter, the reader will be able to:

- Identify the characteristics of a profession.
- Evaluate nursing's current status as a profession.
- Describe the barriers that slow the professionalization of nursing.
- Discuss factors that influence professional socialization.
- Differentiate between accountability, autonomy, and shared governance as characteristics of professional practice.
- Describe the relationship between professional socialization and participating in professional nursing associations.

PROFILE IN PRACTICE

Peter A. White, BSN, MEd, RN
Master's Degree/Nurse Practitioner Student
College of Nursing, Arizona State University
Tempe, Arizona

Professional socialization is something I must crave, like some people and their relationship with chocolate! I say this because of my decision to change careers in 1991 by taking on the challenge of becoming a professional nurse, hence being socialized into a second profession. I had enjoyed my 20-year career in counseling psychology but reached a point where working only in the area of mental health with individuals was no longer fulfilling enough for me to sustain the energy required of that profession. Coincidentally, many of the individuals I was seeing in

counseling had chronic diseases, such as diabetes, cancer, COPD, and cardiovascular diseases, that impacted their anxious or depressive state in ways to which I was naïve. Not knowing the effect their medical illness could have as it manifested as anxiety or depression was very frustrating to me. After taking some time off to reflect on what I wanted to do with my professional life, I realized I could not stray too far from the central question, "Just who am I, now?" It didn't take long to figure out that the human service professions were what "I was put here for." I had always appreciated looking at my patients from a holistic perspective of the body, mind, and spirit. I knew for certain I would have to be in a profession I believed in, one where my values and the profession's values would interface like two strands of DNA. It was my lack of understanding of human physical functioning that led me to take this exciting journey into nursing with the goal of becoming a nurse practitioner eventually.

What I recall of my undergraduate nursing student years is the transformation of what I had already known, and was currently learning and experiencing, into a professional identity. This new identity combined the best of what I could offer the people I would care for with the strength and support of the nursing process, nursing theory, and nursing research. Nursing diagnosis helped to bring my new professional identity into focus. I did not have the luxury of merely stating, "Mr. Johnson has COPD." My challenge was to help Mr. Johnson learn new ways to cope with his impaired gas exchange, identify any knowledge deficits he might have

about this illness, and counsel him in his plan to quit smoking and adapt to his illness. This approach would require me to view any person I cared for as a nurse from a holistic and a chronological perspective, with short- and long-term goals—another plus for how I like to approach these challenges.

Many of my views and appreciation of the ability of people to adapt that I had gained in my prior profession carried over into nursing. My new profession has given me additional new appreciation for the act of caring for others: we nurses will have even greater effect when we consider the individual's physical, social, cultural, and emotional environments as we provide care. Nurses practice health promotion, disease prevention, and the care of individuals with altered health states. No human being is simply his or her diagnosis. The profession of nursing has taught me to consider each patient and his or her reaction to illness, if present, within that person's environment as the best way to provide care for those in need.

How does someone go from being a regular person—student, son, daughter, clerk— to being a professional nurse? Each person must acquire values, skills, behaviors, and norms appropriate to nursing practice. This process of learning and incorporating these aspects of a profession into individual professional identity is termed *socialization*. Socialization to professional nursing is an interactive process that begins in the educational setting and continues throughout one's nursing career.

The first socialization occurs in the basic nursing program. The socialization process is again activated at each of the following junctures: (1) when the new graduate leaves the educational setting and begins professional practice; (2) when the experienced nurse changes work settings, either in a new organization or

within the same organization; and (3) when the nurse undertakes new roles, such as assuming a leadership role or returning to school. Socialization, whether the first to be experienced or a later change in place or role, involves personal changes as a new professional self-identity is formed. These changes, like other kinds of change, can be both exciting and stressful, and may evoke strong emotional reactions and inner conflict as old patterns are replaced with new perspectives, values, behaviors, and skills.

To understand socialization to professional nursing practice it is helpful to examine the status of nursing as a profession. An exploration of these concepts will facilitate an understanding of the professional status of nursing and the process of socialization to professional nursing practice.

Nursing as a Profession

Nursing's roots are firmly anchored in service to others—individuals, groups, and communities. Since the days of Florence Nightingale, nurses have entered nursing to help people and serve the health care needs of society. This service orientation is evident in the Nightingale Pledge, which has been spoken by millions of nurses since the late 1800s. Dedication to duty is reflective of nursing's evolutionary links from holy orders (Birchenall, 1998). The pledge concludes with "devote myself to the welfare of those committed to my care." But is devotion and caring sufficient for nursing to call itself a profession? This question has stimulated discussion, debate, and controversy within health care and related disciplines. The ongoing debate about what nursing *is* and *is not* is timely and essential as the profession delineates its place within the emerging new order of health care delivery (Koerner & Burgess, 1997).

Social scientists and leaders in nursing have worked for several decades to define what constitutes a profession. A *profession* is defined as an occupation that meets specified criteria beyond that of occupation. Although the terms occupation and profession are often used interchangeably, it is important to understand the critical differences between the two concepts. A *profession* is characterized by prolonged education that takes place in a college or university and results in the acquisition of a body of knowledge based on theory and research. Values, beliefs, and ethics relating to the profession are an integral part of the educational preparation. By definition, a professional is *autonomous* in decision making and is *accountable* for his or her own actions. Personal identification and commitment to the profession are strong, and individuals are unlikely to change professions. In contrast, craft and trade *occupations* are characterized by technical skills learned through on-the-job apprenticeships. The training does not incorporate, as a prominent feature, the values, beliefs, and ethics of the occupation. Workers are supervised, and ultimate accountability rests with the employer. Thus, commitment from individuals may vary, and the rate of job changes may increase.

There are two models that can assist in addressing the question of what constitutes a profession (Catalano, 1996). The *process model* is the first. It proposes a continuum, with *position* (a group of tasks assigned to an individual) at one end of the continuum and *profession* at the other. With the process approach there is the expectation of advancement along the continuum until professional status is achieved. This would apply to a full range of positions—trash collectors, computer operators, psychologists, or nurses. But the process model does not provide criteria to aid in determining placement along the continuum. With the process model, identification as a profession is primarily dependent on the public's perception that profession status has been achieved. The second model focuses on traits or characteristics deemed to be important to professional status, such as service to the public, demonstrated competency, and accountability (Catalano, 2000). As scholars and researchers have attempted to describe a profession, several definitions have emerged. Each definition addresses the nature of knowledge and its application, values, and characteristics that symbolize a profession.

CHARACTERISTICS OF A PROFESSION

In response to concerns about the quality of educational programs in medical schools, particularly admission standards and curriculum, the Carnegie Foundation issued a series of papers. Abraham Flexner's (1910) classic paper was part of this series and served as the catalyst for reform of medical education in the United States and Canada. Flexner's recommendations were supported by the American Medical Association and the American Public Health Association. Their collective efforts, along with the willingness of members of the medical community to

TABLE 3-1 **Characteristics of a Profession**

Characteristic	Kelly & Joel (1999)	Houle (1980)	Bixler & Bixler (1959)	Greenwood (1957)
Knowledge	Uses well-defined and well-organized body of knowledge that is intellectual and describes phenomena of concern	Mastery and use of theoretical knowledge Role distinctions that differentiate professional work from that of other vocations	Uses well-defined body of specialized knowledge at the intellectual level of higher learning	Uses a systematic body of knowledge
Mission	Enlarges body of knowledge and subsequently imposes on its members the lifelong obligation to remain current	Concept of mission open to change Capacity to solve problems	Continuously enlarges body of knowledge; uses scientific method to improve education and service	
Education	Entrusts the education of its practitioners to institutions of higher education.	Formal training	Prepares practitioners in institutions of higher learning	
Social construct	Applies body of knowledge in services that are vital to human welfare; tradition of seasoned practitioners shaping skills of newcomers to role	Service to society Public acceptance	Applies knowledge through services that are vital to human and social welfare	Sanctions of the community
Autonomy	Functions autonomously in formulation of professional policy and in monitoring of its practice and practitioners.	Autonomous practice; credentialing system to certify competence	Functions autonomously in formulating professional policy and controlling professional activity	Professional autonomy
Accountability	Guided by a code of ethics that regulates the relationship between professional and client.	Ethical practice Legal reinforcement of professional standards Penalties against incompetent or unethical practice		Ethical codes of conduct
Culture	Distinguished by presence of specific culture, norms, and values that are common among its members Attracts individuals of intellectual and personal qualities who exalt service above personal gain and who recognize their occupation as their life work	Creation of subculture	Attracts individuals who exalt service above personal gain and who recognize their chosen occupation as their life work	Professional culture
Compensation	Strives to compensate its practitioners by providing freedom of action, opportunity for continuous professional growth, and economic security	Continued seeking of self-enhancement by its members	Compensates practitioners by providing freedom of action, opportunity for continuous professional growth, and economic security	

embrace a major reorientation of medical education, led to changing the face of medicine within a 10-year period, strengthened medicine as a profession, and raised its status in the eyes of the public (Schwirian, 1998).

Flexner also studied other disciplines, and in 1915 he published a list of criteria he believed were characteristic of all true professions. He viewed the intellectual aspect as central to professions. According to Flexner, a true profession

- Is basically intellectual (as opposed to physical), with high responsibility.
- Is based on a body of knowledge that can be learned.
- Is practical (applied) rather than theoretical.
- Can be taught through the process of professional education.
- Has a strong internal organization of members.
- Has practitioners who are motivated by altruism (the desire to help others).

Since Flexner's work in 1915, additional authors have modified and amplified criteria of a profession. The works of Greenwood (1957), Bixler and Bixler (1959), Houle (1980), and Kelly and Joel (1999) are summarized in Table 3–1.

A specified body of knowledge and altruism are the most widely acknowledged characteristics of a profession. A professional possesses unique knowledge, and members of the profession acquire this knowledge through a significant period of training. Group members "profess" to be knowledgeable in an area that is not known by most people but which society needs. Members also are invested with a service ideal, *altruism.* Nursing actions convince the public that members are not self-serving but use knowledge to benefit the public. Society then grants autonomy or control to the profession to set its standards and regulate practice (McCloskey & Maas, 1998).

Professionalization of Nursing

Professionalization is the process through which an occupation achieves professional status. The status of nursing as a profession is important because it reflects the value society places on the work of nurses and the centrality of this work to the good of society (Strader & Decker, 1995). Guided by the descriptions of what constitutes a profession, how does nursing measure? At the time criteria were being developed, nursing fell short of professional status in a number of areas. For example, most nursing education programs were based in hospitals and reflected an apprenticeship model rather than being in institutions of higher education. Nursing research was in its infancy, thereby offering little toward the identification of a unique body of knowledge that would improve nursing practice and education. In addition, autonomous nursing practice was relatively uncommon, and there was no formalized code of ethics.

In contrast, today most nursing education programs are based in institutions of higher education. There is an expanding body of knowledge derived from systematic research. Opportunities for autonomous practice are expanding, and there is a well-defined code of ethics. Areas still needing attention include nursing's control of policies and activities that affect the delivery of nursing care. This has become more evident as health care delivery has undergone dramatic organizational, financial, and personnel changes that individually and collectively affect how, what, and where nursing is practiced. In this redesigned health care environment nurses are challenged to engage in practice that embodies the social service ideal where clients rather than tasks are given the highest level of importance.

An analysis of nursing's placement along the occupation–profession continuum reveals strengths and challenges. Strengths include (1) a service-to-society mission, (2) the provision of services that are vital to human welfare, and (3) a well-defined code of ethics. Challenges include (1) limited development of nursing theory and a unique body of nursing knowledge, (2) lack of standardization of nursing education, with university preparation still not the minimum entry requirement, (3) variation in members' commitment to their work, and (4) minimal cohesive culture within the nursing community (Schwirian, 1999).

BARRIERS TO PROFESSIONALISM

Autonomy, the freedom to act, is a key characteristic present in all the definitions and is clearly linked to achieving professional status. But autonomy is linked to other characteristics as well. A limited body of scientific knowledge and an incomplete articulation of phenomena unique to nursing are cited as major contributors to the lack of autonomy in nursing practice. Nursing is still viewed by many as a lower level of medical knowledge that should be under the jurisdiction of medicine (Wurst, 1994).

The development of nursing knowledge is fundamental to the professionalization of nursing. The science of nursing is concerned with developing a unified body of knowledge that includes skills and methodologies for applying that knowledge (Chinn & Kramer, 1999). Until the 1980s, knowledge by definition was empirically based, focusing exclusively on objective, observable data and an analytical, linear line of reasoning. Since that time, there has been growing awareness that exclusive reliance on empirical data provides only a partial view of the world and that our knowledge can best be expanded by utilizing multiple approaches to scientific inquiry. Barbara Carper's classic paper (1978) describes four fundamental and enduring patterns of knowing:

- *empirics*—the science of nursing
- *ethics*—moral knowledge component of nursing

- *aesthetics*—the art of nursing
- *personal knowing* in nursing

"The fundamental patterns of knowing remain valuable in that they conceptualize a broad scope of knowing that accounts for a holistic practice" (Chinn & Kramer, 1999, p 4). Thus, nursing knowledge is derived not only from theoretical formulations and scientific research, but also from analysis of personal experiences which contributes to clinical knowledge and expertise. The continued development of a distinct body of knowledge will aid in differentiating nursing from other health professions and provide a stronger basis for practice.

Other factors identified as limiting nursing's autonomy include gender stereotypes and lack of unity. Historically, females have been socialized to shy away from power and assume more subservient roles, which supports a job orientation instead of a professional orientation (Nicolson, 1996). In addition, nursing is fragmented by subgroups, internal dissent related in part to entry into practice, rivalry, and failure to view the professional association as a vital component of the professional culture.

Presentation of self may also act as a barrier to advancing nursing's professional status. For example, "nurses' verbal informality with patients is linked to persistent stereotypic themes that diminish the professional image, shroud the cognitive nature of their work, perpetuate hierarchical relationships between physicians and nurses, and even threaten nurses' therapeutic effectiveness" (Campbell-Heider, Hart, & Bergren, 1994, pp. 212–213). In addition, Campbell-Heider and colleagues argue that current clothing styles and the differential use of titles (doctor for physicians and first name for nurses) further diminish the professional status of nursing.

Other groups that attempt to control nursing, such as organized medicine and health services administration, are well organized, have clearly defined their unique phenomena, and are viewed as having control of a profession that enjoys high status. However, we are reminded that the occupation-profession distinction is largely artificial. The designation of what is professional versus what is occupational is based on tradition and existing mechanisms (unions and academic departments) in an effort to maintain the status quo (McCloskey & Maas, 1998).

Taking a different approach to professionalization, Adams, Miller, and Beck (1996) focus on the individual nurse. Their approach reflects the view of Styles (1982), who maintained that it is the individual and her or his personal presentation that fosters the collective image of nursing.

A MODEL FOR PROFESSIONALISM

Citing lack of consensus among nurses on what behaviors exemplify professional status, Miller (1985) and Miller, Adams, and Beck (1993)

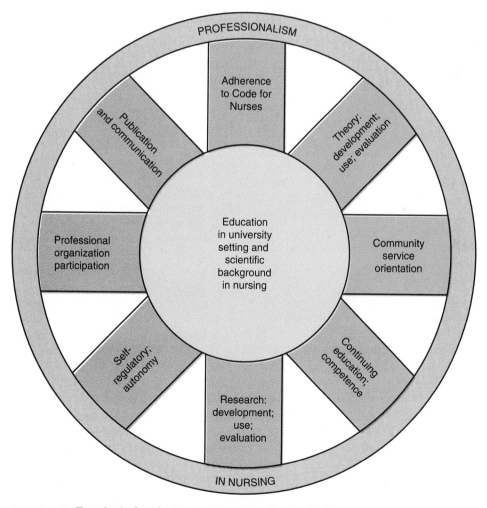

FIGURE 3–1 The wheel of professionalism in nursing. (Reprinted with permission: Wheel of Professionalism in Nursing. Copyright 1984, Barbara Kemp Miller.)

drew from common definitions of a profession and to these added behaviors expressed in key nursing documents such as the American Nurses Association's *Nursing: A Social Policy Statement* (1995) and *Code for Nurses* (1985). Barbera Miller's "wheel of professionalism" is presented in Figure 3–1. The basic education of a professional, occurring in a university setting with emphasis on the scientific basis of nursing, is at the hub of the wheel. The eight spokes extending from the hub represent behaviors deemed essential to achieving, maintaining, and expanding professionalism in the individual nurse.

Professional Nursing Practice

Florence Nightingale (1860), in her clear and direct manner, stated that the goal of nursing is to "put the patient in the best condition for nature to act upon him." This essence of nursing practice continues to be reflected in contemporary nursing. In the revised *Social Policy Statement* developed by the ANA (1995), four essential features of contemporary nursing practice are identified:

1. Attention to the full range of human experiences and responses to health and illness without restriction to a problem-focused orientation.
2. Integration of objective data with an understanding of the subjective experience of the patient.
3. Application of scientific knowledge to the process of diagnosis and treatment.
4. Provision of a caring relationship that facilitates health and healing.

VALUES OF THE PROFESSION

Knowledge and skills and ethical grounding of the nurse directly affect the quality of care provided (Fagermoen, 1997). The profession's values give direction and meaning to its members, guide nursing behaviors, are instrumental in clinical decision making and influence how nurses think about themselves. Although skills change and evolve over time, core values of nursing persist and are communicated through the ANA's *Code for Nurses* (ANA, 1985). With licensure as a registered nurse, each nurse accepts responsibility for practicing nursing consistent with these values. The code for nurses with associated ethical principles is summarized in Table 3–2 (Fargotstein, 2000). Note that philosophical ethical principles and concepts of interpersonal relationships are reflected, either directly or indirectly, in all of the canons. The ethical principles are those most directly reflected in the respective canons.

Weis and Schank (2000) developed and tested an instrument based on the ANA's *Code for Nurses* that measured professional nursing values. Each of 44 items was a short descriptive phrase reflecting a specific code statement and its interpretive commentary. With a sample of 599 respondents, *caregiving* was the major professional nursing value identified.

When nurses were asked to provide a description of a patient care situation that would exemplify what was meaningful in nursing, *altruism* (unselfish concern for or devotion to the welfare of others) was identified as the overall philosophy that guided practice. Human dignity was further identified as a core value, with linking values of recognition of the client as an individual, empathetic understanding, and reciprocal trust (Fagermoen, 1997).

Thus, service to society has remained a central value of nursing, and nursing's consistent provision of service to benefit the public has earned the public's trust. A key component in preserving this trust is accountability. *Accountability* is the state of being responsible and answerable for one's own behavior. This is explicit in the ANA's *Code for Nurses* (1985): "The nurse assumes responsibility and is accountable

TABLE 3–2 Code for Nurses with Associated Ethical Principles

Code Canons	Ethical Principles	Ethical/Therapeutic Concepts Addressed
1. The nurse provides services with respect for human dignity and uniqueness of the client, unrestricted by considerations of social or economic status, personal attributes, or the nature of the health problem.	• Autonomy • Veracity (truth-telling) • Justice (distributive)	• Dignity and worth of client • Respect • Advocate for client rights • Interpersonal connectedness
2. The nurse safeguards the client's right to privacy by judiciously protecting information of a confidential nature.	• Confidentiality	• Trust within the nurse-client relationship. • Anonymity (research or nonclinical purposes)
3. The nurse acts to safeguard the client and the public when health care and safety are affected by the incompetent, unethical, or illegal practice of any person.	• Beneficence • Nonmaleficence (avoid doing harm)	• Advocate for client well-being • Legal obligations (Standards, Nurse Practice Act)
4. The nurse assumes responsibility and accountability for individual nursing judgments and actions.	• Fidelity (loyalty) • Beneficence	• Collaboration in nurse-client relationship • Accountability/Responsibility
5. The nurse maintains competence in nursing.	• Beneficence	• Accountability/Responsibility • Competency
6. The nurse exercises informed judgment and uses individual competence and qualifications as criteria in seeking consultation, accepting responsibilities, and delegating nursing activities to others.	• Beneficence	• Collaboration • Responsibility
7. The nurse participates in activities that contribute to the ongoing development of the profession's body of knowledge.	• Autonomy (client) • Informed consent • Privacy	• Client advocacy in research process
8. The nurse participates in the profession's efforts to implement and improve standards of nursing.	• Fidelity	• Values (professional; personal) • Standards of Care
9. The nurse participates in the profession's efforts to establish and maintain conditions of employment conducive to high-quality nursing care.	• Autonomy (professional)	• Values (professional)
10. The nurse participates in the profession's efforts to protect the public from misinformation and misrepresentation and to maintain the integrity of nursing.	• Beneficence • Nonmaleficence • Veracity	• Values (professional) • Integrity (professional)
11. The nurse collaborates with members of the health professions and other citizens in promoting community and national efforts to meet the health needs of the public.	• Justice (distributive) • Beneficence	• Collaboration • Values (professional; societal)

From Fargotstein, B. P.: Unpublished manuscript. Tempe, Arizona, 1999.

for individual nursing judgments and actions." Accountability extends to self, the client, the employing agency, the profession, and the public. The ANA's *Standards of Clinical Nursing Practice* (1998) describe both the what and how of professional nursing. *Standards of care* are the "what" and describe a competent level of nursing care through use of the nursing process. *Standards of professional performance* are the "how" of nursing, with eight standards describing a competent level of behavior in the professional role. Each standard is accompanied by criteria that permit measurement of performance and characterize competent, professional practice. These standards are listed in Table 3–3. Further elaboration of professional nursing responsibilities can be found in the standards of care for the various specialty practices.

RESPONSIBILITY

Areas of responsibility within nursing's role are constantly being affected by changes in the larger health care arena. Johnson, Friend, and MacDonald (1997) describe a "sense of displacement" as nurses experience a shift to new areas of responsibility while relinquishing some of the more traditional ones. They identify emerging professional nurse responsibilities as

- Establishing and maintaining partnership relationships with client and family.
- Caring and creating healing space by spending non-task-related time with clients.
- Using time and skills to build trust and work collaboratively.
- Understanding and appreciating client stories and experiences with health and illness as they affect their lives.
- Learning through reflection on self and practice.
- Encouraging the active collaboration of client and family in choosing their own care.
- Sharing work responsibilities in a mindful way.
- Informing clients of treatment choices, and teaching self-care and responsibility for their own health.
- Serving as a mentor to different levels of health care providers.

ACCOUNTABILITY

By virtue of the ANA's *Standards of Clinical Nursing Practice* and the state nurse practice acts, society holds nurses and those under their supervision accountable for their actions. The nurse has a responsibility to demonstrate sound judgment, critical thinking, and competence in the caregiver role. In the supervisory role, the nurse must ensure that only competent health care workers be allowed to care for clients and is obligated to take action against those whose knowledge or skill is questionable. While a task can be delegated, accountability remains with the nurse.

TABLE 3–3 Standards of Clinical Nursing Practice

Standards of Care
Assessment
Diagnosis
Outcome identification
Planning
Implementation
Evaluation

Standards of Professional Performance
Quality of care
Performance appraisal
Education
Collegiality
Ethics
Collaboration
Research
Resource utilization

Data from American Nurses Association. (1998). *Standards of clinical nursing practice.* Washington, DC: Author.

Another demonstration of nursing's accountability is through formulating policies, controlling its activities, and advocating professional issues in the political system. Nursing organizations have developed standards of practice for general and specialty nursing care, with each set of standards addressing professional accountability. *Legal accountability* occurs through licensing procedures, certification, and disciplinary actions that are established and implemented by state boards of nursing. These measures support the public trust that safe, effective practice will be the standard of practice. In the political arena, nurses demonstrate their commitment to service to others by becoming increasingly involved in advocating for health care legislation that strengthens nursing practice, protects the public, and offers choice to consumers.

AUTONOMY

A further reflection of the public's trust in the nursing profession is the responsibility to be self-governing or autonomous. *Autonomy* is independence or the freedom to act. It implies control over practice and is exemplified by the profession being invested with responsibilities for nursing education, development of policies and standards that guide practice, and oversight to ensure competent practice.

Autonomy involves independence on the part of the nurse, a willingness to take risks and be accountable for actions. However, autonomy in nursing practice must be balanced with interdependence, since health care is a multidisciplinary endeavor and several disciplines contribute to total client care. Koerner and Burgess (1997) caution that "Focusing on nursing as an autonomous profession rather than as an essential player in an interdependent team misses the richness of relationships with our health care colleagues" (p. 5). They assert that this focus serves to negate the integrative and cooperative roles that nursing provides for the entire health care team.

Socialization to Professional Nursing

Socialization is the process of becoming, of acquiring knowledge and skills and internalizing attitudes and values specific to a given social group. Much of the literature on socialization has focused on child development and the influence of the family on the child's socialization. This process occurs through role modeling and the reinforcement of socially relevant behaviors. Increased attention is now being given to *adult socialization,* the process by which individuals develop new behaviors and values associated with roles they assume as an adult. With assistance from others, individuals learn necessary behaviors, values, norms, and skills to successfully assume new roles.

Socialization to professional nursing is the process of learning the skills, roles, and values of the profession, with the outcome being the development of a professional identity. It represents a complex process by which a student or practicing nurse acquires the knowledge, skills, and a sense of occupational identity. It involves the internalization of the values and norms of the profession in the individual's own behavior and self-concept. It is taking the values and norms and making them part of who you are as a nurse. "In the process a person gives up the societal and media stereotypes prevalent in our culture and adopts those held by members of the profession" (Cohen, 1981). The individual's conception of what it means to be a nurse and to act as a nurse occurs initially through education and is then extended into the work setting.

SOCIALIZATION THROUGH EDUCATION

Learning any new role may be a challenging and anxiety-producing task. As adults, individuals have developed competencies in various previously learned roles. The choice to learn a new role returns the adult to novice status, one of limited or no knowledge of new role expectations.

Initial Socialization. Professional socialization through education is the pathway to learning new roles within the culture of nursing. Initial socialization to nursing occurs in the educational setting and is subsequently transferred to the practice setting. Howkins and Ewens (1999) sought to understand how nursing students make sense of the socialization process. Through their research they identified three themes relating to how a student's role identity changes and develops during his or her education. The first theme, "development of the graduate practitioner," focuses on awareness of having more knowledge, perspective, confidence, reflective thinking, political awareness, and being able to think critically. The second theme, "gaining a better understanding of own role," focuses on continuing refinement of role components. The third theme, "adopting a less polarized view," is characterized by no longer seeing roles as having rigid boundaries and reveals "the development of graduate practitioners who understand their own role while becoming less rigid in their thinking" (p. 47).

The socialization process experienced by baccalaureate nursing students was described by Reutter and colleagues (1997). The setting for the study was a large university that offered a 4-year baccalaureate nursing program. The development of the students was tracked longitudinally, and their experiences were described as follows:

Year 1: Learning the Ideal. Students begin to internalize new values, focusing on caring and holistic individualized practice. Students are more passive as learners, and while they can delineate professional values, they are unable to describe how these values play out in the practice setting.

Year 2: Confronting Reality. Students place greater emphasis on the application of theory and are more aware of their limited knowledge base and scope of responsibilities. This results in greater feelings of inadequacy but increased appreciation of organizational skills, time management, and the uniqueness of patient situations. With limited confidence they seek validation and are vulnerable to feedback.

Year 3: Becoming Comfortable with Reality. Activities are focused on fine-tuning their art of nursing, role-making and role-taking, modifying behaviors of the role, and moving from "ideal" to "optimal" care delivery.

Year 4: Extending Beyond Reality of Student Practice. Increasing focus is placed on skills of the real world, greater initiation in seeking out experiences to increase confidence, and a broadening of their view of nursing to include political action strategies, the health care system, and public awareness of nursing's expanding role (Reutter et al., 1997).

Resocialization. Returning to school represents a role transition and triggers a new socialization process as new role expectations are synthesized and a new professional. identity is established. Malcolm Knowles's (1970) classic work on adult education defined the "art and science of how adults learn" as *andragogy.* According to Knowles, adult learners

- Exhibit self-direction and self-responsibility.
- Demonstrate a readiness to learn that is oriented toward problem solving.
- Have acquired experience that serves as a resource for learning.
- Have shifted from learning with postponed application to learning with immediate application.
- Strive for self-esteem and self-actualization.

This model is particularly applicable to the nurse who returns to school for an additional degree. Most RNs who return to school continue their employment and must balance concurrent roles of nurse, student, parent, and significant other, to name a few. While challenging, multiple roles can provide new rewards and a positive synergy that might not be experienced from a single role (Curry, 1997).

Historically, educational programs have not been known for their accommodation of the nurse as student. RN students came with a nursing role identity, but little recognition was given to the expertise the nurse possessed, and there was a tendency to force adherence to an educational model most appropriate for beginning nursing students. A "returning-to-school syndrome" (Shane, 1983) was described as beginning positively and with excitement about increasing knowledge and skills, but then turning to conflict, anger, and resentment that could continue even after graduation. It was thought that this response occurred because old knowledge and rules were no longer valid, and the new was not yet accepted.

Learning any new role requires embracing change. The struggle between the old and new may cause anxiety and tension related to being a novice again or fear of failure and fear of unknowns. While nursing has not been successful in reaching agreement about the education needed for entry into professional practice, there has been success in developing educational models that facilitate movement from one level of preparation to another in a relatively "user-friendly" way (McBride, 1999). With increased recognition and appreciation of what the RN student brings to the educational setting, and working to provide program structures that acknowledge the need to balance multiple roles, the RN educational experience can be positive and growth producing. If resocialization through education is fully effective, the student (basic and RN) leaves the educa-

tional program with changes in attitudes and behavior that reflect an integration of the values and norms of the expanded scope of the professional practitioner.

Throwe and Fought (1987) used the eight stages of Erikson's (1950) developmental theory to assess RN students' resocialization. For each of the eight stages, examples of role-resisting and role-accepting behaviors may be observed as the RN student progresses through the resocialization process. A role-resisting behavior of keeping physically isolated from classmates, as opposed to a role-accepting behavior of being involved with classmates, is an example cited for the trust/mistrust stage. For the initiative guilt stage, an example cited of role-resisting behavior is waiting for the instructor to set priorities, while a role-accepting behavior may be effectiveness in time management. With the successful accomplishment of these developmental tasks, the RN student achieves consistent role enactment. The student's knowledge base is strengthened, new options are explored, and problem solving is more creative. The student is ready to try out new roles.

SOCIALIZATION TO THE WORK SETTING

Education is only the initial process in socialization. The professional nursing role learned in the educational setting must now be transferred and modified to fit the workplace. Thus the continuum of socialization extends as resocialization begins.

The socialization process is built around role theory (see Chapter 4). Individuals learn behaviors that accompany each role by two simultaneously occurring processes: (1) interaction involving groups and significant others in a social context and (2) learning through role-playing, identification, modeling, instruction, observation, trial and error, and role negotiation (Hardy & Conway, 1988). Adding to the complexity of this process is the "should be," or ideal presented in the educational setting, and the "what is," or reality of the actual practice environment. Faculty and staff have the obligation of helping students understand the logic and rationale for any discrepancies that may exist (Coudret et al., 1994).

Kramer's Resocialization Model. One of the best-known models of resocialization in nursing is Kramer's *Reality Shock: Why Nurses Leave Nursing* (1974). She describes fears and difficulties new graduate nurses experience in adapting to the work setting and refers to feelings of powerlessness and ineffectiveness as *reality shock*. Reality shock results from a conflict between a new graduate's knowledge and skills acquired in the educational program and the reality of the behaviors required in the actual work setting. New graduates progress through four stages before feeling comfortable in the professional role.

Stage one focuses on *mastery of skills and routines*. New graduates feel inadequate and frustrated, and as a result tend to focus on the mastery of essential skills. A potential problem here is that the nurse may become fixated on technical skills and fail to see other important aspects of client care, such as emotional needs.

Stage two is *social integration*. The new nurse's major concern is getting along with co-workers and fitting into the work group. Conflict occurs when a new nurse strives to maintain high ideals and standards learned in the educational setting and at the same time avoid alienating co-workers.

Stage three is *moral outrage*. During this stage incongruities among roles in the work setting cause the new nurse to feel angry, frustrated, and inadequately prepared. Determining priorities is a challenge.

In stage four, *conflict resolution*, new nurses either give up or compromise their values and behaviors or successfully integrate them into the professional and bureaucratic systems. This results in one of four possible outcomes. The new nurse either (1) finds work situations that are more compatible with her or his beliefs, or

leaves nursing altogether, or (2) accepts the values of the bureaucracy and gives up values gained in the educational program and just tries to fit into the organization, or (3) yields to the organization, with the focus on survival, or (4) learns to use values of both the profession and the organization to influence positive change in the system. Kramer terms this fourth outcome *biculturalism* and considers it the healthiest and most successful resolution.

Following the publication of Kramer's work, educational programs and employers, primarily hospitals, began to examine methods that could reduce reality shock in the transition from student to professional. For example, students were encouraged to gain experience outside of school settings as nursing assistants or nurse externs during the summer, school breaks, and weekends. In addition, educational programs began to pair students with preceptors so that they could work closely with a practicing RN. In the work setting, longer orientation programs provided an opportunity for smoother transitions. Preceptor programs were also offered to allow the new nurse to work alongside an experienced nurse. Commitment, creativity, and collaboration among educational programs and employers are key factors in facilitating the new graduate's successful socialization into the professional nursing role.

SOURCES OF LEARNING: SOCIALIZING AGENTS IN EDUCATION AND PRACTICE

Educational programs and employers can assist in clarifying role expectations and decreasing conflict through the use of role models, preceptors, and mentors. If these socializing agents were placed along an involvement continuum, one end would be anchored by role models (least involvement) and the other end would be anchored by mentors (most involvement). Despite the somewhat blurred boundaries and functions of these roles, each has an important part to play in the nurse's socialization process.

A *role model* is someone to copy, emulate,

and admire. Role models are usually experienced, competent nurses who exemplify excellence in practice. Effective qualities of role models include compassion, caring, and an empathetic approach to care delivery, approachability, flexibility, professional competence, and power (Fitzpatrick, While, & Roberts, 1996). Learning through role modeling occurs primarily through observation. Little contact is needed, and for this reason it is usually viewed as a passive process—the student or new nurse observes the behaviors of the role model and copies those behaviors they choose to incorporate into their own professional identity. The availability of role models in practice is a key influence on professional socialization.

Students may also adopt one another as role models and differentiate between peers who are becoming "good" nurses and those who are less effective in their care delivery. These peer role models facilitate learning by sharing experiences, knowledge, and clinical expertise, providing emotional support, and assisting with psychomotor skills. Students are most influenced by a combination of positive and negative versus positive-only modeling. Nonexemplars (negative role models) are used to reaffirm their own ideals about what they want (and don't want) to become (Reutter et al., 1997). Use of skills in observing and judging and developing the ability to differentiate between effective and ineffective care delivery are critical skills for competent professional practice (Parathian & Taylor, 1993). New graduates are also aware of both positive and negative role models and consciously structure their interactions after positive role models (Benner, Tanner, & Chelsa, 1996). Role models may also be preceptors and mentors.

Preceptors are experienced members of a clinical staff who work one-on-one with students or new graduates to provide guidance and supervision for a predetermined amount of time. More specifically, a *preceptor* models behavior, fosters independence and skill development, aids in application of theory, promotes socialization to the work setting, and helps build competence and confidence in the student or new graduate (Letizia & Jennrich, 1998; McGregor, 1999). Preceptors may function in more than one role. Roles identified as being intrinsic to effective preceptors include change agent, educator, in-service provider, mentor to peers, needs assessor, and resource person (Dusmohamed & Guscott, 1998). Benefits are evident for preceptors as they build knowledge and skills through teaching, learn with the student or new graduate, and feel they are making a contribution to the profession. These benefits contribute to preceptors voicing a renewed sense of pride in nursing (McGregor, 1999). Stress may result from demands on preceptors that exceed their available time and resources. Typically nurses add the preceptor role to their other regular clinical responsibilities. In addition, some preceptors may not have preparation in teaching and evaluation, which are key responsibilities within the role. Active agency support is essential in sustaining effective preceptors.

Mentors take on an even more powerful role in the socialization process. *Mentoring* is defined as a "supportive and nuturing relationship between an experienced professional . . . and an aspiring protégé" (Owens, Herrick, & Kelley, 1998, p. 78). The mentor is generally older and willing to share experiences that may be beneficial to the protégé. The mentor takes a personal interest in helping an individual over a period of time to develop the knowledge and skills needed to realize the protégé's full potential and major life goals (Fuszard & Taylor, 1995).

Identification of a mentor does not occur automatically but requires a proactive approach from both the potential mentor and the protégé in search of a mentor. Certain individual characteristics are necessary before mentoring can occur. These include a mutual attraction with sharing of similar views and common interests, respect, altruism, belief in the other's potential, capacity to work hard, integrity, mastery of concepts and ideas, unselfish gifts of time, energy and trust, and a willingness for self-disclosure (Stewart & Krueger, 1996). "Successful mentoring requires active participation in the relationship with equal responsibility for its success for both mentor and protégé, along with institutional and collegial support" (Owens et al., 1998, p. 22).

A review of the literature confirmed six essential features of mentoring. First is a teaching-learning process in which the protégé can benefit from the mistakes and successes of the mentor and avoid adverse situations. Second, a reciprocal role exists, with the protégé gradually shifting from dependence on the mentor in the beginning to increasing independence and autonomy with a balanced two-way, give-and-take between mentor and protégé. Third, nurses who have been mentored experience greater career development, position advancement, productivity, and development of a "nursing gestalt." Fourth, a knowledge or competence differential exists between mentor and protégé. Fifth, a mentoring has a duration of several years. Sixth, there is a resonating phenomenon—those who have been mentored will mentor others in the future as a way of expressing gratitude for their own experience (Stewart & Krueger, 1996). Mentoring does not just happen. The benefits of mentoring are significant and make the demands on time and energy worthwhile. Unfortunately, not every nurse has the benefit of having a mentor during each career change.

～ Socialization and Career Development

Career development extends over time, with the process beginning when the new graduate enters the work setting and proceeding at varied rates along a career path. Two models of career development in nursing are presented here. The stages of one model lead to an increased level of responsibility (Dalton, Thompson, & Price, 1977); the stages of the other lead to a higher level of clinical expertise (Benner, 1984).

DALTON'S LONGITUDINAL MODEL

Dalton and colleagues described a four-stage model of career development that builds on prior knowledge and experience:

Stage 1. The nurse learns to perform routine duties competently and to use both formal and informal channels of communication. Ideally, the nurse works with an experienced preceptor who also serves as a role model. A problem occurs when the organization does not permit enough time to master this stage.

Stage 2. The individual develops a reputation as a competent nurse, often in an area of clinical specialty. Again, adequate time is needed in this stage to master this level of expertise.

Stage 3. The nurse assumes responsibility for others. The nurse may take on multiple roles, such as informal mentor, manager, supervisor, or coordinator.

Stage 4. The nurse assumes the roles of manager and innovator of ideas to influence the direction of the organization. Relationships are developed inside and outside the organization. Individuals in stage 4 think more broadly about the organization and feel comfortable in exercising power and taking a position with which others may disagree. Only a small percentage of nurses achieve this level of career development, either by choice or because of limits on the number of positions available.

BENNER'S NOVICE-TO-EXPERT MODEL

Five stages or levels of proficiency in nursing care delivery are identified in the novice-to-expert model (Benner, 1984). These stages re-

TABLE 3-4 **From Novice to Expert**

Stage 1: Novice (No experience)

- Learns objective information, with tasks being broken down into steps.
- Knowledge is context-free and can be understood without experience.
- Practice is based on theoretical knowledge, rules, and procedures.
- Rules determine actions that are limited and inflexible.
- Dependent on and has total confidence in those with greater expertise.
- Inability to use discretionary judgment.

Stage 2: Advanced Beginner

- Clinical situation presents as set of tasks that must be completed.
- Patient appears as perplexing collection of problems/conditions for action.
- Work shaped by concern to organize, prioritize, and complete tasks.
- Assessment is more a task rather than a structure to direct clinical care.
- Fragmented or partial grasp of patient condition; absorbed in biological needs and feels unable to attend to psychosocial needs of patient/family.
- Attention and energies focused on inventory of things to do, all of which are relevant.
- Respects and relies on judgment of nurse experts and defers complex clinical observations and decision making to those with greater expertise.
- Aware of their partial grasp; anxiety makes them more vigilant in their care.
- Preceptor involvement helps them fit disjointed pieces together, see patterns, validate observations, weigh and balance competing concerns, appreciate immense variation in individual responses and tailoring of care, and analyze situations that did not go well.

Stage 3: Competent (1-2 years in similar job situation)

- Checklist approach now seen as inadequate.
- Struggles to learn to "read" the situation.
- Improved time management, efficiency, organizational ability, and technical skills; performance more fluid and coordinated.
- Ability to prioritize and anticipate demands and engage in anticipatory planning.
- Meshing theoretical and clinical knowledge.
- Able to alter protocols and standards of care to meet particular patient/family needs.
- Suffering of patient more apparent; "conscious repersonalization" of patient/family.
- Increased diagnostic reasoning with ability to make a clinical case for action to physicians.
- Emotional responses become more informative and guiding.
- Co-workers now recognized as fallible.
- Precepting by proficient to expert nurse very beneficial for refining ability to "read" situation.

Stage 4: Proficient (3-5 years with similar patient populations)

- Increasingly accurate grasp of situation and when missing has a vague sense of uneasiness/discomfort.
- Actively interprets direction of change.
- Can recognize when the situation is not normal.
- Able to recognize early warning signs and notice when patient condition is sufficient to warrant redefinition and change in actions.
- Knows what things can wait and what cannot.
- Growing sense of nursing concerns and difference from medical concerns.
- Learning to be engaged in clinical situation and be connected with patient/family in ways that are helpful.
- Challenges information given but does not take into account all variations that might occur.
- Greater trust in emotional responses to guide attentiveness and consultation with others.
- Most likely will lead to "expert."

Table continued on following page

TABLE 3–4 From Novice to Expert *Continued*

Stage 5: Expert

- Management of multiple tasks simultaneously with skill in performance, timing, and anticipation evident; "thinking in action."
- Grasp of the big picture with ability to go beyond immediate clinical situation with sense of future and recognition of anticipated trajectories.
- Attuned to situation that allows responses to be shaped by mindful reading of patient responses without recourse to conscious deliberation.
- Recognition and assessment language is so linked with actions and outcomes that they become obvious; may have difficulty explaining how they know something.
- Expanded "peripheral vision"—sensing needs of other patients in area and capabilities of nurses assigned to their care.
- Concern for revealing and responding to patients as persons, respecting their dignity, caring in ways that preserve personhood, protecting when vulnerable, helping patient to feel safe in alien environment.
- Working to preserve integrity of close nurse-patient relationship.
- Learning to orchestrate actions in relation to working with others to minimize being overburdened and seeing that all possible resources are brought to bear in difficult situations.
- Expert mastery of technology and expert caring provide prudent and critical view of technology.
- Compelled to take strong positions/moral stands with other nurses and physicians to get what they believe patient needs.

Data from Benner, P. A., Tanner, C. A., & Chelsa, C. A. (1996). *Expertise in nursing practice: Caring, clinical judgement, and ethics.* New York: Springer.

flect changes in three general aspects of skilled performance. First, there is movement from reliance on abstract principles to the use of past concrete experiences as paradigms. Second, there is change in the learner's perception of the demand situation in which the situation is seen less and less as a compilation of equally relevant bits and more and more as a complete whole in which only certain parts are relevant. And third, there is change from being a detached observer to an involved performer, engaged in the situation. Benner also identified 31 different competencies that are evident in clinical practice. She organized the competencies into seven domains of nursing practice:

1. The helping role
2. The teaching-coaching function
3. The diagnostic and patient monitoring function
4. Effective management of rapidly changing situations
5. Administration and monitoring of therapeutic interventions and regimens
6. Monitoring of (and ensuring the quality of) health care practices
7. Organizational and work role competencies

This classic model addresses changes that occur across the seven domains of nursing practice as the inexperienced nurse moves from being a novice (stage 1) to an expert practitioner (stage 5). Characteristics of each of the five stages are presented in Table 3–4.

Environmental Factors That Influence Socialization

Recall that socialization is the adaptation to changing roles and is a continuing, interactive, lifelong process. Each role change may produce stress and conflict whether or not the nurse is experienced. To facilitate successful socialization to nursing roles in the workplace, an awareness and understanding of environmental factors that may enhance or constrain professional nursing practice is helpful.

PROFESSIONALS IN A BUREAUCRATIC ENVIRONMENT

Nursing education focuses on the skills, behaviors, and values of the profession. Once in the work setting, the nurse's goal is to put the profession's values into practice. This may be a significant challenge if the setting is highly bureaucratic and not supportive of professional practice. In a bureaucratic organization, decision making takes place above the level of the practitioner. Under these circumstances, conflict between the practitioner and the bureaucracy is inevitable.

Providing care to clients is complex and requires individuals with differing areas of expertise. An essential dimension is the concept of collegial teams. Outcomes can be improved with shared decision making and mutual trust for the clinical abilities of doctors and nurses. However, the use of titles for physicians while overlooking titles of other care providers in an organizational culture may contribute to status discrepancies. Campbell-Heider and colleagues (1994) call for a new paradigm in nursing leadership to transform the typically hierarchical

hospital organization into more engaging structures that encourage professional advancement and empowerment of nurses.

In an organization where decision making occurs at the level of the practitioner, conflict is reduced. Characteristics of professional and bureaucratic organizations are summarized in Table 3–5. The nurse must learn how to balance the values of both the profession and the organization. Successful blending of these role conceptions will facilitate the socialization process and decrease the amount of perceived stress and conflict. The strong service ideal inherent in nursing sometimes helps to mediate the effects of clashes between professional and bureaucratic values.

SUCCESSFUL NURSING ORGANIZATIONS

During the nursing shortage of the 1980s, some hospitals were successful in attracting and retaining professional nurses when most hospitals were having great difficulty recruiting sufficient nursing staff (Scott, Sochalski, & Aiken, 1999). These facilities were referred to as "magnets" because of their ability to attract and retain professional nursing staff. Because of the significant nurse shortage, a formal study was conducted to identify what made these hospitals so successful. Three areas were examined: (1)

TABLE 3–5 Characteristics of Professional and Bureaucratic Organizations

Bureaucratic	Professional
Hierarchical power with centralized decision making	Knowledge-based power with decentralized decision making
High formalization	Low formalization
Work performed according to division of labor	Work performed according to professional norms
Uniformity of product emphasized; work standardized	Uniqueness of client emphasized; work unstandardized
Routine tasks	Nonroutine tasks
Service to organization	Service to client and profession
Achievement of organizational goals	Loyalty to profession

leadership characteristics of nursing administrators, (2) professional attributes of staff nurses, and (3) the environment that supported professional practice. Hospitals were selected using these criteria: nurses considered them a good place to practice nursing, they had low turnover and vacancy rates, and they were located in a region where there was significant competition for nursing services.

Leadership is critical to the establishment and maintenance of a cohesive and efficient work culture. In their review of the research on magnet hospitals, Scott and colleagues (1999) extracted nursing administrator attributes that were most prevalent in the studies. These leader attributes include the following:

- Visionary and enthusiastic
- Supportive and knowledgeable
- Maintains high standards and high staff expectations
- Values education and professional development
- Highly visible to staff nurses; having a presence
- Responsive to concerns and maintains open communication
- Actively involved in state and national professional organizations.

Staff nurses working within magnet hospitals were also studied. Professional practice attributes of the staff nurses included:

- Ability to establish and maintain therapeutic nurse-patient relationships
- Nurse autonomy and control
- Presence of collaborative nurse-physician relationships at the level of patient care units

To practice as professionals, nurses must have control over the practice environment so that clinical judgments and interventions can reflect the uniqueness of each client. Scott and colleagues defined *autonomous nursing practice* as "full command of expert knowledge and allow[ing] for accountability and authority in de-

cision making" (Scott et al., 1999, p. 11). They address two dimensions of autonomy: organizational and clinical. *Organizational autonomy* relates to the environment in which nurses participate in clinical decision making that guides the unit and organization. *Clinical autonomy* relates to the nurses' scope of practice for which they are accountable. Among the most significant factors in explaining job satisfaction and productivity were autonomy and staff involvement in decision making.

The complexity of care delivery makes collaboration essential. "Twenty-first century learning in nursing may not be about competition as much as coalition building, resource acquisition, and transforming expectations" (Pesut, 1998, p. 37). Open communication and dialogue among peers and other health care providers allow nurses to validate clinical judgments according to standards of professional practice. Collaborative nurse-physician relationships at the level of patient care units are fostered when nurses and doctors have mutual respect for each other's knowledge and competence and a shared concern for provision of quality patient care (Scott et al., 1999).

The magnet hospital findings are consistent with earlier work by Porter-O'Grady (1986), who identified five key issues involved in creating a professional practice climate. The nurse must have

- The freedom to function effectively.
- A sense of support from peers and leaders.
- Clear expectations of the work environment.
- Appropriate resources to practice effectively.
- An open organizational climate.

A number of contemporary client care delivery models have been developed to facilitate the practice of nursing as a professional discipline. While specific organizational designs may vary, all can be classified as professional governance models when they have a focus on autonomy of, and accountability for, nursing practice.

There are three structural approaches to professional governance (Porter-O'Grady, 1987). The *councilor model* uses elected councils to structure the governance processes of staff and management. Councils on practice, quality assurance, and education are composed primarily of practicing nurses, with management having minority representation. These councils make decisions related to clinical practice. Management has a management council, with clinical staff having minority representation. It is in this council that decisions regarding system operations are made.

The *congressional model* consists of a president and cabinet of officers who are elected from the staff of the organization and who oversee the operations. Cabinet members are a mixture of clinical and management representatives. There may be equal representation from each group or, consistent with the belief that the organization is a clinical service, it may be weighted with more clinical representatives. Committees, often chaired by cabinet officers, are empowered with certain responsibilities and accountabilities and report back to the cabinet.

The *administrative model* is perhaps the least professionally structured. Although a management and clinical forum are the basic structural units, each forum is more typically aligned in a hierarchical fashion, and the nurse executive often has a mechanism for vetoing considerations of the various decision-making groups.

Shared governance models are effective in empowering staff nurses with increased responsibility for clinical decisions (Ludemann, Lyons, & Block, 1995). In addition, in successful system integration, commitment to shared governance and point-of-service decision making contribute to the success of systems that have been redesigned (Aikman et al., 1998).

Additional research on factors related to socialization of nurses in today's health care environment is needed. The diverse needs of the learner, multiple roles of students, processes and strategies that best facilitate role transition, effectiveness of role models and preceptors in the socialization process, and resocialization for RNs returning to school are some issues deserving attention.

Professional Associations

A *professional association* is "an organization of practitioners who judge one another as professionally competent and have banded together to perform social functions which they cannot perform in their separate capacity as individuals" (Merton, 1958, p. 50). Professional organizations provide a structure for the exercise of autonomy and accountability to ensure that quality services will be provided by competent professionals.

Associations can be classified as one of two main types: broad-purpose associations and specialty associations. The ANA and its affiliation with the International Council of Nursing (ICN), the National League for Nursing (NLN), and the National Student Nurses Association (NSNA) are examples of broad-purpose associations.

AMERICAN NURSES ASSOCIATION

Mission. By caring for nurses who care for America, the ANA works to unite all registered nurses in order to advance the profession. Areas of focus include improving health, promoting standards and availability of health care services for all people, fostering high standards for nursing and professional practice advocacy, stimulating and promoting the professional development of nurses, and advancing their economic and general welfare. Core values include leadership, standard of excellence, integrity/honesty, stewardship, knowledge, response to change, and the right to health care.

Origin. Founded in 1896 by a group of representatives from nursing school alumnae associations and named the Nurses' Associated Alumnae of the United States and Canada. Became the ANA in 1912.

Membership. Professional association for RNs in the United States, with constituent nursing associations in all 50 states, the District of Columbia, Guam, and the Virgin Islands. Only about 10% of all RNs belong to the ANA. Because the ANA represents every RN, it is critical that all nurses become active, contributing members.

Programs
- Created a national labor entity, United American Nurses, to support state nurses associations in their organizing and collective bargaining efforts.
- Provides specialty certification of RNs.
- Accredits continuing education programs.
- Maintains government relation activities.
- Develops standards for nursing practice.
- Promotes economic and general welfare, research, and priorities for human rights.
- Publishes scope and standards for 22 areas of nursing practice (nurse administrators, advanced practice, college health, diabetes, forensic, home health, correctional, parish, rehabilitation, informatics, gerontological, professional development, addictions, general clinical, acute care nurse practitioner, developmental disabilities and mental retardation, genetics, oncology, otorhinolaryngology, pediatric, psychiatric-mental health, and respiratory).
- Publishes *Code for Nurses* (professional code of ethics).

Official Journal. *American Journal of Nursing*

Web Site. www.nursingworld.org

INTERNATIONAL COUNCIL OF NURSES

Mission. To lead societies of the world toward better health through working together to harness the knowledge and enthusiasm of the entire nursing profession. Committed to advocacy for patients, helping people to help themselves and doing for people what they would do unaided if they had the necessary strength. Determined that science will remain the servant of compassion and ethical caring that includes meeting emotional needs.

Origin. Begun in 1899 as a federation of national nurses associations. Was the first and widest reaching international organization of health professionals. Currently represents nurses in more than 120 countries.

Programs
- Focuses on leadership for change and negotiation.
- Ongoing initiative for development of the international classification for nursing, a common language to be used worldwide for practice, education, research, and management that would permit comparison of nursing data across clinical populations, settings, and geographic areas to document outcomes of nursing interventions.
- Sets and enforces standards for nursing education through member associations to ensure that nursing is recognized as a profession.
- Has proposed universal guidelines for basic and specialty practice to aid professionals working in different regions of the world.
- Focuses on fair and equitable compensation and other work benefits for nurses worldwide. Serves as resource to member associations; represents nurses and nursing within the International Labor Organization.

Web Site. www.icn.ch

NATIONAL LEAGUE FOR NURSING

Mission. To advance quality nursing education that prepares the nursing workforce to meet the needs of diverse populations in an ever changing health care environment.

Origin. Begun in 1893 as the American Society of Superintendents of Training Schools for Nurses. Formed to establish and maintain universal standards of training for nursing. Became the National League of Nursing Education (NLNE) in 1912, and, along with two other organizations, formed the National League for Nursing in 1952. At that time, the organization assumed responsibility for accrediting nursing education programs.

Programs

- Accredits practical, diploma, associate, baccalaureate, and master's nursing programs in the United States and its territories through the National League for Nursing Accrediting Commission (NLNAC).
- Provides testing services for nursing schools ranging from preadmission through graduation, and certification examinations for specialty nursing groups and health care institutions.
- Publishes books and journals and presents workshops and conferences related to nursing education and practice.

Membership. Agency membership, with 2,000 nursing schools and health care agencies, and individual membership.

Official Journal. *Perspectives in Nursing and Health*

Web Site. www.nln.org

NATIONAL STUDENT NURSES ASSOCIATION

Mission. To provide nursing students practice in self-governance, advocate for student rights and rights of patients, and take collective, responsible action on vital social and political issues.

Origin. Begun in 1952 with the assistance of the ANA and NLN to prepare students for eventual participation in professional nursing organizations.

Programs

- Offers opportunities to learn and practice leadership skills through self-governance model, Mid-Year Career Planning Conference, and annual convention.
- Discounts on products and services designed especially for nursing students.

Membership. Open to students in all nursing programs leading to registered nurse licensure.

Official Journal. *Imprint*

Web Site. www.nsna.org

Examples of specialty focused professional organizations are the American Association of Colleges of Nursing (AACN) and Sigma Theta Tau International.

AMERICAN ASSOCIATION OF COLLEGES OF NURSING

Mission. Dedicated exclusively to baccalaureate and higher-degree nursing education programs, to serve the public interest by assisting deans and directors to improve and advance nursing education, research, and practice.

Origin. Begun in 1969 with 121 member institutions. Today represents 550 schools of nursing at public and private universities and senior colleges nationwide.

Programs

- Publishes and disseminates essentials of baccalaureate education, core standards for master's degree curricula for advanced practice nursing, and guidelines defining essential clinical resources for nursing education, research, and faculty practice.

- Maintains government relations focusing on advancing public policy on nursing education, research, and practice; secures federal support for nursing education and research; shapes legislative and regulatory policy affecting nursing school programming; and ensures continuing financial assistance for nursing students.
- Created the Commission on Collegiate Nursing Education (CCNE) in 1996 to accredit baccalaureate and master's degree programs.

Membership. Schools of nursing offering a baccalaureate higher degree, with the nursing dean or other chief administrative nurse serving as representative to the AACN.

Official Journal. *Journal of Professional Nursing*

Web Site. www.aacn.nche.edu

SIGMA THETA TAU INTERNATIONAL

Mission. A nursing honor society that fosters, develops, and connects nurse scholars and leaders worldwide to improve health care worldwide.

Origin. Founded in 1922 by six nursing students at Indiana University to advance the status of nursing as a profession through recognition of the value of scholarship and importance of excellence in practice. Name is from initials of three Greek words *storage, tharos,* and *time,* meaning love, courage, and honor. Currently has 383 chapters located on college and university campuses in 78 countries and territories.

Programs
- Funds nursing research through grants and scholarships. Holds annual research-oriented educational programs.
- Maintains an electronic library which includes on-line services of *The Online Jour-*

nal of Knowledge Synthesis for Nursing and the Registry of Nursing Research.
- Houses the International Leadership Institute, which seeks to develop and advance nurses as leaders.

Membership. By invitation to baccalaureate and graduate nursing students who demonstrate excellence in scholarship and the potential for leadership, and to community leaders who demonstrate exceptional achievement in nursing.

Official Journal. *Journal of Nursing Scholarship*

Web Site. www.nursingsociety.org

The ANA's *Code for Nurses* (1985) reminds nurses of their obligation to participate in knowledge development, implementation and improvement of standards, establishment and maintenance of conditions of employment, and protection of the public from misinformation and misrepresentation. Nursing associations provide a structure for participation and empower nurses to engage in the advancement of nursing and improve health care services to the public.

As nursing continues to expand and specialize, many nurses have chosen to join a specialty practice organization that most closely represents their clinical area of expertise. These include organizations representing maternal-child, community, medical-surgical, and mental health nursing specialties. Other specialty organizations focus on the areas where nurses work, such as the emergency department, operating room, and critical care. A listing of specialty organizations can be found at the web site www.springer.com.

What are the benefits of belonging to a professional organization? Membership in the ANA and specialty practice organizations provides nurses with the opportunity to play an active role in the present and future of nursing. It is through these professional organizations that nurses are elected to represent their peers as standards of practice are revised, policies are formulated, and issues affecting nursing practice and the public's health are addressed. Membership in professional associations benefits both the individual and the profession of nursing. Recognition of expertise through certification, collective bargaining to improve salary and working conditions, lobbying to influence laws affecting nursing, and promoting state laws that will ensure quality care are some of the initiatives undertaken by these organizations. To increase the effectiveness of professional associations as official representatives of nurses, more nurses must become active by becoming members, attending meetings, and participating in the organizational activities. Through active participation, nurses become a powerful collective of professionals. It is through participation in and support of professional associations that nurses can amplify their impact on nursing care delivery and the health of the nation.

KEY POINTS

- Socialization is an interactive, dynamic, lifelong process.
- Socialization to professional nursing includes internalizing its attitudes, behaviors, skills, and values.
- The ANA's *Code for Nurses* identifies the professional values of nursing; these should be evident in the delivery of nursing care.
- The status of nursing as a profession can be analyzed using criteria for professions as indicators.
- Actions of individual nurses contribute to the public's collective image of nursing.
- Accountability is the cornerstone to maintaining the public's trust in nursing.
- Models of socialization identify the progression that occurs as one learns new roles in professional practice.
- Nurses in practice and education serve as role models, preceptors, and mentors to guide new practitioners in their socialization to roles and responsibilities, and assist in the development of career paths.

- Environmental factors influence the delivery of professional nursing care.
- Autonomy is a critical factor in attracting and retaining nurses in work settings.
- Participation in professional organizations is one of the defining attributes of being a professional nurse.
- Professional organizations benefit the individual nurse, the profession, and the public.

CRITICAL THINKING EXERCISES

1. Select one set of criteria for a profession from Table 3–1 and use it to analyze nursing's status as a profession. Give concrete examples of how nursing fulfills each criterion, or identify improvements that must be made.

2. List five ways to advance your own level of professionalism.

3. Identify characteristics of what you *want to be* and *don't want to be* as a nurse and compare them with the values in the *Code for Nurses.*

4. Describe your nursing role model and explain why you have selected that nurse. How did this role model influence your nursing practice? What, if any, impact did this role model have on your decision to return to school for further nursing education?

5. Talk with a nursing faculty, a hospital nurse recruiter, and a clinical nurse administrator about strategies they use to address "reality shock."

6. Use the Internet to compare and contrast the mission, purpose, and services of two professional organizations.

REFERENCES

Adams, D., Miller, B. K., & Beck, L. (1996). Professionalism behaviors of hospital nurse executives and middle managers in 10 western states. *Western Journal of Nursing Research, 18*(1), 77–88.

Aikman, P., Andress, I., Goodfellow, C., LaBelle, N., & Porter-O'Grady, T. (1998). System integration: A necessity. *Journal of Nursing Administration, 28*(2), 28–34.

American Nurses Association. (1985). *Code for nurses with interpretative statements.* Kansas City, MO: Author.

American Nurses Association (1995). *Nursing: A social policy statement*. Washington, DC: Author.

American Nurses Association. (1998). *Standards of clinical nursing practice* (2nd ed.). Washington, DC: Author.

Birchenall, P. (1998). Professional and educational directions. In M. Birchenall & P. Birchenall (Eds.), *Sociology as applied to nursing and health care* (pp. 174–194). London: Harcourt Brace.

Benner, P. A. (1984). *Novice to expert*. Menlo Park, CA: Addison-Wesley.

Benner, P. A., Tanner, C. A., & Chelsa, C. A. (1996). *Expertise in nursing practice: Caring, clinical judgement, and ethics*. New York: Springer.

Bixler, G. K., & Bixler, R. W. (1959). The professional status of nursing. *American Journal of Nursing, 59,* 1142–1147.

Campbell-Heider, N., Hart, C. A., & Bergren, M.D. (1994). Conveying professionalism: Working against old stereotypes. In B. Bullough & V. Bullough (Eds.), *Nursing issues for the nineties and beyond* (pp. 212–231). New York: Springer.

Carper, B. A. (1978). Fundamental patterns of knowing in nursing. *Advances in Nursing Science, 1*(13), 13–23.

Catalano, J. T. (1996). *Contemporary professional nursing*. Philadelphia: Davis.

Catalano, J. T. (2000). *Nursing now: Today's issues, tomorrow's trends*. Philadelphia: Davis.

Chinn, P. L., & Kramer, M. K. (1999). Theory and nursing: Integrated knowledge development (5th ed.). St. Louis: Mosby.

Cohen, H. A. (1981). *The nurse's quest for professional identity*. Menlo Park, CA: Addison-Wesley.

Coudret, N. A., Fuchs, P. L., Roberts, C. S., Suhrheinrich, J. A., & White, A. H. (1994). Role socialization of graduating student nurses: Impact of a nursing practicum on professional role conception. *Journal of Professional Nursing, 10,* 342–349.

Curry, B. D. (1997). Coping with returning to school. In R. K. Nunnery (Ed.), *Advancing your career: Concepts of professional nursing* (pp. 16–38). Philadelphia: Davis.

Dalton, G. W., Thompson, P. H., & Price, R. L. (1977). The four states of professional careers: A new look at performance by professionals. *Organizational Dynamics, 6,* 9–42.

Dusmohamed, H., & Guscott, A. (1998). Preceptorship: A model to empower nurses in rural health settings. *Journal of Continuing Education in Nursing, 29,* 154–160.

Erikson, E. (1950). *Childhood and society*. New York: Norton.

Fagermoen, M. S. (1997). Professional identity: Values embedded in meaningful nursing practice. *Journal of Advanced Nursing, 25,* 434–441.

Fargotstein, B. P. (2000). *Ethical foundations for code for nurses*. Unpublished manuscript.

Fitzpatrick, J. A., While, A. E., & Roberts, J. D. (1996). Key influences on the professional socialisation and practice of students undertaking different pre-registration nursing education programmes in the United Kingdom. *International Journal of Nursing Studies, 33,* 506–518.

Flexner, A. (1910). *Medical education in the United States and Canada*. New York: Carnegie Foundation for the Advancement of Teaching.

Flexner, A. (1915). Is social work a profession? *School Society, 1,* 901.

Fuszard, B., & Taylor, L. J. (1995). Mentorship. In B. Fuszard, *Innovative teaching strategies in nursing* (2nd ed., pp. 200–208). Gaithersburg, MD: Aspen.

Greenwood, E. (1957). Attributes of a profession. *Social Work, 2*(3), 45–54.

Hardy, M. E., & Conway, M. E. (1988). *Role theory: Perspectives for health professionals*. New York: Appleton-Century-Crofts.

Houle, C. O. (1980). *Continued learning in the professions*. San Francisco: Jossey-Bass.

Howkins, E. J., & Ewens, A. (1999). How students experience professional socialization. *International Journal of Nursing Studies, 35,* 41–49.

Johnson, B., Friend, S., & MacDonald, J. (1997). Nurses' changing and emerging roles with the use of unlicenced assistive personnel. In S. Moorhead & D. G. Huber (Eds.), *Nursing roles Evolving or recycled?* (pp. 78–89). Thousand Oaks, CA: Sage.

Kelly, L. Y., & Joel, L. A. (1999). *Dimensions of professional nursing* (8th ed.). New York: McGraw-Hill.

Knowles, M. (1970). *The modern practice of adult education: From pedagogy to andragogy*. Chicago: Follett.

Koerner, J., & Burgess, C., S. (1997). Nursing's role and functions in a seamless continuum. In S. Moorhead & D. G. Huber (Eds.), *Nursing roles: Evolving or recycled?* (pp. 1–14). Thousand Oaks, CA: Sage.

Kramer, M. (1974). *Reality shock: Why nurses leave nursing*. St. Louis: Mosby.

Letizia, M., & Jennrich, J. (1998). A review of preceptorship in undergraduate nursing education: Implications for staff development. *Journal of Continuing Education in Nursing, 29,* 211–216.

Ludemann, R. S., Lyons, W., & Block, L. (1995). A longitudinal look at shared governance: Six years of evaluation of staff perceptions. In K. Kelly (Ed.), *Health care work redesign* (pp. 234–250). Thousand Oaks, CA: Sage.

McBride, A. B. (1999). Breakthroughs in nursing education: Looking back, looking forward. *Nursing Outlook, 47,* 114–119.

McCloskey, J. C., & Maas, M. (1998). Interdisciplinary team: The nursing perspective is essential. *Nursing Outlook, 46,* 157–163.

McGregor, R. J. (1999). A preceptored experience for senior nursing students. *Nurse Educator, 24*(3), 13–16.

Merton, R. (1958). The functions of the professional association. *American Journal of Nursing, 58*(1), 50–54.

Miller, B. K. (1985). Just what is a professional? *Nursing Success Today, 2*(4), 21–27.

Miller, B. K., Adams, D., & Beck, L. (1993). A behavioral inventory for professionalism in nursing. *Journal of Professional Nursing, 9,* 290–295.

Nicolson, P. (1996). *Gender, power and organizations: A psychological perspective.* London: Routledge.

Nightingale, F. (1860). *Notes on nursing: What it is and what it is not.* New York: Appleton.

Owens, B. H., Herrick, C. A., & Kelley, J. A. (1998). A prearranged mentorship program: Can it work long distance? *Journal of Professional Nursing, 14,* 78–84.

Parathian, A. R., & Taylor, F. (1993). Can we insulate trainee nurses from exposure to bad practice: A study of role play in communicating bad news to patients. *Journal of Advanced Nursing, 18,* 801–807.

Pesut, D. J. (1998). Twenty-first century learning. *Nursing Outlook, 46,* 37.

Porter-O'Grady, T. (1986). *Creative nursing administration: Participative management into the 21st century.* Rockville, MD: Aspen.

Porter-O'Grady, T. (1987). Shared governance and new organizational models. *Nursing Economics, 58,* 50–54.

Reutter, L., Field, P. A., Campbell, I. E., & Day, R. (1997). Socialization into nursing: Nursing students as learners. *Journal of Nursing Education, 36,* 149–155.

Schwirian, P. M. (1998). *Professionalization of nursing: Current issues and trends* (3rd ed.). Philadelphia: Lippincott.

Scott, J. G., Sochalski, J., & Aiken, L. (1999). Review of magnet hospital research. *Journal of Nursing Administration, 29*(1), 9–19.

Shane, D. (1983). *Returning to school: A guide for nurses.* Englewood Cliffs, NJ: Prentice Hall.

Stewart, B. M., & Krueger, L. E. (1996). An evolutionary concept analysis of mentoring in nursing. *Journal of Professional Nursing, 12,* 311–321.

Strader, M. K., & Decker, P. J. (1995). *Role transition to patient care management.* Norwalk, CT: Appleton & Lange.

Styles, M. (1982). *On nursing: Toward a new endowment.* St. Louis: Mosby.

Throwe, A. N., & Fought, S. G. (1987). Landmarks in the socialization process from RN to BSN. *Nurse Educator, 12*(6), 15–18.

Weis, D., & Schank, M. J. (2000). An instrument to measure professional nursing values. *Journal of Nursing Scholarship, 32*(2), 201–204.

Wurst, J. (1994). Professionalism and the evolution of nursing as a discipline: A feminist perspective. *Journal of Professional Nursing, 10,* 357–367.

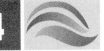

4

Professional Nursing Roles

JOAN L. CREASIA, PhD, RN

OBJECTIVES

At the completion of this chapter, the reader will be able to:

- Discuss the theoretical foundations of personal and professional roles.
- Differentiate between structural-functional and symbolic interaction perspectives of nursing roles.
- Discuss the impact of the multiple roles experienced by the professional nurse.
- Analyze common role stressors as they relate to the role of the nurse.
- Describe selected roles commonly assumed by the professional nurse and the responsibilities associated with each.

PROFILE IN PRACTICE

Deborah Williamson, MSN, RN, CNM
College of Nursing Midwifery Faculty Practice
Medical University of South Carolina,
Charleston, South Carolina

After graduating from nursing school in 1972, I worked as a community health nurse at an inner-city neighborhood health center in Rochester, New York. All of the Ob-Gyn care for the health center was provided by a group of obstetricians and a nurse midwife. This was the first opportunity I had to work with a nurse midwife. I was impressed by her knowledge, her clinical skills, and her independent mode of practice. My primary area of interest, even then, was in the health care of women. Nurse midwifery provided an avenue for specialization in my area of interest. I also saw nurse midwifery as a way to become a primary care provider. I wanted to be the

person responsible for managing the care of the women in my practice. I wanted to do the clinical exams and necessary procedures. I enjoyed the mental challenge of problem solving that exists in clinical nurse midwifery. Most important, I wanted to provide health care that was sensitive to the needs of women.

My first practice after completion of nurse midwifery school was a major influence on the rest of my career. I practiced in a rural community with three family physicians. The similar philosophy of care made the practitioners cohesive and enhanced the community's sense of being cared for by the practice. I learned about continuity of care, the importance of recognizing your own limits, and the importance of follow-up. On a personal level, I experienced the intense relationships that come from living and providing health care in a small town. The sense of connectedness that comes from sharing the joy of birth is powerful, and the bond established is forever.

Being a midwife means being part of the community, whether you practice in a small town or in the city. Birth is a family affair—it's not unusual to know the mother and several generations of her family by the end of the postpartum period. After practicing for more than 20 years, I can honestly say there is nothing I would rather do than practice midwifery. I feel lucky to have chosen a career that I have loved and have always felt was challenging.

I enjoy the challenge of clinical practice. But there are other challenges in the practice of midwifery. The ongoing political struggles to have

nurse midwifery recognized as part of the mainstream of the American health care system is exhausting. Midwifery attracts ardent supporters and fanatical opposition. The players are physicians, nurses, and administrators. The role of supporter or oppressor is different from practice to practice. However, uniformly, women and their families are ardent supporters of nurse midwifery care.

Another major challenge of practice is the blending of one's personal and professional life. The irregular hours and the physical and emotional fatigue take their toll on family members. To be a midwife requires a family that is supportive of the career. But I can also say that my children and my husband are proud when we're out and a parent shows me the child that I helped deliver. The radiance of this interaction is a mixture of the loving parent-child relationship and a special bond that formed between the parents and myself at the time of childbirth.

In today's rapidly changing health care environment, the nursing role is becoming less traditional and increasingly diverse. As the professional disciplines are called on to provide expanded and more diverse health care services in a wide variety of settings, the traditional structure of provider roles is being challenged. Nursing is responding to this challenge by examining the nature of the professional role, identifying its component parts, and adapting it to better meet the needs and changes of a dynamic health care system.

This chapter focuses on role-taking in nursing by examining the theoretical foundations of roles, the types of roles nurses commonly assume, the impact of multiple roles, and common role stressors. Finally, selected nursing roles and associated responsibilities are discussed.

Theoretical Foundations of Roles

Roles are the primary mechanisms that drive the social system (Parsons, 1951). Individuals assume roles that define their position in society. Although the terms *role* and *position* are often used interchangeably, it is important to differentiate between the two. *Roles* are sets of patterned behaviors unique to a given position and may be reflective of personal, social, or occupational domains. The behavior patterns are manifested in the performance of duties and tasks and the assumption of certain responsibilities. *Position*, on the other hand, denotes status or a place within a specified context or setting, such as a health care organization. An organizational chart is used to illustrate the placement of positions within the organization and to depict vertical and horizontal relationships. Thus, roles are classifications of behavior, whereas positions are classifications of people (Biddle, 1979).

The expected behaviors of those who occupy a social position determine how a person in a given role should act. A *social position* refers to an identity that is widely known and held by persons who behave in a characteristic way. Roles, then, are associated with social positions and are shaped by the expectations of others in an individual's social network, often referred to as *socializing agents* (Biddle, 1979). Either explicitly or implicitly, socializing agents communicate the values and norms that are associated with a given role. Over time, the values and norms are assimilated by the person assuming that role and develop into a behavior pattern.

Roy's adaptation model for nursing identifies the *role function mode* as a social mode that focuses on the roles a person occupies in society (Roy & Andrews, 1999). According to Roy, a *role* is derived from a set of expectations about how persons occupying different positions behave toward one another. The particular complex of roles a person holds simultaneously is that person's *role set*. Role function is influenced by the concepts of *role clarity* and *social integrity*—the need to know who one is in relation to others so that one can act according to role expectations.

The context in which the social position exists also contributes to role expectations. *Context* refers to the environment in which the role is enacted and may be defined as a setting (e.g., community), an organization (e.g., hospital), or a social situation (e.g., discussion group). Although a person could theoretically hold an identical position in all three contexts (e.g., nurse), it is clear that the expected behavior patterns would vary markedly. Thus, role behaviors are limited by the physical, environmental, or temporal boundaries of the context.

In applying these concepts to the role of professional nurse, the expected behaviors or roles of the nurse are determined by the nurse's social position and the context in which nursing care is delivered. "Individuals enact roles mainly according to their personal knowledge of the role, the behavior modeling they have witnessed, the sets of expectations of others interacting with the role, and the social structure in which the role is being expressed" (Christman, 1991, p. 210).

ROLE THEORIES AND PARADIGMS

There are two competing theoretical perspectives that may be used to analyze roles. The first perspective is the *structural-functional* paradigm, which links the individual to the social structure and focuses on the division of labor within that context (Hardy & Conway, 1988). "The assumption exists that the division of labor in a given society is an expression of its state of development . . . the more developed a society, the more complex are its structures, and thus, the more differentiated are the components of the labor force" (Lambert & Lambert, 1999, p. 172). The structural-functional perspective includes formal prescriptions for actions that result in appropriate behavior. For example, this perspective might focus on the formal prescriptions for action found in policy and procedure manuals and the job description of a nurse who holds a staff nurse position in a large teaching hospital.

An additional assumption of the structural-functional perspective is that norms and values attached to the position are handed down from generation to generation (Berger & Luckman, 1966), but as the social structure changes over the years, the values and norms of a given position adapt to that change. For example, when the length of stay in hospitals was much longer than it is today, it was the norm for nurses to implement the teaching plan after the client had sufficiently recovered from the acute stage of illness. Nurses valued client teaching and viewed it as an important dimension of the nursing role. As resource-driven care resulted in shortened lengths of stay, the norm was altered.

	TABLE 4–1 **The Structural-Functional Perspective and Symbolic Interaction Perspective Compared**	

Structural-Functional Perspective	Symbolic Interaction Perspective
Roles are shaped by the social structure	Roles are shaped by the interaction of people in the social system
Formal prescriptions for action determine role behavior	Responses of others determine role behavior
Role behaviors are influenced by traditional norms and values but can adapt to changes in the system	Role behaviors are validated or altered by responses of others in the role constellation

Teaching plans and strategies were adapted to accommodate early discharge, and although nurses still valued client teaching, they modified their belief that teaching must occur before discharge. Today, referral to a community rehabilitation program or home health agency may be initiated to continue the teaching plan after discharge.

The second perspective is the *symbolic interaction* paradigm, which focuses on the interaction between people in the social system. Specifically, the meaning that is given to acts and symbols forms the basis on which behaviors are selected and roles are constructed. For communication to be effective, symbols must have the same meaning for each person in the interaction (Hardy & Conway, 1988). Mutual understanding of the meaning of symbols controls role-related behavior by either supporting or suppressing it. The responses of others serve to validate behavior. "To understand a role from the symbolic interactionist perspective, the counter-role must be understood. Every role is oriented toward one or more existing roles" (Lambert & Lambert, 1999, p. 173). This perspective explains the concept of professional socialization of nurses who learn the role of the professional nurse by observing other nurses' actions, understanding the meaning of their actions, and responding to their reactions. More specifically, a new graduate who is oriented to a position with a preceptor learns the staff nurse role by observing the preceptor's actions and

responding to the preceptor's feedback through alteration of the new graduate's own performance (Godinez et al., 1999).

In nursing, both perspectives are valid. Many nurses function in highly structured settings. A great deal of formalization exists in the form of policies, procedures, job descriptions, evaluation mechanisms, classification systems, and so forth. Thus the structural-functional perspective can be a useful approach for analyzing the formalized aspects of a nurse's role. As nurses assume caregiver and administrative roles, they interact with a variety of people, known as their *role constellation* or *role partners*. As the symbolic interaction perspective suggests, meaning is assigned to the various interactions between people in the role constellation as perceived by those individuals. This perspective is useful for analyzing the interdependent nature of nursing roles and the process of acquiring behaviors specific to a given nursing role. A comparison of the structural-functional and symbolic interaction perspectives is presented in Table 4–1.

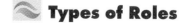 **Types of Roles**

Examination of the content of roles reveals that they are derived from personal, social, and occupational domains. Nurses commonly assume positions in all three domains, often simultaneously. For example, a nurse may be a mother or father, a leader in a civic organization, and a nurse educator. Although these roles are not mutually exclusive, they reflect a primary orientation to what we refer to as our personal life, social life, and occupational life.

In most societies the social structure consists of positions that are reciprocal; that is, they are dependent on one or more persons for appropriate enactment of the role. Such positions include the roles of mother, father, wife, husband, teacher, nurse, breadwinner, politician, and so forth. Each of these positions brings to mind an image of the person assuming the role, along with an associated set of expected behaviors, and of other people in the social system who are critical to the enactment of the role. Thus the nurse who holds positions in all three domains develops behavior patterns for each role and interacts with a wide range of people with whom interdependent relationships are established. The result is a complex pattern of overlapping social positions and roles, each demanding certain behaviors and relationships that are unique.

The Professional Nursing Role

How do these concepts apply to the role of the professional nurse? Neither perspective alone can fully accommodate the range of roles nurses commonly assume. Nurses most often provide services within a formal structure or system. In

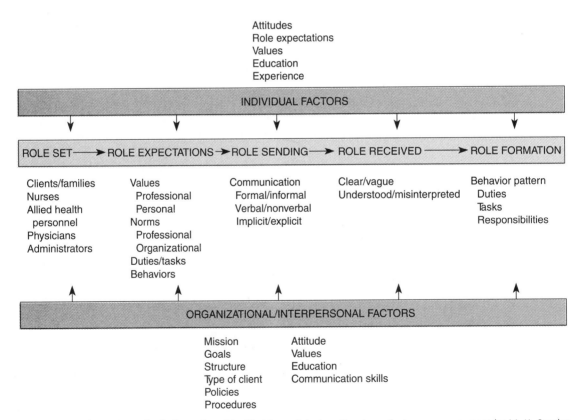

FIGURE 4–1 The process of role formation. (Modified from *Role transition to patient care management* by M. K. Strader & P. J. Decker. © 1995. Reprinted by permission of Prentice-Hall, Inc. Upper Saddle River, N.J.)

addition, the role is defined by the context or setting within which it is enacted and by the formalized role prescription designed by the organization. The structural-functionalist perspective on roles is useful to explain nursing's unique contribution to health care within the formal structure of the health care delivery system. However, the nursing role is a reciprocal one, since it is interdependent with others in the role constellation, such as clients and families, physicians, and ancillary health care personnel, for its enactment. The symbolic interaction perspective is useful in explaining these relationships. The nurse's own role expectations and the expectations of individuals in the role constellation influence the formation of behavior patterns specific to the professional nursing role. Persons in the role constellation communicate their expectations by sending messages that condemn some behaviors and endorse others. Figure 4–1 combines the structural-functional and symbolic interaction perspectives to illustrate the formation of the nursing role. Role formation is influenced by the characteristics of the organization (structural-functional), the characteristics and traits of the individual nurse, and the interactions of the nurse with others in the role set (symbolic interaction).

As previously mentioned, the performance of duties and tasks and the assumption of certain responsibilities form the pattern of behaviors that characterize the professional nurse. The professional role is unique, however, because it is influenced by a *code of ethics* that helps to shape professional behavior and frame role expectations. For instance, the nurse is expected to provide high-quality nursing care "with respect for human dignity and the uniqueness of the client, unrestricted by considerations of social or economic status, personal attributes, or the nature of the health problem" (American Nurses Association [ANA], 1985, p. 1). ANA's code of ethics also specifies dimensions and responsibilities of the role, such as accountability, advocacy, competence, delegation, and collaboration. Because nurses are licensed, there are also legal dimensions to the role, as specified in state nurse practice acts. These influences add to the complexity of the professional nursing role by identifying multiple subroles and dimensions of the role that are bounded by organizational, ethical, and legal constraints.

Impact of Multiple Roles

People in today's society typically assume multiple roles, and nurses are no exception. A woman may be a wife, mother, daughter, daughter-in-law, student, teacher—the list goes on. Similarly, a man may be a husband, father, son, son-in-law, brother, and sportsman and still hold several occupational roles. In addition, each may participate in religious or civic organizations by assuming membership or leadership roles that demand a different set of role behaviors.

Often, multiple roles are assumed within different contexts. However, it is possible to assume multiple roles within the same context. Such is the case with the professional nurse, who may be a caregiver, case manager, teacher, advocate, and so forth. When the same person holds several roles with a similar focus, those roles are referred to as *subroles*. Each subrole may be equally critical to the focal role, or one may be more dominant. For instance, a staff nurse who practices in a setting that employs a number of nonprofessionals to assist with nursing care might see management and supervision of these caregivers as the dominant subroles. As the number and type of roles and subroles held by an individual increase, the risk of role strain also increases.

ROLE STRESS AND STRAIN

Role stress and strain are common phenomena among individuals who hold multiple roles. *Role stress,* generated by the social structure, is said to exist when role obligations are vague, irritating, conflicting, or unrealistic. These conditions are external to the individual, but they may result in role strain, an internal response. *Role strain* is described as an emotional reaction to role stress that may be experienced as feelings of frustration, anxiety, irritability, or distress. When an individual encounters major difficulty in meeting role obligations, role strain is apt to occur (Hardy & Conway, 1988).

What conditions are likely to contribute to role stress and strain in nursing? Hardy and Conway (1988) have identified a number of factors, including changes in the organization and delivery of health care, the generation of new nursing roles, economic conditions that result in redefining patient-provider relations, and technological advances. As a result of one or more of these factors, nurses may experience feelings of frustration or anxiety as their role perception and competence are threatened. However, the severity of role stress and strain is individually determined and is dependent on the perceptions of the person assuming the role. This premise was supported in a study of registered nurses (RNs) returning to school (Dick & Anderson, 1993). The investigators found that taking on the additional role of student did not increase the level of stress and strain when the nurses perceived that they had control over their professional career and support from family and colleagues. Personality characteristics were found to partially explain role strain in another sample of RNs returning to school (Lengacher, 1993). Neuroticism, described as feelings of depression, inadequacy, or a poor self-image, was the strongest predictor of role strain among RNs in this study.

A study of multiple-role stress was conducted with a sample of mothers who were enrolled in an associate degree nursing program (Gigliotti, 1999). The only significant finding in this study was the relationship between the age of the woman and role stress. Role involvement in women age 37 and older resulted in a significant level of multiple-role stress.

The existence of multiple subroles as necessary components of the focal role is another factor that is tied to role stress and strain. In a sample of undergraduate nursing faculty, Lott, Anderson, and Kenner (1993) found that the existence of multiple roles (i.e., nurse, clinician, teacher, advisor, committee member, researcher) was the most prevalent cause of role strain reported by that group. Next were multiple demands on time, followed by multiple role relationships, each with different role obligations. Role stress and strain were manifested by feelings of frustration, anger, inappropriate emotional responses, anxiety, forgetfulness, and fatigue. Although the sample for this study was nursing faculty, staff nurse roles also involve multiple subroles, multiple demands on time, and multiple role relationships that are likely to generate role stress and strain.

COMMON ROLE STRESSORS IN NURSING

Role conflict, role ambiguity, role incongruity, and role overload are stressors common to nursing. These stressors may be generated by the changing health care environment in which the nursing role is enacted and by a myriad of personal and professional factors. A brief discussion of each of the stressors follows.

Role Conflict. When role expectations within or among roles are incompatible with one another, *role conflict* may result. An early study by Corwin (1961) identified alienation in nurses who had both a high professional and a high bureaucratic orientation. This phenomenon has become known as the professional-bureaucratic conflict, whereby organizational norms and values dictate behaviors that may be in conflict with professional norms and values. The result is a strain that, if not reconciled, can result in a response known as *burnout,* an overwhelming inability to adapt to or deal with stressors. Kramer (1974) addressed a similar issue when she discussed *reality shock,* the impact felt by recent nursing graduates who assume positions in highly bureaucratic settings. Selected personality variables, moral behavior, and role concept are some of the factors found to explain professional and bureaucratic role orientations of professional nurses.

The nurse in middle management is also a prime candidate for role conflict due to incompatible expectations of staff and administration, such as those identified by Langenfeld (1988). Areas of potential conflict are evident when the manager is expected to "operate from a management perspective, seeing the broad picture in terms of impact for the entire institution" (p. 79) (management expectation) and to "understand problems from the employee's point of view, creating 'win-win' situations" (p. 78) (employee expectation). Additional areas of possible role conflict include the base of loyalty (e.g., the organization versus the profession) and the cost-quality dichotomy in terms of what is ideal and what is realistic.

Several studies of role conflict in the 1980s focused on RNs returning to school for an advanced degree. The RN probably held a job, had personal and family responsibilities, and, in addition, assumed the role of student. Behavior patterns for each role were already established, and now a new role was being added. It was hypothesized that expected behaviors associated with the new role would compete with the established behavior patterns and result in role conflict. Contrary to these notions, Campaniello (1988) found that for a sample of RNs returning to school, the occupancy of multiple roles did not increase their perceived role conflict. For this group, the role of parent more than any other role was a major source of conflict. In another study of RNs returning to school, personality orientation explained the lack of role conflict (Rendon, 1988). The findings suggested that when interpersonal orientation was compliant, rather than detached or aggressive, there was role congruence rather than conflict. Areas of stress and dissatisfaction identified by this group related mostly to economic burdens and disruptions of social and family life.

Multiple role stressors were also identified in a study of nursing faculty. Oermann (1998) found that full-time clinical faculty in associate degree and baccalaureate nursing programs experienced a significantly higher degree of role strain than did part-time faculty, and that the level of student (sophomore level) generated the highest level of role strain for baccalaureate program faculty. Faculty reported considerable role overload, that is, having too many expectations associated with their clinical teaching position. They also identified three types of role conflict: *interrole conflict,* in which job demands interfered with personal responsibilities; *intersender conflict,* which manifested itself in an inability to satisfy all work-related constituents (e.g., students, patients, clinical agency personnel); and *intrasender conflict,* or the incompatible demands of the role itself (e.g., needing to maintain clinical competence without time to do so).

Role Ambiguity. When role expectations are unclear, the stressor is termed *role ambiguity* or *role confusion.* Possibly more problematic for nurses than role conflict, "ambiguity for nurses has been related to their diversity of role partners, the lack of clarity in role expectations, and to an uncertainty as to how to initiate subroles of the nursing role" (Hardy & Conway, 1988, p. 202). In addition to these factors, the uncertainty associated with professional practice contributes greatly to role ambiguity. Clinical decision making is one example of uncertainty in which action is taken, possibly based on incomplete information, without certain knowledge of the outcome. While health care organizations may be designed to minimize structurally generated ambiguity, professionals are expected to deal with role ambiguities related to their area of expertise and scope of practice (Hardy & Conway, 1988).

Although role ambiguity has been identified as a construct separate from role conflict, much of the role-related research examining role conflict also measures role ambiguity. In several studies of nurses and organizations, the findings indicated that role ambiguity is more detrimental to role performance, satisfaction, and commitment than is role conflict (Hardy & Conway, 1988). Health care organization and workforce redesign initiatives that are currently under way provide fertile ground for continued role ambiguity in nursing. For example, Neal, Brown, and Rojjanasrirat (1999) described role confusion that resulted when the role of case coordinator was implemented on a psychiatric unit. This confusion was attributed to the lack of clear distinction between the roles of staff nurse and case coordinator, perhaps because the case coordinator often assumed three roles in a given week (charge nurse, staff nurse, and case coordinator). The extent of role overlap between the newly instituted role of care coordinator, clinical nurse specialist, social worker, and unit coordinator also contributed to role confusion, ambiguity, and frustration among staff in a study reported by Smith-Blair and colleagues (1999).

Role Incongruity. *Role incongruity* occurs when values are incompatible with role expectations. We can take as an example a staff nurse who spends much of the time supervising and directing nonprofessional caregivers as a dominant subrole. If the nurse's value system embraces the belief that nursing care should be provided by a nurse rather than by nonprofessionals, there is a potential for role strain due to role incongruity.

Role transition, the process of assuming and developing a new role, is a form of role incongruity that is familiar to nurses. In a classic work, Kramer and Schmalenberg (1977) describe the professional socialization of the graduate nurse who, on assuming a new social position in a health care organization, must assimilate the values and norms of that position as set forth by the organization. A problem arises when these are not in concert with the values and norms the nurse was exposed to as a student. To further complicate the issue, the new graduate must learn the professional nurs-

ing role and internalize professional norms and values. Hardy and Conway (1988) note, however, that the strain resulting from role incongruity in this situation may be a prerequisite to learning a new role and may actually facilitate it. When successful transition into the nursing role occurs, it is marked by a sense of role mastery and a feeling of well-being.

It is important to realize that issues related to role incongruity, role transition, and role mastery are not unique to the new graduate. Experienced nurses face the same issues when they are assigned precipitously to an unfamiliar patient care unit or work site. With little opportunity to identify role expectations and clarify values in this new situation, the nurse may experience an increased level of role stress and strain. Murray (1998) reported that nurses who changed from a hospital-based practice to home care nursing described feelings of anxiety, incompetence, and lack of skills to provide care in the home. Formella and Bahner (1999) described the process of role transition in a group of patient care vice presidents who became a cohesive work group after system integration of their individual organizations. "Conditions that may influence the quality of the [role] transition experience and the consequences of transitions are meanings, expectations, level of knowledge and skill, environment, level of planning, and emotional and physical well-being" (Schumacher & Meleis, 1994, p. 119).

Role Overload. Finally, when too much work is expected in the allotted time or the role becomes too complex, *role overload* is experienced. This is a common problem for nurses that may be attributed to structural, contextual, or role-related factors. Consider, for example, the nurse who practices in an acute care hospital. Since the beginning of the cost-containment effort in 1983, hospitalized patients as a group are much more acutely ill. Coupled with changes in staffing patterns, the rapid advances in technology, and additional consumer expectations, hospital-based nurses have more responsibilities today than ever before. They often carry a caseload of patients who are more acutely ill and who have very complex care requirements. In addition, they may have to oversee the work of nonprofessionals or professionals who are unfamiliar with the setting, and they may also be required to perform a variety of nonnursing tasks. By the time the shift is over, nurses are often exhausted, frustrated, and distressed that the quality of care they were able to deliver was less than optimal. The problem is not exclusively that of staff nurses; nurse executives in hospitals also experience a high level of role overload.

Role overload is a serious problem in other health care settings as well. As hospitalized patients are discharged earlier, the use of home health services is escalating. Like hospital-based nurses, home health nurses also oversee unlicensed personnel and coordinate the acquisition and delivery of health care services to the client. Their caseload is increasing in both size and complexity as home care becomes more intense and technologically oriented. With the advent of managed care and increased government involvement in health care financing, the amount of paperwork also increases, expanding the nurse's role responsibilities and demanding greater amounts of time.

STRATEGIES FOR RESOLVING ROLE STRESS AND STRAIN

The appropriate strategies for resolving stress and strain are situation specific and are influenced by the availability of resources, the flexibility of the setting, and/or the position of the nurse in the organization. Consider, for example, a middle manager who seeks to resolve role overload by delegating some managerial functions to an assistant. This strategy can also be used at the staff nurse level to delegate nonnursing functions to available personnel. However, it may be that human resources are not sufficient to delegate part of the workload to

others. In that case, it becomes necessary to set priorities to make the workload more manageable, with the recognition that less important tasks will not get done.

Modifying contextual or structural conditions is another strategy for relieving role stress and strain. Contextual and structural conditions that may be modified include the setting in which care is delivered, the organization of nursing care delivery, and the control and allocation of resources in the form of money, space, time, materials, or personnel. As these conditions are favorably modified, there is an indirect effect on the type and intensity of role strain experienced.

Role redefinition is a more direct strategy for relieving role strain due to role conflict, ambiguity, or overload. This may be accomplished on either a formal or an informal basis. That is, the role may be redefined in writing, or it may be negotiated with others. Although a change in the formal job description is more permanent, negotiating changes in the role is usually a more immediate solution. This latter strategy, derived from the symbolic interactionist perspective, involves mutual understanding between role partners, which results in reprioritizing role expectations, reallocating the workload, and redefining adequate role performance.

Rewriting the job description so that expectations are clearly presented is perhaps the best strategy for reducing role ambiguity. Defining the range of a person's tasks, duties, and responsibilities will diminish the extent to which blurred or overlapping position boundaries can exist. This strategy is especially important when new position titles are bestowed or old roles are blended or combined. Other solutions for reducing role ambiguity include setting one's own performance expectations in writing and sharing them with the supervisor for approval, or developing written goals and objectives as part of the performance appraisal mechanism. However, given the rapidly changing health care environment, accepting ambiguity and uncertainty as a fact of life may be the least stressful approach.

Integrating the demands of multiple roles into a larger and meaningful whole and eliminating some of the demands of these roles are both effective strategies for reducing role conflict. For instance, a nurse who works full-time and maintains home and family responsibilities is at risk for role conflict when additional roles are added, such as the role of student (Curry, 1997). Role integration for this nurse may consist of making adjustments in ongoing roles to make the role set more manageable. If this same nurse also has been active in community volunteer work, suspending involvement in those activities can reduce role conflict further. These adjustments involve changing the behavior pattern associated with specific roles to a set of behaviors that is more realistic, given the situation. A frequent roadblock to using this strategy is that it usually involves changing the expectations of oneself, a notion that presents major difficulties for some people.

Avoiding situations that conflict with one's value system is the best strategy for reducing the stressful effects of role incongruity. For example, if a nurse's value system opposes the use of extraordinary means to prolong the life of terminally ill clients, it might be extremely stressful for that nurse to work in the intensive care unit of a large medical center. In that situation, requesting a transfer to another unit is highly recommended. If that cannot be accomplished, negotiating or redefining the role might be an alternative strategy for reducing the level of stress. However, if no middle ground can be reached, assuming a position where role expectations are more compatible with the values of the nurse may be the only recourse.

A theory describing successful role integration, a process by which multiple roles are meaningfully organized into a larger whole, was formulated by Hall, Stevens, and Meleis (1992) through a study of women with multiple roles. *Role integration* reflects the interaction of the individual and the environment on a day-to-day basis, incorporating several distinct roles in a variety of contexts. Nurses who experience a manageable level of role stress and strain may be more successful at integrating multiple roles, thereby feeling less fragmented and frustrated.

Analyzing Professional Nursing Roles

Professional nurses assume a number of roles and subroles concurrently as they seek to provide comprehensive care to clients in a variety of health care settings. A useful conceptualization of the role of the nurse as described by McClure (1989) divides it into two subroles: caregiver and integrator. *Caregivers* attend to clients' needs and *integrators* coordinate other specialized services as clients' needs warrant. The nurse, drawing from the functional, cognitive, and affective domains, uses a combination of skills, abilities, knowledge, judgment, attitudes, and values to develop and implement a plan for nursing care. As role theory suggests, nursing care is modified by the setting in which care is delivered and by the subrole(s) assumed by the nurse. For example, a nurse practicing as a case manager in a community setting may use a different set of competencies than a nursing case manager in an acute care hospital. Similarly, a nurse manager of a community-based prenatal clinic uses different competencies than a dialysis nurse practicing at the same site. The model depicted in Figure 4–2 illustrates these relationships. Nursing competencies derived from the functional, cognitive, and affective domains are selected and modified by the role the nurse assumes and the setting in which care is delivered.

The theoretical perspectives of roles discussed earlier in this chapter are useful in analyzing the caregiver and integrator facets of the nursing role. With the reader keeping in mind that the setting in which care is delivered tends to shape the content of the role, the following section describes selected roles that nurses may assume and identifies some specific responsibilities associated with each.

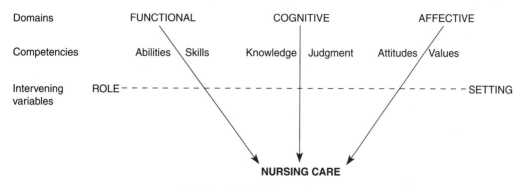

FIGURE 4–2 Model for nursing care.

CAREGIVER

An essential feature of nursing practice is the provision of a caring relationship that facilitates health and healing (ANA, 1995). Thus, a fundamental nursing role is that of caregiver (i.e., helping the client and modifying situations that support illness and impede health). Nurses provide care within three types of nursing systems: wholly compensatory, partly compensatory, and supportive/educative (Orem, 1995). Appropriate nursing actions are selected to provide complete care for the client who is totally dependent, either physically or psychologically; to provide partial care, when the client cannot fully assume self-care; and to provide supportive/educative care to assist clients in attaining or maintaining the highest possible level of health. The goal of nursing is to move clients toward responsible self-care at the highest point on the health-illness continuum of which they are capable.

With the client viewed as a biopsychosocial system, caregiving is directed toward addressing identified physiological, psychological, social, and spiritual needs. The nurse draws from a repertoire of skills derived from the functional, cognitive, and affective domains to develop nursing interventions appropriate to the caregiver role. Subsumed within the caregiver role are a number of subroles (e.g., teacher, coun-

selor, advocate), some of which are subsequently discussed in greater depth.

Role Responsibilities. McClure (1989) described the caregiver role as meeting the following client needs: dependency, comfort, monitoring, therapeutic, and educational. The dimensions of nurse caring include respectful deference to others, assurance of a human presence, positive connectedness, professional knowledge and skill, and attentiveness to the other's experience (Wolf et al., 1994). Consumers defined quality nursing care as having nurses who were concerned about them and demonstrated caring behaviors, were competent and skilled, communicated effectively with them, and taught them about their care (Oermann, 1998).

Whether the client is defined as the individual, family, or community, nursing care proceeds along similar lines. Selecting competencies derived from the cognitive, functional, and affective domains and using the nursing process, the nurse

- Assesses the client.
- Analyzes the data.
- Identifies the nursing diagnoses.
- Develops the nursing care plan.
- Implements the plan.
- Evaluates the outcomes.

Nursing responsibilities can include the provision of direct nursing care or the delegation and supervision of care to other caregivers. Subsumed in the caregiver role are various components of the integrator role, including coordinating the efforts of the multidisciplinary health team, teaching, counseling, discharge planning, and referral. The nurse also makes use of self by exhibiting caring behaviors such as empathy, comfort, respect, and compassion.

TEACHER

As clients attempt to execute complex treatment regimens in an effort to cope with chronic disease over extended periods of time, the nurse in both inpatient and outpatient settings frequently assumes the role of teacher. A component of the caregiver role, teaching is also a primary focus of specialized positions such as that of diabetic educator, cardiac rehabilitation nurse, or wound care specialist. In addition to teaching patients how to live with an existing condition, nurses are also involved in teaching for health promotion and disease prevention.

Health teaching is the process whereby information is imparted to individuals, families, and groups for the purpose of altering cognitive, affective, or psychomotor behavior. A goal of health teaching is to assist individuals in attaining and maintaining healthful lifestyles and practices by preventing, promoting, or modifying a number of health-related behaviors. Thus teaching activities are aimed at promoting self-care behaviors, such as adherence to a prescribed treatment regimen, maintenance of a healthful lifestyle, and appropriate use of health care services (Redman, 1997). It is important for the nurse to have a thorough understanding of the teaching-learning process to facilitate successful client teaching (see Chapter 18).

Role Responsibilities. The nurse may either assume an active teaching role or coordinate the teaching efforts of others. When the nurse as-

sumes the active role of teacher, responsibilities include:

- Identifying teaching-learning needs
- Assessing the client's motivation and readiness to learn
- Developing educational goals and objectives with the client
- Planning the teaching-learning experience
- Providing information using appropriate teaching strategies
- Evaluating the outcomes of the teaching-learning interaction

When several disciplines are involved in educating the client, the nurse may serve as coordinator of the multidisciplinary team. Responsibilities include:

- Referring teaching-learning needs to appropriate disciplines
- Scheduling teaching sessions to enhance learning
- Reinforcing information provided by others
- Evaluating outcomes

CLIENT ADVOCATE

The role of client advocate is one that lies at the heart of nursing's value system. When the nurse assumes the advocacy role, the primary emphasis is on safeguarding and advancing the interests of the client (Wisdom, 2000) and supporting the client emotionally, physically, spiritually, and socially. The advocacy role has moved from its original focus on treatment choices to include prevention, detection, diagnosis, survivorship, long-term care, and terminal care (Morra, 2000). Advocacy is based on mutual understanding between nurses and clients as human beings, taking into account our common needs and our common rights.

The role of client advocate has three major themes: (1) protector of the client's self-determination, (2) mediator between the client and persons in the client's environment, and (3) actor on the client's behalf (Nelson, 1988). The nurse may provide materials necessary for informed decision making, encourage clients to make health care choices that are congruent with their value system, or act directly on behalf of the client to protect human dignity. Thus, the client advocate runs the risk of conflict with others in the client's personal or health care environment.

Role Responsibilities. Within each component of the advocacy role, specific responsibilities have been identified. As protector of the client's self-determination, the nurse assists the client in making autonomous and informed decisions by

- Ensuring that relevant information is available to the client.
- Helping the client examine and prioritize values and goals.
- Supporting the client in whatever decision is made.

As mediator between the client and the environment, the nurse is responsible for

- Coordinating health care services.
- Clarifying communication between the client and community, family, other disciplines, and/or medical services.
- Explaining the roles and relationships between various health care providers.

As one who acts on the client's behalf, the nurse may intervene directly by

- Altering the environment to safeguard the client's welfare.
- Protecting the client against receiving inadequate care.
- Championing the client's rights in the health care, social, and political arenas.

QUALITY IMPROVEMENT COORDINATOR

Providing care that is comprehensive and of high quality has long been a basic value of nursing. Assessing the quality of care in nursing and other disciplines has been difficult, in part because quality of care is an evolutionary concept that is multidimensional, value laden, dynamic, and changing in response to consumer expectations and technological advances. In addition, many studies lack scientific rigor. Despite these and other shortcomings, efforts to evaluate the quality of care have gained momentum in recent years because of the increased involvement of the government in health care financing, the concern for accountability arising out of the consumer movement, the proliferation of health care organizations and providers, and the swift pace of advances in health care technologies.

As a result, many health care organizations have created a position whose responsibility it is to monitor and improve quality of care within the realm of TQM (total quality management), CQI (continuous quality improvement), or QA (quality assurance), or a combination of these approaches. Although one individual or department may be responsible for measuring and improving quality throughout the organization, nurses in various positions within the organization often assume responsibilities of quality improvement as a nursing subrole. Emphasis is placed on improving the system rather than focusing on isolated events. A factual, ongoing, problem-solving approach is used, and statistical trends and variations from the norm are examined (ANA, 1994a).

Role Responsibilities. Quality management requires that a structured process be used to focus on a particular problem, respond to an opportunity, or design a new process (Maddox, 1999). Individuals across the organization are incorporated into the process of evaluating quality, and the nurse may be the coordinator of these activities. Specific responsibilities of the quality improvement coordinator include designing and implementing studies, reviewing findings, making recommendations for improvement, and coordinating the reevaluation effort.

The first step in evaluating nursing care quality is to identify values that define high-quality care. Standards of nursing practice serve as one source of these values, and to make them explicit, structure, process, and outcome indicators must be identified, along with measurable criteria for each (ANA, 1994a). A team may assist with selecting criteria for evaluation, setting standards of care against which actual performance will be judged and identifying measures to use for data collection. How the study proceeds from this point depends on how the evaluation program is designed. Frequently it is the responsibility of the quality improvement coordinator to develop a method of sampling, identify a time frame for the study, and determine the frequency of monitoring. At the end of the study the evaluator tabulates the data and compares actual performance against the performance standard. If remedial action needs to be taken, the quality improvement coordinator may be responsible for identifying possible courses of action, developing the plan, and setting a time for reevaluation.

MANAGER/EXECUTIVE

All nurses function as managers to some extent, and the roles of nurses who occupy management positions in health care organizations vary in breadth, scope, and homogeneity. Positions whose roles are primarily management include clinical manager (head nurse), nursing supervisor, clinical director, and vice president for nursing. Other positions, such as staff nurse and assistant clinical manager, are usually mixed. That is, the position includes aspects of the caregiver role as well as the management role.

Nursing management positions demand a diversity of behaviors and strategies for effective role enactment. The set of expected behaviors depends on the perspectives of the people in the role constellation, the placement of the position on the organizational chart, and the relevant issues with which it is concerned. Nurses at higher levels of management are involved with issues such as resource allocation and labor relations, and they make liberal use of problem-

solving and decision-making skills. These nurse executives must be flexible, creative, action oriented, and knowledgeable in both business and clinical affairs (Williams, 1998). On the other hand, staff nurses who manage and supervise nonprofessional caregivers as a primary nursing subrole use strategies related to personnel management but do not necessarily deal with issues related to the broader organization, such as finances.

The nurse in first-level and middle management has experienced a substantial expansion in scope of responsibility and accountability in recent years. It was predicted that by the year 2000, hospital-based nurse managers would have responsibility for more than one unit, participate in hospitalwide strategic planning, set goals, and plan for the effective and efficient use of human, material, and financial resources (Barrett, 1990). This prediction has definitely become reality.

Role Responsibilities. Because of the variety of management positions in nursing, it is difficult to come up with a single set of responsibilities that would apply equally. Not only are manager roles highly differentiated within a single organization, but manager roles at the same administrative level can vary across organizations. Some of the responsibilities outlined here may be relevant to positions in middle management, such as clinical manager or head nurse. Others are more relevant to nurses in upper-level management. In general, the responsibilities of a nurse manager can be classified as those related to managing the organization and those related to managing people. Litwin and colleagues (1997) and Porter-O'Grady (1997) identified several dimensions of the nurse manager role, some of which are listed here:

- Strategic planning and controlling
  Establishing operating goals and objectives
  Initiating and managing change

Managing data to support planning and decision making

Developing policies, procedures, and standards of care

Managing a budget

- Managing human resources

    Determining staffing standards

    Measuring productivity

    Hiring personnel

- Developing human resources

    Evaluating performance

    Coaching and counseling staff

    Delegating effectively

    Resolving conflicts

    Promoting team building

    Facilitating communication, both formally and informally

    Monitoring interpersonal relations within and between departments

    Serving as a role model and mentor for future managers

- Enhancing quality

    Enforcing organizational policy

    Implementing professional standards

    Serving as a clinical resource

    Developing and monitoring expected client care outcomes

When asked to identify role factors of nurse executives, 40 nurse executives and 56 colleagues identified the role of "leader" as the most important and the one that the nurse executive performs best. Nurse executives spent the most time in the role of "disturbance handler," which was focused on resolving patient care problems, and they found the role of "entrepreneur" to be the most satisfying. Other roles that they assumed were "liaison," "spokesperson," "resource allocator," and "negotiator" (Fosbinder et al., 1999).

RESEARCHER

The ANA's *Code of Ethics* specifies that the nurse participate "in activities that contribute to the ongoing development of the profession's body of knowledge" (ANA, 1985, p. 1), and the *Standards of Clinical Practice* identifies research utilization as one of the professional performance core competencies (ANA, 1998). In concert with these mandates, nurses are assuming an increasingly active role in research. In recent years some hospitals and other health care delivery organizations have created the position of nurse researcher. Typically, a doctorally prepared nurse assumes this role for the purpose of coordinating institutional approval of research studies, writing grants, and directing research programs. In addition, the researcher spearheads the involvement of clinical nurses in the research process. The expanding body of research builds the theoretical basis for nursing practice and assists in the understanding of specific client issues related to health and illness, nursing issues related to the professional nursing role, and a broad range of health care delivery issues.

Role Responsibilities. The responsibilities of the nurse researcher vary according to the level of research expertise and, frequently, level of education (Stotts, 1997). Baccalaureate nursing programs prepare nurses with a basic understanding of the research process so that graduates can apply research findings to their practice. Master's programs prepare nurses to critique research and to implement changes in practice based on research data. Doctoral programs prepare nurse scientists for the beginning researcher role (American Association of Colleges of Nursing [AACN], 1998).

Although not every nurse might participate fully in the research process, all nurses should be consumers of research. As consumers, nurses must critically evaluate research studies for their quality and relevance to nursing and apply the findings to their clinical practice. For those who wish to take a more active role in research, responsibilities include identifying nursing problems for study, serving as a member of a research team, participating in nursing research under the guidance of a senior investigator, and directing the scientific investigation of nursing problems.

The research process serves as a framework for identifying specific responsibilities related to the researcher role:

- Identifying the problem
- Reviewing related literature
- Formulating hypotheses
- Determining a suitable research design
- Delimiting the setting and sample
- Selecting and testing measures for data collection
- Collecting data
- Analyzing data and interpreting the results
- Reporting findings

A senior nurse researcher can be fully involved in the entire research process, whereas less experienced nurses can participate in selected activities under the direction of the senior investigator.

CONSULTANT

As nurses develop specialized areas of expertise, they are often called on to serve as consultants. A *consultant* is one who draws from personal expertise to advise others, validate current practices, identify problems, or provide specialized knowledge. The consultant may serve as a resource person for the purpose of providing the client with choices for decision making, or may be asked to identify a problem and prescribe a solution (Sebastian & Stanhope, 1999). Consultants can be contracted for such varied services as assisting with research design and data analysis, evaluating new health care products, advising health care professionals and other caregivers on complex client care procedures, designing and evaluating new programs, developing curricula for nursing education, or reviewing records for legal cases. In addition, nurse consultants also serve as expert witnesses in legal cases involving malpractice, environmental hazards, pharmaceuticals, equipment design, and so forth. A nurse who wishes to start

a consultation business should develop a business plan that describes the service, identifies the marketing approach, determines the financial requirements, and provides a tool for evaluating success (Papp, 2000).

Role Responsibilities. To ensure its success, marketing must be a major component of the consultant role. This is especially critical for nurses who are in independent practice. Marketing involves identifying the groups that can use the consulting service and then developing a market mix. Defining the service, promoting the service, identifying the place where the service will be delivered, and setting a price are essential to a successful consulting business.

Contracting is a second major responsibility of this role. Contracting should be a formal process that involves outlining the services to be performed, identifying the outcomes, determining a time frame, and negotiating a fee. If expenses such as transportation, lodging, food, and supplies are to be paid by the contractor, it should be so indicated in the contract. A well-written contract serves as a legal document and protects the nurse consultant against possible negative developments (Scott & Beare, 1993). It is recommended that legal counsel be obtained to review the contract to guard against unforeseeable problems. Depending on the terms of the contract, specific activities of the consultant may include:

- Providing information
- Training/educating others
- Identifying issues
- Solving problems
- Proposing solutions
- Counseling others

INFORMATICS NURSE

A relatively new role in nursing is that of the informatics nurse. Activities involved in identifying, naming, organizing, grouping, collecting, processing, analyzing, storing, retrieving, or managing data and information for nursing and health care are termed *nursing informatics.* The American Nurses Credentialing Center (ANCC) describes informatics nursing practice as encompassing the full range of activities that focus on the methods and technologies of information handling in nursing. "Informatics nursing practice includes the development, support and evaluation of applications, tools, processes and structures" (ANCC, 1999, p. 4). The informatics nurse is a nurse specialist who is uniquely trained to integrate computer science, information science, and nursing science (Delaney, Mehmert, & Johnson, 1997). "The work of the informatics nurse can involve any and all aspects of information systems: theory formulation, design, development, marketing, selection, testing, implementation, training, maintenance, evaluation, and enhancement" (ANCC, 1999, p. 4).

Nursing informatics supports the practice of all nursing specialties through the handling of information and spans both clinical and nonclinical domains. The informatics nurse may be at the patient's bedside, teaching in academia, employed by vendors, managing hospital information systems, conducting research, and developing software. The nurse may function as a member of a health informatics team to develop integrated systems that serve the information needs of multidisciplinary health care providers. It is important to have a nurse on this team to ensure that the integrated system meets the information needs of practicing nurses.

Role Responsibilities. The role of the informatics nurse involves activities related to nursing/health care information systems. These include but are not limited to

- Designing or implementing nursing informatics applications in nursing practice.
- Analyzing and evaluating information requirements for nursing practice.
- Evaluating computer and information technologies for their applicability to nursing practice problems.

- Developing and teaching theory and practice of nursing informatics.
- Consulting and conducting research in the field of nursing informatics.
- Collaborating with specialists from nursing and other disciplines in the creation of applications for informatics theory and practice.
- Developing strategies, policies, and procedures for introducing, evaluating, and modifying information technology applied to nursing practice (ANA, 1994b).

CASE MANAGER

The role of the professional nurse case manager emerged as an outgrowth of the need for cost-effective and high-quality care in an increasingly complex health care system. "The case manager (CM) integrates clinical and management skills with professional and financial accountability to ensure that needed health care resources are accessible and available at a reasonable cost" (Haddock, 1997, p. 144). The focus of the case manager role is to mediate client goals or outcomes resulting from activities of interdisciplinary professional care providers. The base of power lies in the fact that these outcomes in turn direct the dollars.

Case management may refer to a system, a process, a role, a technology, or a service. Molloy (1994) described three models of case management: reimbursement based (e.g., third-party payers), social welfare based (e.g., government-funded programs), and hospital or agency based (e.g., hospital or home health programs). Whatever the model of case management, the goals are the same: to ensure continuity of care, cost containment, appropriate and timely intervention, and smooth transition across the care continuum (More & Mandell, 1997). Case management is a way to balance the needs of clients and their families with those of the health care industry and society.

As case manager, the nurse uses interpersonal skills and professional expertise to ensure coordinated and cost-effective care alternatives throughout the course of treatment. A key factor in the case management approach is the identification of outcomes that are specific and time based. This approach facilitates continuous tracking of the client and ongoing evaluation of progress toward expected outcomes, including postdischarge outcomes.

Role Responsibilities. The case manager is responsible for assessment, coordination, integration, and evaluation of effectiveness and efficiency of health services. Embedded in the role of case manager are the subroles of manager, consultant, advocate, clinician, researcher, and educator. Seven basic components of the case manager role have been identified by Rossi (1999, p. 12):

- Assessment and collection of data
- Organization of data and planning
- Service planning and resource identification
- Counseling, education, and advocacy
- Coordination and referral
- Implementation and linkage of patient to needed services
- Reassessment and monitoring

Increasingly, hospitals and home health care agencies are using clinical pathways (also called critical paths) as tools to designate what care should be provided for a given health problem within a specified time frame. These tools are useful to the case manager for coordinating and integrating client care and for determining the effectiveness and efficiency of care through analysis of variance reports. The case manager is accountable for achieving outcomes within an appropriate length of stay, using resources efficiently, and establishing standards of care.

Third-party payers and managed care organizations are fully aware of the value of using the case management system to ensure high-quality and cost-effective care. In these models, the case manager monitors the care provided, serves as a gatekeeper by either approving or denying care, as professional expertise warrants, or sug-

gests alternatives that might be more cost-effective. A more in-depth discussion of case management is presented in Chapter 7.

ADVANCED PRACTICE ROLES

As it is currently used, *advanced practice nursing* is an umbrella term that includes nurse practitioners, clinical nurse specialists, certified nurse midwives, and certified nurse anesthetists. Advanced practice nurses (APNs) have a specialized body of knowledge and expanded practice skills acquired through study at the graduate level. They work with individuals, families, and communities to assess health needs, provide and manage care, and evaluate the outcomes of that care. APNs are certified by one of the recognized specialty organizations or the American Nurses Credentialing Center, and their practice is regulated by the state nurse practice act.

Certified nurse midwives (CNMs), approximately 7,400 in number, provide prenatal and women's health care; deliver babies in hospitals, homes, and birthing centers; and provide follow-up postpartum care (ANA, 1997). The American Association of Colleges of Nursing reports that there are 35 graduate nursing programs preparing nurse midwives (AACN, 2000).

Certified RN anesthetists (CRNAs) administer anesthesia for all types of surgery in a variety of settings such as operating rooms, dental offices, and outpatient surgical centers. There are more than 25,000 CRNAs in the United States, and it is estimated that they administer more than 65% of all anesthetics (ANA, 1997). They are the sole providers of anesthetics in 85% of rural hospitals. There are 35 graduate nursing programs that prepare nurse anesthetists (AACN, 2000).

Clinical nurse specialists (CNSs), about 58,000 in number, provide care in a variety of clinical specialties in both inpatient and outpatient settings (ANA, 1997). Specialty areas may be defined in terms of a population (e.g., pediatrics), setting (e.g., critical care), pathology (e.g., diabetes), type of care (e.g., rehabilitation), or type of problem (e.g., pain) (National Association of Clinical Nurse Specialists, 1998). The CNS role is multidimensional and includes direct care, consultation, education, research, administration, and other administrative components. Currently 143 master's programs prepare clinical specialists (AACN, 2000).

Nurse practitioners (NPs) provide primary care related to health promotion and disease prevention within an area of specialization in both urban and rural settings. Numbering more than 60,000 (Running et al., 2000), they conduct physical examinations, diagnose and treat common acute illness, provide immunizations, manage chronic conditions, and teach lifestyle modifications for healthy living. There are 305 master's programs that produced 6,500 graduates in 1999. More than 50% of these graduates were in the family nurse practitioner specialty (AACN, 2000).

Although the roles of nurse midwives and nurse anesthetists are separate and distinct, clinical nurse specialists and nurse practitioners often have blurred or overlapping roles. In a study of CNS and NP role components, Williams and Valdivieso (1994) found that both groups of nurses were involved in education, consultation, administration, and research, but CNSs spent a greater amount of time in those activities than did NPs. On the other hand, NPs spent 63% of their time in direct practice, whereas CNSs spent 33% of their time in direct practice. The overlap of roles may be partially due to the fact that more similarities than differences are evident in the graduate educational programs of these two groups. Since 1990, when the NP and CNS advanced clinical practice councils of the ANA merged, consolidation of NP and CNS graduate educational programs into a combined NP/CS program has become increasingly common. The result is the emergence of combined roles such as acute care nurse practitioner (ACNP) or psychiatric clinical specialist/nurse practitioner.

Traditionally, CNSs practiced in acute care settings and NPs practiced in outpatient settings. CNSs were valued for their clinical expertise and NPs were valued for their role as primary care providers. Selected characteristics from each of these roles are incorporated into the combined role, but their relative emphasis is different. For example, the primary ACNP role of direct care is a secondary role of the CNS. And the primary CNS role of education and staff support is a secondary role for the ACNP (Norsen et al., 1997).

Role Responsibilities. Whatever the clinical focus of their work, APNs are expected to

- Identify individuals, families, or communities at risk.
- Plan and advocate for cost-effective, high-quality care.
- Provide care or manage systems of care.
- Manage acute and chronic health states.
- Assist clients in regaining and maintaining optimal health.
- Prescribe and manage pharmacological interventions.
- Serve as mentor and consultant for other nurses.
- Consult and collaborate with other health professionals.
- Evaluate health programs for populations at risk.
- Participate in professional, organizational, and legislative activities.
- Participate in research to improve client outcomes.
- Develop new cost-effective interventions (ANA, 1994b).

Comment

Nursing's contribution to health care is illustrated by the nature and diversity of nursing roles. Although the roles described in this chapter do not constitute an exhaustive list, they are representative of the roles nurses commonly assume. As the health care system continues to change, it is anticipated that additional nursing roles will emerge.

KEY POINTS

- The practice of nursing involves assuming a number of diverse roles, some of them simultaneously, in a variety of settings.
- Role theory is useful in understanding the professional nursing role and the problems generated by the social system in which the nurse practices.
- The need to assume multiple roles in nursing can result in role stress and strain.
- Strategies to modify role stress and strain are situation specific.
- An examination of nursing roles reveals their diversity and complexity.
- In the caregiver role, the nurse assists clients in modifying situations that support illness and impede health.
- The teaching role focuses on assisting individuals in attaining and maintaining healthy lifestyles.
- In the role of client advocate, the nurse protects the client, mediates between the client and the environment, and acts on the client's behalf.
- As quality improvement coordinator, the nurse coordinates activities to improve the system of care delivery.
- Managerial roles in nursing may be enacted at different levels of the organization and thus vary in content, scope, and responsibility.
- Among the responsibilities associated with the research role are identification of nursing problems for study and application of published research findings to practice.
- The nurse consultant contracts with interested parties to provide services derived from a specialized area of expertise.
- The informatics nurse is involved in the acquisition and management of health care information.
- As case manager, the nurse uses professional expertise to ensure coordinated and cost-effective care alternatives throughout the course of treatment.
- Advanced practice nurses (nurse practitioners, nurse midwives, nurse anesthetists, and clinical nurse specialists) have a specialized body of knowledge and expanded practice skills acquired through study at the graduate level.

CRITICAL THINKING EXERCISES

1. Select a nursing role of your choice and:
   a. Analyze it according to the symbolic-interactionist perspective and the structure-functionalist perspective.
   b. Describe the role stressors that may be an integral part of the role.
   c. Identify strategies that can be employed to reduce role strain.

2. Identify the sources of role conflict that you are currently experiencing. How can you reduce the impact of this conflict? What can others do?

3. Describe a situation where you experienced role overload. What were the consequences? How did you resolve the situation? Formulate additional strategies that might have been useful.

4. Describe a situation related to the professional nursing role where role incongruity might be an issue for you. What alternatives can you identify that could result in a satisfactory resolution?

5. Speculate how advanced practice nurses might best be used in your clinical setting. What would be the benefits for the patients? How would the organization benefit from their practice?

REFERENCES

American Association of Colleges of Nursing (1998). *Position statement on nursing research*. Washington, DC: Author.

American Association of Colleges of Nursing. (2000). *Enrollment and graduations in baccalaureate and graduate programs in nursing*. Washington, DC: Author.

American Nurses Association. (1985). *Code of ethics with interpretative statements*. Kansas City, MO: Author.

American Nurses Association. (1994a). *Implementation*

of nursing practice standards and guidelines. Washington, DC: Author.

American Nurses Association. (1994b). *The scope of practice for nursing informatics.* Washington, DC: Author.

American Nurses Association. (1995). *Nursing's social policy statement.* Washington, DC: Author.

American Nurses Association. (1997). Advanced practice nursing: A new age in health care. [On-line]. Available: http://www.nursingworld.org/readroom/fsadvprc.htm

American Nurses Association. (1998). *Standards of clinical nursing practice* (2nd ed.), Washington, DC: Author.

American Nurses Credentialing Center. (1999). *Informatics nurse certification catalog.* Washington, DC: Author.

Barrett, S. (1990). *AONE national nurse manager study.* Chicago: American Hospital Association.

Berger, P., & Luckman, T. (1966). *The social construction of reality.* New York: Free Press.

Biddle, B. J. (1979). *Role theory: Expectations, identities and behaviors.* New York: Academic Press.

Campaniello, J. A. (1988). When professional nurses return to school: A study of role conflict and well-being in multiple-role women. *Journal of Professional Nursing, 4*(2), 136–140.

Christman, L. (1991). Perspectives on role socialization of nurses. *Nursing Outlook, 395,* 209–212.

Corwin, R. (1961). The professional employee: A study of conflict in nursing roles. *American Journal of Sociology, 66*(6), 604–615.

Curry, B. D. (1997). Coping with returning to school. In R. K. Nunnery (Ed.), *Advancing your career: Concepts of professional nursing* (pp. 16–38). Philadelphia: Davis.

Delaney, C., Mehmert, P., & Johnson, D. (1997)). The evolving role of the informatics nurse. In S. Moorhead & D. G. Huber (Eds.), *Nursing roles: Evolving or recycled?* (pp. 59–77). Thousand Oaks, CA: Sage.

Dick, M., & Anderson, S. E. (1993). Job burnout in RN-to-BSN students: Relationships to life, stress, time commitments, and support for returning to school. *Journal of Continuing Education in Nursing, 24*(3), 105–109.

Formella, N. M., & Bahner, J. (1999). Role transition for patient care vice presidents: From a single entity to a system focus. *Journal of Nursing Administration (29)*4, 11–17.

Fosbinder, D., Parsons, R. J., Dwore, R. B., Murray, B., Gustafson, G., Dalley, K., & Forderer, L. H. (1999). Effectiveness of nurse executives: Measurement of role factors and attitudes. *Nursing Administration Quarterly, 23*(3), 52–62.

Gigliotti, E. (1999). Women's multiple role stress: Test-ing Neuman's flexible line of defense. *Nursing Science Quarterly, 12*(1), 36–44.

Godinez, G., Schweiger, J., Gruver, J. & Ryan, P. (1999). Role transition from graduate to staff nurse: A qualitative analysis. *Journal for Nurses in Staff Development, 15*(3), 97–110.

Haddock, K. S. (1997). Clinical nurse specialists: The third generation. In S. Moorhead & D. G. Huber (Eds.), *Nursing roles: Evolving or recycled?* (pp. 139–149), Thousand Oaks, CA: Sage.

Hall, J. M., Stevens, P. E., & Meleis, A. I. (1992). Developing the construct of role integration: A narrative analysis of women clerical workers' daily lives. *Research in Nursing and Health, 15,* 447–457.

Hardy, M. E., & Conway, M. E. (1988). *Role theory: Perspectives for health professionals* (2nd ed.). Norwalk, CT: Appleton & Lange.

Kramer, M. (1974). *Reality shock.* St. Louis: Mosby.

Kramer, M., & Schmalenberg, C. (1977). *The path to biculturalism.* Wakefield, MA: Contemporary Publishing.

Lambert, V. A., & Lambert, C. E. (1999). Role theory and effective role acquisition in the health care system. In J. Lancaster (Ed.), *Nursing issues in leading and managing change* (pp. 171–192). St. Louis: Mosby.

Langenfeld, M. L. (1988). Role expectations of nursing managers. *Nursing Management, 19*(6), 78, 80.

Lengacher, C. A. (1993). Development of a predictive model for role strain in registered nurses returning to school. *Journal of Nursing Education, 32*(7), 301–308.

Litwin, R., Beauchesne, K., & Rabinowitz, B. (1997). Redesigning the nurse manager role: A case study. *Nursing Economics, 15*(1), 191–203.

Lott, J. W., Anderson, E. R., & Kenner, C. (1993). Role stress and strain among nondoctorally prepared undergraduate faculty in a school of nursing with a doctoral program. *Journal of Professional Nursing, 9*(1), 14–22.

Maddox, P. J. (1999). Quality management in nursing practice. In J. Lancaster (Ed.), *Nursing issues in leading and managing change* (pp. 453–481), St. Louis: Mosby.

McClure, M. L. (1989). The nurse executive role: A leadership opportunity. *Nursing Administration Quarterly, 13*(3), 1–8.

Molloy, S. P. (1994). Defining case management. *Home Healthcare Nurse, 12*(3), 51–54.

More, P. K., & Mandell, S. (1997). *Nursing case management: An evolving practice.* New York: McGraw-Hill.

Morra, M. E. (2000). New opportunities for nurses as patient advocates. *Seminars in Oncology Nursing, 16*(1), 57–64.

Murray, T. (1998). Using role theory concepts to understand transition from hospital-based nursing practice to home care nursing. *Journal of Continuing Education in Nursing, 29*(3), 105–111.

National Association of Clinical Nurse Specialists. (1998). *Statement on clinical nurse specialist practice and education.* Glenview, IL: Author.

Neal, J., Brown, W., & Rojjanasrirat, W. (1999). Implementation of a case coordinator role: A focused ethnographic study. *Journal of Professional Nursing, 15*(6), 349–355.

Nelson, M. (1988). Advocacy in nursing: A concept in evolution. *Nursing Outlook, 36*(3), 136–141.

Norsen, L., Fineout, E., Fitzgerald, D., Horst, D., Knight R., Kunz, M. E., Lumb, E., Martin, B., Opladen, J., & Schmidt, E. (1997). The acute care nurse practitioner: Innovative practice for the 21st century. In S. Moorhead & D. G. Huber (Eds.), *Nursing roles: Evolving or recycled?* (pp. 150–169). Thousand Oaks, CA: Sage.

Oermann, M. (1998). Role strain of clinical nursing faculty. *Journal of Professional Nursing, 14,* 329–334.

Oermann, M. (1999). Consumers' descriptions of quality health care. *Journal of Nursing Care Quality, 14*(1), 47–55.

Orem, D. E. (1995). *Nursing: Concepts of practice* (5th ed.). St. Louis: Mosby.

Papp, E. M. (2000). Starting a business as a nurse consultant: Practical considerations. *American Association of Occupational Health Nurses Journal, 48*(3), 136–144.

Parsons, T. (1951). *The social system.* New York: Free Press.

Porter-O'Grady, T. (1997). Process leadership and the death of management. *Nursing Economics, 15*(6), 286–293.

Redman, B. K. (1997). *The practice of patient education* (8th ed.). St. Louis: Mosby.

Rendon, D. (1988). The registered nurse student: A role congruence perspective. *Journal of Nursing Education, 27*(4), 172–177.

Rossi, P. (1999). *Case management in health care.* Philadelphia: Saunders

Roy, C. (1989). The Roy adaptation model. In Riehl-Sisca, J.P., *Conceptual models for nursing practice* (3rd ed., pp. 105–114). New York: Appleton-Century-Crofts.

Roy, C., & Andrews, H. A. (1999). *The Roy adaptation model* (2nd ed.). Stamford, CT: Appleton & Lange.

Running, A., Calder, J., Mustain, B., Foreschler, C. (2000). A survey of nurse practitioners across the United States. *The Nurse Practitioner, 25*(6), 15–16, 110–115.

Schumacher, K. L., & Meleis, A. I. (1994). Transitions: A central concept in nursing. *Image: Journal of Nursing Scholarship, 26*(2), 119–127.

Scott, L. D., & Beare, P. G. (1993). Nurse consultant and professional liability. *Clinical Nurse Specialist, 7*(6), 331–334.

Sebastian, J. G., & Stanhope, M. (1999). Consultation as a tool for change. In J. Lancaster (Ed.), *Nursing issues in leading and managing change* (pp. 585–607). St. Louis: Mosby.

Smith-Blair, N., Smith, B. L., Bradley, K. J., & Gaskamp, C. (1999). Making sense of a new nursing role: A phenomenological study of an organizational change. *Journal of Professional Nursing, 15,* 340–348.

Stotts, N. A. (1997). Nurse researchers: Who are they, what do they do, and what challenges do they face. In J. C. McCloskey & H. K Grace (Eds.), *Current issues in nursing* (5th ed., pp. 41–44). St. Louis: Mosby.

Strader, M. K., & Decker, P. J. (1995). *Role transition to patient care management.* Norwalk, CT: Appleton & Lange.

Williams, C. A., & Valdivieso, G. C. (1994). Advanced practice models: A comparison of clinical nurse specialist and nurse practitioner activities. *Clinical Nurse Specialist, 8*(6), 311–318.

Williams, M. B. (1998). *Changing roles and relationships in nursing and health care.* St. Louis: Green.

Wisdom, K. (2000). Nursing roles in the health care delivery system. In K. K. Chitty (Ed.), *Professional nursing: Concepts and challenges* (3rd ed., pp. 246–274). Philadelphia: Saunders.

Wolf, Z. R., Giardino, E. R., Osborne, P. A., & Ambrose, M. S. (1994). Dimensions of nurse caring. *Image: Journal of Nursing Scholarship 26*(2), 107–111.

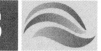

5

Client Systems

GAIL O. MAZZOCCO, EdD, RN

OBJECTIVES

At the completion of this chapter, the reader will be able to:

- Identify and describe the elements of general systems theory.
- Apply general systems theory to the assessment of the individual, family, community, or population.
- Analyze data; plan, implement, and evaluate nursing care based on the general systems model.

PROFILE IN PRACTICE

Jacqueline Snelson, MSN, CRNP
Family Nurse Practitioner
Friendsville Office, Garrett Medical Group
Friendsville, Maryland

I am a nurse practitioner and the only primary health care provider in a rural town in western Maryland. Our clients and local health care providers are members of an interdependent community system. I utilize all parts of that system to ensure that the health needs of individuals and families are met. In a single week, I sent flu suffers to the pharmacy, consulted the hospice nurse about a patient and her family, referred a patient to the librarian for help with a computer search on coping with menopause, contacted a dentist about a young mother with a toothache, and called the rescue squad to transport a seriously ill woman from my office to a regional hospital. I got updates on this woman's condition from the members of the local church prayer chain, who also visit my office. I will have most of the facts about this client before the surgeon mails me his discharge summary.

I am just a single element in the system that promotes the health of the entire community. The Head Start program and public schools have a fluoride rinse program for preventing dental decay. The County Health Department arranges for WIC and Healthy Start services to ensure that children come into this world with a chance for success. The same organization provides funding for breast and cervical cancer screening. The Department of Social Services helps families obtain Medicaid funding and provides pharmacy assistance for the needy. The Community Action Agency helps meet nutritional needs for families and the elderly. While these formal programs are significant, it is often the informal subsystem of families and friends who recognize problems and take actions toward solutions. It is only when I look at the combined efforts of the entire community system that I begin to understand how complex systems work to improve health.

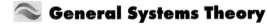

Introduction

Certain historical periods encourage all of us to take a serious look at the direction in which we are heading. This is one of those times. As nurses consider the directions in which the profession might best move, we do so in conditions of uncertainty. What are the unique roles of the nurse today and how might they best be demonstrated? To what degree do those roles contribute to care that is both compassionate and cost-effective? Many nurses have come to believe that the current emphasis on cost containment precludes either competent or compassionate care. Obviously, we must identify a method of providing care that allows us to successfully combine humanistic and scientific perspectives in a single model. Moreover, given the interdisciplinary nature of health care, that approach must be usable by all health professionals. General systems theory meets these requirements. This chapter focuses on three types of client systems: individuals, families, and communities or populations at risk. All three are typical of living systems, since they are goal directed and display complex behaviors.

General Systems Theory

General systems theory was developed in response to the tendency of modern science to explain complex phenomena by dividing them into their component parts. While that approach worked reasonably well in the physical sciences, it was less successful when it was used to explore behavior. With the assistance of a number of other scientists, von Bertalanffy (1956) developed general systems theory as a new analytical approach—one that is based on integration and holism.

"General systems theory is a set of related definitions, assumptions, and propositions which deal with reality as an integrated hierarchy" (Miller, 1978, p. 9). Systems theory focuses on each system as a whole but pays particular attention to the ways in which its parts or subsystems work together. This perspective makes systems theory especially helpful in recognizing patterns and dealing with complexity (Tonges & Madden, 1993). Because it is so widely applicable, systems theory also has the potential to improve communication between the members of the health team. These general attributes make systems theory particularly helpful to nurses.

In spite of changes in the health care delivery system, most nurses continue to use the medical model as they provide care to individuals and families. When a problem is identified as physiological in origin, most of us use this body systems approach to health care. A client's health problems are identified and treated based on a health history, physical examination, and diagnostic tests. The specific body system that is malfunctioning is then treated in an attempt to improve the client's health status. While education and social support are often included in the treatment plan, they are generally supportive services.

Consider the effect of this approach on the most common of clients, a 71-year-old man who is hospitalized with signs of dementia.

While his immediate problems are certainly related to his neurological and mental status, effective long-term management is rarely the result of intervention with either of those systems. In fact, focusing on these systems may even result in repeated admissions to the hospital. Most nurses are all too familiar with this expensive and dysfunctional pattern.

A general systems model examines the individual holistically even as it considers the elements that compose the system. The nurse who uses systems theory evaluates the individual, family, or community as an aggregate and simultaneously considers the relationship between parts. For that reason, the theory can serve as the foundation for a comprehensive assessment and analysis of human systems. Because the theory is general, information is easy to share with nurses in a variety of settings, as well as with other health professionals.

SYSTEMS TERMINOLOGY

A *system* may be defined as a group of objects whose parts work together toward a specific goal (Hall & Fagin, 1968). *Input,* in the form of matter, energy, and information, enters the system and is used by the system's parts or *subsystems* in a process known as *throughput.* The system then releases matter, energy, and information into the environment as *output.* While most of the output remains in the environment, part of it returns to the system as *feedback.* This operation allows a nonliving system to monitor itself in an attempt to move closer to a steady state known as *equilibrium.* Living systems attempt to achieve a less static state, sometimes referred to as *homeostasis* or *dynamism.* Every system is surrounded by a *boundary* that separates it from the environment and determines what enters the system (Fig. 5–1). The environment can also be subdivided into a *suprasystem,* the next larger grouping of which the system is a part. Beyond that is a series of larger and more complex systems. An individual is a system because he or she takes in matter, energy, and information in the form of food, fluids, oxygen, data, and sensations and then uses biological, psychological, and sociocultural subsystems to process that input. The individual

---

Box 5–1 Systems Terminology

Boundary   The separation between the system and what lies outside. The boundary also determines what enters and leaves the system.

Entropy   The tendency toward disorder or chaos.

Environment   All larger systems that either influence or are influenced by the system under study.

Equilibrium   A steady state.

Feedback   Output that is returned to the system and that allows it to monitor itself over time in an attempt to move closer to a steady state known as equilibrium or homeostasis.

Homeostasis   A condition of balance within the range of normal.

Input   Matter, energy, and information that enter a system.

Negentropy   The tendency toward order.

Output   Matter, energy, and information that leave a system.

Subsystems   The subparts of the system.

Suprasystem   The next larger organized entity of which a system is a part.

System   A group of elements that interact with one another in order to achieve a goal (von Bertalanffy, 1956).

Throughput   The process by which the system processes input and releases it as output.

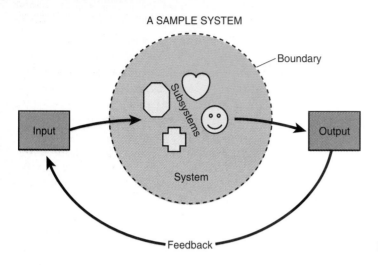

FIGURE 5-1 A sample system.

then returns matter, energy, and information to the environment in the form of both physical and psychosocial behaviors. Some of that output returns to the human system as feedback, which allows the individual to determine how well he or she is functioning. The amount of feedback that is accepted is partially controlled by the individual, who can decide what to allow in and what to exclude. In the human, a boundary extends beyond the skin to an area of personal space and separates the individual system from that of the family, which is usually the individual's suprasystem.

COMMON CHARACTERISTICS OF ALL SYSTEMS

Each system has common characteristics that influence its ability to operate. The first of these is system structure and function. Structure refers to a system's visible physical parts, whereas function represents those activities that a system carries out to achieve its goals. Structure and function are not separate entities. Rather, they are so closely related that a change in one causes a change in the other (Turner, 1998). For example, a person has physical structures that process all input. Those structures include relatively complex nervous and endocrine systems that work together to coordinate both physical and psychosocial behaviors. A structural change in the nervous system alters the way in which the individual functions.

A second characteristic is related to *boundary permeability*. Each system is surrounded by a boundary, which may range from being completely open to the environment to being completely closed to it. However, few systems are found at the extremes, since most require a moderate amount of environmental input in order to function. Without that input, a system becomes increasingly disordered, or entropic. For example, the parents of a schoolage child receive input from the school indicating that their 9-year-old has difficulty reading. A family whose boundary is open reviews the information and takes steps to correct the situation. A family with a less permeable boundary may discount or ignore the information and allow the situation to deteriorate.

Finally, systems are hierarchically arranged in increasing levels of complexity (Leddy & Pepper, 1998). In other words, there is an organizational scheme in which simple systems precede those that are more complex. As a result, most systems are a part of larger, more complex systems (*suprasystems*) and contain smaller, simpler systems (*subsystems*). For example, a family is part of a community, and that community is

THE FAMILY IN THE COMMUNITY

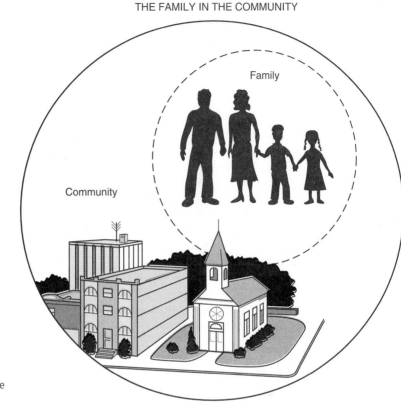

FIGURE 5–2 The family in the community.

part of a state or region. However, the family also has individual members who function as individual systems themselves (Fig. 5–2). Surrounding the system is the environment, which is composed of all those elements that have an impact on the system being studied. While it may be more accurate to think of the environment as a series of increasingly complex systems, it generally is simpler to view it as a single unit.

SPECIAL CHARACTERISTICS OF BEHAVIORAL SYSTEMS

The generalizations that have been made thus far apply to all systems, closed or open, living or nonliving. However, the nurse is primarily concerned with living or behavioral systems. These systems have some additional characteris-

tics that reflect their vital natures. The characteristics presented here are those that are traditionally a part of systems theory. In the next section, we will review some recent challenges to these notions.

Perhaps because it has the physical and chemical characteristics of life, a behavioral system operates as more than just a collection of specialized subsystems. As they work together to achieve system goals, the subsystems become an efficient and functional unit. Therefore a living system performs as a unified whole rather than as merely the sum of its parts (Byrne & Thompson, 1978). Common purpose is the fuel for this cooperative effort.

Because common purpose is so important, a living system must be goal directed. The specific goal varies with the system, but goals direct the function and structure of every system. An individual, as a complex behavioral system, may select and later alter some goals. Those alterations require the individual to overcome the forces that operate to maintain the system's status quo.

A living system continually takes in matter, energy, and information from the environment and never reaches true equilibrium. Instead, a human works toward *homeostasis,* a condition of balance within the range of normal (von Bertalanffy, 1956). To maintain that balance, a living system must adapt to environmental changes. Homeostatic regulators must sometimes be overcome in order to stimulate alterations in the system's internal processes and to change its level of functioning (Kast & Rosenzweig, 1981). This process is not easy, particularly when the system's goals and those of the environment are at odds. For example, an individual may be totally committed to life in a small town where employment is unavailable. If he or she is to survive economically, it may be necessary to move to a less desirable location. In spite of the environmental pressure, that move may be impossible if the individual cannot change his or her level of functioning.

Fortunately, a living system is always open to the environment (Lindberg, Hunter, & Kruszewski, 1998). The continual intake of new matter, information, and energy, when combined with feedback, provides ample opportunity for a system to become aware of the need to change its goals. Equally important, input allows the system to become increasingly complex and organized. This increasing organization is called *negentropy.* The ability to absorb input is essential both for system growth and for goal achievement. In fact, living systems will become disordered, or entropic, if they are unable to obtain sufficient input.

A final characteristic that is also related to goal achievement is *equifinality.* This refers to living systems' ability to reach the same goal from different initial conditions and by different routes (von Bertalanffy, 1956). It was difficult for systems theorists to explain how open systems, which began with differing resources and in different environments, could achieve similar goals. Von Bertalanffy suggested that this ability results from the dynamic interaction of the subsystems involved, which allows creative approaches to goal achievement.

Systems Theory and the Individual

Systems theory can help the practicing nurse deliver humane, clinically proficient health care. However, that goal will be reached more easily if the nurse keeps several suggestions in mind. These hints will help both new and experienced users of systems theory avoid some of the pitfalls that can result when any theory is applied in a practical setting.

First, it is best to work with the system that seems to be the source of the problem. The divisions between subsystem, system, and suprasystem are sometimes arbitrary. For example, in a tightly knit or fused family, the family group may carry on some functions that commonly belong to the individual. Infants and small children are very dependent on their families for basic needs. In these and similar cases, it may be difficult to decide where the individual ends and the family begins. In such situations, it is usually best to focus on the system in which the problem resides.

Second, systems theory is a general theory that can be used across disciplines. As a result, the approach is especially helpful in dealing with problems broadly and in focusing on the relationship between subsystems. It works best as a general guide rather than as a blueprint for nursing action.

AN APPROACH TO ASSESSMENT

The following case study is used to illustrate the application of systems theory throughout the nursing process.

Sara Warmly is a 16-year-old high school student who lives in a small city located about 100 miles from a major metropolitan area. Sara lives with her 14-year-old brother Matt and their parents, Bill (aged 41) and Jane (39), in a six-room apartment located on the upper floors of a two-family house. All four of Sara's grandparents, two aunts (Bill's sisters), and several cousins live nearby. The family belongs to a local church but attends services only once or twice a year. Both Bill and Jane work outside the home, Bill as an auto mechanic and Jane as a teacher's aide in a local elementary school. All of the family members participate in a variety of athletic activities (basketball, bowling, volleyball, and soccer); they are involved in few other community activities.

While the family has faced what they define as the "usual problems with teenagers," until recently they had no serious problems. In February, Sara began spending most of her spare time at her boyfriend Tim's home. She frequently ate dinner there, and arrived home after 11 p.m., her schoolnight curfew. Bill and Jane had always been concerned about the relationship between Sara and Tim, primarily because Tim is 21 years old. He dropped out of high school when he was 16 and has worked at a local automobile body shop since then. In April, Jane learned that Sara had 11 unexcused absences from school. Sara and her parents met with the school administrator and developed a plan to control the problem. Then, in July, Sara came to her parents and told them that she was 4 months pregnant and that she and Tim wanted to get married.

Sara and her mother visited a local obstetrician who had a reputation for being both competent and sympathetic to teens. The visit to the doctor went well. Sara's health was excellent and her pregnancy was progressing normally. Sara had no preexisting health problems or exposure to teratogenic substances. She did not smoke and denied using alcohol or illicit drugs. Her EDC was set by dates as January 18; she was 5 feet 8 inches tall and weighed 135 pounds. In addition to prescribing vitamins and discussing nutrition, the obstetrician referred Sara and her family to the local teen pregnancy support center, run cooperatively by the school system and the health department.

Sara, Tim, and Jane went to the support center and gathered information about available resources. Jane spoke with a counselor there about the pair's plans to marry and her strong objection to their plans, but neither Sara nor Tim felt that they needed counseling. Rather, they believed that, once they were married, all would be well.

Assess the Individual's Input. Input includes the quantity and quality of matter, energy, and information that cross the individual's boundary. Assume that Sara is the primary client.

Sara eats at home or at Tim's most of the time. She consumes a varied diet, eats some "junk food," denies using alcohol or illegal drugs, and receives active support from her family. She has several good female friends, but has seen them less often as her relationship with Tim has become more serious. Sara watches MTV and enjoys a number of situation comedies. She is willing to use community resources but does not perceive her pregnancy as a problem.

Assess the Individual's Output. The individual's observable behaviors, both physical and psychosocial, are output. These include what we commonly call signs and symptoms.

Sara has had no health problems. She attended school irregularly during the spring but was a star on the high school volleyball team during the last academic year. She told her parents of her pregnancy only after her fourth month, is sexually active, and has never used contraception. Sara indicated that she didn't think that she would become pregnant, but wasn't upset by it.

Consider the Individual's Throughput Mechanisms. The way in which subsystems process matter, energy, and information is suggested by system output and the relationship between input and output. For example, an individual may have signs or symptoms of illness, such as shortness of breath or edema (output), or may be losing weight in spite of eating adequately (imbalance between input and output).

Sara's height and weight suggest that she is able to metabolize the food she eats. The fetus is doing well and was normal according to a sonogram. While Sara does not have any difficulty completing her schoolwork, her frequent absences have put her at risk of failing her junior year. That, combined with her lack of concern about her condition, suggests a throughput problem with her behavioral subsystems.

Assess the Individual's Feedback Mechanisms. Output that the system uses in order to monitor itself is known as feedback. Problems with the sensory subsystem, such as poor hearing, may make it impossible for some feedback to reenter the system. A client may have difficulty monitoring his or her own behavior when an accurate perception of feedback is frightening or would require a change in a valued behavior. For example, a 39-year-old man who has a strong family history of heart disease may ignore episodes of chest pain (feedback) because he is afraid of having a myocardial infarction.

Sara has no problems with seeing or hearing and seems to respond appropriately to feedback from those systems. She shows no physical signs of anxiety, which might reflect concern about her pregnancy. Sara did note the signs of pregnancy and did not ignore the feedback that suggested a change from her prepregnancy condition.

Assess the Individual's Boundary. A boundary must be selectively permeable if a system is to function adequately. Selective permeability refers to the boundary's ability to determine specifically what matter, energy, and information can enter or leave the system. In some instances, system boundaries completely break down. Physiologically, boundary failure is often the re-

sult of the failure of a subsystem. For example, when one's kidneys fail, the entire system loses the ability to control some output. Psychosocial boundary failures are more difficult to describe. Certainly the schizophrenic client who cannot tell where he or she ends and the outside world begins has a problem with boundary integrity.

Sara has no problems with allowing physiological input to cross her boundary. Although she attends to her parent's concerns, she seems to exclude some of the information that they provide to her. These include their concern about her youth, her limited income, and a variety of other issues.

Assess the Individual's Environment. The environment includes both the immediate suprasystem (usually the family) and the larger world. In some instances, problems that seem to belong to the client are actually problems with resources in the larger environment. Since the difficulty did not begin within the client, its solution is apt to be found in the environment from which the problem arose.

The environment includes a number of resources. The teen pregnancy support program is both a resource itself and a method to identify other support services. The school and the church may also be able to provide some additional help. The degree to which Sara, Tim, and the family are willing to use those services will determine how helpful those resources are to them.

Assessment and Analysis Are Reciprocal Activities. As data are gathered, they are interpreted and analyzed. The specific questions one asks in the assessment stage are, to some degree, determined by an analysis of previous answers. Therefore, while assessment and analysis are generally described separately, they actually occur almost simultaneously.

ANALYSIS

Analysis is the process of drawing inferences based on the raw data that have been gathered. Analysis is not simple, since it requires the nurse to apply knowledge and experience to a particular client. In fact, the ability to combine knowledge and experience, as well as client and sensory cues, into a unified sense of the client's condition is the mark of a skilled nurse (Benner, Tanner, & Chesla, 1992). It is clear that in spite of the challenges involved, a holistic analysis is essential to the provision of competent nursing care.

Healthy functioning requires the client to meet both biological and psychosocial goals. The individual's subsystems should operate together in a way that contributes to goal achievement. As a first step in the process of analyzing data, the nurse should describe and evaluate the interaction between the subsystems.

In order to maintain a steady state (sometimes called homeostasis), the individual must balance the matter, energy, and information that enter the system with that leaving the system. A disparity between input and output may suggest a problem with maintaining a steady state. A number of physiological and psychological difficulties, such as fluid volume excess or deficit, ineffective breathing patterns, and some appetite disorders, fall into this category. In some instances, internal processes are working so inefficiently that they prevent effective use of environmental input. As a second step in analysis, the nurse should indicate how well the client is able to maintain homeostasis.

Finally, any individual must adapt to internal and external changes. That process requires energy, which must be imported or diverted from other system activities. The final step in analysis requires the nurse to describe how well the individual is adjusting to internal and environmental changes.

Sara's biological subsystems are functioning well, although pregnancy will present a challenge to her cardiovascular, reproductive, and endocrine systems. There is no obvious reason to expect that she should have problems, although youth alone increases the risk for premature birth. The greatest challenges that Sara faces appear to be psychosocial. She is in the process of developing her own identity and will now be responsible for another person. She seems to have some difficulty seeing the real challenges that she faces, a common adolescent characteristic. On the other hand, she was willing to ask for and accept help from her family, and has also been willing to consider help from outside the family. However, her greatest challenges to her ability to adapt lie in the future.

PLANNING, IMPLEMENTATION, AND EVALUATION

Planning, implementation, and evaluation are considered together in this section. Because systems theory is general, the following suggestions apply to all three of these phases. The focus of this section is on the nurse as a member of the health care team. Since the use of an interdisciplinary team should improve care while it decreases cost, it is likely to be used increasingly in the future. For this reason, every nurse needs to work cooperatively with other health professionals. General systems theory is an effective vehicle by which to reach that end because of its holistic nature.

Because a general systems approach is the basis for many theoretical approaches to care, the method can be used effectively by a team of health care professionals who have differing educational and clinical backgrounds. The client and the team cooperatively determine which problems are amenable to intervention, and develop goals and objectives that focus on those problems. The group identifies the roles of each member, executes the plans that have been developed, evaluates success or failure, and alters the plan as needed.

There are four characteristics of open systems that are particularly helpful to those who are planning, implementing, and evaluating care. These are holism, equifinality, a steady state, and adaptation.

Holism. Focusing on the whole individual, holism emphasizes the uniqueness of that individual. While nursing has almost universally emphasized the need for individualized client care, personalized care occurs relatively rarely in practice settings. Systems theory reminds us to develop plans that address the client as a whole rather than as a collection of illnesses. In fact, if the health care team does not consider the client as a whole, it is likely that planning and intervention will be less than effective.

Equifinality. A second characteristic allows providers to be flexible in responding to a client's unique needs during the development and implementation of plans of care. *Equifinality* suggests that a client's health care goals may be reached by a number of different routes. Therefore planning and implementing care can be an accommodative process—one that meets the needs of the client, effectively uses the skills of team members, and recognizes a range of approaches to meet those needs.

Steady State. Planning and implementation should attempt to maintain or improve homeostatic mechanisms. A client who has unmet health needs often has difficulty maintaining a stable energy supply. This may occur either because the demands that are made on his or her system require increased energy or because normal energy sources (food, oxygen, etc.) are insufficient. Therefore the team and client should develop, implement, and evaluate plans that attempt to reduce energy needs or to increase available energy, both biological and physiological.

Adaptation. Maintaining homeostasis does not preclude adapting to new circumstances. Many common health problems require increased energy merely to maintain a steady state. Positive changes, such as gathering new information or altering habit patterns, require even more energy. Adapting to internal or environmental change means that energy must either be imported by the system or transferred from some other activity. Plans that center on adaptation or change should always include some consideration of whether the energy required for that change is available. If this is not done, goals that focus on these areas are likely to fail.

Sara needs both time and further assessment in order to deal with her problems and their sources. It is likely that the process will involve her family, obstetrician, the school, and an interdisciplinary team from the teen center.

The nursing process is one of those approaches that has its roots in systems theory. Systems concepts provide support for the sequential steps of assessment, analysis, planning, implementation, and evaluation. The inexperienced student can use systems theory as he or she learns about the nursing process. Meanwhile, the experienced practitioner can apply the concepts in the workplace in a flexible, realistic way. Whether this means working independently or with a health care team, it increases the likelihood that the client will be a part of a health care system that is both humane and scientifically sound.

APPLIED RESEARCH

While recent research that directly applies general systems theory concepts to the individual and family is limited, there have been a variety of past attempts to support or refute the theory (Fawcett, 1995; Reed, 1993; Silva, 1986). Systems theory does serve as a foundation for many nursing theorists. For example, Johnson, King, Orem, Rogers, and Neuman all base their theoretical models, at least in part, on general systems theory.

Recent researchers have not focused much attention on the type of grand theory that the systems approach reflects. Rather, current nursing research explores mid-range nursing theories, which, according to Merton (1968, p. 39), lie "between the minor but necessary working hypotheses that evolve in abundance in day-to-day research and the all-inclusive systemic efforts to develop [a] unified theory." This approach allows one to test specific elements of systems theory and prove or disprove those elements. One such mid-range theory is Brook's theory of intrapersonal perceptual awareness, which focuses on throughput and output as the authors attempt to categorize those factors essential to making effective clinical decisions (Brooks & Thomas, 1997). Other systems-based theories include Liehr and Smith's psychological adaptation and resilience (1999).

Finally, there has been some elaboration on systems theory itself. Both complexity theory and chaos theory are directly based on general systems. However, these newer approaches differ from systems theory in their assumptions, particular in regard to linearity, equifinality, and homeostasis. Specifically, both assume that systems are nonlinear, and thus actions result from a complex interplay of factors. Those factors may result in multifinality, in which systems that begin at very similar states reach very different outcomes. Finally, living systems do not reach homeostasis but come to a dynamic state that is often restless and unpredictable and can encourage system change (Warren, Franklin, & Streeter, 1998). One nursing model that reflects this approach is the nonlinear quality health outcomes model of Mitchell and colleagues, which is broad enough to provide a framework for research at the system level (Mitchell, Ferketich, & Jennings, 1998).

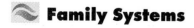 **Family Systems**

Most of us are born into, live out our lives, and die within families, and may limit our analysis

to the quirks of our own families. General systems theory provides a framework that helps the nurse assess other families, identify their relevant patterns, and plan, implement, and evaluate family interventions. General systems theory is sufficiently broad to accommodate the perspectives of a number of family theorists. It is also relatively apolitical (Wellard, 1997) and so may be helpful in situations that require a neutral viewpoint.

As family systems change, so do the definitions of the family. The family may be seen as "a small social system and primary reference group made up of two or more persons . . . who are related by blood, marriage, or adoption or who are living together by agreement over a period of time" (Murray & Zentner, 1997, p. 143). It is a living system in which there is "a series of interlocking . . . subsystems [where] a change in one part will produce a change in another" (Bowen, 1974). The family system takes in matter, energy, and information as input, processes it, and either retains it or releases it into the environment as output. The family uses feedback to determine whether it is meeting its goals and evaluates activities as simple as monitoring a savings account balance or as complex as monitoring a child. Every family has a boundary, but because it is emotional rather than physical, it may be difficult to identify. Finally, the family exists within an environment, usually the community (Fig. 5–3).

AN APPROACH TO ASSESSMENT

The same case study that was presented in the section on individual assessment can be used as the basis for family assessment, and provides an example of how one can alter the definition of a system.

Assess the Family's Input. A family obtains most of its matter, energy, and information from the community. Resources include a range of assets that strengthen a family's ability to

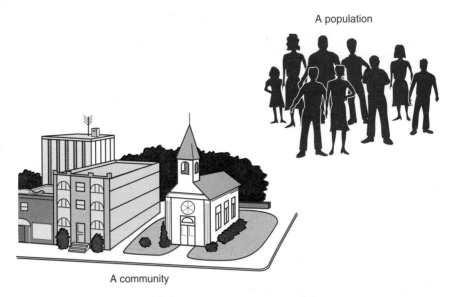

FIGURE 5–3 Communities versus populations.

cope, whereas stressors reflect insufficient assets and demands that diminish family resources.

The family has sufficient income for day-to-day activities. However, they do not own their own home, and their occupations suggest that they have limited assets. They have two teenage children, as well as a number of family members living close by. They may have some friends who share their interest in sports, although that fact is not clear. The family has health insurance through Bill's place of employment. However those benefits do have a family deductible requirement of $250 annually.

Assess the Family's Output. Every family demonstrates a range of observable behaviors to the community and to each other. The activities in which the members participate and the home where they live reflect family resources and values. Families develop both functional and dysfunctional patterns of behavior as they attempt to resolve problems and reduce tensions.

The Warmlys belong to a church but rarely attend. Family members all participate in sports activities. Sara has been especially active in school-based sports. The Warmlys took their children to the pediatrician regularly, and both children's immunizations are up to date. The children have had annual sports physicals. Neither Bill nor Sara visit their family physician regularly, but they do see him when they are ill. Jane last saw her gynecologist 3 years ago. The children see a dentist at school for preventative care, but their parents get dental care only when they have a problem. Jane and Bill have told Sara's aunts about the pregnancy but haven't yet told her grandparents.

Assess the Family's Throughput Mechanisms. The way a system processes information is suggested by the relationship between the system's input and output. However, there are specific issues that directly influence system functioning. Each of these should be considered individually.

The first of these are family set factors. Set factors are those enduring family characteristics that predispose a family to behave in a particular way. They include religion, educational level, socioeconomic class, ethnocultural background, and values. The nurse should pay particular attention to the relationships between these characteristics, since many of them are interconnected. For example, education, socioeconomic class, and values tend to reflect and may predict one another.

The second consideration is family structure. Over the past 25 years, the idea of what constitutes a family has changed dramatically. Family arrangements include a broad range of married, single-parent, and multiadult households, with or without children (Stanhope & Lancaster, 1996). Structural elements include the family composition, value systems, communication network, role system, and power structure (Friedman, 1997).

A third issue is family developmental stage. Developmental theorists suggest that families change in predictable ways over time (Friedman, 1997). These normal changes result from internal and environmental experiences that typically occur as a family matures. Until quite recently, developmental stage was based on childbearing and child-rearing responsibilities such as those described by Duvall (1977).

Because some families do not include children, theorists have also described less-child-oriented stages that can apply to all families. Generally, these stages focus on the following: (1) physical safety, (2) the formation and development of a family identity, (3) increasing family integration (coping with family crises effectively), and (4) maintaining community ties (Murray & Zentner, 1997). Regardless of the approach used, the nurse must attempt to determine whether the family is carrying out the functions that are appropriate to its developmental stage.

A final issue, strongly influenced by structure, is family functioning, or the way the family operates as a unit. Family functioning includes an analysis of its ability to carry out those activities that are traditionally its responsibility, including family communication, decision making, and family role execution. Roles refer to behaviors that are socially defined and expected of an occupant of a particular position or status. Each member of the family typically has a number of roles (Clark, 1999). Since roles within a family significantly influence how the family functions, much information about how a family operates can be obtained by assessing those roles.

Family structure, developmental stage, roles, communication, and decision-making patterns collectively influence the way a family works together. Although a weakness in one area may be compensated for by strengths in another, a family with multiple weaknesses often suffers from severely compromised functioning. A systems approach is a practical way to consider how these factors together influence family functioning. At least one assessment tool, the Feetham Family Functioning Survey, measures the ability of the family to function as an open system. This tool has demonstrated both reliability and validity (Roberts & Feetham, 1982).

The Warmlys are a working-class nuclear family composed of two parents and their children. Both parents are high school graduates, and Bill attended trade school as well. Developmentally, they are a family with teenagers. The family is working on the tasks of maintaining open communication, and balancing teenage freedom with responsibility. The latter task is a current challenge. In addition, Sara has challenged the family by asking them to deal with tasks that are usually a part of the launching stage.

Assess the Family's Feedback Mechanisms. Although individuals commonly use both physical and psychosocial data as they evaluate themselves, families primarily use psychosocial measures. In some families, goal accomplishment is determined mainly by external measures of success, such as income or status, whereas other families measure success internally, based on personal values. Families differ in their responses to evidence that they are not meeting their goals, and they may change their behavior or their goals, or both.

The Warmlys believe that success isn't measured by money. Instead, family unity, hard work, and physical activity are their measures of success. Although they don't often attend church, Bill and Jane believe in God and try to live good lives. While the children have, until now, lived according to their parent's values, Sara is currently questioning some of those values. Matt has little to say on the topic.

Assess the Family's Boundary. Although an individual's boundary may be easy to identify, a family's boundary is defined not only by position but also by norms, values, attitudes, and rules (Clemen-Stone, McGuire, & Eigsti, 1998). That border may surround only the family members who live in the home, or it may include other, not so obvious members. Boundaries vary in both permeability and integrity. One of the functions of a boundary is to exclude matter, energy, and information that the system does not need or want. In some families, that function is severely compromised. If substances that could be harmful to members are allowed to enter freely, then the boundary is not functioning effectively.

The Warmly nuclear family includes four members. However, both Bill and Jane live near their own parents, have keys to their parents' homes, and interact with them often. Jane and Bill welcome their children's friends into their home, but Tim has been a rare guest. Generally, Sara goes to Tim's home, and Matt's friends rarely visit him at home.

Assess the Family's Environment. Normally, the community in which the family lives is con-

sidered to be the suprasystem. Many of the family's resources must be obtained from the suprasystem. Often a family's developmental stage helps to determine what resources are most significant to its members. An elderly family may be particularly concerned about health care services but very little about schools, whereas a family with growing children may have different priorities. A mixed-age community requires a balance of services that can meet the needs of all residents.

The Warmlys live in a mixed-age community that has a range of health care and social services. Public transportation is limited, although some door-to-door transportation is available for the elderly and disabled. Generally, residents drive private cars, and children who live a distance from school are bused to school. There are a variety of sports programs for children, a mall with a multiscreen theater, and a new YMCA with an indoor swimming pool and an ice hockey rink.

ANALYSIS

Analysis is the process of making sense of the information about the family that has been gathered. A nurse must make inferences that are based on adequate data and arise from a combination of experience and a strong knowledge base. Although many of us have developed unique approaches to analysis, a family's ability to achieve family goals and to maintain homeostasis through adapting to change and managing environmental stressors are two outcomes on which to base nursing inferences.

A functioning family should be able to meet its goals successfully. These goals include both the responsibilities that the society asks of any family and those more personal decisions about how time, money, and energy should be spent. Set factors, developmental stage, communication, decision-making patterns, and roles influence a family's functional patterns. It is essential to use the gathered data as a basis for describing how well the family is functioning and to draw conclusions about why a family is or is not successful in achieving its goals.

A second measure of a functional family is its ability to maintain homeostasis. To do so, it must take in sufficient matter, energy, and information to balance that which it uses with that which it returns to the community. Since it is the boundary that regulates what enters and leaves the system, a family that is relatively closed to its environment may have difficulty obtaining what it needs to maintain a dynamic balance. On the other hand, a family may give so much to the community that it has insufficient energy to meet its own needs. A large disparity between input and output suggests that a family is having difficulty maintaining its balance. When a family requires significant community support and still has difficulty functioning, something may be wrong with its internal processes. Stressors such as illness or a developmental or role change may demand increased resources or may impair a family's ability to effectively use the resources it has. Any family must be able to adapt to a variety of changes. The nurse should begin by focusing on the family's specific developmental stage. Each stage brings with it predictable family challenges that require the use of adaptive energy. In addition, there are environmental stressors with which the family must cope. Because of the environment's unpredictability, these stressors may require a surplus of adaptive energy. A combination of developmental and environmental stressors may tax the resources of even the most functional family.

Until recently, the Warmlys had been meeting their family goals, as defined by both society and themselves. Now their daughter's school problems and pregnancy have made them question that success. However, in spite of these challenges, the family has demonstrated some real developmental strengths as they have dealt with their problems. The parents have supported their daughter and reached out to community resources. After a period of acute stress, the family has been able to communicate even when members have had real differences. Family members have not isolated themselves from one another, and some members of the extended family have provided support to the Warmlys. Family roles are changing. Sara the daughter is about to become Sara the mother and perhaps wife. These changes will alter Sara's parent's roles as well as those of her brother.

In view of their problems, and in spite of their strengths, this family is in a state of imbalance. The stressors that they face would unbalance almost any family but need not destroy them. If the family is able to build on its strengths and use community resources effectively, the family may regain its balance. There are, however, a number of unpredictable factors in this situation, which make predicting its outcome difficult. They include Sara's youth, her boyfriend, about whom we know little, as well as those intangible factors that operate in all families.

PLANNING, IMPLEMENTATION, AND EVALUATION

Planning, implementation, and evaluation are based on family needs and represent the action segments of the nursing process. They give the nurse who is working with a family the opportunity to cooperatively and thoughtfully develop, carry out, and evaluate the process. Because the three steps are so closely connected that they are often reciprocal, they are discussed together here. As is true for the individual, this process requires cooperation between family, health team members, and community resources.

A systems approach to planning, implementation, and evaluation has some unique features. Because the family is goal directed, its participation is essential to achieve health-related goals The family should clearly identify the goals its members are willing to pursue and, with the health team, determine how to meet them (Clemen-Stone et al., 1998). While the nurse may be aware of particular strategies that may be helpful, a range of possible approaches, any of which may achieve the goal, should be considered (equifinality). This requires the active participation of the family, the health team, and other resource people.

Nursing actions should focus on supporting or improving the family's homeostatic mechanisms. When a family is overwhelmed by demands, it is often helpful to identify and reduce the number of stressors with which the members are dealing. The family may have to alter its behavior in order to return to or maintain a steady state. It is during periods of stress that the family has the opportunity to experiment with new approaches to solving problems in order to make permanent adaptations. The nurse should encourage healthy changes that increase family stability.

In addition, the nurse may help the family adapt to change or increase the permeability of its boundary. Increasing boundary permeability has a dual purpose: to help the family identify external resources and then help them to actually use them (Miller & Janosik, 1980). A wide range of coping strategies may be used in the process (Box 5–2).

Finally, because systems theory is especially useful to examine the relationship between subsystems, research that explores the relationship between family members may suggest effective strategies for specific families. For example, past studies that explore feedback between mother and child (Anderson, 1981) or mothers' perceptions during childbirth (Mercer, Hackley, & Bostrom, 1983) support the use of general systems theory in family-centered maternity settings. Unfortunately, further confirmatory research studies have not been undertaken.

Community/Population Systems

Many people think of a community as an environment with physical or political boundaries. Community health nursing, however, defines the term more broadly to reflect concern with the health of groups or populations of individuals (Clark, 1999). Communities are composed of population groups—collections of individuals with shared characteristics (Clemen-Stone et al., 1998). These population groups may be defined by the areas in which they live (inner city, suburb) but are more commonly composed of subgroups of the general population (the elderly, schoolage children). Although community health nursing is concerned about improving the health of the entire population, it is especially concerned about groups that are at special

---

Box 5–2 Increasing Family Coping

WITHIN THE FAMILY
1. Family support
2. Family humor
3. Sharing of experiences
4. Redefining the problem
5. Shared problem solving
6. Role flexibility

OUTSIDE THE FAMILY
1. Seeking information
2. Maintaining community relations
3. Seeking support, both social and spiritual

Adapted from *Family nursing: Research, theory, and practice* by Friedman, M. M. © 1996. Reprinted by permission of Prentice-Hall, Inc., Upper Saddle River, N.J.

risk for illness. Figure 5–3 illustrates both a traditional community and a population group.

ASSESSMENT

The primary reason to assess a community is to identify and change factors that influence its health status. This process requires the nurse, often in concert with others, to gather data from a variety of sources in order to develop an accurate and comprehensive picture of the group involved. This may seem overwhelming even to an experienced community health nurse. A systematic approach can help to make the process more manageable.

Assess the Community's Input. The matter, energy, and information to which the community has access influences its health status. This includes health care and non-health care resources from both public and private sources. For example, while the elderly have more chronic illnesses than other age groups, they also have access to health care provided by the federal government and access to a potent political action group, the American Association of Retired Persons (AARP). Newspapers, radio, and television reflect and shape community opinion, whereas state and national policy help to determine community resources.

Assess the Community's Output. A community's goals and the degree to which they are achieved represent its output. Regardless of the unique features of the population, two goals are almost always present. All groups work to ensure their own survival and to achieve self-fulfillment for themselves and for their members. Demographic, morbidity, and mortality statistics describe a community's characteristics as well as its health outcomes. These data help to identify illness patterns or public health problems that are unique to the group. For example, in some communities osteoporosis is a serious problem, whereas other communities are more concerned about teenage pregnancy.

Assess the Community's Throughput Mechanisms. Throughput refers to the ways in which a community processes its input, including the ways that information is communicated between members. For example, are there formal communication networks, or do informal systems predominate? Are there newspapers or newsletters? What recreational and other interactional opportunities are there? Does the population take advantage of them?

Health and health-related programs may be provided by the community itself, the state, or the nation. These programs may treat existing disease or may attempt to ensure that a group remains healthy, both physically and emotionally. In either case, social services, programs, and activities are targeted at specific geographical regions and population groups.

Assess the Community's Feedback Mechanisms. Every community has the opportunity to evaluate its own goal achievement, especially in the area of health. Healthy groups should attempt to realistically evaluate feedback that relates to their health goals and then make an effort to respond to the data appropriately. This may require an entire community to change its behavior.

Assess the Community's Boundary. Some communities have clearly defined boundaries that are determined by age, gender, socioeconomic status, or place of residence. These boundaries may be defended rigidly or loosely, depending on the purposes of the community. It is essential that boundaries allow necessary matter, energy, and information to enter and that they exclude that which is unnecessary.

Assess the Community's Environment. Because communities are not self-sufficient, they depend on their environment to function effectively. This dependence on others requires negotiation and cooperation in both the private and the public sectors. However, some groups have abundant resources within their community and are therefore less dependent on the external environment. Most community nursing texts contain survey tools that include the preceding information. These tools may be helpful to those who undertake a community assessment.

DATA ANALYSIS

The purpose of analyzing population data is to identify group health needs. To do this, the nurse must draw conclusions about the data that have been gathered. There are a number of approaches to data interpretation that can facilitate the inferential process. In any case, the community involved must be an active participant in the process. A systems approach is particularly helpful in identifying the relationships between subsystems. Begin by reviewing the data in each category and summarizing the information, describing both strengths and weaknesses and supporting your conclusions with statistical evidence. The second step is to identify gaps, omissions, or inconsistencies in the data and gather additional information as needed.

Inferences about community health problems are then described based on the collected data. This process generally involves comparing the amassed data with the data of the larger population or by using measures that reflect a desired group outcome or goal. The last step is to develop a priority list to indicate the order in which problems should be addressed.

PLANNING, IMPLEMENTATION, AND EVALUATION

The same skill and knowledge that help the nurse plan, implement, and evaluate care with the individual and the family are used with larger populations. However, some special abilities are essential to the community health nurse. One person alone rarely resolves a group health problem. Instead, it requires the concerted action of all those who are concerned about health. As a result, the nurse must work cooperatively with other professional groups as well as with governmental and voluntary agencies and organizations. This cooperative planning requires patience, negotiation, compromise, and more patience. The outcome is a plan that reflects group input and is therefore more likely to be successfully implemented. It may, however, be quite different from the one the nurse originally envisioned.

Evaluation is the weak link in many population-focused health plans. Because planning and implementation require so much energy, there is often little inclination to rework those steps when they are ineffective. Therefore evaluation should begin early in the process, when alterations are simpler and less costly. However, because many population-focused plans address complex problems, it remains necessary to measure long-term outcomes despite the difficulty involved.

In spite of the challenges inherent in addressing population-based health problems, it can be an extremely rewarding process for the nurse. It encourages the development of new skills that can be used to help clients in a wide variety of settings. More important, the process can have a tremendous impact on the health of population groups, the state, and the nation.

KEY POINTS

- Systems theory is especially useful to nursing because it focuses on the whole but pays particular attention to the way the parts work together.

- Systems theory is a broadly applicable interdisciplinary approach that can be used by nurses in most settings, with all types of clients, and by all members of the health care team.

- Systems theory is applicable in all phases of the nursing process and is particularly useful in the analysis of data.

- The case study illustrates how general systems theory can serve as a useful framework for assessing and providing care for individuals and families.

- Care for communities and populations at risk can be accommodated within the general systems theory framework.

CRITICAL THINKING EXERCISES

1. Discuss the major advantages of using general systems theory as a basis for client care. What, if any, are the disadvantages?

2. What element do chaos theory and complexity theory add to general systems?

3. How do the following concepts apply to the family in which you were raised: input, throughput, output, boundary, environment, homeostasis, and suprasystem.

4. Select an individual client, and
  a. Use general systems theory as a framework for assessment and data analysis.
  b. Describe your findings according to the principles and concepts of general systems theory.

5. One of the most challenging parts of family assessment is assessing the family's throughput. Describe a family (your own or other) in terms of its set factors, structure, developmental stage, and functioning. How might that family process information?

6. Compare and contrast the use of systems theory to assess, plan, implement, and evaluate care with a population group and a geographical community.

REFERENCES

Anderson, C. (1981). Enhancing reciprocity between mother and neonate. *Nursing Research, 30*(2), 89–93.

Benner, P., Tanner, C., & Chesla, C. (1992). From beginner to expert: Gaining a differentiated clinical world in critical care nursing. *Advances in Nursing Science, 14*(3), 13–28.

Bowen, M. (1974). *Bowen on triangles.* Workshop monograph, Washington, DC: Georgetown University, Center for Family Learning.

Brooks, E. M., & Thomas, S. (1997). The perception and judgement of senior baccalaureate student nurses in clinical decision making. *Advances in Nursing Science, 19*(3), 50–69.

Byrne, M., & Thompson, L. (1978). *Key concepts for the study and practice of nursing* (2nd ed.). St. Louis: Mosby.

Clark, M. J. (1999). *Nursing in the community.* Stamford, CT: Appleton & Lange.

Clemen-Stone, S., McGuire, S. L., & Eigsti, D. G. (1998). *Comprehensive family and community health nursing: Family, aggregate, and community practice* (5th ed.). St. Louis: Mosby.

Duvall, E. M. (1977). *Marriage and family development* (5th ed.). Philadelphia: Lippincott.

Fawcett, J. (1995). *Analysis and evaluation of nursing theories.* Philadelphia: Davis.

Friedman, M. (1997). *Family nursing: Research, theory and practice.* Norwalk, CT: Appleton & Lange.

Hall, A. D., & Fagin, R. E. (1968). In W. Buckley (Ed.), *Modern systems research for the behavioral scientist,* (pp. 81–92). Chicago: Aldine.

Kast, F., & Rosenzweig, J. (1981). General systems theory: Applications for organizations and management. *Journal of Nursing Administration, 81*(8), 32–40.

Leddy, S., & Pepper, J. M. (1998). *Conceptual bases of professional nursing* (3rd ed., pp. 165–200). Philadelphia: Lippincott.

Liehr, P., & Smith, M. J. (1999). Middle-range theory: Spinning research and practice to create knowledge in the new millenium. *Advances in Nursing Science, 21* (4), 81–91.

Lindberg, J. B., Hunter, M. L., & Kruszewski, A. Z. (1998). *Introduction to nursing* (3rd ed., pp. 94–97). Philadelphia: Lippincott.

Mercer, R., Hackley, K., & Bostrom, A. (1983). Relationship of psychosocial and perinatal variables to perception of childbirth. *Nursing Research, 32,* 202–207.

Merton, R.K. (1968). *Social theory and social structure.* New York: Free Press.

Miller, J. (1978). *Living systems.* New York: McGraw-Hill.

Miller, J., & Janosik, E. (1980). *Family focused care.* New York: McGraw-Hill.

Mitchell, P. H., Ferketich, S., & Jennings, B. M. (1998). Quality health outcomes model. *Image: Journal of Nursing Scholarship, 30*(1), 43–52.

Murray, R. B., & Zentner, J. P. (1997). *Health assessment and promotion strategies throughout the life span* (6th ed., pp. 141–196). Stamford, CT: Appleton & Lange.

Reed, K. (1993). Adapting the Neuman systems model for family nursing. *Nursing Science Quarterly, 6*(2), 93–97.

Roberts, C., & Feetham, S. (1982). Assessing family functioning across three areas of relationships. *Nursing Research, 31,* 231–235.

Silva, M. (1986). Research testing nursing theory: State of the art. *Advances in Nursing Science, 9*(1), 1–11.

Stanhope, M., & Lancaster, J. (1996). *Community health nursing: Process and practice for promoting health* (4th ed.). St. Louis: Mosby.

Tonges, M., & Madden, M. J. (1993). "Running the vicious cycle backward" and other system solutions to nursing problems. *Journal of Nursing Administration, 23*(1), 39–44.

Turner, S. L. (1998). The family. In J. L. Leahy & P. E. Kizilay (Eds.), *Foundations of nursing practice* (pp. 366–383). Philadelphia: Saunders.

von Bertalanffy, L. (1956). General systems theory. In B. D. Ruben & J. Kim (Eds.), *General systems theory and human communication* (pp. 7–16). Rochelle Park, NJ: Hayden.

Warren, K., Franklin, C., & Streeter, C. L. (1998). New directions in systems theory: Chaos and complexity. *Social Work, 43*, 357–372.

Wellard, S. (1997). Constructions of family nursing: A critical exploration. *Contemporary Nurse: A Journal for the Australian Nursing Profession, 6*(2), 78–84.

Theories and Frameworks for Professional Nursing Practice

JOAN L. CREASIA, PhD, RN

OBJECTIVES

At the completion of this chapter, the reader will be able to:

- Distinguish between a concept, a theory, a conceptual framework, and a model.
- Identify and define the four central concepts of nursing theories.
- Compare and contrast the main precepts of selected theories of nursing.
- Examine criteria for evaluating the utility of a specific nursing theory for its relevance to practice, education, or research.
- Identify theories from related disciplines that have application to nursing.

PROFILE IN PRACTICE

Jacqueline Fawcett, PhD, RN, FAAN
College of Nursing,
University of Massachusetts-Boston
Boston, Massachusetts

I earned my baccalaureate degree in nursing from Boston University (BU) in 1964 and worked as an operating room staff nurse during that summer. My first exposure to a nursing discipline–specific theory occurred during my nursing course work at BU. I learned Orlando's theory of the deliberative nursing process and have continued to find this simple yet elegant nursing theory of great utility in assisting patients, colleagues, and students to express their immediate needs for help.

I began teaching in a small hospital-based diploma nursing program in Connecticut in January 1965. I have continued to teach nursing ever since, first at the University of Connecticut for 6 years, with interruptions for my master's degree

in parent-child nursing and my PhD in nursing, then at the University of Pennsylvania for 21 years, and now at the University of Massachusetts in Boston.

During my master's program at New York University (NYU), I was introduced to theory-guided nursing practice. The clinical courses in parent-child nursing emphasized the application of theory to the nursing of childbearing women and their families, well children, and children with acute and chronic illnesses. At that time, knowledge about nursing discipline–specific conceptual models and theories was limited. The NYU nursing faculty, my classmates, and I worked hard to adapt crisis theory to nursing situations, and to

115

explore the applicability of developmental theories and family theories to nursing situations. I immediately recognized the benefit of using theories to guide nursing practice—I finally had found a way to organize my thinking and my practice. Indeed, I finally knew what to say and do and the reasons for what I was saying and doing when I interacted with a patient!

When I returned to the University of Connecticut after earning my master's degree in 1970, my faculty colleagues and I began to design and implement a new curriculum based on crisis theory. We extended the original theory to encompass physiological as well as psychological events (see White, 1983; Infante, 1982).

I returned to NYU 2 years later and entered the "brave new world" of Martha Rogers's conceptual system, now called the science of unitary human beings, which was my first exposure to a comprehensive nursing discipline–specific conceptual model. Given my strong interest in theory-guided nursing practice, I was very attracted to Rogers's work. I rapidly immersed myself in the course work that led to my dissertation research, which was based on my extension of Rogers's conceptual system to the family (see Fawcett, 1975, 1977). My course work sensitized me to the need to use nursing discipline–specific conceptual models and theories to guide not only nursing practice but also nursing research. Furthermore, the course work sensitized me to the reciprocal relationship between research and conceptual models and between practice and conceptual models. I realized that conceptual models inform research and practice, and research findings and the results observed in practice in turn inform revisions in the conceptual model.

I returned to the University of Connecticut in 1975 and completed all requirements for the PhD degree in 1976. I began to teach nursing research courses and had the opportunity to develop courses in contemporary nursing knowledge and the relation of theory and research. The latter two courses became the focus of my scholarly work and the underlying reason for my passion about nursing.

I was recruited by the University of Pennsylvania (Penn) in 1978 and had the honor of teaching the subject matter of my scholarly work in a new nursing doctoral program. Throughout all the years at Penn and now at the University of Massachusetts in Boston, my teaching has informed my scholarly work and my scholarly work has informed my teaching. My books about analysis of nursing models and theories (Fawcett, 2000) and the relationship of theory and research (Fawcett, 1999) are the direct result of my students' requests for more information and more examples about the use of nursing discipline–specific conceptual models and theories.

Since 1979, I have used Roy's adaptation model to guide my empirical research, which has focused on women's responses to cesarean birth and on functional status in normal life transitions and serious illness. I have found Roy's model to be a very useful guide for my research and for the nursing practice that stems from the findings of the research.

Much of my current work focuses on helping nurses understand the connection between research and practice (see Fawcett, 2000, chap. 18). I am firmly convinced that all nurse clinicians also are nurse researchers, because the nursing practice process (assessment, labeling, goal setting, implementation, evaluation) is the same as the nursing research process (collection of baseline data, statement of the problem and hypotheses, experimental and control treatments, data analysis). I also am firmly convinced that the parallels between the nursing practice process and the nursing research process are most readily understood when both nursing practice and nursing research are guided by a nursing discipline–specific conceptual model or theory. The challenge is to assist nurses in practice to recognize that clinical information is research data, and to report the effects of nursing practice in ways that will help other nurses and other health professionals and policymakers understand how nursing practice benefits the health of humankind.

"Theory is the poetry of science. The poet's words are familiar, each standing alone, but brought together they sing, they astonish, they teach."

● *Levine, 1995, p. 14*

Theories and conceptual frameworks consist of the theorist's words brought together to form a meaningful whole. Theories and frameworks provide direction and guidance for structuring professional nursing practice, education, and research. In practice, theories and frameworks help nurses to describe, explain, and predict everyday experiences, and they also serve to guide assessment, intervention, and evaluation of nursing care. In education, a conceptual framework provides the general focus for curriculum design and guides curricular decision making. In research, the framework offers a systematic approach to identifying questions for study, selecting appropriate variables, and interpreting findings. The importance of theory in building a body of nursing knowledge is emphasized by Chinn and Jacobs (1987), who state, "Nursing theory ought to guide research and practice, generate new ideas, and differentiate the focus of nursing from other professions" (p. 145). Figure 6–1 illustrates these relationships.

Many nurse theorists have made substantial contributions to the development of a body of nursing knowledge. Offering an assortment of perspectives, the theories vary in their level of abstraction and their conceptualization of the client, health and illness, and nursing. From a historical perspective, nursing theories reflect the influence of the larger society and illustrate increased sophistication in the development of nursing ideas. Table 6–1 presents a chronology of events related to the development of nursing theories.

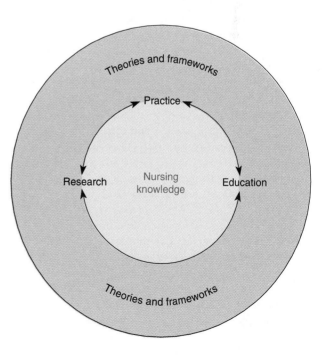

FIGURE 6–1 Relationship between theories and frameworks and nursing education, research, and practice.

TABLE 6-1 History of Nursing Theory Development

Events	Year	Nurse Theorists
	1860	Florence Nightingale Described nursing and environment
	1952	Hildegard E. Peplau Nursing as an interpersonal process: patients with felt needs
Scientific era: nurses questioned purpose of nursing	1960	Faye Abdellah (also 1965; 1973) Patient-centered approaches
	1961	Ida Jean Orlando Nurse-patient relationship; deliberative nursing approach
Process of theory development discussed among professional nurses	1964	Ernestine Weidenbach (also 1970; 1977) Nursing: philosophy, purpose, practice, and art
	1966	Lydia E. Hall Core (patient), care (body), cure (disease)
	1966	Virginia Henderson (also 1971; 1978) Nursing assists patients with 14 essential functions toward independence
Symposium: theory development in nursing	1967	Myra Estrin Levine (also 1973) Four conservation principles of nursing
Symposium: nature of science and nursing	1968	
Dickoff, James, and Weidenbach published "Theory in a Practice Discipline" in *Nursing Research*		
Symposium: nature of science in nursing	1969	
First nursing theory conference		
Second nursing theory conference	1970	Martha E. Rogers (also 1980) Science of unitary man: energy fields, openness, pattern, and organization
Consensus on nursing concepts: nurse/nursing, health, client/patient/individual, society/environment	1971	Dorothea E. Orem (also 1980; 1985) Nursing facilitates patients' self-care
Discussion on what theory is: the elements, criteria, types, and levels, and the relation to research	1971	Imogene King (also 1975; 1981) Theory of goal attainment through nurse-client transactions
NLN required conceptual frameworks in nursing education	1973	
Borrowed theories from other disciplines	1974	Sister Callista Roy (also 1976; 1980; 1984; 1989; 1999)
Expanded theories from other disciplines		Roy's adaptation model: nurse adjusts patient's stimuli (focal, contextual, or residual)
		Betty Neuman Health care systems model: a total person approach

TABLE 6-1 **History of Nursing Theory Development** *Continued*		
Events	**Year**	**Nurse Theorists**
Recognized problems in practice and developed theories to test and use in practice	1976	Josephine Paterson and L. Zderad Humanistic nursing

Second nurse educator conference on nursing theory	1978	Madeleine Leininger (also 1980; 1981)
		    Transcultural nursing
		    Caring nursing

Articles on theory development in *ANS, Nursing Research,* and *Image*	1978 1979	Jean Watson (also 1985) Philosophy and science of caring; humanistic nursing
Books written for nurses on how to critique and develop theory, and describing application of nursing theories	1980	Dorothy E. Johnson Behavioral system model for nursing
Graduate schools of nursing develop courses in how to analyze and apply nursing theories		
Research studies in nursing identified nursing theories as framework for study	1981	Rosemarie Rizzo Parse (also 1987) Man-living-health: a theory of nursing
Numerous books published on analysis, application evaluation, and/or development of nursing theories	1982–present	

Modified from Christensen, P. J., & Kenney, J. W. (1995). *Nursing process: Application of conceptual models* (4th ed.). St. Louis: Mosby.

Terminology Associated with Theoretical Perspectives

To understand the structure of nursing knowledge, it is necessary to define the main components of theoretical perspectives. The most fundamental component of a theory is a *concept,* which is defined as a word or phrase that summarizes the essential characteristics of a phenomenon (Fawcett, 1999). Attributes or characteristics of concepts distinguish one from another and bring forth a mental image of the phenomenon being described (Rodgers & Knafl, 2000). Since a concept is an abstract representation of the real world, it is important to realize that concepts embedded in a theory represent the theorist's perspective of reality (Keck, 1998). The fact that a theorist's perspective may be different from that of the reader does not invalidate the theory. Rather, a different perspective offers an alternative way of viewing the world of nursing.

For a theory to exist, concepts must be related to one another. Theoretical statements, also called *propositions,* describe a concept or the relationship between two or more concepts (Fawcett, 1999). One theoretical statement, or several theoretical statements taken together, can constitute a theory. A *theory,* then, is a statement or a group of statements that describe, explain, or predict relationships between concepts. Theories represent abstract ideas rather than concrete facts (Alligood, 2000) and may be broad or limited in scope, thus varying in their ability to describe, explain, or predict.

There are four levels of theoretical thinking (Higgins & Moore, 2000). *Metatheory,* or the theory of inquiry, is the most abstract. *Grand theories* are composed of relatively abstract concepts and relationships that establish and substantiate the discipline's identity and boundaries. *Middle-range theories* encompass a limited number of concepts that are relatively concrete and more easily tested (Barnum, 1998). They are sufficiently specific to guide research and practice yet sufficiently general to cross multiple clinical populations. *Micro-range theories* consist of one or two concepts, and their application is limited to a particular event or a set of working hypotheses or propositions (e.g., practice theory). Grand theories enable the development of middle-range and micro-range applications that have sufficient detail to be used in practice (Alligood & Marriner-Tomey, 1997).

A theory is based on a set of *assumptions* (statements commonly held to be true) that cannot be empirically tested (Chinn & Kramer, 1995). Assumptions may be either implicitly or explicitly stated by the theorist. Assumptions that are implicit require the reader to infer their existence, as in Orem's self-care deficit theory, where it must be presumed that individuals desire self-care. Assumptions that are explicit, on the other hand, are in the form of clear statements, as in Johnson's behavioral system model, which describes an individual as a set of behavioral subsystems.

A *conceptual framework* serves as a guide for the generation of new middle-range theories by providing an orienting scheme or worldview that helps focus our thinking (Fawcett, 1999). A conceptual framework may be visualized as an umbrella under which many theories can exist. The major distinction between a conceptual framework and a theory is the level of abstraction, with a conceptual framework being more abstract than a theory. The term conceptual framework is often used interchangeably with *conceptual model,* although the term model is generally used to refer to a graphic illustration of theoretical relationships. Without attempting to justify the classification of individual theoretical perspectives included in this chapter, the term to which each is most commonly referred (i.e., theory, model, or framework) is used.

Components of Nursing Theories

A *nursing theory* is a relatively specific and concrete set of concepts and propositions that purports to account for or characterize phenomena of interest to the discipline of nursing (Fawcett, 1999). Four central concepts of interest to the discipline of nursing are person, environment, health/illness, and nursing. *Persons* are the recipients of nursing care and include individuals, families, and communities. *Environment* refers to the surroundings of the client, internal factors affecting the client, and the setting where nursing care is delivered. *Health and illness* describe the client's state of well-being. *Nursing* is the discipline from which client care actions are derived. These concepts, taken together, comprise the *metaparadigm* of nursing (Alligood, 1997). Most nursing theories define or describe these central concepts, either explicitly or implicitly. In addition to these concepts, many theories include assumptions about the nature of the client and the environment, theoretical statements describing the relationships between the major concepts, and definitions of concepts specific to a particular theory.

In keeping with this organizational scheme, descriptions of the theoretical perspectives presented in this chapter include a brief overview, the theory's basic assumptions about the individual and the environment, definitions of health and illness, a description of nursing, including the goal of nursing, and definitions of concepts and subconcepts specific to each theory. Some theories are more amenable to this scheme than others because of their degree of specificity or stage of development. When the needed information is not explicitly detailed by the theorist, inferences are made based on what seems to be implicitly stated. Because most of the theories are quite global, condensing them into discrete and somewhat restrictive categories obscures some of the true essence of the relationships. The reader is encouraged to consult the primary source to gain a full appreciation of the depth, scope, and extent of the relationships put forth.

 Overview of Selected Nursing Theories

Theories and frameworks selected for inclusion in this chapter are those that exemplify the evolution of nursing from early times (e.g., Nightingale) to more recent ones (e.g., Parse), as illustrated in Table 6–1.

> "Exploring a variety of nursing theories ought to provide nurses with new insights into patient care, opening nursing options otherwise hidden, and stimulating innovative interventions. But it is imperative that there be variety—for there is no global theory of nursing that fits every situation."
>
> ● *Levine, 1995, p. 13*

NIGHTINGALE'S ENVIRONMENTAL THEORY

Florence Nightingale conceptualized disease as a reparative process and described the nurse's role as manipulating the environment to facilitate and encourage this process. Her directions regarding ventilation, warmth, light, diet, cleanliness, variety, and noise are discussed in her classic nursing textbook *Notes on Nursing,* first published in 1859.

Brief Overview. The environment is critical to health, and the nurse's role in caring for the sick is to provide a clean, quiet, peaceful environment to promote healing. Nightingale's intent was to describe nursing and provide guidelines for nursing education.

Assumptions About the Individual. Individuals are responsible, creative, in control of their lives and health, and desire good health.

Environment. The environment is external to the person but affects the health of both sick and well persons. One of the chief sources of infection, the environment must include pure air, pure water, efficient drainage, cleanliness, and light.

Health and Illness. Health is described as a state of being well and using one's powers to the fullest. Illness or disease is the reaction of nature against the conditions in which we have placed ourselves. Disease is a reparative mechanism, an effort of nature to remedy a process of poisoning or of decay.

Nursing. Nursing is a service to mankind intended to relieve pain and suffering. Nursing's role is to promote or provide the proper environment for patients, including fresh air, light, pure water, cleanliness, warmth, quiet, and appropriate diet. The goal of nursing is to promote the reparative process by manipulating the environment.

Key Concepts. Environment refers to conditions external to the individual that affect life and development (i.e., ventilation, warmth, light, diet, cleanliness, and noise). Nightingale (1859/1946) identified three major relationships: the environment to the patient, the nurse to the environment, and the nurse to the patient. Examples of these follow.

- The need for light, particularly sunlight, is second only to the need for ventilation. If necessary, the nurse should move the patient "about after the sun according to the aspects of the rooms, if circumstances permit, [rather] than let him linger in a room when the sun is off" (p. 48).
- Nursing's role is to manipulate the environment to encourage healing. Nursing "ought to signify the proper use of fresh air, light, warmth, cleanliness, quiet, and the proper selection and administration of diet" (p. 6).
- The sine qua non of all good nursing is never to allow a patient to be awakened,

intentionally or accidentally. "A good nurse will always make sure that no blind or curtains should flap. If you wait till your patient tells you or reminds you of these things, where is the use of their having a nurse?" (p. 27).

- Variety is important for patients to divert them from dwelling on their pain. "Variety of form and brilliancy of color in the objects presented are actual means of recovery" (p. 34).

PEPLAU'S INTERPERSONAL PROCESS

Hildegard Peplau published *Interpersonal Relations in Nursing* in 1952. In this book she described a partial theory for nursing practice. The book described the phases of the interpersonal process in nursing, roles for nurses, and methods for studying nursing as an interpersonal process. Numerous papers were published over the years, and her book was reprinted in 1988.

Brief Overview. The focus of Peplau's model is on the goal-directed interpersonal process. "Psychodynamic nursing is being able to understand one's own behavior to help others identify felt difficulties, and to apply principles of human relations to the problems that arise at all levels of experience" (1952, p. xiii). The interpersonal relationship "has a starting point, proceeds through definable phases and, being time-limited, has an end point" (1992, p. 4).

Assumptions About the Individual. The individual is an organism that lives in an unstable equilibrium and "strives in its own way to reduce tension generated by needs" (1952, p. 82).

Environment. Although the environment is not explicitly defined, it can be inferred that the environment is the "existing forces outside the organism and in the context of culture" (1952, p. 163).

Health and Illness. Health is a "word symbol that implies forward movement of personality and other ongoing human processes in the direction of creative, constructive, productive, personal, and community living" (1952, p. 12). By implication, illness is a condition that is marked by no movement or by backward movement in these areas.

Nursing. Nursing is a therapeutic interpersonal process because it involves the interaction between two or more individuals who have a common goal. For individuals who are sick and in need of health care, it is a healing art. Six nursing roles emerge in the various phases of the nurse-patient relationship: stranger, resource person, teacher, leader, surrogate, and counselor.

Key Concepts. The nurse-patient relationship consists of four phases:

- *Orientation:* The patient seeks professional assistance with a problem. The nurse and patient meet as strangers, and recognize, clarify, and define the existing problem.
- *Identification:* The patient learns how to make use of the nurse-patient relationship and responds selectively to people who can meet his or her needs; the patient and nurse clarify each other's expectations.
- *Exploitation:* The patient takes advantage of all available services. The nurse helps the patient to maintain a balance between dependence and independence and to use the services to help solve the current problem and work toward optimal health.
- *Resolution:* The patient is free to move on with his or her life as old goals are put aside and new goals are adopted. The patient becomes independent of the nurse, and the relationship is terminated.

HENDERSON'S COMPLEMENTARY-SUPPLEMENTARY MODEL

Virginia Henderson viewed nursing as an art and a discipline separate from medicine. In *The Nature of Nursing* (1966), she wrote that the "unique function of the nurse is to assist the individual, sick or well, in the performance of those activities contributing to the health or its recovery (or a peaceful death) that he would perform unaided if he had the necessary strength, will, or knowledge" (p. 15).

Brief Overview. The nurse's role is that of a substitute for the patient, a helper to the patient, and a partner with the patient. Fourteen basic patient needs constitute components of nursing care.

Assumptions About the Individual. The mind and body being inseparable, a person must maintain physiological and emotional balance. An individual requires assistance in order to achieve health and independence or a peaceful death. Individuals will achieve or maintain health if they have the necessary strength, will, or knowledge (p. 15). The individual and family should be viewed as a unit.

Environment. The environment is "the aggregate of all the external conditions and influences affecting the life and development of an organism" (1978, p. 829).

Health and Illness. Health is a quality of life basic to human functioning. Although not specifically stated, health seems to be equated with independence. Conversely, it can be inferred that illness is a lack of independence.

Nursing. Nursing has a unique function to assist sick or well individuals in a supplementary or complementary role. The goals of nursing are to help the individual gain independence as rapidly as possible and to promote health (1971).

Key Concepts. Fourteen basic patient needs constitute the components of nursing care (1966):

1. Breathe normally.
2. Eat and drink adequately.
3. Eliminate body wastes.
4. Move and maintain a desirable position.
5. Sleep and rest.
6. Select suitable clothes.
7. Maintain the body temperature within normal range by adjusting clothing and modifying the environment.
8. Keep the body clean and well-groomed to protect the integument.
9. Avoid dangers in the environment and avoid injuring others.
10. Communicate with others in expressing emotions, needs, fears, or opinions.
11. Worship according to one's faith.
12. Work in such a way that there is a sense of accomplishment.
13. Play or participate in various forms of recreation.
14. Learn, discover, or satisfy the curiosity that leads to normal development and health and use the available health facilities.

ROGERS'S SCIENCE OF UNITARY HUMAN BEINGS

First presented in *An Introduction to the Theoretical Basis for Nursing* in 1970, Martha Rogers's conceptualizations, dating back to the 1960s, evolved into the current science of unitary human beings. She posited that humans are dynamic energy fields who are integral with the environment and who are continuously evolving. She viewed nursing as a science and art that focuses on the nature and direction of human development and human betterment. Nursing scholars who subscribe to Rogers's theory are committed to continuing her work.

Brief Overview. The individual is viewed as an irreducible energy field who is integral with the environment. The nurse seeks to promote symphonic interactions between humans and their environments.

Assumptions About the Individual. The individual is a unified irreducible whole, manifesting characteristics that are more than, and different from, the sum of his or her parts, and is continuously evolving irreversibly and unidirectionally along a space-time continuum. Pattern and organization of humans are directed toward increasing complexity rather than maintaining equilibrium. The individual "is characterized by the capacity for abstraction and imagery, language and thought, sensation and emotion" (1970, p. 73).

Environment. The environment is an irreducible pandimensional energy field identified by pattern and integrated with the human energy field (1994). The individual and the environment are continually exchanging matter and energy with one another, resulting in changing patterns in both the individual and the environment.

Health and Illness. Health and illness are value-laden, arbitrarily defined, and culturally infused notions. They are not dichotomous but are part of the same continuum. Health seems to occur when patterns of living are in harmony with environmental change, whereas illness occurs when patterns of living are in conflict with environmental change and are deemed unacceptable.

Nursing. A science and an art, nursing is unique in its concern with unitary human beings as synergistic phenomena. The science of nursing should be concerned with studying the nature and direction of unitary human development integral with the environment and with evolving descriptive, explanatory, and predictive principles for use in nursing practice. The new age of nursing science is characterized by a synthesis of fact and ideas that generate principles and theories (1994). The art of nursing is the creative use of the science of nursing for human betterment (1990). The goal of nursing is the attainment of the best possible state of health for the individual who is continually evolving by promoting symphonic interactions between humans and environments, strengthening the coherence and integrity of the human field, and directing and redirecting patterning of both fields for maximum health potential.

Key Concepts. The concepts describe the individual and environment as energy fields that are in constant interaction. The nature and direction of human development form the basis for the principles of nursing science:

- *Energy field:* The fundamental unit of the living and nonliving. Energy fields are dynamic, continuously in motion, and infinite. They are of two types:
  - *Human energy field:* More than the biological, psychological, and sociological fields taken separately or together; an irreducible, indivisible, pandimensional whole identified by pattern and manifesting characteristics that cannot be predicted from the parts.
  - *Environmental energy field:* An irreducible, indivisible, pandimensional energy field identified by pattern and integral with the human field.
- *Openness:* Continuous change and mutual process as manifested in human and environmental fields.
- *Pattern:* The distinguishing characteristic of an energy field perceived as a single wave.
- *Principles of nursing science:* Principles postulating the nature and direction of unitary human development; also called principles of homeodynamics, which are as follows:
  - *Helicy:* "The continuous, innovative, probabilistic, increasing diversity of human and environmental field patterns

characterized by repeating rhymicities" (1989, p. 186).

- *Resonancy:* "The continuous change from lower to higher frequency wave patterns in human and environmental fields" (1989, p. 186). The process of change is one of increasing diversity.
- *Integrality:* Replacing the earlier concept of complementarity, integrality is "the continuous mutual human and environmental field process" (1989, p. 186).

OREM'S SELF-CARE DEFICIT THEORY OF NURSING

The foundations of Dorothea Orem's theory were introduced in the late 1950s, but it was not until 1971 that the first edition of *Nursing: Concepts of Practice* was published. The second, third, fourth, and fifth editions were published in 1980, 1985, 1991, and 1995, respectively, and show evidence of development and refinement of the theory. Orem focuses on nursing as deliberate human action and notes that all individuals can benefit from nursing when they have health-derived or health-related limitations for engaging in self-care or the care of dependent others. Three theories are subsumed in the self-care deficit theory of nursing: the theory of nursing systems, the theory of self-care deficits, and the theory of self-care (1995).

Brief Overview. The individual practices self-care, a set of learned behaviors, to sustain life, maintain or restore functioning, and bring about a condition of well-being. The nurse assists the client with self-care when there is a deficit in his or her ability to perform.

Assumptions About the Individual. The individual is viewed as a unity whose functioning is linked with the environment and who, with the environment, forms an integrated, functional whole. The individual functions biologically, symbolically, and socially.

Environment. The environment is linked to the individual, forming an integrated system. It is implied that the environment is external to the individual.

Health and Illness. Health, which has physical, psychological, interpersonal, and social aspects, is a state in which human beings are structurally and functionally whole or sound (1995). Illness occurs when an individual is incapable of maintaining self-care as a result of structural or functional limitations.

Nursing. Nursing involves assisting the individual with self-care practices to sustain life and health, recover from disease or injury, and cope with their effects (1985). The nurse chooses deliberate actions from nursing systems (see below) designed to bring about desirable conditions in persons and their environments. The goal of nursing is to move a patient toward responsible self-care or meet existing health care needs of those who have health care deficits.

Key Concepts. The concepts focus on self-care in terms of requisites, demands, and deficits, and delineate the nurse's role in client care:

- *Self-care:* "Activities that individuals initiate and perform on their own behalf to maintain life, health, or well-being" (1995, p. 104).
- *Self-care requisites:* Actions that are known or hypothesized to be necessary to regulate human functioning. Three types:
  - *Universal:* Common to all human beings; concerned with the promotion and maintenance of structural and functional integrity. These include air, water, food, elimination, activity and rest, solitude and social interaction, prevention of hazards, and promotion of human functioning.
  - *Developmental:* Associated with conditions that promote known developmental processes and occurring at various stages of the life cycle.

- *Health-deviation:* Genetic and constitutional defects and deviations that affect integrated human functioning and impair the individual's ability to perform self-care.
- *Therapeutic self-care demand:* Based on the notion that self-care is a human regulatory function; the totality of self-care actions performed by the nurse or self in order to meet known self-care requisites.
- *Self-care agency:* Acquired ability to know and meet requirements to regulate own functioning and development.
- *Self-care deficits:* Gaps between known therapeutic self-care demands and the capability of the individual to perform self-care.
- *Nursing systems:* Systems of concrete actions for persons with limitations in self-care. These actions are of three types (1995):
  - *Wholly compensatory:* The nurse compensates for the individual's total inability to perform self-care activities.
  - *Partly compensatory:* The nurse compensates for the individual's inability to perform some (but not all) self-care activities.
  - *Supportive-educative:* With the individual able to perform all self-care activities, the nurse assists the client in decision making, behavior control, and the acquisition of knowledge and skill.
- *Subsystems of each nursing system:*
  - *Social:* The complementary and contractual relationship between the nurse and the client.
  - *Interpersonal:* The nurse-client interaction.
  - *Technological:* "Diagnosis, prescription, regulation of treatment, and management of nursing care" (1985, p. 160).

KING'S THEORY OF GOAL ATTAINMENT

Although the foundation for her theory was developed in 1964, it was not until the 1971 publication of her book, *Toward a Theory for Nursing,* that Imogene King presented her entire conceptual framework and identified the concepts of social systems, health, perception, and interpersonal relations. The theory was refined in *A Theory for Nursing: Systems, Concepts, Process* (1981), where King identified the focus of nursing as being on people interacting with their environments, leading to a state of health, which is the ability to function in roles. The theory is derived from a systems framework and is concerned with human transactions in different types of environments (1995a).

Brief Overview. The individual is viewed as an open system and as one component of a nurse-client interpersonal system whose interactions lead to the attainment of mutually agreed-on goals.

Assumptions About the Individual. Human beings are open systems in transaction with the environment and are conceptualized as social, sentient, rational, perceiving, controlling, purposeful, action-oriented beings.

Environment. As an open system, it is implied that the individual and the environment interact and that both the internal and external environments generate stressors.

Health and Illness. Health is described as an individual's ability to function in social roles. This implies optimal use of one's resources to achieve continuous adjustment to internal and external environmental stressors. Illness is a deviation from normal, an imbalance in a person's biological structure, psychological makeup, or social relationships.

Nursing. An interpersonal process of action, reaction, and interaction, the nurse and client communicate, set goals, and explore means to achieve those goals. "The domain of nursing includes promoting, maintaining and restoring health, caring for the sick and injured and caring for the dying" (1981, p. 4). The goal of nursing is to help individuals to maintain their health so they can function in their roles. "The goal of the nursing system, as a whole, is health for individuals, health for groups, such as the family, and health for communities within a society" (1995b, p. 24).

Key Concepts. Two sets of concepts are subsumed in the theory, one relating to the parties involved in the nurse-client relationship and the other pertaining to the process of goal attainment:

- Concepts related to the nurse-client relationship:
  - *Personal system:* An individual.
  - *Interpersonal system:* Two or more interacting individuals.
  - *Social system:* Communities and societies.
- Concepts related to goal attainment:
  - *Communication:* The process of giving information from one person to another.
  - *Interaction:* The process of perception between the person and environment or one or more persons, represented by verbal and nonverbal behaviors that are goal directed.
  - *Perception:* An individual's representation of reality.
  - *Transaction:* Observable behavior of individuals interacting with their environment.
  - *Role:* A set of behaviors displayed by the individual, who occupies a given position in a social system.
  - *Stress:* A dynamic state of interaction with the environment to maintain balance for growth, development, and performance.
  - *Growth and development:* "Continuous changes in individuals occurring at molecular, cellular, and behavioral levels" (1981, p. 148).
  - *Time:* A duration between one event and another.

- *Space:* Defined by "gestures, postures, and visible boundaries erected to mark off personal space" (1981, p. 148).

ROY'S ADAPTATION MODEL

Sister Callista Roy has continuously expanded her model from its inception in the 1960s to the present time, building on the conceptual framework of adaptation. She focuses on the individual as a biopsychosocial adaptive system and describes nursing as a humanistic discipline that "places emphasis on the person's own coping abilities" (1984, p. 32). The individual and the environment are sources of stimuli that require modification to promote adaptation.

Brief Overview. The individual is a biopsychosocial adaptive system, and the nurse promotes adaptation by modifying external stimuli.

Assumptions About the Individual. The individual is in constant interaction with a changing environment, and to respond positively to environmental change, a person must adapt. The person's adaptation level is determined by the combined effect of three classes of stimuli—focal, contextual, and residual. The individual uses both innate and acquired biological, psychological, or social adaptive mechanisms and has four modes of adaptation.

Environment. All conditions, circumstances, and influences surrounding and affecting the development and behavior of persons and groups constitute the environment. Having both internal and external components, the environment is constantly changing.

Health and Illness. "Health and illness are one inevitable dimension of a person's life" (1989, p. 106). Health is "a state and process of being and becoming integrated and whole" (Roy & Andrews, 1999, p. 31). Conversely, illness is a lack of integration.

Nursing. An external regulatory force, nursing acts to modify stimuli affecting adaptation by increasing, decreasing, or maintaining stimuli. The goal of nursing is to promote the person's adaptation in the four adaptive modes, thus contributing to health, the quality of life, and dying with dignity (Roy & Andrews, 1999).

Key Concepts. The concepts describe and define adaptation in terms of the individual's internal control processes, adaptive modes, and adaptive level:

- *Adaptation:* The individual's ability to cope with the constantly changing environment.
- *Adaptive system:* Consists of two major internal control processes (coping mechanisms):
  - *Regulator subsystem:* Receives input from the external environment and from changes in the person's internal state and processes it through neural-chemical-endocrine channels.
  - *Cognator subsystem:* Receives input from external and internal stimuli that involve psychological, social, physical, and physiological factors and processes it through cognitive pathways.
- *Adaptive modes:* Ways a person adapts. There are four modes:
  - *Physiological:* Determined by the need for physiological integrity derived from the basic physiological needs.
  - *Self-concept:* Determined by the need for interactions with others and psychic integrity regarding the perception of self.
  - *Role function:* Determined by the need for social integrity; refers to the performance of duties based on given positions within society.
  - *Interdependence:* Involves ways of seeking help, affection, and attention.
- *Adaptive level:* Determined by the combined effects of stimuli:
  - *Focal stimulus:* That which immediately confronts the individual.

- *Contextual stimuli:* All other stimuli present in the environment. These stimuli influence how the individual deals with the focal stimulus.
- *Residual stimuli:* Beliefs, attitudes, or traits that have an indeterminate effect on the present situation.

NEUMAN'S SYSTEMS MODEL

Betty Neuman developed her systems model in 1970 in response to student requests to focus on breadth rather than depth in understanding human variables in nursing problems. First published in 1972, it was refined to its present form and published in *The Neuman Systems Model* (1995). "The Neuman systems model is an open systems model that views nursing as being primarily concerned with defining appropriate actions in stress-related situations (1995, p. 11). Neuman believes that nursing encompasses a wholistic client systems approach to help individuals, families, communities, and society reach and maintain wellness. Neuman's focus on the whole system explains her use of the term "wholistic."

Brief Overview. This theory offers a wholistic view of the client system, including the concepts of open system, environment, stressors, prevention, and reconstitution. Nursing is concerned with the whole person.

Assumptions About the Individual. The client is a whole person, a dynamic composite of interrelationships between physiological, psychological, sociocultural, developmental, and spiritual variables. "The client is viewed as an open system in interaction with the environment" (1989, p. 68). The client is in "dynamic constant energy exchange with the environment" (1989, p. 22).

Environment. Both internal and external environments exist, and the person maintains varying degrees of harmony between them. The environment includes all internal and external factors affecting and affected by the system (1995). Emphasis is on all stressors—interpersonal, intrapersonal, extrapersonal—that might disturb the person's normal line of defense.

Health and Illness. "Health and wellness is defined as the condition or degree of system stability" (1995, p. 12). Disharmony among parts of the system is considered illness. "The wellness-illness continuum implies that energy flow is continuous between the client system and the environment" (1989, p. 33).

Nursing. Nursing is a "unique profession in that it is concerned with all of the variables affecting the individual's response to stress" (1982, p. 14). The major concern of nursing is in "keeping the client system stable through accuracy in both the assessment of effects and possible effects of environmental stressors and in assisting client adjustments required for an optimal wellness level" (1989, p. 34). Nursing goals are determined by "negotiation with the client for desired prescriptive changes to correct variances from wellness" (1989, p. 73).

Key Concepts. The nurse is concerned with all the variables affecting an individual's response to stressors:

- *Stressors:* Tension-producing stimuli that may alter system stability (1995).
  - *Intrapersonal:* Internal stressors (e.g., autoimmune response).
  - *Interpersonal:* External environmental forces in close proximity (e.g., communication patterns).
  - *Extrapersonal:* External environmental forces at distant range (e.g., financial concerns).
- Concepts related to client *system stability:*
  - *Flexible line of defense:* Outer boundary that ideally prevents stressors from entering the system.
  - *Normal line of defense:* Represents a range of responses to environmental

stressors when the flexible line of defense is penetrated; usual state of wellness (1995).
- *Lines of resistance:* Protect the basic structure of the client and become activated when the normal line of defense is invaded by environmental stressors.
- *Interventions:* Purposeful nursing actions that help clients retain, attain, and/or maintain system stability. There are three levels of intervention:
  - *Primary prevention:* Reduces the possibility of encounter with stressors and strengthens the flexible lines of defense.
  - *Secondary prevention:* Relates to appropriate prioritizing of interventions to reduce symptoms resulting from invasion of environmental stressors; protects the basic structure by strengthening the internal lines of resistance.
  - *Tertiary prevention:* Focuses on readaptation and stability. A primary goal is to strengthen resistance to stressors by reeducation to help prevent recurrence of reaction or regression. "Tertiary prevention tends to lead back, in a circular fashion, toward primary prevention" (1989, p. 73).

LEININGER'S CULTURAL CARE THEORY

Drawing from a background in cultural and social anthropology, Madeleine Leininger's contribution to nursing knowledge is related to transcultural nursing and caring. Her book, *Transcultural Nursing: Concepts, Theories and Practice* (1978), presented her conceptual framework for cultural care and health. She continues to explicate the linkages between nursing and anthropology as she identifies and defines concepts such as care, caring, culture, cultural values, and cultural variations (1984, 1991, 1995).

Brief Overview. Transcultural nursing focuses on a comparative study and analysis of different cultures and subcultures in the world with respect to their caring behavior, nursing care, health-illness values, and patterns of behavior, with the goal of developing a scientific and humanistic body of knowledge from which to derive culture-specific and culture-universal nursing care practices (1978).

Assumptions About the Individual. Clients are caring and cultural beings who perceive health, illness, caring, curing, dependence, and independence differently. The social structure, world view, and values of people vary transculturally.

Environment. The environment is a social structure, the "interrelated and interdependent systems of a society which determine how it functions with respect to certain major elements, namely: the political (including legal), economic, social (including kinship), educational, technical, religious, and cultural systems" (1978, p. 61). The environment is the totality of an event, situation, or particular experience that gives meaning to human expression and interaction.

Health and Illness. Perceptions of health and illness are culturally infused and therefore cannot be universally defined. "Health refers to a state of well-being that is culturally defined, valued, and practiced, and which reflects the ability of individuals (or groups) to perform their daily role activities in culturally expressed, beneficial, and patterned lifeways" (1991, p. 48). Worldviews, social structure, and cultural beliefs influence perceptions of health and illness and cannot be separated from them. For example, some cultures perceive illness to be largely a personal and internal body experience, whereas others view illness as an extrapersonal or cultural experience.

Nursing. Nursing is a learned humanistic and scientific profession that focuses on personalized (individual and group) care behaviors, functions, and processes that have physical, psycho-

cultural, and social significance or meaning. The goal of nursing is to assist, support, facilitate, or enable individuals or groups to regain or maintain their health in a way that is culturally congruent, or to help people face handicaps or death (1991).

Key Concepts. Among the core concepts of transcultural nursing theory are:

- *Care:* Phenomena related to assistive, supportive, or enabling behavior toward or for another individual with evident or anticipated needs to ease or improve a human condition.
- *Caring:* Actions directed toward assisting, supporting, or enabling an individual (or group) to ameliorate or improve the human condition or lifeway.
- *Culture:* Values, beliefs, norms, and lifeway practices of a particular group that guides thinking, decisions, and actions in patterned ways.
- *Cultural care:* The cognitively known values, beliefs, and patterned lifeways that assist, support, or enable another individual or group to maintain well-being, improve a human condition or lifeway, or deal with illness, handicaps, or death.
    - *Cultural care diversity:* The variability of meaning, patterns, values, lifeways, or symbols of care that are culturally derived for health or to improve a human condition.
    - *Cultural care universality:* Common, similar or uniform care meanings, patterns, values, lifeways, or symbols that are culturally derived for health or to improve a human condition.
- *Cultural-congruent care:* Assistive, supportive, facilitative, or enabling acts or decisions that fit individual, group, or institutional cultural values, beliefs, and lifeways (1995).
    - *Cultural care preservation or maintenance:* Professional actions and decisions

that help people of a particular culture to retain and/or preserve relevant care values.

- *Cultural care accommodation or negotiation:* Professional actions and decisions that help people of a designated culture adapt to or negotiate with others for a beneficial or satisfying health outcome.
- *Cultural care repatterning or restructuring:* Professional actions and decisions that help a client change or modify their lifeway to improve health while still respecting the client's cultural values and beliefs.

WATSON'S PHILOSOPHY AND SCIENCE OF CARING

Jean Watson's theoretical formulations focus on the philosophy and science of caring, the core of nursing. With the aim of reducing the dichotomy between nursing theory and practice, the framework was first published in 1979 and further developed in Watson's 1985, 1988, and 1994 publications. Watson draws from multiple disciplines to derive carative factors that are central to nursing and describes concepts as they relate to the pivotal theme of caring.

Brief Overview. Caring, a moral ideal rather than a task-oriented behavior, is central to nursing practice and includes aspects of the actual caring occasion and the transpersonal caring relationship. An interpersonal process, caring results in the satisfaction of human needs.

Assumptions About the Individual. Individuals (i.e., both the nurse and the client) are nonreducible and are interconnected with others and nature (1985, p. 16).

Environment. The client's environment contains both external and internal variables. The nurse promotes a caring environment, one that allows individuals to make choices relative to the best action for him or her at that point in time.

Health and Illness. Health is more than the absence of illness, but because it is subjective, it is an illusive concept. "Health refers to unity and harmony within the mind, body, and soul" (1985, p. 48). Conversely, illness is disharmony within the spheres of the person.

Nursing. The practice of nursing is different from curing. It is a transpersonal relationship that includes but is not limited to the ten carative factors described below. The goal of nursing is to help persons attain a higher degree of harmony by offering a relationship that the client can use for personal growth and development.

Key Concepts. The caring relationship and the ten carative factors form the core of nursing and delineate the domain of nursing practice:

- *Transpersonal caring:* An intersubjective human-to-human relationship in which the nurse affects and is affected by the other person (client). Caring is the moral ideal of nursing where there is the utmost concern for human dignity and preservation of humanity (1985).
- *Carative factors* (1979):
  1. Formation of a humanistic-altruistic system of values
  2. Instillation of faith-hope to promote wellness
  3. Cultivation of sensitivity to self and to others
  4. Development of a helping-trust relationship
  5. Promotion and acceptance of the expression of positive and negative feelings
  6. Systematic use of the scientific problem-solving method for decision making
  7. Promotion of interpersonal teaching-learning
  8. Provision for a supportive, protective, and/or corrective mental, physical, sociocultural, and spiritual environment

9. Assistance with the gratification of human needs
10. Allowance for existential-phenomenological forces

In addition to the carative factors, nurses must facilitate clients' development in the area of health promotion through teaching preventive health actions.

JOHNSON'S BEHAVIORAL SYSTEM MODEL

Originally presenting her theory as a paper at Vanderbilt University in 1968, Dorothy Johnson did not personally publish her theory of nursing until 1980. However, her early paper was widely cited, and published interpretations of it appeared in 1974 (Grubbs, 1974) and 1976 (Auger, 1976). Johnson views the individual as a behavioral system that is continually striving for balance. The nurse fosters "efficient and effective behavioral functioning . . . to prevent illness and during and following illness" (1980, p. 207).

Brief Overview. The individual is viewed as a collection of interrelated behavioral subsystems whose response patterns form an organized and integrated whole. The nurse serves as an external regulatory force to preserve and maintain system balance.

Assumptions About the Individual. A behavioral system composed of a set of behavioral subsystems, the individual strives to attain and maintain behavioral system balance, sometimes requiring adaptation and modification to return to a steady state. The individual is characterized by organization, interaction, interdependency, and integration of the parts and elements (subsystems).

Environment. The natural forces impinging on the individual constitute the environment in which the behavioral system exists. There are both internal and external environments, but these are not defined.

Health and Illness. It may be inferred that health is a state of balance in which the behavioral system is self-maintaining and self-perpetuating, and interrelationships between the subsystems are harmonious. Conversely, illness is a state of disorganization and dysfunction of the system.

Nursing. Described as an external regulatory force, the practice of nursing imposes external controls to fulfill the functional requirements of the subsystems. The goal of nursing is "to restore, maintain or attain behavioral system balance and stability at the highest possible level for the individual" (1980, p. 214).

Key Concepts. The concepts describe the individual as a set of subsystems that, together, form a behavioral system:

- *Behavioral system:* Composed of seven behavioral subsystems that are integrated and that characterize each person's life.
- *Behavioral subsystem:* A formed set of behavioral responses that seem to share a common drive but that are modified over time through maturation or learning. The seven subsystems are:
  - *Affiliative:* Security as a consequence of social inclusion, intimacy, and the formation and maintenance of a strong social bond.
  - *Dependency:* Succoring behavior that calls for the response of nurturing and has as its consequence approval, attention, or physical assistance.
  - *Ingestive:* Appetite satisfaction as it is governed by social and psychological considerations.
  - *Eliminative:* Elimination of body wastes as a learned behavior that strongly influences purely biological eliminative acts.

- *Sexual:* Procreation and gratification with responses originating with gender role identity and the broad range of behaviors dependent on one's biological sex.
- *Achievement:* Mastery or control over some aspect of the self or environment; includes intelligence, physical, creative, mechanical, care-taking, and social skills.
- *Aggressive:* Protection and preservation of self and society within the limits imposed by society.

PARSE'S THEORY OF HUMAN BECOMING

Rosemarie Rizzo Parse developed a philosophical model that focuses on the inseparable concepts of man-living-health as nursing's concern. Taking an existential approach, she derived three principles that center on the idea of man-living-health always moving toward greater diversity and "becoming" (1981).

Brief Overview. Always in the process of becoming, man-living-health are inseparable. Nursing is a human science that focuses on man and health.

Assumptions About the Individual. The individual is an open being, coexisting with the environment. Man freely chooses meaning in situations and bears responsibility for decisions. As life progresses, individuals become more complex and diverse, forming new patterns of relating.

Environment. The environment is inseparable from the individual. Both man and the environment interchange energy, unfold together toward greater complexity and diversity, and influence one another's rhythmical patterns of relating (1995).

Health and Illness. Health is an open process of becoming and is a rhythmically coconstituting process of the man-environment interrelationship. Illness is not the opposite of health

but rather a pattern of man's interrelationship with the world (1981). Both health and illness are lived experiences.

Nursing. A human science, nursing focuses on man as a living unity and man's participation in health experiences. The goal of nursing is to illuminate and mobilize family (human) interrelationships.

Key Concepts. The concepts are incorporated into three major principles that focus on meaning, rhythmicity, and cotranscendence. Within each principle, succeeding concepts build on preceding ones.

- *Meaning:* Arises from man's interrelationship with the world and refers to happenings to which we attach varying degrees of significance.
  - *Imaging:* A process that structures the meaning of an experience.
  - *Valuing:* A process of confirming cherished beliefs.
  - *Languaging:* Expressing valued images.
- *Rhythmicity:* The movement of man and environment toward greater diversity.
  - *Revealing-concealing:* Disclosing of some aspects of self and hiding of others all at once.
  - *Enabling-limiting:* The result of making choices. In choosing, one is both enabled in some things and limited in others.
  - *Connecting-separating:* A simultaneous process. Connecting with some phenomena results in separating from others.
- *Cotranscendence:* The process of reaching out beyond the self.
  - *Powering:* A process of moving toward all future possibilities.
  - *Originating:* Creating unique ways of living; distinguishing self from others.
  - *Transforming:* An ongoing process of change; moving toward greater diversity by transcending the present.

TABLE 6-2 Comparison of Theoretical Perspectives

Theory/Model	Nursing	Environment	Health	Person
Nightingale's environmental theory	Intended to relieve pain and suffering and restore health by manipulating the environment	Conditions external to the person that affect both sick and well persons	State of well-being; using one's power to the fullest	One who is in control of own life and health, and desires good health
Peplau's interpersonal process	Therapeutic interpersonal process	Existing forces outside the organism	Forward movement of ongoing human processes and personality	An organism that lives in an unstable equilibrium and strives to reduce tension generated by needs
Henderson's complementary-supplementary model	Functions to assist sick or well individuals in a supplementary or complementary role	The aggregate of all external conditions affecting life and development	Quality of life basic to human functioning	An entity whose mind and body are inseparable and who requires assistance to achieve health, independence, or a peaceful death
Rogers's science of unitary human beings	Science and art; the art of nursing is the creative use of science for human betterment	Pandimensional energy field integral with the human energy field	Patterns of living in harmony with the environment	A unified irreducible whole; more than and different from sum of parts
Orem's self-care deficit theory	Involves assisting individuals with self-care practices	Linked to the individual, forming an integrated system	State in which humans are structurally and functionally whole	A unity who functions biologically, symbolically, and socially and whose functioning is linked with the environment
King's theory of goal attainment	Process of action, reaction, and interaction	Interactive with the individual	Ability to function in social roles	Open system in transaction with the environment who is social, sentient, rational, perceiving, controlling, purposeful, and action-oriented
Roy's adaptation model	An external regulatory force that modifies stimuli affecting adaptation	Internal and external conditions that surround and affect individuals	State and process of being and becoming an integrated and whole person	A biopsychosocial adaptive system that is in constant interaction with a changing environment
Neuman's systems model	Concerned with variables affecting the individual's response to stress	Internal and external factors affecting and affected by the individual	Optimal system stability	A whole person; a dynamic composite of physiological, psychological, sociocultural, developmental and spiritual variables

TABLE 6-2 **Comparison of Theoretical Perspectives** *Continued*				
Theory/Model	**Nursing**	**Environment**	**Health**	**Person**
Leininger's cultural care theory	Culturally congruent care behaviors, functions, and processes that have physical, psychocultural, or social significance	The interrelated, interdependent systems of a society	State of well-being that is culturally defined	Caring, cultural beings who perceive health, illness, caring, curing, dependence, and independence differently
Watson's philosophy and science of caring	Transpersonal caring relationship that includes use of ten carative factors	Internal and external variables	Unity and harmony within mind, body, and soul	An entity that is nonreducible and is interconnected with others and nature.
Johnson's behavioral system model	External regulatory force aimed at restoring, maintaining, or attaining system balance	Natural forces, internal and external, that impinge on the individual	State of balance; interrelationships between the subsystems are harmonious	A behavioral system composed of a set of behavioral subsystems
Parse's theory of human becoming	A human science that focuses on man as a living entity	Inseparable from the individual	An open process of becoming; a lived experience	An open being, coexisting with the environment; become more complex and diverse as life progresses

Application to Nursing Practice

"Utilization of nursing theory, applied in nursing practice, provides a framework for a nursing approach and guides the critical thinking process of reasoning and decision making for nurses to practice in an organized manner" (Alligood & Marriner-Tomey, 1997, p. 11). It is evident that the nursing theories and frameworks discussed here offer a variety of perspectives for application to clinical practice. For example, some are process oriented and dynamic, such as Peplau's interpersonal process, King's theory of goal attainment, Rogers's science of unitary human beings, and Parse's human becoming. Others are more outcome oriented, such as Roy's adaptation model, Johnson's behavioral system model, and Orem's self-care deficit theory. Rogers's and Neuman's models focus on the wholeness of the individual and conceptualize nursing as one component of the individual's life process. King's theory is directed toward the interaction between the nurse and the client, who are inseparable. Leininger, Nightingale, and Henderson developed humanistic perspectives, since they focus on personalized, individualized care for all. Johnson and Roy conceptualize the nurse as an external regulator whose function is to promote system balance or adaptation. Orem views the nurse as one who assists the individual with self-care practices when the individual is unable to effectively care for himself or herself. A comparison of the theoretical perspectives discussed in this chapter is presented in Table 6-2.

Most of the nursing theories and frameworks presented in this chapter are too extensive to be used in their entirety in a given nursing care situation. For example, Orem describes three types of nursing systems, but for a client who is in the intensive care unit and on life support, only the wholly compensatory nursing system is relevant. Similarly, with Neuman's three levels of prevention, only clients with symptoms resulting from invasion of environmental stressors are appropriate recipients of secondary prevention. However, the theories can guide nursing assessment in terms of what questions to ask and what areas to assess. For instance, a nurse using Roy's adaptation model would assess the biological, psychological, and social aspects of the client. Similarly, the nurse who uses Johnson's behavioral system model would assess the seven subsystems for evidence of system balance or imbalance. The type of client, the setting where care is delivered, and the goal of nursing are what influence the selection of an appropriate theoretical framework for practice. The more specific theories can be readily adapted for use in a practice setting. The more global theories may better serve as frameworks for research, the findings of which can then be applied to practice.

Evaluating the Utility of Nursing Theories and Frameworks

Not all theories and frameworks are equally comprehensive or equally useful in every situation; nor are they meant to be, as discussed in this chapter. The definition of the client and the setting where care is delivered limit the utility of some of the theories and frameworks presented here. To be useful in practice, a theory must work in a specific setting. "A nursing theory should structure the work, giving the practicing nurse a frame of reference from which to view patients and from which to make patient care decisions" (Barnum, 1998, p. 80). Its concepts must be operationalized in ways that promote application and facilitate nursing activities in that setting. It is important to examine a theory's utility for the intended use and the consistency of its internal structure. The value and logi-

cal structure of a theory can be evaluated by asking questions proposed by Fawcett (1989, 1993, 1995) and Barnum (1998), such as:

1. Are the assumptions inherent in the theory clearly stated?
2. Does the model provide adequate descriptions of all four concepts of nursing's metaparadigm?
3. Are the relationships between the concepts of nursing's metaparadigm clearly explained?
4. Is the theory stated clearly and concisely?
5. Are there conflicting views within the structure of the theory?
6. Can relationships between concepts be tested in research (i.e., observed and measured) and applied to practice?
7. Does the theory lead to nursing activities that meet societal expectations (social congruence)?
8. Does the theory lead to nursing activities that are likely to result in favorable client outcomes (social significance)?
9. Does the theory include explicit rules for use in practice, education, or research (social usefulness)?

Theories from Related Disciplines

Several nursing theories derived their conceptual basis from theories developed by related disciplines and adapted to specific situations. Many of these theories are useful and relevant to nursing in their original form. For example, systems theory (von Bertalanffy, 1956) is useful as an approach to assess individuals, families, and communities, as described in Chapter 5. General adaptation syndrome, a theory of adaptation to stress, describes three phases of adjustment to stress: alarm reaction, stage of resistance, and stage of exhaustion (Selye, 1974, 1982). This theory can be applied to clients who are suffering not only psychological or social stress, but physiological stress as well. Theories of coping have been developed by Lazarus and Folkman (1984) and by McCubbin and Patterson (1981), who agree that coping is the process that leads to adaptation. For clients experiencing an intense level of stress, nursing interventions designed to promote and support the coping process can be derived from the relationships specified by this theory. Both coping and adjustment are embedded in Duvall's (1977) stages of family life and developmental tasks, which can serve as the framework for delivering age-specific or situation-specific nursing interventions. Aguilera (1970, 1998) provides a theory and framework for successful resolution of a crisis situation.

These theories are only a sample of those developed by related disciplines that can be useful to nursing. One or more of these theories can serve as a framework for designing interventions for clients throughout the life cycle, developing and implementing research studies, and framing educational curricula. In combination with nursing theories, there is a wide array of theoretical perspectives in various stages of development from which to choose.

KEY POINTS

- A theory is a group of statements that describe the relationship between two or more concepts.
- The main components of nursing theories are persons, environment, health/illness, and nursing.
- Nightingale's theory focuses on nursing's role in manipulating the environment.
- Peplau's theory centers on the interpersonal process in nursing.
- Henderson identifies 14 basic patient needs that constitute the components of nursing care.
- According to Rogers, the nurse seeks to promote coherence between individuals and their environments.
- As specified by Orem, when there is a deficit in the client's own ability for self-care, the nurse assists the individual with self-care practices.

- King conceptualizes the nurse and the client as components of an interpersonal system who seek to attain mutually agreed-on goals.
- Roy's theory describes the client as a biopsychosocial adaptive system and the nurse as one who modifies stimuli to promote adaptation.
- Three levels of nursing intervention—primary, secondary, and tertiary prevention—are specified in Neuman's systems model.
- Leininger's theory centers on providing culturally congruent nursing care.
- Watson identifies the caring relationship and 10 carative factors that form the core of nursing.
- Johnson's theory describes the nurse as an external regulatory force whose goal is to restore behavioral system balance.
- Parse describes nursing as a human science that focuses on man and health.
- The more specific theories, in whole or in part, can be readily adapted for use in any practice setting.
- The more global theories may better serve as frameworks for research, the findings of which can then be applied to practice.
- Theories from related disciplines also have relevance to nursing practice, education, and research.
- All theories have the potential to make substantial contributions to the nursing profession by enhancing the development of a unique body of nursing knowledge.

CRITICAL THINKING EXERCISES

1. "An individual is in constant interaction with the environment." Apply this statement to the client in each of the following settings and discuss the implications for nursing practice:
   a. A community mental health clinic
   b. An intensive care unit
   c. An extended care facility
   d. A well-baby clinic

2. How do Florence Nightingale's ideas apply to nursing practice in the current health care system?

3. Defend or refute the following statement: "We should have only one nursing theory, rather than several, to guide education, practice, and research."

4. Compare and contrast the definitions of health and illness in two nursing theories, citing similarities and differences. Which one of these is most reflective of your own definitions of health and illness?

5. What is your personal philosophy of nursing? Which of the theoretical perspectives of nursing presented in this chapter is most closely aligned with your philosophy of nursing?

6. Identify the nursing theory or model that would be most useful to you in your practice and explain why.

REFERENCES

Abdellah, F. G., Beland, I. L., Martin, A., & Matheny, R. (1960). *Patient centered approaches to nursing.* New York: Macmillan.

Abdellah, F. G., & Levine, E. (1965). *Better patient care through nursing research* (3rd ed.). New York: Macmillan.

Abdellah, F. G., Beland, I. L., Martin, A., & Matheny, R. (1973). *New directions in patient centered nursing: Guidelines for systems of service, education, and research.* New York: Macmillan.

Aguilera, D. C. (1970). *Crisis intervention: Theory and methodology.* St. Louis: Mosby.

Aguilera, D. C. (1998). *Crisis intervention: Theory and methodology* (8th ed.). St. Louis: Mosby.

Alligood, M. A. (1997). Models and theories: Critical thinking structures. In M. A. Alligood & A. Marriner-Tomey (Eds.), *Nursing theory: Utilization and application* (pp. 31–45). St. Louis: Mosby.

Alligood, M. A. (2000). Nursing theory: The basis for professional nursing. In K. K. Chitty (Ed.), *Professional nursing: Concepts & challenges* (3rd ed, pp. 246–274). Philadelphia: Saunders.

Alligood, M. A., & Marriner-Tomey, A. (Eds.). (1997). *Nursing theory: Utilization and application.* St. Louis: Mosby.

Auger, J. R. (1976). *Behavioral systems and nursing.* Englewood Cliffs, NJ: Prentice Hall.

Barnum, B. J. S. (1998). *Nursing theory: Analysis, application, evaluation* (5th ed.). Philadelphia: Lippincott.

Chinn, P. L., & Jacobs, M. K. (1987). *Theory and nursing: A systematic approach* (2nd ed.). St. Louis: Mosby.

Chinn, P. L., & Kramer, M. K. (1995). *Theory and nursing: A systematic approach* (4th ed.). St. Louis: Mosby.

Christensen, P. J., & Kenney, J. W. (1995). *Nursing process: Application of conceptual models* (4th ed.). St. Louis: Mosby.

Dickoff, J. J., James, P. A., & Weidenbach, E. (1968). Theory in a practice discipline, II. Practice-oriented research. *Nursing Research, 17,* 545–554.

Duvall, E. M. (1977). *Marriage and family development* (5th ed.). New York: Lippincott.

Fawcett, J. (1975). The family as a living open system: An emerging conceptual framework for nursing. *International Nursing Review, 22,* 113–116

Fawcett, J. (1977). The relationship between identification and patterns of change in spouses' body images during and after pregnancy. *International Journal of Nursing Studies, 14,* 199–213.

Fawcett, J. (1989). *Analysis and evaluation of conceptual models of nursing* (2nd ed.). Philadelphia: Davis.

Fawcett, J. (1993). *Analysis and evaluation of nursing theories.* Philadelphia: Davis.

Fawcett, J. (1995). *Analysis and evaluation of conceptual models of nursing* (3rd ed.). Philadelphia: Davis.

Fawcett, J. (1999). *The relationship of theory and research* (3rd ed.). Philadelphia: Davis.

Fawcett, J. (2000). *Analysis and evaluation of contemporary nursing knowledge: Nursing models and theories.* Philadelphia: Davis.

Grubbs, J. (1974). An interpretation of the Johnson behavioral system model. In J. P. Reihl & C. Roy (Eds.), *Conceptual models for nursing practice* (pp. 160–197). New York: Appleton-Century-Crofts.

Hall, L. (1966). Another view of nursing care and quality. In M. K. Straub, (Ed.), *Continuity of patient care: The role of nursing.* Washing003ton, DC: The Catholic University Press.

Henderson, V. (1966). *The nature of nursing: A definition and its implications for practice, research, and education.* New York: Macmillan.

Henderson, V. (1971). Health is everybody's business. *Canadian Nurse, 67,* 31–34.

Henderson, V., & Nite, G. (1978). *The principles and practice of nursing.* New York: Macmillan.

Higgins, P. A., & Moore, S. M. (2000). Levels of theoretical thinking in nursing. *Nursing Outlook, 48*(4), 179–183.

Infante, M. S. (Ed.). (1982). *Crisis theory: A framework for nursing practice.* Reston, VA: Reston Publishing.

Johnson, D. E. (1980). The behavioral system model for nursing. In J. P. Reihl & C. Roy (Eds.), *Conceptual models for nursing practice* (2nd ed., pp. 207–215). New York: Appleton-Century-Crofts.

Keck, J. (1998). Terminology of theory development. In A. Marriner-Toomy & M. R. Alligood (Eds.), *Nursing theorists and their work* (4th ed., pp. 16–24). St. Louis: Mosby.

King, I. (1971). *Toward a theory for nursing.* New York: Wiley.

King, I. (1975). A process for developing concepts for nursing through research. In P. J. Verhonick (Ed.), *Nursing Research* (Vol. 1, pp. 25–43). Boston: Little, Brown.

King, I. (1981). *A theory for nursing: Systems, concepts, process.* New York: Wiley.

King, I. (1995a). A systems framework for nursing. In M. A. Frey & C. L. Sieloff (Eds.), *Advancing King's systems framework and theory of nursing* (pp. 14–21). Thousand Oaks, CA: Sage.

King, I. (1995b). The theory of goal attainment. In M. A. Frey & C. L. Sieloff (Eds.), *Advancing King's systems framework and theory of nursing* (pp. 23–32). Thousand Oaks, CA: Sage.

Lazarus, R. S., & Folkman, S. (1984). *Stress appraisal and coping.* New York: Springer.

Leininger, M. (1978). *Transcultural nursing: Concepts, theories and practice.* New York: Wiley.

Leininger, M. (Ed.). (1984). *Care: The essence of nursing and health.* Thorofare, NJ: Slack.

Leininger, M. (1991). *Culture, care, diversity and universality: A theory of nursing* (NLN Publication No. 15-2402). New York: National League for Nursing.

Leininger, M. (1995). *Transcultural nursing: Concepts, theories, research, and practice.* Columbus, OH: McGraw-Hill.

Levine, M. (1967). The four conservation principles of nursing. *Nursing Forum, 6,* 45–49.

Levine, M. (1973). *Introduction to clinical nursing* (2nd ed.). Philadelphia: Davis.

Levine, M. E. (1995). The rhetoric of nursing theory. *Image: Journal of Nursing Scholarship, 27*(1), 11–14.

McCubbin, H. I., & Patterson, J. M. (1981). *Family stress: Resources and coping.* St. Paul: University of Minnesota Press.

Neuman, B. (1982). *The Neuman systems model: Application to nursing theory and practice.* Norwalk, CT: Appleton-Century-Crofts.

Neuman, B. (1989). *The Neuman systems model* (2nd ed.). Norwalk, CT: Appleton & Lange.

Neuman, B. (1995). *The Neuman systems model* (3rd ed.). Norwalk, CT: Appleton & Lange.

Neuman, B. M., & Young, R. J. (1972). A model for teaching total person approach to patient problems. *Nursing Research, 21,* 264–269.

Nightingale, F. (1946). *Notes on nursing: What it is and what it is not.* Philadelphia: Stern. (Original work published 1859)

Orem, D. E. (1980). *Nursing: Concepts of practice* (2nd ed.). New York: McGraw-Hill.

Orem, D. E. (1985). *Nursing: Concepts of practice* (3rd ed.). New York: McGraw-Hill.

Orem, D. E. (1991). *Nursing: Concepts of practice* (4th ed.). St. Louis: Mosby.

Orem, D. E. (1995). *Nursing: Concepts of practice* (5th ed.). St. Louis: Mosby.

Orlando, I. J. (1961). *The dynamic nurse-patient relationship.* New York: Putnam.

Parse, R. R. (1981). *Man-living-health: A theory of nursing.* New York: Wiley.

Parse, R. R. (1995). *Illuminations: The human becoming theory in practice and research.* New York: National League for Nursing.

Peplau, H. (1952). *Interpersonal relations in nursing: A conceptual frame of reference for psychodynamic nursing.* New York: Putnam. (Reprinted in 1988 by Macmillan and in 1991 by Springer.)

Peplau, H. (1992). Interpersonal relations: A theoretical framework for application in nursing practice. *Nursing Science Quarterly, 5,* 13–18.

Rodgers, B. L., & Knafl, K. A. (2000). *Concept development in nursing: Foundations, techniques and applications.* Philadelphia: Saunders.

Rogers, M. E. (1970). *An introduction to the theoretical basis of nursing.* Philadelphia: Davis.

Rogers, M. E. (1989). Nursing: A science of unitary man. In J. P. Reihl-Sisca (Ed.), *Conceptual models for nursing practice* (3rd ed., pp. 181–188). Norwalk, CT: Appleton & Lange.

Rogers, M. E. (1990). Nursing: Science of unitary, irreducible, human beings. Update 1990. In E. A. M. Barrett (Ed.), *Visions of Rogers' science-based nursing* (pp. 5–11). New York: National League for Nursing.

Rogers, M. E. (1994). Nursing science evolves. In M. A. Madrid & E. A. M. Barrett (Eds.), *Rogers' scientific art of nursing practice* (NLN Publication No. 15-2610, pp. 3–9). New York: National League for Nursing.

Roy, C. (1984). *Introduction to nursing: An adaptation model* (2nd ed.). Englewood Cliffs, NJ: Prentice-Hall.

Roy, C. (1989). The Roy adaptation model. In J. P. Reihl-Sisca (Ed.), *Conceptual models for nursing practice* (3rd ed., pp. 105–114). Norwalk, CT: Appleton & Lange.

Roy, C., & Andrews, H. A. (1999). *The Roy adaptation model.* Stanford, CT: Appleton & Lange.

Selye, H. (1974). *Stress without distress.* Philadelphia: Lippincott.

Selye, H. (1982). History and the present status of the stress concept. In I. A. Goldberger & S. Breznitz (Eds.), *Handbook of stress: Theoretical and clinical aspects.* New York: Free Press.

von Bertalanffy, L. (1956). General systems theory. In B. D. Ruben & J. Kim (Eds.), *General systems theory and human communication* (pp. 7–16). Rochelle Park, NJ: Hayden.

Watson, J. (1979). *Nursing: The philosophy and science of caring.* Boston: Little, Brown.

Watson, J. (1985). *Nursing: Human science and health care.* Norwalk, CT: Appleton-Century-Crofts.

Watson, J. (1988). *Nursing: Human science and human caring—A theory of nursing.* New York: National League for Nursing.

Watson, J. (1994). *Applying the art and science of human caring.* New York: National League for Nursing.

Weidenbach, E. (1964). *Clinical nursing: A helping art.* New York: Springer

Weidenbach, E. (1970). Nurses' wisdom in nursing theory. *American Journal of Nursing, 70,* 1057–1062.

White, M. B. (Ed.). (1983). *Curriculum development from a nursing model: The crisis theory framework.* New York: Springer.

7

Case Management: A Nursing Role

SHARON W. UTZ, PhD, RN, AND PAMELA A. KULBOK, DNSc, RN

OBJECTIVES

At the completion of this chapter, the reader will be able to:

- Analyze professional nursing roles and settings for case management:
- Compare terms such as case management, disease management, and care management.
- Examine the process of nursing care management to delineate new and unique aspects of the nursing process.
- Identify the knowledge base necessary for nursing care management as a basis for career planning.
- Apply the concept of levels of prevention and the process of resource analysis/utilization to the health problem of alcoholism.

PROFILE IN PRACTICE

Kathryn K. Ward, BSN, RNC
MSN Student, University of Virginia
Charlottesville, Virginia

This is an exciting time for the nursing profession as we embark on a new century. As providers of patient care, change will continue to be the operative word. We must embrace this challenge and treat it as an opportunity to continue to advance our role in the delivery of health care.

Case management is a term with many connotations, usually defined by the agency or institution that employs this level of care. It is not a new role to nursing, as public health nurses first provided case management many years ago. Since obtaining my BSN, I've had two positions with the title. While the concept has been similar, the practice has been somewhat different. In

the former position I provided care across an episode, and in my current position I follow patients across the continuum of care. The scope of practice includes, but is not limited to, coordinating care and resources needed, advocating, integrating and procuring services considered necessary, and being fiscally responsible to provide quality care in a cost-effective manner. With episodic care there is always an eventual termination of services, and this is usually time related. For example, in home health care, when specific objectives have been met or when a patient is no longer homebound, services will be discontinued. In inpatient settings, the time of discharge from the facility will automatically terminate the service. In contrast, following patients across the continuum of care could and usually does include the provision of both inpatient and outpatient care for as long as needed or until death.

Although this may sound overwhelming and not what we typically see at the bedside, it is an inherent part of who we are and what we do everyday as nurses. Case management requires a sound basis of clinical knowledge to support decisions and match appropriate services to client needs. The demands placed on case managers are a direct reflection of the degree of chronic illness in our society and the immense needs of those populations. We have the responsibility and opportunity to provide our patients with the best possible resources to meet their needs for a productive, quality lifestyle individualized to their desired goals and capabilities.

Having been in nursing for more than 25 years, I have seen multiple changes in the health care system. Change has been the only consistent thing over time; however, it has advanced our roles and provided us with unique opportunities. I urge you to accept the baton each time it's handed to you and take the opportunity to make a difference in the lives of your patients and your profession.

The evolution of new forms of managed health care, such as health maintenance organizations (HMOs) and preferred provider organizations (PPOs), brought with it new roles for nurses. One role that has increased in recent years is that of nurse case manager. Although there are many job titles for this general role (such as care manager, care coordinator, outcomes manager, and others), there are common components that can be described to help nurses understand and prepare for this important role in the health care system.

This chapter begins with selected definitions of case management, then provides background information on the health care system and roles for case managers across the continuum of care. The process of case management is examined within the broader framework of the nursing process. One segment of the case management process, resource analysis and utilization, is examined in depth, using the health problem of alcoholism as the example. Finally, the areas of knowledge needed by case managers are briefly described to provide a guide for nurses to plan their career development consistent with emerging case management roles.

Definition of Case Management

Nurses have been involved in aspects of case management since the earliest days of nursing in the United States, when pioneers such as Lillian Wald followed patients to their homes to deal with their complex health and social needs (Heinrich, 1983). Case management has also been consistently visible in the mental health system, where psychiatric nurses and social workers often follow patients from hospitalization to long-term community-based care. These early forms of case management make it clear that the underlying ideas and indeed the need for case management are not new. However, the recently emerging forms of case management reflect the differences in the current health care system from the previous forms. As positions for case managers have increased in health care systems, the need to define and clarify the role has also increased.

As with any newly emerging role, that of case manager has evolved, with many different forms and descriptions. In one insightful description, Powell (1996) notes that the role of case manager is in its adolescence, "complete with identity crisis, and a growing awkward form" (p. 309). In recent years, many leaders in nursing have provided descriptions and definitions of case management to enhance understanding of the role and to lay the foundation for educating and certifying case managers.

In 1992 American Nurses Association (ANA) published *Case Management by Nurses,* in which case management is described as a "paradoxically simple, yet complex concept" (Bower, 1992, p. 3). Bower notes that the term *case management* can simultaneously describe "a system, a role, a technology, a process and a service" (p. 4). The role of case manager is described as that of actively coordinating care, and the case manager as one who has both the authority and the accountability to provide and obtain needed services. The case manager has in-depth skills and knowledge to manage the care of a client population, including both direct and indirect care components.

The Case Management Society of America (CMSA) is another professional group that has published a definition of case management. CMSA members include a variety of health care providers, with the majority being nurses. It defines case management as follows:

> Case management is a collaborative process which assesses, plans, implements, coordinates, monitors and evaluates options and services to meet an individual's health needs through communication and available resources to promote quality cost-effective outcomes (Case Management Society of America, 1995, p. 8).

The "official" definitions of the ANA and CMSA have been fleshed out in numerous books that can help nurses prepare for this important role. One of the most comprehensive definitions has been provided by Bower and Falk:

> Case management is a clinical system that focuses on the accountability of an individual or group for coordinating a patient's care (or group of patients)

across an episode or continuum of care; ensuring and facilitating the achievement of quality, clinical and financial outcomes; negotiating, procuring, and coordinating services and resources needed by the patient and family; intervening at key points (or significant variances from the anticipated plan of care) for individual patients; addressing and resolving consistent issues that have negative quality or cost impact; and creating opportunities and systems to enhance outcomes (1996, p. 164).

Although these three definitions are different in some ways, their similarities are helpful to those trying to understand exactly what nursing case management might look like. The common themes that emerge from these definitions are (1) there is a broad responsibility for providing comprehensive services to individuals, groups, or populations of patients across boundaries in the health care delivery system (often referred to as the continuum of care); (2) the case manager has a high level of responsibility and skills in the clinical realm and is also "system savvy"— able to make the system work for patients and families who need care; (3) collaboration with other health care professionals is essential; and (4) there is a focus on both the quality of the service and cost-effectiveness in the delivery of care.

THE CONTEXT AND APPLICATIONS OF NURSING CARE MANAGEMENT

Health care delivery in the United States has undergone a major transformation. Less than a decade after national efforts to legislate health care reform failed, managed care initiatives have taken root, and state-by-state regulation of health care heralds more turbulent change in the near future. One major driving force in health care is upwardly spiraling costs. Spiraling health care costs are a direct result of scientific advances and technology, inappropriate use of services, and the increasing need for services by the aging American population (Cohen & Cesta, 1997). At the same time, both consumers and providers are demanding increased attention to quality care and satisfaction. These consumer trends are fueled in large part by market competition and the use of business strategies to make health systems more accountable to multiple stakeholders, among them consumers, providers, employers, and insurers (Conrad & Shortell, 1997). In the year 2000 we are on the brink of realizing a patients' bill of rights, designed to protect health care consumers by balancing countervailing demands for cost control, assurance of quality, and improved access to health care.

Managing Health Across the Continuum of Care: From Managing Costs to Managing Care to Managing Health

Health care delivery in the United States is moving toward a system of "managed health" (Conrad & Shortell, 1997; Shortell, Gillies, & Devers, 1995). This pathway began in the 1970s with federal health care financing initiatives to manage costs, including the HMO movement and Medicare reimbursement policies designed to reduce catastrophic health care costs. The diagnosis-related groups (DRG)/ prospective payment system restricted hospital admissions, limited length of stay, and ultimately increased the acuity of home care patients (Dieckmann, 1994). Initial strategies for managing costs gave rise to a broader focus on the management of financial and clinical systems.

The term managed care (or managed health care) emerged with several accepted uses and meanings. *Managed care* describes restructured health care organizations, such as HMOs, which were designed to control costs for purchasers of care by measures such as insurance benefit limitations or exclusions, prepaid health plans, prospective payment methods, and fee schedules (Williams & Torrens, 1993). Managed care also represents a broad system-oriented approach that attempts to control costs, ensure quality, and improve access to health care (Powell, 2000). However, the dominant characteristic of managed care is the use of financial incentives and management controls designed to direct patients to efficient providers of appropriate care, in cost-effective treatment settings (Lee, 1993; Powell, 2000).

Managed health is a conception of health care delivered through integrated health systems that are learning to move "from managing costs to managing care to managing health" (Conrad & Shortell, 1997, p. 36) (Fig. 7–1). The essence of managed health is health promotion, disease prevention, and health maintenance of populations across the full continuum of care. Health management integration is generally intended when the term disease management is used. Disease management refers to clinical care and supportive self-management for individuals with specific chronic conditions. However, confusion regarding emphasis on health or disease will continue to exist as long as labels such as disease management are used.

Integrated health systems require active partnering between the public and private sectors of the American health care enterprise (Baker et al., 1994). At its core, public health is a population-based practice that utilizes the science of epidemiology and the philosophical principles of social justice to apply scientific knowledge to improve the health of the public—to manage health. The successful transformation of health care delivery from a medical model to a health

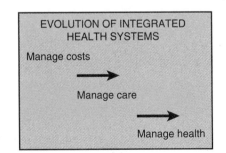

FIGURE 7–1 Evolution of integrated health systems.

system depends on integrating the guiding principles of public health with evolving financial and clinical management systems.

Until recently, the hospital was regarded as the center of health care service delivery. The success of ventures directed toward managing health depends on the integration of hospitals and public or private sector health care providers into networks of organized, community-oriented health care and social service delivery systems. The ultimate goal is to establish an entire continuum of care—from health promotion and self-care to hospice care or long-term care—to maximize effective outcomes across episodes of illness and pathways to wellness (Shortell et al., 1995) (Fig. 7–2). The maximum potential of integrated health systems will be realized when these systems accept accountability for meeting the needs of people in their local communities. The shift from concern focused solely on "covered lives" to broader accountability for the population is critical (Conrad & Shortell, 1997).

CONTINUUM OF CARE

The *continuum of care* is often described as an array of acute or chronic care services ranging from in-home and community-based services to institutional services. In-home services include visiting nurse/home care, pediatric home care, home infusion therapy, hospice, homemaker-home health aide, chore services, and Meals on Wheels. Community services include assisted living/custodial care, respite care, geriatric day care, sheltered workshops, congregate meals, senior citizens, community mental health, legal and protective services. Institutional services are provided by institutions, including the acute care hospital, chronic care and subacute care hospital, rehabilitation facility, and intermediate and skilled nursing facility.

The continuum of care also encompasses health promotion and disease prevention services. These services can be formal self-help and social support groups as well as informal networks of families and friends. Health promotion and disease prevention services are not as well known but are proliferating in many communities. Some managed care systems such as HMOs and PPOs provide regular health education and screening programs to their beneficiaries. Newly forming health systems may also offer free health promotion programs and educational material to the general population or groups of clients with specific diseases or conditions (e.g., diabetes or other chronic conditions). When health systems offer health pro-

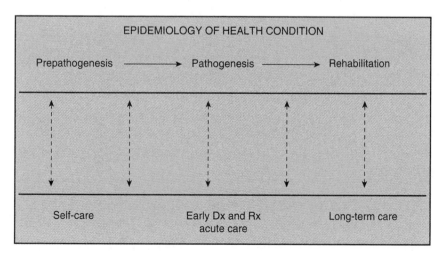

FIGURE 7–2 Continuum of care.

motion programs they are generally accepting accountability for meeting the needs of people in their local communities. Shortell et al. (1995) defined this strategy as "community benefit."

Disease prevention, health promotion, and accountability for meeting the needs of the community are not new models of care for professional nurses. These are essential concepts in baccalaureate and master's level nursing curricula (American Association of Colleges of Nursing 1996, 1998). The Pew Health Professions Commission (1991) reinforced the overarching importance of knowledge and skill in the areas of health promotion and community or population-oriented care for all health care practitioners. Professional nurses are positioned to take a leadership role in implementing managed health systems by using the strategies outlined in this chapter to ensure access, contain costs, and improve the quality of client outcomes.

 ## The Process of Case Management

One of the best ways to understand case management is to examine exactly what the profes-

sional nurse does in the process of case management. Nurses at all levels of practice are familiar with the nursing process, a generic term describing the commonly used steps in clinical problem solving. The steps in this process are generally understood to include assessment, diagnosis, planning, intervention, and evaluation of outcomes. The case management process fits within the overall framework of the nursing process but has additional, more specialized components. The nursing process and the case management process are compared in Table 7–1.

CASE FINDING, SCREENING, AND ASSESSMENT

The first phase of the nursing process for the case manager involves identifying the health needs or problems of individuals and populations and selecting those who need case management (case selection). Many nurses are already skilled in the first step of the nursing process for individuals, the assessment phase, in which the health status of the patient or client is examined. Communication skills are essential to assess individual patients and families and to communicate with other health professionals. The skills of physical examination and interpre-

---

TABLE 7–1 Comparison of Nursing Process and Case Management Process

Nursing Process	Case Management Process
Assessment	Case finding, screening, and assessment
Diagnosis	Interdisciplinary diagnosis
Planning	Planning and outcome projection
Implementation	Implementation, service planning and resource analysis/allocation
Evaluation	Final evaluation and follow-up
Documentation and data collection	Documentation for clinical records, utilization management, and outcomes

From Utz, S. W., & Kulbok, P. A. (1999). Managing care through advanced practice nursing. In J. Lancaster (Ed.), *Nursing issues in leading and managing change.* St. Louis: Mosby.

tation also come into play. Although this is a part of what the case manager does, often the case manager focuses on groups or populations of patients and the subsequent determination of common needs across the group. When the focus is at the group or program level, this phase is often referred to as a needs assessment. Two essential skills for this phase are knowledge of the population and skill in collecting and analyzing data at the individual and group level. For example, for the case manager specializing in geriatric services, a thorough knowledge of questionnaires useful with elderly populations is necessary to choose a screening tool to be administered to elderly patients admitted to a care system or enrolled in the health care plan. The result of screening is to determine which level of care is needed for each individual entering the program of care. The screening process is used to determine those with the most complex needs who can benefit from being assigned a case manager. This process is also called case selection (Powell, 2000). Those with more simple, predictable health conditions can be followed with routine clinical pathways or standard protocols, such as those for surgical procedures such as joint replacement or vascular surgery.

It has been noted that although everyone deserves well-coordinated care, not everyone needs a case manager. There are a number of target groups that are more likely to need case managers, including those who:

- have frequent or recent hospital or emergency department admissions.
- are elderly.
- live alone.
- have limited finances.
- have a high-need medical diagnosis or DRG.
- are substance abusers.
- have complex chronic illnesses (physical and mental).
- have complicated social and economic problems.

- are unable to follow a prescribed medical regimen.
- have cultural or religious perspectives significantly different from the health care team's.
- have suffered major life-changing health events (e.g., traumatic injury) or significant loss of health, or have unrealistic expectations for their health situation (Cohen & Cesta, 1997; Flarey & Blancett, 1996; Powell, 2000).

It should be noted here that many screening instruments have been developed to help the case manager with the initial screening of some populations For example, the Praplus (Pacala & Boult, 1997) was developed to screen groups of elderly and identify existing and potential health needs. The well-known Medical Outcome Study instrument, the Short-Form 36 (SF-36) (Ware, 1995), is often used both as a screening tool and as a way of tracking progress in many patient populations. Such instruments can be an efficient way to make "initial cuts" within a population and identify which individuals may need further assessment.

When the initial screening and case selection is completed, the case manager has a list of those needing more in-depth assessment. At this time, clinical expertise is required to complete a focused yet comprehensive assessment of health status and factors affecting health and self-care. This case management nursing assessment has been described by Powell as "the critical pivot around which the nursing case management revolves" (2000, p. 416). The assessment is the foundation for subsequent actions by the case manager as well as other health care providers. Specific categories for an in-depth assessment have been identified by numerous authors of textbooks on case management (Cesta, Tahan, & Fink, 1998; Cohen & Cesta, 1997; Powell, 2000). The most common components are often familiar to nurses: health history, demographic factors, socioeconomic factors, cultural perspectives, financial situation, environmental factors, and functional level. For each practice setting and patient population, the case manager must tailor the specific assessment process to obtain adequate information to determine whether case management is needed or not. Early identification of all relevant problems allows the case manager to develop a plan that considers the many complex factors that impinge on health, and to offer care that addresses both the presenting problems and the underlying causes and prevents future complications or problems.

PROBLEM IDENTIFICATION/DIAGNOSIS

The second phase of the case management process, like the nursing process, results in a clear, concise statement of the identified problems or diagnoses to be addressed. There are some unique aspects of the diagnostic process in case management. As with many nursing roles, the case manager role requires that the nurse engage in a dialogue with patients and families about the identified problems and potential approaches. Patient and family knowledge of the identified problems is the starting point for decisions about care. Without a foundation of understanding about what the individual and family desire and find acceptable, all subsequent plans will be incomplete and potentially useless. Whether the case manager is operating from the care provider's or the payer's perspective, having agreement on what the problems are, what is desirable, and what is possible allows further negotiation about the specifics of the care to be delivered and received.

Another factor that affects diagnosis within a case management framework is the interdisciplinary focus. More so than many other nursing roles, case management requires a strong partnership with professional colleagues and an approach that incorporates the perspectives of physicians, therapists, social service experts, the payers, and others. The call for interdisciplinary approaches has sometimes led nurses to believe that it was no longer appropriate to use nursing language, such as nursing diagnoses, because it might create barriers to working with other health care professionals. In contrast, this point of view has never kept physicians from using medical language, assumed to be essential for all health care professionals. Nurses should be cognizant that the "strength of the multidisciplinary effort is that all disciplines are clear about what they can contribute" (McCloskey & Bulechek, 1994, p. 56). Nurses are accountable for diagnosing and addressing patient problems according to the nurse practice act in the state in which they practice. The use of nursing language, such as a nursing diagnosis, makes it clear what the focus of the nurse is upon and helps provide documentation for addressing patient problem areas.

In recent years, nurses have worked to develop standardized vocabularies for use in practice, education, and research. Many nurses who have used these standardized languages have found them helpful for describing what nurses do and for documenting the specifics of nursing care. Two examples of standardized language are the North American Nursing Diagnosis Association's list of nursing diagnoses (1999–2000; currently under revision by the Nursing Diagnosis Extension and Classification group), and the Omaha Nursing Problem List (Martin & Scheet, 1992). While both are useful, they differ in emphasis. As examples, sample categories in the NANDA classification system are Ineffective Airway Clearance and Chronic Pain. Sample categories in the Omaha problem list are Neighborhood/Workplace Safety and Neglected Child/Adult.

PLANNING AND OUTCOME PROJECTION

The planning phase of the case management process is not unlike the familiar nursing care plan; however, case management requires some specific elements. The goal of the planning phase is to help individuals and groups of patients achieve optimal health, self-care, and control over their lives. During this phase the case manager takes the information gleaned during the assessment process and develops a plan that is mutually agreeable to the client, the payer, and the health care providers. To do this well, the case manager must be able to prioritize existing problems, anticipate ways to prevent additional problems, and customize a plan of care, given all the existing individual and environmental factors. The process requires thinking about long- and short-term goals and formulating these broad goals into specific outcomes that can be tracked and measured. An "ideal plan" must be developed and negotiated with the clients and the payers, often in the form of an agreement or contract. The plan is constructed using the best available information, yet the case manager needs to be aware that she or he may have to fall back on a plan B if the first plan does not work out. An example might involve planning for an elderly person to go to a family member's home after surgery but having an arrangement with an extended care facility in case the family member is not able to provide adequate care.

Projecting outcomes is one of the areas of case management that is new to many nurses and is a crucial component of the process. Flarey and Blancett (1996) note that "to be effective, all case management systems must be outcome driven. They must be designed to move the patient through the process of care delivery toward the attainment of defined outcomes. Outcomes must be clearly defined and measurable" (p. 9). Many tools already exist to aid case managers in developing a plan and projecting desired outcomes. Some of these tools include nationally established guidelines for care, such as those published by the National Guideline Clearing House (1999), published on-line through a collaboration of the Agency for Health Care Research and Quality, the American Medical Association, and the American Association of Health Plans. Standardized guidelines provide rapid sources for evidence-based practice recognized nationwide. Other sources may be local, regional, or agency-specific clinical pathways, guidelines, and protocols, which present approaches agreed upon by clinicians and payers for the care of patients with particular medical or nursing diagnoses, with projected outcomes and time frames.

In previous decades, outcomes that were collected in standardized databases included such items as medical diagnoses at admission and discharge, types of medical treatments, and cause of death. In recent years, other outcomes have become recognized as important to both consumers and payers of health care. Among such outcomes are quality of life and ability to function. The popularity of the Medical Outcome Study Short-Form (SF-36) (Ware, 1995) is a reflection of this trend toward measuring outcomes of health care in a more comprehensive way. Outcomes may be at the individual clinical level (e.g., patient able to return home after surgery, with functional level increased within a specified time frame) or at the group level (e.g., more people referred for screening mammograms) or at the system level (e.g., decreased costs of care for a group that previously made high-cost visits to the emergency department for nonurgent care).

One of the most useful sources for delineating outcomes for nurse case managers to be published in recent years is *The Nursing Outcome Classification* (NOC) (Johnson, Maas, & Moorhead, 2000). The NOC represents a comprehensive listing of outcomes that are sensitive to nursing care, organized into categories, and coded for computerization. The NOC is derived from the work of hundreds of nurses, organized by the Iowa Center for Nursing Classification with funding from the National Institute for Nursing Research. The NOC was published for use by nurses and other health care providers to aid in measuring results of care. A few examples of nursing outcomes are

Circulation Status, Cognitive Ability, Body Image, and Dignified Dying.

IMPLEMENTATION, SERVICE PROVISION, AND RESOURCE ALLOCATION

During the implementation phase, the plans are put into practice, and skillful management of the right services customized to fit the patient/family is carried out. This is the phase during which the case manager has the responsibility to see that the best care is provided using appropriate, cost-effective resources. Depending on the role of the case manager, she or he may provide direct care or may direct others to carry out the plan.

One of the important functions of the case manager during this phase is to utilize resources in the community to complement and supplement those of the patient, family, and health care providers. Being able to tap valuable resources in the community is a skill that must be acquired for successful case management, and thus is examined in the next section in detail. The health problem of Alcoholism is offered as an example of the application of resource analysis across the continuum of care.

COMMUNITY RESOURCE ANALYSIS: A BASIC TOOL FOR EFFECTIVE NURSING CARE MANAGEMENT

Understanding and knowing how to use community resources is an essential competency for practice as a nursing care manager. Kulbok and Utz (1999) reviewed several authoritative sources to determine what areas of knowledge are needed to prepare nursing care managers. There was consensus that knowledge related to the system of care coordination and service delivery is fundamental. Cary (2000) characterized this knowledge domain for case management as "care resources for clients within institutions and communities; facilitating the development of new resources and systems to meet clients needs" (p. 385). Knowledge of existing resources and of

gaps in health care resources evolves from community/public health nursing specialty content.

Conducting an analysis of community resources is important for successful nursing care management, although it is not typically delineated as a stage in the process of managing care. Powell (2000) identifies *service planning and resource allocation* as a step in the stage of *development and coordination of the case plan.* Powell (2000) states that allocating resources requires knowledge of public and private organizations, including services provided by the client's medical insurance and "informal" resources when insurance is not available or inadequate to meet the client's needs. In the process of care management, the implementation stage of the nursing process is expanded to include *implementation, service planning, and resource allocation;* resource allocation "requires the nurse to be well-informed about resources in the community at large—from local to the national level" (Utz & Kulbok, 1999, p. 447).

Information about access, affordability, and availability of community resources across the continuum of care must be utilized in developing a plan for care management. Access refers to dimensions of the continuum of care that indicate the potential or actual entry of a population or groups into the health care sycontinuum of care that indicate the potential or actual entry of a population or groups into the health care system and subsumes issues of affordability and availability. The dimensions of access include direct factors, such as the client's insurance benefit package or eligibility requirements, and indirect factors, such as distance to the facility, the availability of transportation, the cost of lost work time, and other time-related factors such as lead time, travel time, waiting time, and conflicts in time schedule.

Other dimensions of access that indirectly affect access to services include the subjective beliefs and prior experiences of consumers (positive or negative). Discrimination by race, gender, socioeconomic status, age, or mental status and the quality of provider-consumer relationships can also indirectly affect access to care. Organizational characteristics such as limited hours of operation, fragmented services, and lack of appropriate health care providers have a direct impact on access to care.

Nurse care managers require community resource information about the full continuum of care and equity of access that spans all levels and intensity of care, including primary, secondary, and tertiary levels of prevention. Levels of prevention, as originally described by Leavell and Clark (1965), were derived from the science of epidemiology to guide public health practice (Table 7–2). The application of any

preventive measure corresponds to the natural history of health and illness. Primary preventive measures are directed toward "well" individuals in the prepathogenesis period to promote health and to provide specific protection from disease. Secondary preventive measures are applied to diagnose or to treat individuals in the period of disease pathogenesis. Tertiary prevention addresses rehabilitation and the return of people with chronic illness to a maximal ability to function. Basic knowledge of the natural history of health and illness and levels of prevention can be used to guide analysis of a specific population to identify community resources that exist

TABLE 7–2 Levels of Application of Preventive Measures in the Natural History of Disease

The Natural History of Any Disease of Man				
Prepathogenesis Period		Period of Pathogenesis		
Primary Prevention		Secondary Prevention		Tertiary Prevention
Health Promotion	Specific Protection	Early Diagnosis and Prompt Treatment	Disability Limitation	Rehabilitation
Health education	Use of specific immunizations	Case-finding measures, individual and mass	Adequate treatment to arrest the disease process and to prevent further complications and sequelae	Provision of hospital and community facilities for retraining and education for maximum use of remaining capacities
Good standard of nutrition	Attention to personal hygiene	Screening surveys		
Adjusted to developmental phases of life	Use of environmental sanitation	Selective examinations	Provision of facilities to limit disability and to prevent death	Education of the public and industry to utilize the rehabilitated
Attention to personality development	Protection against occupational hazards	**Objectives:**		
		To cure and prevent disease processes		
Provision of adequate housing, recreation, and agreeable working conditions	Protection from accidents	To prevent the spread of communicable diseases		As full employment as possible
Marriage counseling and sex education	Use of specific nutrients	To prevent complications and sequelae		Selective placement
Genetics	Protection from carcinogens	To shorten period of disability		Work therapy in hospitals
Periodic selective examinations	Avoidance of all allergens			Use of sheltered colony

From Leavell, H. F., & Clark, E. G. (1965). *Preventive medicine for the doctor in his community: An epidemiologic approach.* New York; McGraw-Hill. Reproduced with permission of The McGraw-Hill Companies.

Box 7–1 Application: Community Resources for Clients with Alcohol-Related Health Problems

Service planning and resource allocation for alcohol-related disorders requires a two-pronged approach to analysis: (1) clarifying disease progression from the prepathogenic or prealcoholic stage to extreme pathogenesis with manifest alcohol-induced disorders (e.g., gastritis, cirrhosis, malnutrition); and (2) describing existing treatment options from early identification and treatment to maintenance monitoring. When the nurse case manager has a clear idea of the natural history of disease (e.g., alcoholism), it is possible to identify community resources for care across the continuum of disease progression.

The model of treatment options for alcoholism rehabilitation (Table 7–3) provides a useful example of community resource knowledge necessary for nurse case managers to meet the needs of clients with alcohol-related health problems. Early identification of potential or actual alcohol-related problems most often occurs in community-based settings through formal and informal referral mechanisms. A nurse case manager who works with substance abuse problems will know existing resources and gaps in resources in the local community. The case manager provides essential coordination to facilitate early identification and entry into the appropriate care facility and subsequent transition across the stages of care, from initial treatment to maintenance and follow-up. The nurse case manager is able to create necessary linkages because of knowledge of the community, including referral sources, patterns of use of services, transition patterns between levels of care, and sociodemographic characteristics of the users.

across the continuum of care. Box 7–1 describes the application of resource analysis to the health problem of alcoholism; Table 7–3 lists the treatment options.

Once the analysis of the resources of the community has been completed and appropriate resources have been tapped by the care manager, another component of the case manager's role during implementation is to monitor the care and the interim outcomes, in order to keep things on track or to make adjustments. Case managers typically monitor for variances from the expected pattern, and systematically collect data about the types and frequency of variances, for the purpose of solving individual and system problems. A variance is defined as a deviation

TABLE 7–3 Model of Treatment Options for Alcoholic Rehabilitation

Identification: Churches, business community, medical center (MC), emergency department, social services, mental health services, physician offices

Entry: Private treatment facility, medical center—inpatient (medically unstable), mental health facility—outpatient or inpatient

Initial treatment: Detoxification, inpatient rehabilitation, outpatient rehabilitation

Maintenance: Long-term rehabilitation facility, halfway house, sheltered living, independent living facility

Follow-up: Alcoholics Anonymous, job finding—social services, churches, other community involvement, vocational training

From Hulton, L. (1994). Community resource analysis for alcoholism. Unpublished manuscript.

from the expected care and lack of attaining an outcome within the expected time frame (Tahan & Cesta, 1996). The most common categories of variances are (1) patient/family variances, such as unexpected physical complications or family problems; (2) practitioner variances, such as a specialist not being available or practice patterns that do not fit the population; (3) institution or system variances, such as unavailability of a therapy on the weekend or poorly sequenced testing that delays treatment decisions; and (4) community variances, such as lack of available beds in extended care facilities or lack of mobile meals to support individuals during home recovery (Cohen & Cesta, 1997; Powell, 2000).

To document the care provided during the implementation phase, the case manager and other care providers can benefit from documenting with standardized languages that are nationally recognized and coded for computerization. Examples of standardized languages for recording nursing actions include the Nursing Intervention Classification (NIC) and the Omaha Nursing System interventions list (Martin & Scheet, 1992). Each of these languages provides commonly accepted terms for nursing actions that can provide clear communication between health professionals about the kind of care provided. Using such an approach allows for computer coding and subsequent tracking of interventions for purposes of comparing results of care across time and across individuals and groups of patients.

In summary, the implementation phase of case management requires that the care manager monitor the care given with an eye to balancing quality care with appropriate available resources across the care continuum. It is essential that the nurse case manager have sufficient clinical knowledge of the population of patients to be served and of available resources so that she or he can skillfully implement care as well as guide others. Additional responsibilities lie in monitoring and analyzing variances in order to solve individual and system problems. The use of standardized nursing language enhances the case manager's ability track interventions and outcomes.

FINAL EVALUATION AND FOLLOW-UP

The final phase of the case management process, that of evaluation and follow-up, is one that is new to many nurses, and indeed to the health care system overall. During this phase the case manager reviews the ultimate results of care provided to individuals and to groups of patients. The value of this analysis is self-evident: it provides the final pieces of information about the effectiveness of a plan of care and an overall program of care for special populations. The setting in which the case manager is employed will influence the extent and purpose of this evaluation. If the case manager follows patients across the continuum of care from hospital to home, the information will be quite comprehensive and informative to the caregivers as well as to payers. In other situations, the case manager's role may be limited to one small area of the overall continuum, such as managing an acute episode within the walls of the hospital. Regardless of the client or agency to whom the case manager reports, key aspects of the evaluation include comparing projected outcomes with actual outcomes of care, analyzing costs, and determining what changes may be needed to enhance both quality and cost-effectiveness of the service provided.

DOCUMENTATION AND DATA ANALYSIS

Documentation of case management, like other forms of nursing care, is important to communicate the plan of care as well as provide a record of events and a legal document. Case managers need to be skillful and efficient to complete the extensive documentation that is used for individual care and for system-level reports. An additional challenge related to documentation of case management is the multidisciplinary nature of the care. Within the context of many providers of care, it is even *more* important that the case manager be clear and explicit about nursing actions and use recognizable, standardized language. It has previously been noted that "compelling legal reasons make it essential that patient records reflect what actions were taken by which health professional" (Utz, 1998). It should be noted again that all phases of the case management process are strengthened by the use of standardized languages and computerization of information. Whereas physicians have for decades been using coded systems such as the International Disease Classification System (ICD) to collect statistics about diseases, and the Current Procedural Terminology (CPT) codes to submit bills for treatments, similar languages for nursing have only become available within the last 20 years (McCloskey & Bulechek, 1994). Computer software companies are just beginning to make these available for documentation systems, thus allowing nurses to quickly and easily document in standardized ways to allow comparisons of all phases of care across time, across health care systems, and indeed across national or international boundaries (Clarke, 1998; Joel, 1998).

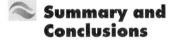 **Summary and Conclusions**

Professional nurses are challenged to manage care with limited resources in the ever changing and dynamic context of health care delivery. Often it is the nurse who is responsible for coordinating services for clients as they transition from one level and type of care to another, such as from home to hospital or ambulatory care, or from a skilled nursing home or rehabilitation facility to home care. The process of case management described in this chapter is used by the nurse case manager to achieve the five "rights" or outcomes of care: the *right* care at the *right* time by the *right* provider in the *right* setting for the *right* price (Bower, 1992).

It is clear within the nursing literature that a defined knowledge base is needed for nurses who wish to move into case manager roles. Kulbok and Utz (1999) presented a summary of the current consensus about areas of knowledge that are needed for case management and the types of certification available for those who wish to confirm their competence. Cary (1996) has itemized the necessary areas of knowledge as follows:

- The health care financial environment and payer requirements
- Clinical skills and the maturity to direct sequencing of care, considering quality
- Discharge planning for ideal timing and quality
- Management skills at the clinical and system levels
- Teaching, counseling, and educator skills
- Program development and evaluation, including quality improvement techniques
- Legal issues

This list underscores the need for ongoing education and a strong clinical foundation as the basis for the role. The article by Kulbok and Utz (1999) provides the reader with additional details about education and certification of case managers.

As we indicated earlier in this chapter, not all patients may need comprehensive case management, but all patients do deserve to have their care well coordinated. Case management is a logical extension of the clinical problem-solving process. Basic knowledge of nursing case management, an understanding of health needs across the continuum of care, and an emphasis on health promotion and disease prevention are regarded as essential content for professional nursing practice. Because many hospitals today are reinventing themselves as "health systems," responsive to the health needs of local communities, the nurse case manager is well positioned to lead the multidisciplinary team and health care consumers toward the "right" outcomes of care.

KEY POINTS

● Although the role of case manager began with public health nurses in the early 1900s, today case managers are found in a variety of health care settings.

● The successful case manager must be flexible and willing to continually embrace new and better approaches in caring for patients and families because of rapid changes in the health care system.

● Historically nurses have focused on comprehensive, patient-focused care, and therefore are in a strong position to contribute their expertise to enhance the quality and cost-effectiveness of care through case management.

● The health care system should include the entire continuum of care—from health promotion and self-care to long-term care or hospice—while maximizing effective outcomes across both episodes of illness and pathways to wellness.

● The continuum of care encompasses a wide array of services both formal and informal, ranging from in-home and community-based services to those of acute and rehabilitative institutions.

● The case management process builds on the nursing process by expanding the focus to groups and populations and by adding elements such as outcome projection, resource analysis, follow-up, and outcome analysis.

● Although everyone deserves to have well-coordinated care, not everyone needs a case manager.

● Case management is most likely to be needed by target groups with complex health problems or complex social and financial circumstances.

● A strong partnership with professional colleagues is essential to the success of the case manager who works closely with physicians, social workers, and a variety of therapists to achieve optimal health and quality cost-effective care.

● Multidisciplinary care is most effective when all disciplines can articulate and document their individual contributions to successful outcomes.

● Standardized nursing language is useful in demonstrating and documenting the contributions that nurses make to all phases of case management.

● Knowledge of community resources from the local to the national level is essential to assure coordination and delivery of quality care.

● Nurse case managers need to identify health care resources in the community that are accessible, affordable, and available to their clients.

● As with any other role for nurses, positions for case managers may require differing levels of expertise within a variety of settings.

● Areas of knowledge needed for case managers are well described in the nursing literature and are evident in established certification processes.

● Professional nurses are positioned to take a leadership role in the health care system as case managers who help ensure access to, contain costs of, and promote optimal health outcomes.

CRITICAL THINKING EXERCISES

1. The role of the nurse case manager is evolving at a unique pace in various regions of the country. Describe your personal experiences with or observations of the role of case manager.

a. Indicate the region of the country, type of agency, clinical specialty focus, and formal or informal application of the case management process.

b. Compare and contrast your experiences and observations with those of your classmates or professional peers.

2. Interview BSN-prepared nurses in at least two different clinical specialty areas and settings (institution-based and community-based) about the role of nurse case manager, its evolution, and its implementation.

a. What job title is used to describe this role in each setting?

b. Compare and contrast relevant duties and responsibilities across settings.

c. How are health promotion and disease prevention incorporated into these case manager roles?

3. Using the community resource analysis of alcohol-related problems as a guide, identify treatment options across the continuum of care in your local community for a common chronic illness (e.g., diabetes, pediatric asthma) of interest to you.

4. In your opinion, is managed health a realistic option in the current health system in your community? Provide evidence and a logical argument to support your position.

5. Analyze one "best" case management and one "worst" case management scenario from your professional experience. Applying stages of the process of case management from this chapter, discuss why the "best" case was optimally managed and how the "worst" case can be improved.

REFERENCES

American Association of Colleges of Nursing. (1996). *The essentials of master's education for advanced practice nursing. Report from the Task Force on Essentials of Master's Education for Advanced Practice Nursing.* Washington, DC: Author.

American Association of Colleges of Nursing. (1998). *The essentials of baccalaureate education for professional nursing practice.* Washington, DC: Author.

Baker, E. L., Melton, R. J, Stange, P. V., Fields, M. L. Koplan, J. P., Guerra, F. A., & Satcher, D. (1994). Health reform and the health of the public: Forging community health partnerships. *Journal of the American Medical Association, 272,* 1276–1282.

Bower, K. (1992). *Case management by nurses.* Washington, DC: American Nurses Association.

Bower, K., & Falk, C. (1996). Case management as a response to quality, cost, and access imperatives. In E. M. Cohen (Ed.), *Nurse case management in the 21st century.* St. Louis: Mosby.

Cary, A. (1996). Case management. In M. Stanhope & J. Lancaster (Eds.). *Community health nursing* (4th ed., pp. 357–374). St. Louis: Mosby.

Cary, A. H. (2000). Case management. In M. Stanhope & J. Lancaster (Eds.), *Community health nursing* (5th ed., pp. 380–399). St. Louis: Mosby.

Case Management Society of America. (1995). *Standards of practice for case management.* Little Rock, AR: Author.

Cesta, T., Tahan, H., & Fink, L. (1998). *The case manager's survival guide.* St. Louis: Mosby.

Clarke, J. (1998). The international classification for nursing practice. In J. McCloskey & H. Grace (Eds.), *Current issues in nursing* (5th ed.). St Louis: Mosby.

Cohen, E., & Cesta, T. G. (1997). *Nursing case management: From concept to evaluation* (2nd ed.). St. Louis: Mosby.

Conrad, D. A., & Shortell, S. M. (1997). Integrated health systems: Promise and performance. *Frontiers of Health Services Management, 13*(1), 3–40.

Dieckmann, J. L. (1994). Home health administration: An overview. In M. H. Harris (Ed.), *Handbook of Home Health Care Administration* (pp. 3–13) Gaithersburg, MD: Aspen.

Flarey, D. L., & Blancett, S. S. (1996). Case management: Delivering care in the age of managed care. In D. Flarey & S. Blancett (Eds.), *Handbook of nursing case management.* Gaithersburg, MD: Aspen.

Heinrich, J. (1983). Historical perspective on public health nursing. *Nursing Outlook, 31*(6), 317–320.

Johnson, M., Maas, M., & Moorhead, S. (Eds.). (2000). *The nursing outcome classification* (2nd ed.). St. Louis: Mosby.

Joel, L. A. (1998). From NANDA to ICNP. *American Journal of Nursing, 98*(7), 7.

Kulbok, P. A., & Utz, S. W. (1999). Managing care: Knowledge and educational strategies for professional development. *Family & Community Health, 22*(3), 1–11.

Leavell, H. F., & Clark, E. G. (1965). *Preventive medicine for the doctor in his community: An epidemiologic approach.* New York: McGraw-Hill.

Lee, J. L. (1993). A history of care modalities in nursing. In K. Kelly (Ed.) & M. Maas (Chair of the Board), *Managing Nursing Care: Promise and Pitfalls. Series on Nursing Administration, 5:* 20–38.

Martin, K., & Scheet, N. (1992). *The Omaha system: Applications for community health nursing.* Philadelphia: Saunders.

McCloskey, J. C., & Bulechek, G. M. (1994). Standardizing the language for nursing treatments: An overview of the issues. *Nursing Outlook, 42*(2), 56–63.

McCloskey, J. C., & Bulechek, G. M. (Eds.). (2000). *Nursing interventions classification.* St. Louis: Mosby.

National Guideline Clearing House. (1999). Washington, DC. Retrieved Aug. 11, 1999, from the World Wide Web: http://www.guideline.gov

North American Nursing Diagnosis Association. (1999–2000). *Nursing diagnoses: Definitions and classification.* Philadelphia: Author.

Pacala, J. T., &. Boult, C. (1997). *Praplus screening of older populations.* Minneapolis: University of Minnesota Medical School, Department of Family Practice and Community Health.

Pew Health Professions Commission. (1997). *Healthy America: Practitioners for 2005, an agenda for action for U.S. Health Professional Schools.* San Francisco: Pew Memorial Trust.

Powell, S. K. (1996). *Nursing case management: A practical guide to success in managed care.* Philadelphia: Lippincott-Raven.

Powell, S. K. (2000). *Nursing case management: A practical guide to success in managed care* (2nd ed.). Philadelphia: Lippincott-Raven.

Shortell, S. M., Gillies, R. R., & Devers, K. J. (1995).

Reinventing the American hospital. *The Milbank Quarterly, 73,* 131–160.

Tahan, H. A., &. Cesta, T. G. (1996). Evaluating the effectiveness of case management plans. In D. I. Flarey & S. S. Blancett (Eds.), *Handbook of nursing case management* (pp. 184–193). Gaithersburg, MD: Aspen.

Utz, S. W. (1998). Computerized documentation of case management: From diagnosis to outcomes. *Nursing Case Management, 3,* 247–254.

Utz, S. W., & Kulbok, P. A. (1999). Managing care through advanced practice nursing. In J. Lancaster (Ed.), *Nursing Issues in Leading and Managing Change.* St. Louis: Mosby.

Ware, J., Kosinski, M., Bayliss, M., McHorney, C., Rogers, W., Raczek, A. (1995). Comparison of methods for the scoring and statistical analysis of SF-36 health profile and summary measures: summary of results from the Medical Outcomes Study. *Medical Care, 33*(4Suppl), AS264–279.

Williams, S. J., & Torrens, P. R. (1993). *Introduction to health services.* New York: Delmar.

8

Leadership and Management Strategies

MARY GUNTHER, PhD, RN

OBJECTIVES

At the completion of this chapter, the reader will be able to:

- Compare and contrast leadership and management.
- Describe the personal attributes of leaders and managers.
- Analyze the functions and roles assumed by leaders and managers.
- Discuss classical and modern theories of leadership and management.
- Discuss strategies used by successful leaders and managers.

PROFILE IN PRACTICE

Kim Massey, MSN, RN
Director, Pediatric Administration
University of Tennessee Medical Center
Knoxville, Tennessee

After obtaining my BSN, I worked as a staff nurse in a very busy pediatric intensive care unit. For 3 years I concentrated on expanding my clinical knowledge and technical skills and learned a tremendous amount from the experienced staff in the unit. I began working as a charge nurse and eventually became assistant head nurse. Six years after starting my career I was promoted to head nurse. It took me only 2 weeks to resign, but my supervisor refused to accept my resignation. She supported and encouraged me and never took no for an answer. It was in the head nurse role that I really learned what leadership was all about. My BSN knowledge base assisted in fulfilling my role, but I knew I needed additional education.

I completed a master's degree in nursing and decided to take a clinical leadership role in another state. I worked as an emergency/trauma staff nurse educator for a few months before becoming hospital trauma coordinator. I had to gain credibility from the medical and nursing staff by participating in the clinical aspects of patient care before I could begin didactic instruction and change time-honored practices. This was a completely new experience, as I had responsibility for a combined adult and pediatric program but no line authority. However, since I did not have to keep detailed personnel records and could concentrate on improving clinical skills, I had more freedom to be creative.

After a few years, I was appointed clinical instructor at the University of South Florida. Teaching new students was like a breath of fresh air— all that fresh enthusiasm for the profession!

Since then I have returned to an administrative role and now provide leadership for nurses and physicians as well as some social workers, dietitians, clerical staff, and technicians. I have learned throughout my career that in order to be an effective leader, you need the following: a desire to improve yourself or the ways things are being done, dissatisfaction with the status quo, lots of energy, an ability to think out of the box, discipline, self-direction, a view of change as opportunity and challenge, a desire for lifelong learning, and a persistent sense of humor.

Although there is increasing agreement that you cannot be one without being the other, some authors continue to differentiate between leaders and managers. The difference lies in not only *what* these people do, but also *how* they do it. You lead people, you manage things. Whereas *leaders* achieve goals through motivation of people, *managers* accomplish work through control of resources. Curtin (1997) states that managers provide structure and context, to which leaders add vision, integrity, stimulation, and commitment. Flarey (1997) views *leadership* as an art involving determination, dreams, innovation, and charisma, whereas *management* is a science about discipline and methodology. *Management* is an assigned role frequently rewarding competence; *leadership* is an attained position resulting from individual personality characteristics (Murphy-Ruocco, 1997). In a descriptive study of nurses, Manfredi (1996) noted:

> In executing the managerial role, the nurse manager is responsible for maintaining the unit in a steady state, upholding policies, managing the budget, and maintaining morale. In executing the leadership role, the nurse manager must be a visionary, anticipate the future, challenge the present, take risks, introduce innovations, and motivate staff toward goal achievement (p. 315).

Major differences between leadership and management identified in the literature are summarized in Table 8–1.

In today's world of flattened hierarchical structures, leadership is expected to emerge from an expansion of managerial responsibilities

TABLE 8–1 Leadership versus Management

	Leadership	Management
Form	Art	Science
Power base	Expert and referent power	Legitimate, reward, and coercive power
Source	Attained role	Assigned role
Style	Transformational	Transactional
Function	Motivate people by:	Regulate resources by:
	Facilitating	Planning
	Coordinating	Organizing
	Communicating	Directing
	Mentoring	Coordinating
		Controlling

(Lehmann, 1996; Murphy-Ruocco, 1997; Spitzer, 1996), but it is also critical that staff nurses develop leadership competencies, as they have a major impact on the perception of the quality of care and the organization's effectiveness (Krejci & Malin, 1997). Most authors agree that both leadership and management can be learned, although Mintzberg (1997) cautions:

> Management, meaning also leadership, is not some technical skill, like calligraphy. It cannot be picked up in a classroom; it is a practice that grows from experience (which can then be helped by certain classroom activities). Leadership has to be earned, by showing an ability to inspire people and move organizations. And it grows out of a deep understanding of the situation being managed (p. 14).

Because of the massive breadth and depth of the subject, this chapter can provide only an elementary overview of leadership and management. Following a description of each, the terms leadership and management are used interchangeably unless otherwise noted. The reader is encouraged to use this chapter as a starting pont in exploring the theory and practice applications of the role.

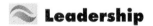

Leadership

Grossman and Valiga (2000) note that more than 350 definitions of leadership can be found in the literature of various disciplines. *Leadership* has been identified as a collection of personality traits, a role, and a process. By far the most frequently cited and most important characteristic of a leader is that of being a *visionary,* which is congruent with the common meaning of one who goes ahead in order to lead others. This forward thinking results in seeing possible futures. A *vision* is the ideal image of a unique future toward which the leader steers the group or organization (Gregory, 1995). Leaders deliberately involve others in their plans of action in order to achieve that future (Parse, 1997; Perra,

2000). Leaders are intelligent, adaptable, creative, energetic, persistent, empathic, and ethical (Crotty, 1995; Flarey, 1996; Goleman, 1998; Murphy-Ruocco, 1997; Spitzer, 1996; Tappen, 2001; Zwingman-Bagley, 1999) while being available, humorous, fair, consistent, decisive, humble, objective, and tough (Trott & Windsor, 1999). Perra's (2000) *integrated leadership practice model* states that self-knowledge, respect, trust, and integrity are the fundamental principles guiding leaders' actions. Open to new ideas while being committed, indeed passionate, about achieving their goals, leaders are confident risk-takers because they possess the ability to see both the whole picture and the individuals involved—the forest *and* the trees.

A leader's role encompasses facilitating, coordinating, communicating, and mentoring in order to get others to work more effectively (Goleman, 1998; Manion, 1997; Porter-O'Grady, 1997a; Taccetta-Chapnick, 1996; Zwingman-Bagley, 1999). Leaders work toward honing their communication skills, maximizing resources, and managing large amounts of information (Bernhard & Walsh, 1995). Nurse leaders interviewed for a descriptive research study stated that their visions of and methods for achieving quality patient care and satisfying work environments came from professional reading, attending professional conferences, and obtaining advanced academic degrees (Manfredi, 1996). It is the nurse leaders' ability to clearly articulate the contribution nursing makes to health care that enables them to obtain the resources needed to realize their vision. They become experts in environmental assessment, strategic planning, program implementation, and outcome evaluation. Kerfoot (2000) notes that the successful nurse leader incorporates nursing's emphasis on the person-environment interaction by demonstrating the interrelatedness of technology (such as medical treatments and electronic records) and the human condition (health). Zwingman-Bagley (1999) identifies four role competencies a leader must develop to be successful: optimizing, surviving, investing, and transforming. In other words, the leader

- makes the most effective use of resources.
- maintains a stated standard of performance.
- develops potential leaders.
- creates a positive environment to overcome barriers to goal attainment.

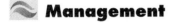

Management

Management is a logical process aimed at controlling the production of services and goods. Paralleling most problem-solving techniques, it includes gathering data, identifying limitations and strengths, creating a plan, taking action, and evaluating results. In order to effectively use these processes, a manager must possess a broad knowledge of the organization's internal and external environments, display political savvy, and accept responsibility for outcomes (Mateo, Frusti, & Newton, 1997). Enthusiastically identifying with the nursing profession and collaborating with hospital administrators, an effective nurse manager conveys to the staff an optimistic understanding of the effects of health care reforms to prevent feelings of powerlessness or victimization (Fosbinder, Everson-Bates, & Hendrix, 2000). While many managers possess the same personal characteristics identified as necessary for leaders to establish successful relationships, the emphasis of this role remains on completing the tasks needed to reach organizational goals. An effective manager is one who is flexible enough to manage both change and the conflict it may engender (Fosbinder, Everson-Bates, & Hendrix, 2000). Traditional roles of the manager include

- obtaining the resources necessary to do the work.
- assigning the work to individuals.
- telling the workers how it is to be done.
- supervising the actual process of work.
- evaluating the outcome.
- rewarding or punishing the workers.

Power

For leaders/managers, *power* (derived from a Latin word meaning "to be able") suggests energetic movement: the ability to obtain resources and influence others, joined with the right to take control of a situation. Power is much more than controlling actions; it is the "manipulation of thoughts, attitude, and social relationships" (Kuokkanen & Leino-Kilpi, 2000, p. 237). Unfortunately, for many nurses working in traditional hierarchical organizations that promote patriarchal and authoritarian leadership styles, power negatively equates with restrictive control (Dixon, 1999; Kuokkanen & Leino-Kilpi, 2000).

Hawks (1991), in an extensive analysis of the concept based in King's (1981) nursing framework, differentiates between *power to* and *power over*, or effectiveness versus dominance. Some degree of both facets of power is inherent in leadership and management. What differs is the origin of such power. The organization grants the right to exert control to specific managers, while leaders earn the right from other group members. *Legitimate, reward,* and *coercive power* are organizationally imposed forms that allow the leader/manager to assume the authority necessary to achieve goals through reward and punishment motivators. A nurse manager exerting these forms of power is guided by standards of practice and care, organizational and unit policies, and administrative disciplinary procedures (Manfredi, 1996). On the other hand, *expert* and *referent* powers emerge from the group being led. Such forms of power express the group's respect for expertise or admiration of personality characteristics and require the nurse manager to share knowledge while obtaining the staff's cooperation and participation in change. While a person may be granted more than one type of power, managers most often function using the imposed types while leaders exert the emergent forms. Differing forms of power granted simultaneously to a manager and a group-appointed leader who do not share a common goal result in conflict and confusion, whereas a balance of power facilitates collaboration (Bernhard & Walsh, 1995; Jennings & Meleis, 1988).

Style

The degree to which a person exerts power, how decisions are made, and what the person values most (relationships with other people or getting the job done) results in a pattern of interaction behavior known as *style* (Bernhard & Walsh, 1995; Valiga & Grossman, 1997). Leadership behavior may be either transactional or transformational. The *transactional leader* is the traditional manager who has a contract with employees wherein rewards and punishments depend on effort and results. The *transformational leader* is a visionary who inspires followers to move beyond their self-interests to increased awareness of the overall organization. As Trott & Windsor (1999) explain, "[T]he transactional leader can be compared to the crisis manager, 'putting out fires' so to speak. The transformational leader on the other hand is the visionary who prevents fires from starting in the first place" (p. 128). Nursing research links both transactional and transformational leader behaviors positively to job satisfaction, outcomes, and perceived effectiveness, and therefore indirectly to the quality of nursing care (Morrison, Jones, & Fuller, 1997; Stordeur, Vandenberghe, & D'hoore, 2000).

As illustrated in Figure 8–1, if the amount of power retained by the leader/manager is placed on a continuum from total to none, the three generic categories of style are authoritative, democratic, and laissez faire.

MANAGEMENT STYLE

The *authoritative* style (also known as *paternalistic* or *bureaucratic*) involves the leader/manager retaining total control, dominating the group, and, often, using fear as a motivator. As Valiga and Grossman (1997) point out, orders are given and obedience is expected. Although such a style obviously results in decreased individual creativity and autonomy, it is useful in times of crisis when there is little or no time for collaborative decision making (Crotty, 1995). The exact opposite of the authoritative style is the *laissez-faire* (also known as *permissive*) style, in which the group has total control and freedom. Indeed, the person supposedly directing the group is so passive and inactive it is difficult to apply the title "leader" or "manager." Unless the group is very mature, this style results in confusion, apathy, and minimal productivity. Somewhere between these two styles lies the *democratic* style (frequently referred to as *collaborative, participative,* or *collegial*). Very successful when implementing change, this style allows group members the opportunity to make suggestions, offer criticism, and take responsibility for mutual decisions. Research studies support the hypotheses of a positive relationship between leader/manager style and staff job satisfaction, productivity, and organizational commitment. Job satisfaction increases as style

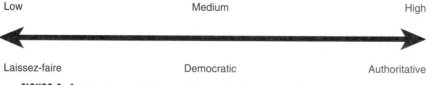

FIGURE 8–1 Continuum of degree of control and corresponding management style.

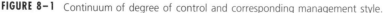

moves toward the participative mode, while both authoritative and laissez-faire styles result in frustration and diminished effectiveness (Laschinger et al., 1999; McNeese-Smith, 1997; Moss & Rowles, 1997).

Leadership and Management Theories

Person, group, and situational characteristics determine the amount of power exerted by the leader/manager (or conversely, the amount of freedom granted to subordinates). Studies of persons successful in this role yield theories about common characteristics and patterns of behavior. Such theories become organizing frameworks for describing, explaining, and predicting how leaders and managers get the work done (Alexander, 1998). Table 8–2 provides a synopsis of selected theories.

CLASSICAL THEORY

The Industrial Revolution resulted in increasing numbers of people working outside their homes and an increase in the size of the groups coordinating efforts to manufacture products. Deciding that a set of rules was necessary to promote efficiency, theorists turned to military and religious organizations as models, resulting in a hierarchical bureaucratic approach to manage-

TABLE 8-2 Synopsis of Leadership/Management Theories

Theory	Proposition
Traitist theories	
"Great man"	Leadership is dependent on genetics and predisposing personality traits.
Emotional intelligence	Emotional competence is measured by self-awareness, motivation, self-regulation, empathy, and social skill in relationships.
Classical management	Eliminating wasteful motion increases productivity.
Motivational theories	
Theory X	Human beings are self-centered, lazy, and unmotivated.
Theory Y	Human beings are interested in others, eager and willing, and motivated by the satisfaction that accepting responsibility brings.
Theory Z	Strong relationships increase commitment, resulting in decreased need for supervision and control.
Herzberg's two-factor theory	Satisfaction and dissatisfaction are separate phenomena on two separate continua and affected by completely different factors.
Situational theory	No one right leadership style fits every occasion.
Fiedler's contingency theory	A leader's style and the amount of control exerted over a group reflects the value placed on either task completion or relationships.
House's path-goal theory	Leaders motivate people by linking execution of a task with subsequent rewards.
Blanchard and Hersey's theory	Styles change, depending on the values of the leader and group member readiness to perform the task.
Transformational leadership	Those doing the work determine the outcomes and decision-making process. The leader's role is to facilitate the expression of that power.

ment. Henri Fayol (1841–1925), a French industrialist known as the "Father of Modern Management," identified the following 14 principles of management, which guided later theories: division of work; authority and responsibility; discipline; unity of command; unity of direction; subordination of individual interests to general welfare; compensation of personnel; degree of centralization; scalar chain; order; equity; retention of personnel; initiative; and esprit de corps (Fayol, 1916/1949).

Traitist Theory. Perhaps the oldest leadership theory is derived from the notion of the *Great Man*. Based in Aristotelian philosophy, it proposes that leadership is the result of both genetics and predisposing personality traits. Some versions of this classical theory presuppose a specific social or economic class (such as royalty or "high society"), while others emphasize charismatic personalities. Concentrating on prescribing the ideal personality and social acceptance necessary for a leader to emerge, these traitist theories ignore the influence of followers, situational circumstances, and the tasks to be directed (Valiga & Grossman, 1997).

Although based more on personality attributes than genetic predisposition, contemporary work on emotional intelligence may fall into the category of traitist theory. In his synthesis of research studies and leadership interviews, Goleman (1998) states that 67% of the competencies essential for successful leadership are emotional. Indeed, in this work a *competence* is defined as a "personal trait or set of habits that leads to a more effective and superior job performance" (Goleman, 1998, p. 16). The five elements constituting emotional intelligence are (1) self-awareness, (2) motivation, (3) self-regulation, (4) empathy, and (5) social skill in relationships (Bellack, 1999; Goleman, 1998; Tappen, 2001).

Emotional intelligence involves a conscious assessment of personal strengths and limitations, the recognition that emotion affects behavior, and the ability to control impulsive reactive be-

havior. Acknowledging the effect of emotions on behavior, sensitivity to others contributes to effective interpersonal relationships. This empathic awareness enables leaders to evaluate the needs, abilities, and values of individuals and groups. Successful leaders display competence in personal, social, and cognitive arenas. They are achievement oriented, self-confident, committed, influential, politically aware, and empathic. They recognize patterns and can envision the future.

Classical Management Theory. Also known as *scientific management,* classical management theory views the organization as a machine and the workers as its moving parts. The theory began with Frederick Taylor, an engineer, who believed that eliminating wasteful motion would increase productivity: the less time it took to do a task, the more times the task could be completed in a day (Taylor, 1947). Once the single best way of doing an activity is determined, it is the manager's role to select and train workers to perform these standardized actions while offering incentives to increase output. Taylor's ideas are the basis of "piecework" (specialization) and the assembly line. This is the original transactional theory, in which productivity is assured by appealing to the workers' best interests, that is, by rewarding effort (usually with money). Alexander (1998) notes that because many health care organizations continue in the machine bureaucracy mode, many traditional nurse managers continue to operate in this paradigm: using a punishment-reward system, controlling processes, and maintaining authority.

MOTIVATIONAL THEORY

Testing the propositions of Taylor's scientific management theory led to the discovery of the *Hawthorne effect,* that is, the realization that workers' behaviors change whenever attention (negative or positive) is given to them. This in turn led to an increased interest in what motivates people to work. As Goleman (1998) notes:

> Except for the financially desperate, people do not work for money alone. What also fuels their passion for work is a larger sense of purpose or mission. Given the opportunity, people gravitate to what gives them meaning, to what engages to the fullest their commitment, talent, energy, and skill (p. 58).

These theories emphasize the role of the organization more than that of the individual leader/manager (Tappen, 2001).

Theory X, Y, and Z. McGregor (1960) proposed that there are two opposing beliefs about human nature. *Theory X* states that people are naturally self-centered, lazy, and unmotivated, whereas *Theory Y* sees people as interested in others, eager and willing, and motivated by the satisfaction accepting responsibility brings. Theory X people are dependent on specific directions, strict rules, and threats of punishment. Rewards are limited to money in the form of continuing paychecks, paid time off, and pay raises. The leader's role is one of controlling close supervision to ensure that the work is ongoing and that rules are obeyed. Theory Y workers choose work that meets their needs of belonging, recognition, and self-actualization. The Theory Y worker, loyal and committed to the organization that provides such rewards, works hard to do his or her share in meeting production goals. The role of the leader is to provide the rewarding environment.

Ouchi (1981) adapted successful Japanese business practices, combined with the humanistic beliefs of Theory Y, to propose a democratic approach to leadership known as *Theory Z*. Decision making is consensual and participative, with the democratic process as the "mechanism for broad dissemination of information and of the values within the organization" (Ouchi, 1981, p. 78). Theory Z encourages long-term employment with slower promotions and broader skill bases to develop strong relation-ships among co-workers. This consistency of organizational culture and commitment to common goals allows autonomy, thus eliminating the need for close supervision and tight control. Managers choose employees based on similarity to their own past experiences. The fusion of work and social life, the desire for peer approval, and personal involvement in consensual decisions motivate the worker. Ouchi noted that these factors, while successful in Japan, do not allow innovation, rapid change, or diversity in management, for "the only way to influence behavior is to change the culture" (p. 88).

Herzberg's Two-Factor Theory. While interviewing engineers and accountants in the early 1950s to determine the sources of motivation, Herzberg (1966) noted that significantly different elements were identified, depending on whether people were asked what they liked or what they disliked about their jobs. This led him to believe that satisfaction and dissatisfaction are not opposite ends of the same continuum but rather two separate phenomena on two separate continua. He called the elements affecting satisfaction *motivational factors* and those affecting dissatisfaction *hygiene factors*. Motivational factors include the nature of the work to be done, achievements and recognition, the amount of responsibility granted, and the opportunity for personal and professional growth. Hygiene factors embody organizational and environmental elements: policies, working conditions, degree of supervision, job security, and salary. Other hygiene factors relate to how working affects one's personal life, such as the shift one works, the distance from home to job, and all the elements that may make it difficult to meet personal and family obligations.

SITUATIONAL THEORY

Situational theory more clearly addresses the interactions between and among the leader's personality, the environment, group members, and the required tasks. However, the emphasis falls on the interplay between the leader and the environment—the amount of control the former exerts over the latter. Simply put, the theory proposes that there is no one right style that fits every situation. Either a leader/manager changes styles as circumstances warrant or the need for change produces a new leader (Bernhard & Walsh, 1995; Hersey & Duldt, 1989; Valiga & Grossman, 1997). The premise is that an organization is an open system that interfaces with other systems. This interaction produces environmental changes to which the leader/manager must react by adapting. Situational styles reflect both the adaptation and the underlying values influencing the leader/manager.

Blanchard and Hersey's Situational Leadership. Choice of style depends on (1) whether the leader is more concerned with the people involved or the task to be completed and (2) the followers' willingness and ability, or readiness, to complete the tasks necessary to achieve the goals. According to Hersey and Duldt (1989), who explored how situational theory guides nurse leaders, there are four main styles: telling, selling, participating, and delegating. When the leader is more concerned with task completion and the members are least ready, *telling* (issuing direct orders) is the appropriate style. The leader retains total control. In situations where the leader is highly task- and relationship-oriented, *selling* (persuading) becomes the style of choice. Leaders who share control with their followers but still value task completion over relationships opt for a *participating* (asking for group input) style. Those who display little interest in either task completion or relationships and thus take little control over goal achievement adopt a *delegating* (placing responsibility on others) style.

Fiedler's Contingency Theory. Fiedler and Chemers (1974) proposed that individual leadership styles are fixed and cannot be changed easily, as they reflect basic values of the individ-

ual. Nevertheless, the amount of control exerted by the leader over the situation is contingent on the relationship with group members, the structure of the task, and position within the organization. The relationship between leaders and group members is the most important variable determining the leader's power, as authority is dependent on group acceptance (Fiedler & Chemers, 1974). Power and influence increase when group members highly trust and accept the leader, as evidenced by their meeting set goals. To do so, group members must understand what the goals are, the steps required to complete the task, and who is responsible for outcomes. The clearer the goal and the fewer ways of achieving it, the more powerful the leader, as detailed instructions carry organizational backing. When the task is unstructured and vague, the leader's power is diminished, "as members can argue they know as much about it as the leader" (Fiedler & Chemers, 1974, p. 66). The organization supports the actions of the leader/manager by granting reward and coercive power. The overall degree of leadership power is determined by rating relationships as good or poor, task structure as high or low, and position power as strong or weak. The most favorable rating includes good relationship, high structure, and strong position power.

House's Path-Goal Theory. In this theory, the leader is more concerned with influencing the expectations of the individual group members than with completing the task at hand. People are motivated to complete a task by their expectation that they will be rewarded for reaching a goal. Leadership behaviors aim at providing support, removing obstacles that might limit the group members' ability to complete the work, and illuminating the connection between task execution (*path*) and reward acquisition (*goal*) (Tappen, 2001). According to House (1971), leaders exhibit a combination of the following styles: directive, supportive, participative, and achievement-oriented. The leader exerts control over the task structure by defining roles, assigning responsibility, consulting group members, and rewarding productivity. Satisfaction increases with decreased role ambiguity and increased feedback. Consequently, the ability to keep the group on the right path in order to meet goals and achieve satisfaction measures leader effectiveness (Bernhard & Walsh, 1995).

TRANSFORMATIONAL LEADERSHIP THEORY

The philosophical assumptions underlying transformational leadership arise not only from motivational theories but also from quantum science, and thus speak to the nonlinearity of change and the subsequent unpredictability of consequences. Transformational leadership involves a shift from viewing organizations as controllable machine bureaucracies to seeing them as complex, adaptive, whole systems (Anderson & McDaniel, 2000). In open systems such as organizations, outcomes of actions depend on the context in which they occur and the people initiating them. Each action alters the original situation: there is a constant state of change. Increasing the number of simultaneous and sequential actions increases the number of possible outcomes. It becomes increasingly difficult to predict which outcome will result from multiple actions. Thus, the function of the leader/manager can no longer be restricted to controlling the parts, but rather must be broadened for coordination of the whole. Dixon (1999) states that "maintaining a sense of stability in unstable environments is the mantra of the 21st century" (p. 17) and can only be achieved through a balance of mind, body, and spirit.

The number of professions involved in the operation of a health care organization intensifies the complexity due to diversity in knowledge, values, and desired outcomes. Interaction between and among these professions defines the organization. Therefore, the system cannot be examined from the perspective of just one profession. Nor can the organization decide what values determine a profession's role in meeting shared goals, as these values are instilled in academic programs and perpetuated by professional organizations (Anderson & McDaniel, 2000). Managing the resultant complexity requires involving all of the relevant professions in decision making. Recognizing that one person's or one group's increase in power does not equal another's loss, transformational leaders work collaboratively with their staff using informal influence strategies rather than positional power to achieve the shared vision (Fullam et al., 1998; Ohman, 1999). Bass (1985) describes a transformational leader as one who is charismatic, able to motivate others, and who has a strong personal value system.

While a participatory management style facilitates the development of transformational leadership, this is not just another theory that *allows* those who do the work to participate in making decisions. Porter-O'Grady (1997b) specifies that because ownership of decisions belongs to those who provide the service, subsequent action cannot be required, managed, or controlled by others. The leadership processes of facilitating and coordinating now depend on the collective decisions of the followers made in light of stated organizational goals. Those doing the work determine the outcomes, and so own both the parts and whole. Such ownership of decision making and outcomes equals power. The leader provides the resources (information, training, and feedback) that facilitate the expression of that power. *Transformational leaders* structure an environment that promotes collaboration, enhances the quality of communication, decreases competition, and coordinates the exchange of information (MacDaniel, 1997). The primary responsibility of the leader is to "rouse people through the sheer power of their own enthusiasm" (Goleman, 1998, p. 196) and thus inspire followers to see beyond the narrow boundaries of their own self-interest by valuing the broader mission and purpose of the organization (Dixon, 1999; Wolf, Boland, & Aukerman, 1994). According to Curtin (1997), this is particularly relevant in health care because all "activities are directly related to the most critical human needs of an especially vulnerable population" (p. 7).

NURSING THEORY

Nurse leaders/managers encounter some difficulties when they attempt to apply traditional product-oriented strategies to a discipline whose central concern is the human being. As Smith (1993) explains:

> Health care organizations exist to provide nursing and health care; this is the "product" of these organizations. Nurses provide the expert knowledge for this "product line." Advanced knowledge about processes that enhance health and well-being are articulated within nursing theories. Therefore, understanding nursing theory is essential to understanding the product delivered by health care organizations (p. 64).

Leadership and management theories derived from nursing conceptual models are based on the philosophical premise that human response patterns are shaped by individual perceptions and experiences (Jennings & Meleis, 1988; Smith, 1993). Within these theories, operational definitions of the central concepts of the profession (person, environment, health, and nursing) guide management practice. *Person* refers to nursing staff, the department of nursing, or the entire organization; *environment* extends to include social, political, and economic influences; *health* encompasses functional efficiency and job satisfaction; while administrative structures and policies embody *nursing* (Brooks & Rosenberg, 1995; Fawcett, 1995; Smith, 1993). Nursing administration literature documents how nursing conceptual models guide the development of

- roles and functions
- practice standards
- classification and documentation systems
- quality indicators
- education plans

Leadership Management Strategies and Competencies

In addition to identifying the principles of management, Henri Fayol identified and defined five primary managerial functions incorporating these roles: planning, organizing, directing, coordinating, and controlling. Over time, descriptions of these functions have been modified by behavioral theories and systems thinking, but they continue to offer guidelines for increasing productivity and effectiveness.

PLANNING

Planning involves deciding in advance the who, what, when, why, and how of the work to be done (Grohar-Murray & DiCroce, 1997; Tappen, 2001). Usually, general information regarding *what* needs to be done *when*, along with guidelines concerning the *who* and *how*, are determined by the organization's goals and resources. These resources include money, people, equipment, and time. An effective nurse manager incorporates unit-specific goals addressing the quality and cost of patient care with both administrative goals and staff development needs. The manager's task then is to create a detailed procedural design using this information. The more information the manager gathers, the better the plan. Planning incorporates

- specifying goals and objectives.
- determining priorities.
- analyzing alternative methods of achieving set objectives.
- choosing a method.
- specifying a time span for implementing the chosen method.
- describing possible barriers, and solutions for overcoming them.
- devising a method of evaluating outcomes (Rowland & Rowland, 1997).

In addition, the manager plans the work of the group by defining the extent of staff participation in decision making, deciding the sequence in which tasks must be completed, determining what skills the staff members must possess, and allocating resources to each step of the plan (Tappen, 1995). This requires not only knowledge of the organization's internal environment, but also a broad overview of external forces such as health care law, economics, standards, and established nursing practice. Crucial to managerial success is the effective use of a major resource—time. Table 8–3 gives some tips on time management.

Strategic Planning. A proactive systematic process, *strategic planning* identifies goals and objectives for a specified time period. A written plan outlines in concise terms who will accomplish what and by when. A dynamic document used to guide daily activities, the plan should be continuously reviewed and revised as needed to meet the goals. Sharing the planning process and reporting progress toward goal attainment with everyone involved increases the likelihood of successfully meeting the stated goals. The assessment phase commences with a review of the organization's mission and vision statement, remembering that *mission* describes the nature of the business while *vision* delineates a management philosophy (Gregory, 1995). Determining goals with these statements in mind ensures congruence with overall organizational goals. A *S-W-O-T* environmental analysis can be useful in setting realistic goals. Start by assessing the organization's internal environment for *strengths* and *weaknesses*, then examine the external environment for *opportunities* and *threats*. Internal strengths and weaknesses may include administrative support, resources (people and money), physical facilities, and staff willingness and ability to implement the program and achieve set goals. External opportunities and threats deal primarily with competitive services offered by other agencies, funding sources, and governmental regulations.

TABLE 8–3 Tips on Time Management

Make to-do lists daily. Spend the first 15 minutes of your day identifying what you want to accomplish. Be realistic, and include uncompleted tasks from the previous day.

Prioritize the activities as of critical importance (must do), moderate importance (should do), or minimal importance (would be nice to do).

Do the most important things first.

Concentrate on one task at a time. Talking on the telephone while you read your mail means you will miss details.

Establish deadlines for completing tasks; enter these onto your appointment calendar.

Do it now! The longer you put it off, the more you will worry about it and the more stress you will feel.

Touch each piece of paper only once. After reading mail either take action, file it, or throw it out!

Keep your workspace clean and uncluttered to avoid feeling overwhelmed by paper.

'Learn to say no if you cannot take on any more projects.

If subordinates need information that is not in your immediate possession in order to complete their assignment, don't volunteer to find it out for them. Tell them whom to call.

Become computer literate; use project management software.

Use your appointment calendar as a diary to record daily activities. This will help when you are writing progress reports.

ORGANIZING

Organizing is the process of identifying the tasks to be accomplished, grouping the necessary responsibilities and activities into discrete units, assigning lines of authority and communication, and developing patterns of coordination between individuals and the organization as a whole (Rowland & Rowland, 1997). It encompasses the creation of vertical and horizontal structures, the chain of command and the division of labor. The underlying premise embraces the belief in the need for a clear chain of command with authority equaling assigned responsibility.

The *vertical structure* (referred to as the hierarchical organization) defines the gradation of superiors and subordinates, including who has authority to direct and who has responsibility to ensure task completion in the nurse manager's absence (for example, assistant head nurse or charge nurse). There are two relationships inherent in the hierarchy: line and staff. Group members in a *line position* have assigned authority and responsibilities; those in a *staff position* provide advice or technical support to line managers. For example, head nurses are in line positions, while clinical nurse specialists and educators usually are considered staff relationships. Although authority and responsibility may be delegated to varying degrees, the manager retains overall accountability. Being *accountable* means that the manager is aware of what is being done and why. That is, the manager is able to provide a rational explanation of actions taken. Although accountability is embedded in the management role and cannot be delegated, it is not synonymous with being indispensable (Mateo, Frusti, & Newton, 1997; Porter-O'Grady & Wilson, 1995).

Horizontal structures separate large tasks into discrete steps and assign responsibility for completion of these increments to the appropriate staff skill level. In this way, the manager defines the formal relationship among staff members through delineation of roles. *Position descrip-*

tions and *policy statements* describe horizontal structures.

DIRECTING

Directing aims at getting the work done by others through initiation and maintenance of actions. Delegating, communicating, training, and motivating are all elements of directing (Rowland & Rowland, 1997). The manager makes work assignments based on the staff members' abilities and learning needs while communicating clear expectations of what needs to be accomplished.

Delegating. *Delegation* entails transferring the authority to perform a selected task in a specific situation to a competent individual while retaining accountability for the outcome (National Council of State Boards of Nursing, 1995). It is the retention of accountability that makes delegating different from "assigning" a task. Delegating is a five-step process:

- Selecting the task.
- Selecting the person.
- Instructing and motivating.
- Maintaining control.
- Assessing performance and outcomes (Hansten & Washburn, 1994).

When working with unlicensed assistive personnel, staff nurses direct patient care through delegation to team members and need to develop the same skills as nurse managers. Managers usually delegate tasks that are routine and of low priority in order to free up their time for more demanding work, tasks required during an emergency, and tasks that need to be completed in their absence. In other situations, managers recognize that delegation promotes the acquisition of problem-solving skills. The leader, however, must be available to teach and assist when a task is delegated to a group member who does not know how to do it. Managers should be consciously aware of why they are delegating the task and why they have chosen that particular group member to be responsible for completing it. The National Council of State Boards of Nursing (1995) advocates using the "five rights of delegation" to facilitate decisions about what can be delegated: the *right task* in the *right circumstances* to the *right person* with the *right direction* under the *right supervision*. Managers should *never* delegate the power to discipline or the responsibility of maintaining the positive attitude of a group.

The primary ingredient of successful delegation lies in selecting a competent nurse or other individual (delegate) whose actual or potential qualifications match the task. The manager owes the individual delegate a detailed explanation of the purpose and expected outcome of the task as well as the amount of authority granted to achieve that outcome. Depending on the nature of the task and the delegate's familiarity with it, the manager includes procedural details and arranges necessary training. It is essential to identify and adhere to reasonable deadlines for both reporting progress and completing the task. Then it is time to let the delegate work without oversupervision. With less structured tasks, the delegate's method may differ from that of the manager. If the results are acceptable, the manager should not redo the task. If the delegate makes a mistake, the manager should take the time to review the process and teach the correct method. Feedback to the delegate includes both a private performance evaluation and public recognition of successful task completion. Successful delegation depends on the manager's confidence that the delegate will succeed.

Communicating. *Communication* is the exchange of information and, more important, meaning between two or more people. Goleman (1998) calls communication the keystone of all social skills, while Flarey (1996) notes it is the power driving others to achieve the vision. Since leaders estimate that they spend 50%–90% of their time communicating in some form, it is appropriate to equate leadership skills with communication skills (Crotty, 1995; Grieshaber, 1993). The use of assertive communication and active listening techniques by the leader facilitates effective interaction with others.

Assertiveness encompasses a clear, honest, and appropriate statement of feelings, needs, and ideas without violating the rights of others. Nonassertive behavior may be either aggressive or submissive. *Aggressive people* demand rather than ask. Frequently defensive or angry, aggressors mount a direct attack in order to gratify their needs and wants. *Submissive people,* on the other hand, hesitate to verbalize their feelings and beliefs. They give in easily to others and therefore seldom if ever get their needs met. *Assertive leaders* express their viewpoints in a positive manner while staying open to suggestions from group members. They are in control of their emotions and understanding of different opinions and viewpoints, acknowledging that others have an equal right to feelings, beliefs, and values. When disagreeing with a statement or denying a request, the assertive leader reacts with an empathic explanation: "I understand that you want/need/believe . . . and I want/need/believe . . . because . . . ." Assertive leaders *actively listen* to the message being conveyed (verbally and nonverbally), seek clarification if uncertain of the message's meaning, and provide feedback concerning specific behaviors and results (Breisch, 1999; Goleman, 1998; Tappen, 1995). Active listeners are capable of letting others voice their opinions without interruption or ridicule. As Blount and Nahigian (1998) note: "Expressed thoughts and feelings can contribute to new meanings more positively than suppressed fears. Openness is essential for productive change" (p. 29).

COORDINATING

Coordinating is the act of maintaining balance among resources by prioritizing and synchronizing activities (Grohar-Murray & DiCroce, 1997). It involves timing of activities, resource allocation, conflict management, and team building. Ensuring that work goes smoothly and that workers cooperate with each other depends on good planning, organizing, and directing. Knowing that no one individual or one discipline works in isolation, health care managers integrate their team into the larger organization.

Conflict Management. *Conflict* is a struggle between two or more persons resulting from a difference in beliefs and value systems, expectations, or interpretation. Unclear roles, ambiguous communication, and competition for resources can contribute to conflict. An inherent element in society, conflict can affect the health of people, their relationships, and organizations. The absence of conflict, however, does not necessarily equate with health. Conflict stimulates interest and increases innovative thinking. As Crowell (1998) points out, "Being too nice to each other will inhibit growth and diminish relationships. Relationships are enhanced and enriched by living through conflict and chaos and reaching the other side, knowing and understanding each other better" (p. 29). Leaders have prime responsibility for managing, not resolving, conflict so that the involved parties are satisfied and their needs met.

Individuals manage conflict through avoidance, accommodation, collaboration, competition, or compromise. Although *avoiding* (not addressing the issue) may intensify the underlying problem, it can also be the appropriate approach when the cost of getting what is wanted is greater than the benefit. This can happen in situations where one player is much more powerful than the other, or the issue itself is relatively unimportant (McElhaney, 1996). McNeese-Smith (1997) notes that staff nurses voice frustration with managers who routinely avoid addressing conflict. Such frustration results in decreased job satisfaction, productivity, and organizational commitment. Sometimes the same circumstances warrant *accommodation*, that is, one player refuses to compete, possibly sacrifices his or her interests, to promote harmony (Dove, 1998). The accommodating person may view this as doing a favor for the other person and expect that person to reciprocate in future interactions. A mutually agreeable solution emerges from *collaboration,* where all views are considered and to some degree incorporated in the new perspective. A lengthy process requiring time and commitment of all group members, it does more to resolve interpersonal differences than the other approaches. The opposite of accommodation is *competition,* where one person loses but not voluntarily. Rather than promoting harmony, competition may result in angry, frustrated group members who will be intent on revenge (Dove, 1998). In a *compromise* everyone gives up something in order to reach an agreement. It can lead to an antagonistic relationship if what each group gives up is not equally valued or if the compromise results in an imbalance of power.

An official form of collaboration and an essential skill for leaders is *negotiation:* a mixture of problem solving and bargaining, of educating and persuading that allows leaders to build rapport and reach consensus (Goleman, 1998; Wyatt, 1999). Negotiation happens in planned sessions rather than during chance encounters. Wyatt (1999) notes that successful negotiation involves 80% planning and 20% action. Good planning predetermines the participants and specific topics for discussion as well as the time, place, and length of the meeting. Necessary leadership behaviors include maintaining emotional control, a willingness to see the other person's point of view, assertive communication, a sensitivity to nonverbal cues; and a deliberate decision to look to the future rather than perpetuate the past (Goleman, 1998; McElhaney, 1996; Wyatt, 1999). The end product of negotiation is a formal agreement, including a written implementation and evaluation plan.

Team Building. Having identified goals and action plans is the beginning of team building. The objective of *team building* is to develop a group that is committed to both the work and to each other. Resulting from members' participation in establishing performance standards and expected outcomes, a high-performance team demonstrates accountability for and ownership of the work; trust in and support of each other; and increased competence and subsequent job satisfaction (Herman & Reichelt, 1998; Pedersen & Easton, 1995). The leader's role in building such teams includes (1) establishing a reliable method of communication, (2) clearly defining responsibilities and decision-making authority for team members, and (3) fostering a sense of trust and willingness to change. To accomplish this, the leader must

- demonstrate an ability to listen to others.
- promote collaboration among members and between teams.
- delegate appropriately (Husting, 1996).

CONTROLLING

A manager sets or adopts standards of performance against which actual performance, as determined by outcomes, is evaluated. When necessary, the manager takes corrective action to adjust variances between the standard and the actual performance. Monitoring the work on an ongoing basis allows the manager to control both processes and outcomes. *Controlling* requires identifying what skills need to be strengthened, motivating others to attain these skills, and providing positive feedback. Specific aspects of controlling include:

- personnel evaluation, discipline, and behavior modification
- resource allocation and inventory
- quality assurance and outcome research programs
- compliance with regulatory and government agency rules

Performance Appraisal. Most organizations have a formal performance appraisal system providing written feedback to each employee on an annual basis. Based on written and published job descriptions, *performance appraisals* include written documentation and face-to-face discussion with the staff member that results in written goals to be achieved within a specified period of time (Rowland & Rowland, 1997; Tappen, Weiss, & Whitehead, 1998). Standards used to evaluate performance need to be clear, objective, known in advance by staff members, and applied consistently, since rewards (e.g., salary increases) and disciplinary actions (e.g., demotion or termination) are attached to the outcomes (Tappen, Weiss, & Whitehead, 1998).

The purpose of a *performance appraisal* is to provide opportunities for personal and professional growth and to ensure the quality of nursing care. A meaningful performance appraisal requires the manager both to observe specific behaviors and to analyze feedback from others. This means attending shift reports and unit meetings, reviewing records and reports, and observing the staff member at the patient's bedside (Manfredi, 1996), as well as collecting information about interactions with other employees, other departments, and the general public. Behaviors then are compared with expectations previously published in written standards, job descriptions, and clinical advancement criteria. Frequently the staff member is asked to come to the evaluation session after having completed a self-assessment of strengths and weaknesses. This helps the manager gain insight into the staff member's perception of his or her own abilities and needs. When variances from expected standards are identified, the nurse manager first must decide if the staff member has developmental issues (e.g., lack of knowledge or opportunities to attain a skill) or actual performance problems (e.g., a conscious refusal to comply with policies and procedures) prior to devising an action plan for improvement (Horvath et al., 1997).

It is important that both the manager and the employee understand that the purpose of a performance appraisal is not punitive but rather is an opportunity for recognizing the staff member's quality of work and identifying areas of future professional development. In this role, the manager is a coach. As Donner, Wheeler, and Waddell (1997) explain:

> *Coaching* is an ongoing, face-to-face process by which the manager and employee collaborate to achieve increased job knowledge, improved skills in carrying out job responsibilities, a stronger and more positive working relationship, and opportunities for personal as well as professional growth for the individual (p. 15).

As such, coaching includes an ongoing assessment of current behaviors, educational counseling, and identification of areas to be developed.

≋ Comment

In today's health care environment, the lines separating managers from leaders are becoming increasingly blurred. Management functions often spill over into the staff nurse role. All nurses are charged with managing resources, redesigning processes, and ensuring quality of patient care at some level. Speaking of the role of nurse leaders and their relationship to staff nurses, Beyers (1999) notes, "[T]he management of this complex and valuable patient care resource is a study of change, of innovation, of chaos, and of values" (p. 592). The complex, dynamic nature of the health care system presents special challenges and exciting opportunities for the nurse leader and manager.

KEY POINTS

- Leadership is the art of motivating others to achieve organizational goals; management is the science of controlling resources.
- A leader's role encompasses facilitating, coordinating, communicating, and mentoring in order to get others to work more effectively.
- The five primary functions of a manager are planning, organizing, directing, coordinating, and controlling.

- Power is the ability to control resources and the right to take control of a situation.
- Style is a pattern of behavior reflecting the exertion of power, decision-making processes, and individual values.
- Leadership and management theories are organizing frameworks for describing, explaining, and predicting how work is accomplished by identifying common characteristics and patterns of behavior.
- Strategic planning is a proactive, systematic process of identifying goals and objectives for a specific time period. It involves an assessment of the strengths and weaknesses of the organization along with opportunities for and threats to goal attainment.
- Organizing encompasses the creation of a chain of command and the division of labor.
- Elements of directing include delegating, communicating, training, and motivating.
- The "five rights of delegation" facilitate decisions about what can be delegated: the *right task* in the *right circumstances* to the *right person* with the *right direction* under the *right supervision*.
- Effective communication necessitates assertive expression and active listening.
- Individuals manage conflict through avoidance, accommodation, collaboration, competition, or compromise.
- A leader builds effective teams by establishing reliable communication methods, clearly defining responsibilities and decision-making authority, and fostering a sense of trust.
- Controlling involves setting standards and evaluating performance as well as correcting variances.

CRITICAL THINKING EXERCISES

1. Write a short paragraph articulating your vision for each of the following:

a. Nursing as a profession
b. Your health care agency
c. Your clinical nursing unit

2. Consider nursing leaders/managers with whom you are familiar. Identify and discuss their style, including forms and sources of power.

3. Identify the leadership/management theory you find most appealing. Discuss how it would guide your practice.

4. You have been charged with the responsibility of starting a new skilled nursing unit in your hospital. Conduct a *S-W-O-T* analysis.

5. You are the manager of a general surgical nursing unit with a staff composed of registered nurses and nursing assistants. Identify tasks that you would delegate to each job classification, and discuss your reasons.

6. It has become increasingly obvious that you and the other registered nurse on your team do not agree about patient care delivery. The two of you work together every day and have equal amounts of power. Discuss how you could use each of the five conflict management styles in this situation.

REFERENCES

Alexander, V. A. (1998). Participative nursing management: A necessity for survival. *Kansas Nurse, 73*(9), 4–5.

Anderson, R. A., & McDaniel, R. R. (2000). Managing health care organizations: Where professionalism meets complexity science. *Health Care Management Review, 25*(1), 83–92.

Bass, B. M. (1985). *Leadership and performance beyond expectations.* New York: Macmillan.

Bellack, J. P. (1999). Emotional intelligence: A missing ingredient? *Journal of Nursing Education, 38*(1), 3–4.

Bernhard, L. A., & Walsh, M. (1995). *Leadership: The key to the professionalization of nursing.* St. Louis: Mosby.

Beyers, M. (1999). The management of nursing services. In L. F. Wolper (Ed.), *Health care administration* (pp. 574–595). Gaithersburg, MD: Aspen.

Blount, K., & Nahigian, E. (1998). How to build teams in the midst of change. *Nursing Management, 29*(8), 27–29.

Breisch, L. R. (1999). Motivate! *Nursing Management, 30*(3), 27–30.

Brooks, B. A., & Rosenberg, S. (1995). Incorporating nursing theory into a nursing department strategic plan. *Nursing Administration Quarterly, 20*(1), 81–86.

Crotty, G. (1995). Myths about leadership. *Tennessee Nurse, 58*(1), 17–18.

Crowell, D. M. (1998). Organizations are relationships: A new view of management. *Nursing Management, 29*(5), 28–29.

Curtin, L. (1997). How—and how *not*—to be a transformational leader. *Nursing Management, 28*(2), 7–8.

Dixon, D. L. (1999). Achieving results through transformational leadership. *Journal of Nursing Administration, 29*(12), 17–21.

Donner, G. J., Wheeler, M. M., & Waddell, J. (1997). The nurse manager as career coach. *Journal of Nursing Administration, 27*(12), 14–18.

Dove, M. A. (1998). Conflict: Process and resolution. *Nursing Management, 29*(4), 30–32.

Fawcett, J. (1995). *Analysis and evaluation of conceptual models of nursing* (3rd ed.). Philadelphia: Davis.

Fayol, H. (1949). *General and industrial management* (Constance Storrs, Trans.). London: Pitman. (Original work published 1916)

Fiedler, F. E., & Chemers, M. M. (1974). *Leadership and effective management.* Glenview, IL: Scott, Foresman.

Flarey, D. L. (1996). Case studies in nursing management. *Seminars for Nurse Managers, 4,* 187–190.

Flarey, D. L. (1997). Management and leadership: Is there a difference? *Seminars for Nurse Managers, 5,* 8–9.

Fosbinder, D., Everson-Bates, S., & Hendrix, L. (2000). Using an interview guide to identify effective nurse managers: Phase II. Outcomes. *Nursing Administration Quarterly, 24*(2), 72–82.

Fullam, C., Lando, A. R., Johansen, M. L., Reyes, A., & Szaloczy, D. M. (1998). The triad of empowerment: Leadership, environment, and professional traits. *Nursing Economics, 16,* 254–257.

Goleman, D. X. (1998). *Working with emotional intelligence.* New York: Bantam.

Gregory, C. S. (1995). Creating a vision for a nursing unit. *Nursing Management, 26*(1), 38.

Grieshaber, L. D. (1993). Managing the emerging organization. *Health Management Quarterly, 15*(4), 25–28.

Grohar-Murray, M. E., & DiCroce, H. R. (1997). *Leadership and management in nursing.* Stamford, CT: Appleton & Lange.

Grossman, S., & Valiga, T. M. (2000). *The new leadership challenge: Creating the future of nursing.* Philadelphia: Davis.

Hansten, R. I., & Washburn, M. J. (1994). The overall

process of delegation. In Hansten, R. I., et al. (Eds.), *Clinical delegation skills: A handbook for nurses* (pp. 1–8). Gaithersburg, MD: Aspen.

Hawks, J. H. (1991). Power: A concept analysis. *Journal of Advanced Nursing, 16,* 754–762.

Herman, J. E., & Reichelt, P. A. (1998). Are first-line nurse managers prepared for team building? *Nursing Management, 29*(10), 68–72.

Hersey, P., & Duldt, B. W. (1989). *Situational leadership in nursing.* Norwalk, CT: Appleton & Lange.

Herzberg, F. (1966). *Work and the nature of man.* Cleveland: World Publishing.

Horvath, K. J., Aroian, J. F., Secatore, J. A., Alpert, H., Costa, M. J., Powers, E., & Stengrevics, S. S. (1997). Vision for a treasured resource. Part 2. Nurse manager learning needs. *Journal of Nursing Administration, 27*(4), 27–31.

House, R. J. (1971). A path goal theory of leader effectiveness. *Administrative Science Quarterly, 16,* 321.

Husting, P. M. (1996). Leading work teams and improving performance. *Nursing Management, 27*(9), 35–38.

Jennings, B. M., & Meleis, A. I. (1988). Nursing theory and administrative practice: Agenda for the 1990s. *Advances in Nursing Science, 10*(3), 56–69.

Kerfoot, K. (2000). TIQ (technical IQ): A survival skill for the new millennium. *Nursing Economics, 18*(1), 29–31.

King, I. (1981). *A theory for nursing: Systems, concepts, process.* New York: Wiley.

Krejci, J. W., & Malin, S. (1997). Impact of leadership development on competencies. *Nursing Economics, 15,* 235–241.

Kuokkanen, L., & Leino-Kilpi, H. (2000). Power and empowerment in nursing: Three theoretical approaches. *Journal of Advanced Nursing, 31*(1), 235–241.

Laschinger, H. K., Wong, C., McMahon, L., & Kaufmann, C. (1999). Leader behavior impact on staff nurse empowerment, job tension, and work effectiveness. *Journal of Nursing Administration, 29*(5), 28–39.

Lehmann, D. M. (1996). Managers versus leaders/managers. *Seminars for Nurse Managers, 4,* 193–194.

MacDaniel, R. R. (1997). Strategic leadership: A view from quantum and chaos theories. *Health Care Management Review, 22*(1), 21–37.

Manfredi, C. M. (1996). A descriptive study of nurse managers and leadership. *Western Journal of Nursing Research, 18,* 314–329.

Manion, J. (1997). Teams 101: The manager's role. *Seminars for Nurse Managers, 5,* 31–38.

Mateo, M. A., Frusti, D. K. & Newton, C. (1997). Management skills in an era of shifting paradigms. *Seminars for Nurse Managers, 5,* 10–17.

McElhaney, R. (1996). Conflict management in nursing administration. *Nursing Management, 27*(3), 49–50.

McGregor, D. (1960). *The human side of enterprise.* New York: McGraw-Hill.

McNeese-Smith, D. K. (1997). The influence of manager behavior on job satisfaction, productivity, and commitment. *Journal of Nursing Administration, 27*(9), 47–55.

Mintzberg, H. (1997). Toward healthier hospitals. *Health Care Management Review, 22*(4), 9–18.

Morrison, R. S., Jones, L., & Fuller, B. (1997). The relationship between leadership style and empowerment on job satisfaction of nurses. *Journal of Nursing Administration, 27*(5), 27–34.

Moss, R., & Rowles, C. J. (1997). Staff nurse job satisfaction and management style. *Nursing Management, 28*(1), 32.

Murphy-Ruocco, M. (1997). Management. In R. K. Nunnery (Ed.), *Advancing your career: Concepts of professional nursing* (pp. 141–154). Philadelphia: Davis.

National Council of State Boards of Nursing. (1995). Delegation: Concepts and decision-making process [On-line]. Available: www.ncsbn.org

Ohman, K. (1999). Nurse manager leadership. *Journal of Nursing Administration, 29*(12), 16.

Ouchi, W. G. (1981). *Theory Z: How American business can meet the Japanese challenge.* Reading, MA: Addison-Wesley.

Parse, R. R. (1997). Leadership: The essentials. *Nursing Science Quarterly, 10*(3), 109.

Pedersen, A., & Easton, L. S. (1995). Teamwork: Bringing order out of chaos. *Nursing Management, 26*(6), 34–35.

Perra, B. M. (2000). Leadership: The key to quality outcomes. *Nursing Administration Quarterly, 24*(2), 56–61.

Porter-O'Grady, T. (1997a). Process leadership and the death of management. *Nursing Economics, 15,* 286–293.

Porter-O'Grady, T. (1997b). Quantum mechanics and the future of healthcare leadership. *Journal of Nursing Administration, 27*(1), 15–20.

Porter-O'Grady, T., & Wilson, C. K. (1995). *The leadership revolution in health care.* Gaithersburg, MD: Aspen.

Rowland, H. S., & Rowland, B. L. (1997). *Nursing administration handbook* (4th ed.). Gaithersburg, MD: Aspen.

Smith, M. C. (1993). The contribution of nursing theory to nursing administration practice. *Image: Journal of Nursing Scholarship, 25*(1), 63–67.

Spitzer, R. (1996). The dynamic of leadership. *Seminars for Nurse Managers, 4,* 185–186.

Stordeur, S., Vandenberghe, C., & D'hoore, W. (2000).

Leadership styles across hierarchical levels in nursing departments. *Nursing Research, 49*(1), 37–43.

Taccetta-Chapnick, M. (1996). Transformational leadership. *Nursing Administration Quarterly, 21*(1), 60–66.

Tappen, R. M. (2001). *Nursing leadership and management: Concepts and practice* (4th ed.). Philadelphia: Davis.

Tappen, R. M., Weiss, S. A., & Whitehead, D. K. (1998). *Essentials of nursing leadership and management*. Philadelphia: Davis.

Taylor, F. W. (1947). *Scientific management*. New York: Harper & Row. (First published in 1911).

Trott, M. C., & Windsor, K. (1999). Leadership effectiveness: How do you measure up? *Nursing Economics, 17*(3), 127–130.

Valiga, T. M., & Grossman, S. (1997). Leadership. In R. K. Nunnery (Ed.), *Advancing your career: Concepts of professional nursing* (pp. 128–139). Philadelphia: Davis.

Wolf, G. A., Boland, S., & Aukerman, M. (1994). A transformational model for the practice of professional nursing. *Journal of Nursing Administration, 24*(4), 51–57.

Wyatt, D. (1999). Negotiation strategies for men and women. *Nursing Management, 30*(1), 22–25.

Zwingman-Bagley, C. (1999). Transformational management style positively affects financial outcomes. *Nursing Administration Quarterly, 23*(4), 29–34.

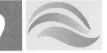

9

The Nursing Practice Environment

BONNIE JEROME D'EMILIA, PhD, MPH, RN

OBJECTIVES

At the completion of this chapter, the reader will be able to:

- Identify changes in the overall health care system and nursing profession.
- Describe the recommendations of the 1997 National League for Nursing Report.
- Discuss how the health care environment is responding to escalating costs of care.
- Describe how health care organizations are restructuring nursing and patient care services.
- Discuss the challenges and opportunities that lie ahead for nursing, and how the nursing profession can meet those challenges.
- Describe the impact of financial forces on nurses as employees in the health care system.
- Describe the American Nurses Association magnet hospital program.

PROFILE IN PRACTICE

Kathryn Chouaf, RN, MSN,
OB/GYN Clinic
University of Virginia Hospital
Charlottesville, Virginia

As a nurse in an Ob/Gyn clinic that provides care primarily to Medicaid and Medicare recipients, as well as the uninsured, I am constantly aware of the effect of the nursing practice environment on the care our clients receive.

The nurses in our clinic have to be aware of how each client's care is being reimbursed and communicate this to the physician staff. For example, Medicaid requires specific paperwork to be filed well in advance for procedures such as tubal ligations, or the procedure is not reimbursed. In that case, either the department absorbs the cost or the client is billed. If a client is uninsured, she may not be able to afford expensive medications such as interferon creams to treat HPV that are not on the hospital's formulary (and thus available for a nominal fee to indigent patients). Since many of the new and very expensive treatments are not available through the hospital pharmacy, these patients frequently have to settle for less effective treatments.

Most of the medical care in our clinic is provided by resident physicians who are rotating among a variety of practice sites as part of their training experience. While the vast majority of these physicians are dedicated and caring, they are often unable to provide continuity, particularly for the obstetrical patients. This is frustrating for both providers and clients, since many of our clients have no primary health care provider, have numerous physical problems that have not been addressed, and may have complex social problems. Nurses in the clinic attempt to address many of these issues and function as de facto case managers, making or suggesting referrals to social workers and other specialty clinics.

Our ability to perform in this case management role is hindered by a number of factors directly related to the practice environment, however. Budget constraints have led to hiring part-time RNs who then face the same difficulty with providing patient continuity as do the residents, and about half of the nursing staff are either unlicensed or are LPNs. There are few opportunities for career growth for a bachelor's-prepared

RN in this clinic, as there is no clinical ladder for outpatient nursing at our institution, causing nurses to leave. The few full-time RNs hired in the past 3 years have either left or have dropped to part-time in order to pursue graduate education in nursing. None of those women expects to return to the clinic in an advanced practice role at the end of her degree.

Nurses could be making even more significant contributions to patient outcomes among our clinic population, but changes are needed at every level. We nurses need to better document our effect on patient outcomes and advocate for nursing practice, the administration needs to recognize and reward nursing's efforts to improve patient care, and fundamental changes in reimbursement that will allow all of our clients access to adequate care are long overdue.

The Health System

Many industrialized countries, such as England and Canada, have centralized systems of health care. In these systems an infrastructure is built which controls the number and location of health care delivery sites and the training, distribution, and reimbursement of providers. In the United States the system of health care can best be described as fragmented: rather than a centralized system, we maintain a patchwork of subsystems that serve different populations with different types of care, paid for by differing sources. As nurses we are an integral part of this complex and fragmented system.

In 1997, the National League for Nursing (NLN) Commission presented its proposal for developing a "workforce for a restructured health care system" (Lamm, 1997, p. 1). The commission concluded that the health care system in the United States is being defined by unsustainable trends such as high costs, poor

outcomes, and maldistribution of resources, which have increased markedly over the past 3 years. The commission recommended that nursing organizations collaborate with other health care–oriented groups to create an action agenda for health care. That agenda should include:

- A major reallocation of resources from acute to community-based primary care and public health.
- A redesign of Medicare and Medicaid.
- Continued efforts at the state level toward providing universal access to primary health care services.
- Health education at the community and occupational level.
- Nursing research that examines the cost-effectiveness of nursing interventions, and the consequences of various staffing and practice models.

The commission went on to enumerate the skills that will be required of nurses working in a new and improved health care system. These include:

- Critical thinking skills
- Relational skills (for collaboration within nursing, with other disciplines, with patients, and with legislators)
- Case management skills
- Primary care skills
- Community focus skills

Nurses are employees (a situation that has recently changed for advanced practice nurses in certain circumstances), and as such we are embedded within the system of health care and subject to its influence in our day-to-day ability to perform our jobs. As nurses who are accountable to our patients for the quality of care we provide, we must be aware of the changes throughout the health care system that may have an impact on our workplace, and thus on the care we provide. We owe it to ourselves to be knowledgeable about outside forces that may affect our ability to get or keep employment, or that may result in improved or worsened staffing, salary, or workplace conditions. One of the most common complaints among health care providers in this era of reform is that decisions are being made by lay people about the provision, reimbursement, and quality of health care. We owe it to our profession to take our place in the decision-making arena, and so we must be aware of the forces, both political and financial, within the health care system that can be expected to affect nurses and nursing practice.

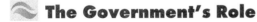 **The Government's Role**

Throughout the history of the United States, the nature of the health care system has changed, and continues to change. In early U.S. history, health and medical care were considered a private and personal matter. This changed drastically with the passage of the Shepard-

Towner Act on Maternity and Infancy in 1921, in which the federal role in health and medical care began with a program of grants to state health agencies for the direct provision of services. Although this act was allowed to die in 1929, its impact was the recognition that the federal government should have a role in protecting the health and welfare of U.S. citizens.

The enactment of the Social Security Act in 1935 marked the first major act of social welfare in this country. Although this act was not intended as a medical insurance act, it did provide federal grants to the states for public health, maternal and child health, services for crippled children, and public assistance for the aged, blind, and families with dependent children. Thus, the role of the federal government in the provision of health care became an accepted fact, which culminated with the 1965 passage of Title XVIII and XIX amendments to the Social Security Act, Medicare and Medicaid. These two programs (see Box 9–1 for descriptions) have changed the face of health care enormously and continue to have a large role in the provision of health care services. Since the advent of Medicare and Medicaid, the federal government's spending on health care as a percentage of total federal government expenditures has increased from 3.3% (in 1960) to 21.1% (in 1997). National health expenditures have risen explosively since the enactment of Medicare and Medicaid, from $41 billion in 1965 to $1 trillion in 1996, with the expectation that total expenditures will reach $2 trillion by 2007 (Ginzberg, 1998). (See Figure 9–1 for a graphic representation of the nation's health care expenditures.) State and local governments, contributors to the Medicaid program, have seen an increase in health spending from 9.7% of total expenditures for 1960 to 14.6% of total expenditures in 1997 (Health Care Financing Administration [HCFA], 1999a).

Since the introduction of Medicare and Medicaid, the health care industry has grown from

Box 9-1 Medicare and Medicaid

MEDICARE

Medicare is the largest public payer of health care, so it dictates how health care is delivered to elderly and disabled persons (coverage for the care of certain disabled persons and people with certain types of kidney disease was added in 1973). Medicare, which is financed by the federal government, consists of two parts. Part A is hospital insurance (HI), which pays for most medically necessary inpatient care, and Part B is supplementary medical insurance (SMI), which pays for most outpatient physician services and various ancillary services that are deemed medically necessary.

HI is provided automatically and without cost to people over age 65 who are eligible for Social Security and Railroad Retirement benefits. In 1999, the HI program provided protection against the costs of hospital and specific other medical care to about 39 million people (34 million aged and 5 million disabled enrollees). HI benefit payments totaled $129 billion in 1999. The HI program is financed primarily through a mandatory payroll tax. Almost all employees and self-employed workers in the United States work in employment covered by the HI program and pay taxes to support the cost of benefits for aged and disabled beneficiaries.

All people eligible for HI are entitled to enroll in SMI on a voluntary basis by payment of a monthly premium. Almost all persons entitled to HI choose to enroll in SMI. In 1999, the SMI program provided protection against the costs of physician and other medical services to about 37 million people. SMI benefits totaled $80.7 billion in 1999. The SMI program is financed through premium payments ($45.50 per beneficiary per month in 2000) and contributions from the general fund of the U.S. treasury. Beneficiary premiums are generally set at a level that covers 25% of the average expenditures for aged beneficiaries. Therefore, the contributions from the general fund of the U.S. Treasury are the largest source of SMI income.

MEDICAID

Medicaid is a federal-state matching entitlement program that pays for medical assistance for certain vulnerable and needy individuals and families with low incomes and resources. Medicaid is the largest source of funding for medical and health-related services for America's poorest people. Although jointly financed by federal and state governments, Medicaid is state administered. Therefore, determinations of eligibility based on income are made by the state, within guidelines promulgated by the federal government. Eligibility requirements and payment rates vary considerably by state.

Data from *Medicare: A brief summary.* (2000). Baltimore, MD: Office of the Actuary, Health Care Financing Administration.

approximately 6% of the gross domestic product (GDP) to over 13%. (The GDP is the total value of goods and services produced in the United States.) In 1997, approximately 81% of the federal government's expenditures went to Social Security, defense, interest on the national debt, and health care services. Although Social Security is the largest component, health care programs are a close second, and the cost of health care services has been rising steadily for the past 30 years, with the rate of health care inflation at least two to three percentage points higher than other sectors of the economy (Whetsell, 1999).

Prior to the enactment of Medicare and Medicaid in 1965, hospitals and physicians

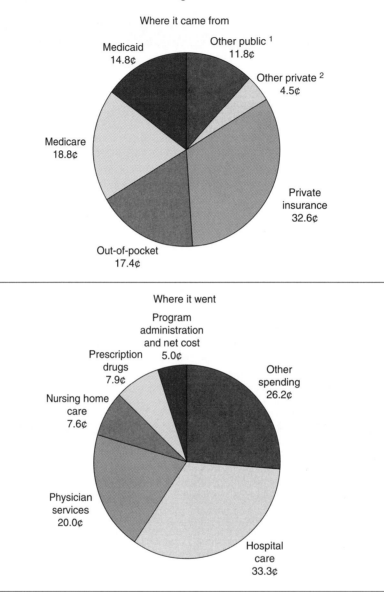

Where it came from

Medicaid
14.8¢

Other public [1]
11.8¢

Other private [2]
4.5¢

Medicare
18.8¢

Private
insurance
32.6¢

Out-of-pocket
17.4¢

Where it went

Program
administration
and net cost
5.0¢

Prescription
drugs
7.9¢

Nursing home
care
7.6¢

Physician
services
20.0¢

Other
spending
26.2¢

Hospital
care
33.3¢

[1] "Other Public" includes programs such as workers' compensation, public health activity, Department of Defense, Department of Veterans Affairs, Indian Health Services, and State and local hospital and school health.

[2] "Other Private" includes industrial inplant, privately funded construction, and non-patient revenues including philanthropy.

NOTE: Numbers shown may not add to 100.00 because of rounding.

NOTE: Other Spending includes dentist services, other professional services, home health, durable medical products, over-the-counter medicines and sundries, public health, research and construction.

SOURCE: Health Care Financing Administration, Office of the Actuary, National Health Statistics Group.

FIGURE 9–1   The nation's health dollar, 1998.

charged for their services, and with few exceptions, insurance companies and individuals paid the full charges for services provided. This type of reimbursement is called fee-for-service. Those individuals who did not have the funds necessary to pay for their care or who were uninsured either found care at primarily public hospitals that provided a large portion of free care or did without medical care.

With Medicare and Medicaid, health services became available to the poor and elderly. By 1967, approximately 30 million people were enrolled in these two programs. In 1997, over 72 million persons, or more than 27% of the population, received care financed through Medicare and Medicaid (Whetsell, 1999). The method of payment for Medicare services at the onset of the program was based on cost reimbursement, so hospitals were paid for the reasonable costs of providing services. Under this formula, higher costs led to higher payments and higher

revenues, and so there was no incentive to provide cost-effective care. Prior to the enactment of Medicare there was a nursing shortage. With the steady reimbursement and increased hospital utilization made possible through the Medicare program, hospitals were able to shift much of the cost of nursing salaries to their Medicare bills, and as employment follows improved wages, the shortage abated.

Throughout the 1970s, hospitals maximized their Medicare reimbursement by adding beds and expanding medical schools. Utilization rose, as did health care costs. From 1973 to 1982, inpatient admissions rose from 31.7 to 36.4 million, patient days rose from 248 to 278 million, and the cost per patient day increased from $102 to $245 (Whetsell, 1999). Other insurers that paid charges rather than costs saw their expenditures grow steadily, with ultimate repercussions at the source of most of this coverage, the employer (Box 9–2). Between 1980

Box 9–2 Employer-Sponsored Insurance

Among the general population 18–64 years old, workers (both full- and part-time) are more likely to be insured than nonworkers. Most Americans rely on their employer for coverage. In 1997, of the 167.5 million nonelderly Americans with private health insurance, 151.7 million belonged to employer-provided health plans. The percentage of Americans who were covered through employment decreased from 69.2% in 1987 to a low point of 63.5% in 1993, and then increased slightly to 64.2% in 1997. The percentage of workers whose employers offered insurance increased from 72.4% in 1987 to 75.4% in 1996, but the proportion of workers who chose to take this coverage fell from 88.3% to 80.1% (Kuttner, 1999), as employees were required to pay more out of pocket costs, or the insurance plans that were offered were inferior to what had been available in the past. According to the U.S. Census Bureau, the tendency to have insurance coverage increases with income level (in 1999 the percentage of people without insurance ranged from 8.3% among households with incomes of $75,000 or more to 24.1% among those in households with incomes of less than $25,000), number of employees in the company (workers in firms with less than 25 employees are least likely to be covered), and more full-time workers are insured than part-time workers (part-time workers had a higher noncoverage rate [22.4%] than full-time workers [16.4%]).

From Mills, R. J. (2000). Current Population Reports, Washington, D.C.: U.S. Department of Commerce, Economics and Statistics Administration, U.S. Census Bureau and 1993, private health insurance costs increased by 218% per enrollee in inflation-adjusted dollars, while the GDP rose by just 17%. The insurance companies passed these increased costs along through annual premium increases to employers. In one year, 1988–1989, employers' health insurance costs rose by 18%. Between 1980 and 1993, employers' spending on health care as a percentage of the total compensation provided to workers increased from 3.7 to 6.6% (Kuttner, 1999).

FOCUS ON COST IN THE MEDICARE PROGRAM

In 1983, in an effort to try to rein in health care costs, Congress adopted the system of prospective payment (PPS) as the mechanism by which Medicare would reimburse hospitals for episodes of inpatient care. This one act, following 10 years of research and planning, changed the way health care was financed, and so had a great impact on the health care system. With the passage of PPS, in which hospitals would get paid based on a patient's diagnosis (Box 9–3), Medicare and the hospital knew in advance that a set amount would be paid, unless the patient developed costly complications requiring unanticipated services or an unexpectedly long length of stay. Many insurance companies, large self-insured employers, and large health systems adopted the PPS as well. Hospitals responded to PPS by cutting staff, reducing inventory, and

monitoring and decreasing length of stay. This led initially to the provision of more cost-effective care, and so profits in the short term rose. Subsequently the government responded by paying hospitals less per discharge than the rate of medical inflation would recommend. Profits dropped substantially, and many hospitals ran deficits, with some forced to close. Patients who were admitted were sicker and discharged sooner to maximize cost-effectiveness in an era of tightening reimbursement. This had and continues to have important implications for the provision of nursing care, both in the hospital and in the growing setting of home care nursing. Nurses were in great demand at this time to facilitate the intensive level of care necessary to accommodate these sicker patients. The result was shortages in 1984–1985 and 1988–1989 (Brewer, 1996). These shortages resulted in the closing of inpatient units, a decrease in services, and an increase in the use of nonprofessionals at the bedside, an issue that still plagues nursing today. Although some of these changes resulted in the provision of more cost-effective care, questions of quality became relevant as the delivery of inpatient care was so drastically changed. Hospitals were able to maintain their nursing workforce in the face of decreased federal reimbursement by shifting the costs of nursing salaries to those payers (private insurance companies or self-paying patients) who paid charges rather than costs of care. This

---

Box 9–3 Prospective Payment System

The prospective payment system (PPS) totally redefined the way hospitals were paid by Medicare for inpatient services. PPS established a per-case payment rate using diagnosis-related groups, a method developed at Yale University. There were 470 DRGs in the system at the onset, and each patient was classified in only one of these groups based on diagnosis, surgical procedure, age, and any complications they might have experienced. Patients in the same DRG were expected to use roughly the same amount of health care resources. Payment rates were based on the cost weight of the DRG as a fixed payment per DRG, regardless of actual costs for services provided.

was a short-term remedy, as these payers soon adopted modified forms of PPS.

THE MEDICARE PROGRAM

Since the advent of PPS, researchers who study the health care system have monitored and evaluated the effect of earlier discharges, decreased length of stay, and the increasing use of ambulatory, outpatient, or home care services for care that would have taken place in a hospital had reimbursement been available. This research focused closely on access, cost, and quality. These three concepts are closely related. As we can see from the preceding discussion, when Medicare changed its reimbursement formula from cost based to prospective payment, the widespread response within the health care system was to cut back on resources, to limit admissions to those most acutely ill, and to decrease length of stay to maximize cost efficiency and so make the most of the reimbursement dollars. If access to inpatient care was to be limited, patients would need to be cared for in other settings, or the nation's overall health status could be expected to decline. Many studies compared health indicators from pre- and post-PPS time periods, but limitations in access to those most acutely ill has not been shown to have negatively affected the nation's health status. Indeed, what has changed in the past 17 years since the initiation of the PPS is our reliance on the hospital as the center for the provision of health care. In 1965, the primary purpose of Medicare enactment was to make health care coverage available to the elderly in a form that was equivalent to that available to the working population. But the working population typically requires acute care services for accidents and injuries (Whitelaw & Warden, 1999). The elderly and disabled populations whose care is financed through Medicare tend to be chronically ill, and so the needs for care are not equivalent to the needs of the average worker in the United States. Hospitalization of the older adult often results in a health status decline that is

unrelated to the progression of the acute problem that led to the admission (Creditor, 1993). The idea that the hospital was to be the primary focus of care delivery was inappropriate for these populations, and the nation is slowly becoming aware of the need for other care settings and other techniques of care management that will be better suited to a chronically ill population. So less attention needs to be given to the idea of reducing inpatient days and hospital admissions and expenditures, and more attention to how to provide optimum care in other more appropriate settings (Whitelaw & Warden, 1999). This has led to an initiative among health care providers and those who pay for care to develop health care delivery systems that are more appropriate for the management of chronic illness or the delay in disability. But our national policy on health care, primarily expressed through the Medicare and Medicaid programs, has been inadequate to this task, owing to its fragmentary nature and lack of primary care, problems that must be resolved before hospital-centeredness can be countered. And although we have focused much attention on governmental health care expenditures for the past two decades, expenditures have continued to grow, primarily because of the growth in the number of Medicare enrollees (Table 9–1) and utilization of services (Whetsell, 1999).

The growth of the Medicare population is expected to crest with the impending retirement of the baby-boom generation. With Americans living longer, the number of Medicare beneficiaries is growing faster than the number of workers paying into the system. By the year 2015, the Medicare trust fund (Part A, or Hospital Insurance) is projected to be insolvent, just as the baby-boom generation begins to retire and enter the system, eventually doubling the number of Americans who are over 65. This fear of the financial collapse of the Medicare system has led to efforts at reform. But this attention has been focused on the Medicare program at the same time that the federal gov-

	TABLE 9-1	Hospital and/or Supplementary Medical Insurance, All Areas, as of July 1, 1966–1998	
Year	All Persons	Aged Persons	Disabled Persons
1966	19,108,822	19,108,822	
1967	19,521,000	19,521,000	
1973	23,545,363	21,814,825	1,730,538
1974	24,201,042	22,272,920	1,928,122
1982	29,494,219	26,539,994	2,954,225
1983	30,026,082	27,108,500	2,917,582
1997	38,444,739	33,629,955	4,814,784
1998	38,824,855	33,802,038	5,022,817

From Medicare enrollment trends 1966–1998. Available at www.hcFa.gov/stats/eNRLTRND.htm

ernment has made a concerted effort to balance the national budget.

One of the results of these two divergent goals was the Balanced Budget Act of 1997 (BBA), which included a 5-year plan for limiting the amount of funding that will be available for Medicare by targeting a $115 billion reduction in Medicare expenditures (Whetsell, 1999). The $115 billion in savings is expected to be generated not by curtailing services but by limiting the increase in payments to providers, including hospitals, physicians, home health services, and skilled nursing providers.

Among payers, growth in public sector spending has slowed since 1991, increasing only 4.1% in 1998. The single most important factor in this decelerating public spending trend in 1998 was Medicare, where the early impacts of the BBA and progress in combating fraud and abuse combined to reduce spending growth from 6.0% in 1997 to 2.5% in 1998 (Levit et al., 2000). Although the rate of growth of Medicare expenditures has decreased, however, the share of public or government spending on health care has increased, passing the $1.0 trillion mark in 1996. This number includes smaller services such as the Department of Defense, the Department of Veterans Affairs, Worker's Compensation, and other programs, but the largest part of these expenditures went

to finance Medicare and Medicaid, totaling $351 billion in health care services in 1996, more than one-third of the nation's total health care bill and almost three-quarters of all public spending on health care (Levit, Lazenby, & Braden, 1998).

ACCESS TO CARE: WHAT ABOUT MEDICAID?

While it is obvious that Medicare increased access to care for the elderly in the United States since its inception (the elderly use four times as much health care as the general population, and per capita expenditures among persons over 80 years old run about 2½ times higher than those for people ages 65 to 69, and seven times higher than for those under 65 [Garber, 1996]), Medicaid has not been as successful in improving the accessibility of care for its beneficiaries. As with all health insurance programs, most Medicaid recipients require relatively small average expenditures per person each year, and a relatively small proportion of recipients incur very large costs. Moreover, the average cost varies substantially by type of beneficiary. The data for 1998, for example, indicate that Medicaid payments for services for 20.6 million children, who constitute 51% of all Medicaid recipients, averaged about $1,150 per child—a relatively small average expenditure per person. For the

8.6 million adults, who compose 21% of recipients, payments averaged about $1,775 per person. However, certain other specific groups have much larger per-person expenditures. Medicaid payments for services for 4 million aged, constituting 11% of all Medicaid recipients, averaged about $9,700 per person; for the 7.2 million disabled, who compose 18% of recipients, payments averaged about $8,600 per person. When expenditures for these high- and lower-cost recipients are combined, the 1998 payments to health care vendors for 40.6 million Medicaid recipients averaged $3,500 per person (HCFA, 2000). Although originally designed to aid the poor, half of all Medicaid expenditures go to support people with incomes above the federal poverty line (Darman, 1991). This is largely a factor of the use of financial loopholes in the Medicaid program to shelter assets of families relying on Medicaid to pay the high cost of nursing home care. Limiting federal assistance to those who are truly needy would result in a cost savings of $200 billion annually but would be unacceptable to the majority of the voting population, who count on entitlement to provide for their present or future care regardless of their level of financial need.

Medicaid is the largest health insurer in the United States in terms of eligible enrollees. The vast majority of these beneficiaries fall outside the employer-based insurance system, and so Medicaid has functioned as a form of safety net for some of our most vulnerable populations. But the enrollees in Medicaid are not as politically savvy as those receiving Medicare, nor can the average citizen suppose that he or she will benefit from Medicaid, as we may hope to benefit someday from Medicare by virtue of longevity. Therefore it has been easier for the government, both at the federal and state level, to manipulate the Medicaid program and to change and limit the number of recipients and the types and amounts of services that can be received by these recipients. A 1994 survey on access to care for Medicaid recipients found that for all of the services included in the survey (medical or surgical care, dental care, prescription drugs, eyeglasses, and mental health care or counseling), Medicaid recipients were about half as likely as the uninsured and about twice as likely as the privately insured to report having difficulty obtaining care (Berk & Schur, 1998). Compared with the uninsured, those with Medicaid were two to four times as likely to have a regular place to obtain medical care, regardless of health status. For those in good or excellent health, there was little difference in access between those privately insured and the Medicaid population. But Medicaid enrollees in fair or poor health were about twice as likely as privately insured individuals in similar health to note an inability to obtain care. Race was also found to be significant, with nonwhites 70% more likely to report difficulty in obtaining medical care than whites. The findings from this study showed that although the vast majority of Americans were able to obtain access to medical care, there was substantial variation across subgroups based on type of insurance coverage. These differences between insured and noninsured persist even if the insurance is publicly or privately funded. But although Medicaid improves access to care, for those with serious health problems the program goes only partway toward providing the same level of care that private insurance provides. As a safety net, then, Medicaid is an imperfect system, and with the wide state variation in levels of eligibility and service provision, where you live can be as significant to your ability to access care as your level of health and functioning.

Although Medicare and Medicaid are both administered at the federal level by the Health Care Financing Administration (HCFA), there is little in common between the two programs. In enacting Medicare, Congress made it clear that the financing of care for the elderly was a federal mandate. But the division of authority between the states and federal government on the administration and funding of Medicaid has resulted in a persistent struggle over how to pay the bills for this population. In 1997 the federal government's contribution was $95.4 billion and the states' contribution—which varied widely, based on each state's per capita income—was $64.5 billion.

Poor people enrolled in Medicaid are more likely to have a usual source of care, to have a higher number of annual ambulatory visits, and to have a higher rate of hospitalization than poor people without Medicaid (Inglehart, 1999). But in 1997, with the passage of the welfare-to-work requirements for persons covered under Temporary Assistance to Needy Families (TANF), a decrease in the Medicaid-eligible population began, which continued into 1998 (Levit et al., 2000). A byproduct of the welfare-to-work legislation is that those persons no longer eligible for welfare may not be aware or advised that they are automatically eligible for Medicaid for 6 months to a year. (Previously there was an automatic link between welfare and Medicaid services, but now one must apply to Medicaid to be declared eligible [Inglehart, 1999]). Anecdotal reports of welfare workers choosing not to advise potential recipients of their eligibility have been rampant in the popular press. It is not known how many Medicaid-eligible families have been denied their rights by lapses in judgment. If the decline in Medicaid enrollment could be explained by a concomitant rise in workers employed in jobs that offered health insurance, this issue would be of no concern. But most former welfare recipients who have found employment are in low-paying jobs that do not provide insurance benefits (Inglehart, 1999). A recent study estimated that 4.7 million children were uninsured despite being Medicaid eligible, or approximately two out of every five uninsured children in the United States (Inglehart, 1999). A study by Families USA, a consumer group, found that the number of low-income parents enrolled in Medicaid in fifteen states had declined by 945,880, or 27%, from January 1996 to December 1999. These states are home to 70% of the uninsured adults under the age of 65 who have incomes less than twice the poverty level, or below $28,300 for a family of three (Pear,

2000). If Medicaid enrollment declines as the number of uninsured increases, there is obviously a connection, in that reductions in Medicaid coverage are fueling an increase in the number of uninsured. In April 2000, President Clinton ordered the states to restore Medicaid benefits to families who were improperly deprived of coverage, but the states' efforts to comply have been slow.

A similar problem faces a new program, the State Children's Health Insurance Program, which authorized the expenditure of $24 billion over 5 years to extend coverage to low-income children who are not already eligible for Medicaid. This program was conceived as a way to protect children whose parents have left the welfare roles for low-paying jobs that do not provide insurance coverage. Congress gave the states leeway in how to use these funds, and so many eligible children have not been located or enrolled because of inadequate outreach or disinterest among the states in increasing their Medicaid expenditures.

States have also tried to manipulate their Medicaid expenditures by using managed care as a means of providing a regular source of care for this population. As defined by Inglehart (1992), the term *managed care* is used broadly to encompass any restriction on the clinical autonomy of physicians and consumer freedom of choice, but its main defining feature is the integration of the financing and delivery of health care services to enrolled members for a predetermined monthly premium. All forms of managed care attempt to control costs by modifying physician practice styles and discouraging the use of medical specialists and nonparticipating physicians. Incentives are geared to saving money through fewer hospital admissions, shorter lengths of stay, the use of less expensive procedures and tests, and the greater use of preventive services (Litman & Robins, 1997). But the Medicaid population tends to have needs that are different from those of the general population. The Medicaid program was not developed in the mode of traditional health insurance. It was developed as a safety net, intended to help those most vulnerable—children, the elderly, the disabled, and those with little or no income or savings—to meet the basic necessities of life. This is a population with multiple needs, high levels of chronic illness, many and varied medical and social problems, and lacking the skill to negotiate a new system of health care that requires gatekeepers and pretreatment authorizations. Deductibles and copayments are two methods used by managed care organizations to limit utilization, but they aren't allowed in most Medicaid programs. And these concepts are meaningless to people with little or no money. Managed care organizations save money by limiting high-tech services and the services of specialists, gaining price concessions from providers, and practicing administrative efficiency. But Medicaid tends to pay so little for its services that many expensive services have already been limited, and are certainly not responsible for the growth of Medicaid expenditures, which can be explained by an increased population of beneficiaries and by the usual means of increasing medical costs—the increased costs of new technology and prescription medications. Managed care savings tend to be maximal in the initial enrollment period but are not seen year after year, and so these programs do not add resources to this population, which is underserved in general, and there is a limit to how much you can squeeze providers by asking for price concessions before they opt out of the market. The use of Medicaid managed care for those populations that use the most care—the disabled, the elderly, and the blind (accounting for 25% of enrollees but 75% of expenditures)—has not proved to provide any cost savings. The only potential saving is in the recruitment of women and children, who account for a small fraction of the Medicaid expenditures already.

THE UNINSURED

The number of people without insurance declined in 1999 for the first time since 1987. In 1999, according to the U.S. Census Bureau,

42.6 million people, or 15.5% of the population, were uninsured. This rise in the insured population, with an estimated 1.7 million person rise in the ranks of the insured, was the result of an increase in the number of persons receiving employer-based coverage. The number of uninsured children (under 18 years of age) was 11.1 million in 1998, or 15.4% of all children. In 1999, this number dropped to 10 million, or 13.9%. Although Medicaid insured 12.9 million poor people in 1999, 10.4 million poor people still had no health insurance, representing about one-third of all poor people (32.4%). Medicaid is the most widespread type of coverage among the poor, with 39.9% (10.4 million) of all poor people covered at some time during the year 1999. This percentage did not change significantly from the previous year. Among the near poor (those with a family income greater than the poverty level but less than 125% of the poverty level), 25.7% (3.1 million people) were without health insurance in 1999. This was a significant decrease from the previous year, and resulted from an increase in the near poor receiving both private insurance and government coverage (Mills, 2000).

In 1998, Cunningham and Kemper studied the ability of uninsured persons to access health care in the Community Tracking Study Household Survey. Consistent with previous studies, this study found that uninsured persons were about twice as likely to report some difficulty getting care (30.8%) as privately insured persons (14.6%) and persons with Medicaid or other state health insurance coverage (16.3%), and more than three times as likely to report difficulty as Medicare beneficiaries (9.5%).

Approximately 90% of the uninsured persons studied in this research who reported difficulty obtaining health care cited the cost of care or lack of insurance as the main reason they experienced difficulty. This measure reflects the financial barriers to care for uninsured persons. Access to care is also influenced by other considerations addressed in this study that may not be directly related to economic factors, such as whether an individual has an identifiable source of primary care, the proximity of health care providers to an individual's place of residence or work, the ease and convenience of seeing health care providers, and the appropriateness of the care setting where services are received.

Consistent with other studies, data from the Community Tracking Study Household Survey showed that uninsured persons nationally were much more likely to be without a usual source of care (32.1%) than persons with insurance coverage, including those with Medicaid and other public insurance. In addition, uninsured persons were only about half as likely as privately insured and Medicare beneficiaries to use a physician's office as their usual source of care, and, along with Medicaid beneficiaries, were more likely to use hospital-based facilities and other clinics. Other problems cited by uninsured persons were inability to obtain medications, treatments, specialized services, and high-tech procedures ordered by physicians. So, even when a health care visit has been made, the follow-up care may not be feasible, for either financial or logistical reasons. Uninsured individuals living in poor urban areas may find that public hospitals and community health centers are convenient and accessible places to obtain medical care. However, excessively long waiting times to see a physician and inability to obtain certain specialty services may result if services for medically indigent persons are rationed in these facilities because of resource constraints. Thus, having a close and identifiable source of care does not necessarily guarantee that all necessary services can be obtained easily. For uninsured persons, cost or lack of insurance is by far the most frequently cited reason given for delaying or not getting needed medical care (90%), and these financial barriers may occur at any step during the care-seeking process, from trying to get into the system (e.g., for an examination and diagnosis) to obtaining highly specialized services or procedures once they are in the system. Much concern has been expressed about the use of hospital emergency departments (EDs) as a source of primary care. This

concern has focused on the higher costs to the health care system compared with nonurgent care provided in community health centers or private physicians' offices. Since hospital ED use is associated with greater difficulty in obtaining care by uninsured persons, this study's findings suggested that reliance on hospital-based facilities, particularly hospital EDs, as sources of care for medically indigent persons resulted not only in higher costs but also in lower access.

Cunningham and Kemper (1998) demonstrated through simulations that expanding private or public health insurance coverage not only would reduce substantially the amount of difficulty that uninsured persons experience in getting medical care but would also result in greater uniformity across communities in the level of difficulty that uninsured persons currently experience. Similar simulations were also conducted for other selected measures (e.g., percentage with no usual source of care, number of ambulatory visits), and the conclusions from these simulations were virtually identical to those stated above. Simulation results for all of the measures showed that access to care for uninsured persons could be improved more effectively by expanding health insurance coverage rather than by improving access to a level similar to that in communities that currently provide the so-called best access to care for uninsured persons. The conclusion of this study was that improved access to care for the uninsured would be more consistently effective by expanding insurance coverage than by increasing the availability of services provided by safety net providers.

ONE SOLUTION: MANAGED CARE

After the failure of the Clinton administration's attempts to pass national health care reform in 1993 and 1994, the health care system and the public turned to the marketplace as the vehicle to address escalating medical costs (Block, 1997). Turning to the market meant turning to managed care, and resulted in a surge in managed care enrollments. This turn has included the creation of large and unyielding health care networks, and so the U.S. health system has been quietly achieving what many (but specifically the health insurers) fought against allowing the government to do with health care reform (Block, 1997). "Managed care organization" is a general term that refers to any type of delivery and reimbursement system that monitors or controls the types, quality, utilization, and costs of health care (Congressional Budget Office [CBO], 1994; Folland, Goodman, & Stano, 1993). Managed care usually involves capitation, a payment arrangement whereby a provider is prepaid a fixed amount of money per person enrolled (usually on a monthly basis) regardless of the amount of services provided or consumed (Folland et al., 1993). Other strategies associated with managed care include utilization review, preadmission certification, and second-opinion requirements. Since the advent of managed care, the structures of managed care organizations have become less restrictive in an effort to appeal to enrollees who may have a choice of several plans in their employment benefit package. Three types of managed care arrangements, health maintenance organizations (HMOs), preferred provider organizations (PPOs), and point-of-service care (POS), will be discussed here.

Health Maintenance Organizations. An HMO is a managed care plan in which a contractual arrangement is made between the providing organization and enrollees: for a prepaid, fixed fee, the organization agrees to provide comprehensive care to enrollees over a specified period of time (Folland et al., 1993). There are several types of HMOs (CBO, 1994; Folland et al., 1993; Office of Technology Assessment [OTA], 1994). These are:

- *Staff model:* Individual physicians are employed by the HMO to provide services to members.
- *Group model:* A group practice is contracted by an HMO to provide care to enrollees.

- *Network model:* Several group practices are contracted to provide care to enrollees.
- *Independent practice association (IPA):* Independent practitioners or small-group practices are contracted by an HMO to provide care to enrollees.

The growing popularity of HMOs is evident from the numbers of persons enrolled: HMO enrollment grew from 6 million members in 1976 to approximately 63 million members in 1997 (Block, 1997; Inglehart, 1992).

Preferred Provider Organizations. Another type of managed care plan, the PPO is a plan whereby the payer (i.e., the insurance company) contracts with certain providers (physicians and hospitals) to deliver care to enrollees; the payer then provides financial incentives to enrollees who receive care from those same providers (Folland et al., 1993). The types of incentives offered to enrollees may include lower coinsurance and deductibles, increased coverage, and lower premiums (Folland et al., 1993). Although payment to providers is made on a fee-for-service basis, payers benefit because contracts for payment are prearranged, and they can often negotiate contracts with providers who discount fees and practice efficiently. Providers who are under contract with payers benefit because the PPO limits enrollees' choices to certain providers unless an enrollee chooses to pay the additional fees associated with a provider who is not under contract with the PPO (Folland et al., 1993).

Point of Service Plan. The POS plan is the fastest growing type of managed care, covering 19% of managed care enrollees in 1996, up from 7% in 1993. These plans allow enrollees a larger choice in providers. Although members are encouraged to use doctors under contract to the plan, they are also allowed to use doctors outside the plan, with certain limitations, for an additional cost. When using an out-of-plan provider, the enrollee is subject to large out-of-pocket expenses in the form of deductibles and copayments, and all provider reimbursement is on a fee-for-service basis. The difference between the PPO and the POS is that the POS plan has a primary care physician to coordinate care, whereas most PPO plans do not (Block, 1997).

Managed care tends to exert an influence on the health care marketplace when penetration reaches at least 20%. At that point, managed care organizations have the clout and the capital to successfully negotiate with providers and affect the way care is provided in a community. Recent attempts to legislate managed care by passing a patient's bill of rights has led to a hotly bipartisan debate over the issue of whether or not a patient has the right to sue a managed care organization for services withheld based on economic rationale that ultimately resulted in health care damages. Although this legislation did not pass the recent session of Congress, a handful of states, including Arizona and Texas, have passed some form of this legislation. The managed care industry argues that such legislation will increase the cost of care without improving the quality, but there is no definitive answer on this divisive issue, and research will have to be undertaken in the states with this legislation as to how costs have been affected by this increase in liability.

Issues Facing Nursing Today

As witnesses and participants to all the upheaval that has been changing the face of the health care delivery system, nurses are uniquely situated to effect change and lead the organizations that provide care in the quest for new and more effective delivery systems. As the front-line workers in health care, we have the opportunity to form links between the needs and demands of our patients and the organizational goals of our workplaces. We also have challenges of our own to face as we enter the 21st century, one of the largest being the looming nursing shortage.

In 1995 the Pew Health Professions Commission predicted that there could be a surplus of 200,000 to 300,000 nurses as acute care hospitals downsized and closed. The commission also predicted that registered nurses would move into other settings such as home care or subacute care, to alleviate the shortage of available acute care positions. Members of the commission suggested that nursing education programs reduce the size of their basic programs and increase the number of master's degree nurse practitioner programs (Pew Health Professions Commission, 1995).

Looking back at these predictions, it is apparent that the effects of limited reimbursement on acute care hospitals were overstated and the expected nursing surplus was an inaccurate prediction. Despite all the changes that took place in third-party reimbursement, the acute care hospital's share of the nation's health care expenditures has dropped only slightly, from 40% to just under 35% (Ginzberg, 1998), with the proportion going to community hospitals rising. As the number of inpatient days fell, the income generated from ambulatory care has increased, so that hospital revenue continues to dominate the health care delivery system (Ginzberg, 1998). Although occupancy rates have decreased to an average of 60%, except for the closing of a few, mostly small, rural hospitals and the affiliations, mergers, and closings of some urban hospitals that were faced with continuing financial losses and lack of new capital, hospitals have not been forced to downsize and close at the rate that was predicted a few years ago. The public does not like to see hospitals close, with the resultant loss of jobs and decreased access to care. The government (at the federal, state, and local level) has made every effort to prevent closures, and except in cases where there was no good financial solution, these have been avoided. Hospitals have chosen to merge and join alliances, but for the most part they have not downsized their nursing staff. Another factor that has an effect on the demand for nurses is that the population is growing, and it is aging, both factors that would increase the demand for care. In the near future the baby-boom generation will become the Medicare population, and as this group of people has been the driving force behind many of our national trends, we can expect it to change the way this population uses health care, as it attempts to get its needs met through our fragmented system. At the same time that the demand for nurses has not decreased as expected, the enrollment of students in nursing programs has decreased substantially. A recent study by Buerhaus, Staiger, and Auerbach (2000) found that the average age of working RNs increased by 4.5 years between 1983 and 1998. This follows a recent report by the American Association of Colleges of Nursing, which found that enrollments in entry-level baccalaureate nursing programs decreased by 4.6% in fall 1999, the fifth consecutive decline in as many years. Additionally, recent data from the National League for Nursing (NLN) indicate declines in enrollments in all types of entry-level nursing programs (Bednash, 2000). Over the next two decades this trend will lead to a further aging of the RN workforce, because most of the RNs working will be between ages 50 and 69 years. Within the next 10 years, the average age of RNs is forecasted to be 45.4 years, an increase of 3.5 years over the current age, with more than 40% of the RN workforce expected to be older than 50 years. The total number of full-time equivalent RNs per capita is forecasted to peak around the year 2007 and decline steadily thereafter as most RNs retire. By the year 2020, the RN workforce is expected to be roughly the same size as it is today, but nearly 20% below projected RN workforce requirements.

The primary factor that has led to the aging of the RN workforce appears to be the decline in younger women choosing nursing as a career during the last two decades. Unless this trend is reversed, the RN workforce will continue to age and eventually shrink, and may not meet projected long-term workforce requirements. As opportunities for women outside of nursing have expanded, the number of young women entering the RN workforce has declined (Buerhaus et al., 2000). These RN shortages are in stark contrast to the oversupply expected by the Pew Health Professions Commission in 1995. Moreover, unlike past shortages, the coming RN shortage will be driven by shifts in the labor market that are unlikely to reverse in the next few years. As shortages develop during the next 20 years, it can be expected that RN wages will rise, and employers will have little choice but to substitute other personnel for RNs. In anticipation of these developments, employers and nursing leaders should begin working together now to plan how best to use increasingly scarce RNs to deliver patient care in the future (Buerhaus et al., 2000).

The continued aging of the RN workforce has important implications for employers. Efforts to restructure patient care delivery must be more sensitive to the needs of older RNs, who are more susceptible to neck, back, and feet injuries and have a reduced capacity to perform certain physical tasks. Also, older and more experienced RNs may have higher expectations of working conditions and require greater autonomy and respect than have typically been accorded (Buerhaus et al., 2000).

Long-term strategies to increase RN supply are needed to avoid a shortage. Although higher wages and better working conditions may attract more women and men to nursing as a career, these effects will occur only slowly and will be limited by the continued expansion of career opportunities for women outside of nursing. Immigration of RNs educated outside the United States is another possible strategy. However, eliminating the projected shortage would require immigration on an unprecedented scale, and such a policy would not be without controversy, such as that which the computer industry is now attempting to resolve.

NURSING CARE DELIVERY SYSTEMS

Faced with the changing needs of consumers of health care, the evolving roles of caregivers, technological advances, and financial constraints, health care organizations are designing their facilities and systems of care delivery. The most efficient and innovative care delivery systems will provide a good fit with the physical layout of the facility and an approach to health care that promotes administrative efficiency, patient and caregiver satisfaction, and the cost-effective use of resources (Guild, Ledwin, Sanford, & Winter, 1994). Strategic management and innovation should include restructuring the delivery of nursing care. There are two basic ways in which these systems can be restructured: job design and system redesign.

Job Design. Job design is a bottom-up approach that focuses on how to shape a particular job to maximize worker productivity (Dienemann & Gessner, 1992). To improve productivity, job enrichment strategies can be used to increase organizational commitment among nurses, allow for differences among positions based on differing uses of technology, support professional nursing; and involve nurses in policy making, strategic planning, and monitoring of quality within the nursing unit (Dienemann & Gessner, 1992).

A popular form of job enrichment is the development of clinical ladders for recognition of clinical expertise and advancement of the staff nurse without requiring a shift away from patient care. Clinical ladders are structures that were developed in the 1970s and 1980s to recognize and reward clinically competent nurses who chose to remain in clinical practice (Hamrick, Whitworth, & Greenfield, 1993). The terms *clinical ladder* and *career ladder* are often used interchangeably, to convey the belief that these models should foster growth and development over one's entire career rather than be limited to a short span of time.

The idea behind the development of clinical ladders was that there were few, if any, advance- ment or promotional opportunities for nurses who wanted to remain in direct caregiver roles. Before the development of clinical ladders, if a nurse wanted to advance within a system, generally the only option was to move into a management role. Therefore ladders were developed to provide more career options for nurses so that nurses who chose to remain clinically active would have a mechanism for being rewarded, recognized, and promoted within an organizational system.

Depending on the philosophy and values specific to the organization, the theoretical framework, process, and compensation associated with advancement vary (Murray, 1993). Nurses who advance on a clinical ladder are typically rewarded with an increase in salary, a new job title, and/or other types of nonmonetary rewards (Murray, 1993). The number of levels for advancement on clinical ladders has been reported to range from as few as one or two to as many as seven or eight, although the majority of organizations have ladders with four levels (Murray, 1993). Advancement is generally based on clinical competence and professional criteria associated with a given level on the ladder. Some organizations have a limited number of slots at each level for which nurses can apply; others do not have quotas.

In most cases, an individual who desires to advance up a clinical ladder generally has to prepare an application for advancement, sometimes called a portfolio, which demonstrates his or her level of practice. A unit, division, department, or some other type of peer review committee usually reviews each applicant's packet. Recommendations for advancement are then made to the appropriate administrative level.

Real benefits have been documented in organizations that have implemented nursing clinical ladders, such as increased nurse job satisfaction, decreased nursing turnover or increased retention, and improved recruitment (Corley et al., 1994; Opperwall et al., 1991; Schultz, 1993). Subjective reports indicate a positive impact on patient care (Schultz, 1993).

SHARED GOVERNANCE. Other methods of job design are the use of shared governance or the development of professional practice models of care. Shared governance is a step toward change from current hierarchical bureaucratic structures used in many health care organizations. This model of care delivery provides a conceptual framework for management styles that promote employee participation in decision making, involvement of employees in governance issues, autonomy in professional practice, and the true attainment of professionalism (Dienemann & Gessner, 1992). Implementation of shared governance requires an institutional investment in improving the nurse's business and collaborative skills, as well as management's clinical, statistical, communication, and motivational skills. The major changes required for shared governance are expanded roles for nurses, allowing staff nurses to work as salaried employees with work hours that are flexibly based on workload demands, job enrichment for nurses, the use of clinical ladders, and support for quality and fiscal control and the enhanced autonomy of the staff nurse (Dienemann & Gessner, 1992). The major drawbacks to shared governance are the high cost of training for both staff nurses and managers, the fact that it is nurse centered and so does not facilitate multidisciplinary collaboration, the high cost of developing information systems to maintain coordination, and the necessary increase in the amount of time nurses spend on committee work rather than direct patient care, which requires an institutional commitment to improve staffing levels (Dienemann & Gessner, 1992).

PROFESSIONAL PRACTICE MODEL. A professional practice model is a framework that reflects the underlying philosophy about the delivery of nursing care within an organization and serves as a guide to nursing care delivery. A professional practice model is usually unique to a particular organization, although aspects of professional practice models can be shared between organizations. Questions that need to be considered when developing a professional practice model include: What elements are essential to the nurse-patient relationship? What is the best method for delivering care to our patients (i.e., primary, team, functional, modular, or case management)? What is the governance structure that best meets the needs of individual nurses and the nursing organization? What rewards and recognitions should be built into the system? What is the management structure that best meets the needs of individuals, groups, and the nursing organization while at the same time remaining consistent with the overall organizational structure? The aspects of professional practice most commonly found to exist in hospitals that support this model of care are threefold: (1) the ability of the nurse to establish and maintain therapeutic relationships with his or her patients, (2) nurse autonomy and control, and (3) the presence of collaborative nurse-physician relationships at the unit level (Scott, Sochalski, & Aiken, 1999). Regardless of the way the patient care delivery system has been designed, a commitment to these three attributes of professionalism is crucial to the maintenance of the professional practice model, and the literature on the magnet hospital program (which will be described in the following section) has demonstrated a positive relationship between these characteristics and improved patient and nurse job satisfaction, and patient outcome (Scott et al., 1999).

System Redesign. System redesign is a top-down approach that involves the redesign of the health care organization from the unit to the larger system. Systems theory views the organization as an open entity and stresses the need for flexibility in adaptation to internal and external environmental demands. The main goal of systems theory is to design systems that enhance productivity while recognizing the presence of multiple competing goals among the workers. This involves the development of a context in which health professionals in all disciplines can act autonomously within a framework of expectations about quality, cost management, and productivity. Professionals are involved in decision making and policy development, but their primary role is the delivery of high-quality health care to consumers.

ONE MODEL: THE MAGNET HOSPITAL PROGRAM

In the early 1980s, prompted by the nursing shortage at that time, a formal investigation of hospitals that appeared successful in their ability to attract and retain nurses was initiated. The first group of 41 magnet hospitals was chosen through a national "reputational" study conducted by the American Academy of Nursing (ANA). This original group of 41 magnet hospitals was found to have a common set of organizational traits that promoted and sustained professional nursing practice. These factors included a flat organizational structure, unit-based decision making, an influential nurse executive, and an investment in the education and expertise of nurses (Aiken, Havens, & Sloane, 2000).

It is increasingly apparent that consumers are concerned about the level of quality in hospitals and health care. In a recent poll, more than 80% of respondents wanted to know how to evaluate the quality of hospital care (Coalition on Health Care, 1998). Although there are several "best hospital" lists, there is little empirical evidence that "best hospitals" provide better clinical outcomes than other hospitals (Chen et al., 1999).

The ANA, through the ANCC, in the early 1990s developed a formal procedure for the subsequent naming of magnet hospitals, called the Magnet Nursing Services Recognition Program. This program is a voluntary form of external professional nurse peer review available to all hospitals. The review includes examination of the extent to which a hospital meets eight standards of care, which are incorporated within the

model of professional practice. Unlike many of the other "best" lists, the magnet hospital program has been studied extensively over the past two decades, and relationships have been found between the processes of nursing practice and outcomes such as job satisfaction, nurse autonomy, control, and relations with physicians (Scott et al., 1999). An additional element of nursing practice found in magnet hospitals is the nurse's ability to establish and maintain therapeutic nurse-patient relationships, a characteristic that is more likely to be found as organizations improve staffing and decrease nurse/patient staffing ratios. In research that examined the effects of reorganization on patient outcomes, Henry (1992) found that nurse turnover was inversely related to patient satisfaction. Grindel and colleagues in 1996 found that quality patient care occurred in practice environments with high degrees of patient satisfaction and nurse job satisfaction.

A study published in the March 2000 issue of the American Journal of Nursing compared a group of ANCC-recognized magnet hospitals with a sample of the original 41 "reputational" magnet hospitals, looking at job characteristics, job outlook, and organizational attributes in relation to patient care. This study provided strong evidence that the ANCC magnet hospital designation process identified hospitals that were as good as, if not better than, the original group of reputationally designated hospitals in providing a high level of nurse job satisfaction and patient satisfaction, both indicators of improved outcomes of care.

The process of applying for magnet status involves three phases. In the first phase, a hospital submits a one-page application form indicating the planned date for submission of the completed application. The ANCC then sends the hospital a booklet with complete instructions for the application process. This second phase consists of responding to and providing supporting evidence for each of the eight required standards of care. This is the phase of the process that involves much intense scrutiny of the organization of nursing care and its delivery, and efforts to shape the organizational structure to that which is specified by the magnet standards. The completed application must be submitted within 2 years of application. Phase three of the process consists of a site visit, which is scheduled following a successful review of the phase two application materials.

OPPORTUNITIES FOR NURSING

Where does the nursing profession stand, given all of the changes in health care? Actually, many of these changes leave the nursing profession in a very favorable position if it capitalizes on opportunities. The nursing profession can take leadership roles in the delineation of health care policy, in public education, and in the provision of a broad-based education for nursing students to facilitate their movement into a variety of positions and health care settings. Above all, nursing must work for the betterment of health care consumers, both individuals and payers, thereby positioning itself to accomplish several important missions.

First, as the health care delivery system continues to look for more efficiency in the delivery of health care, nurses must be able to document their contribution to the health care delivery system through patient outcomes. Groups have begun to document the cost-effectiveness of care provided by advanced practice nurses (Brown & Grimes, 1993); these activities must continue, and nursing must clearly communicate to consumers and payers the message that nurses can and do provide cost-effective care. The development of methodologies to delineate the revenue-generating aspects of nursing is imperative.

The need to demonstrate nursing's ability to improve the quality of care goes hand in hand with the need to document cost-effectiveness. However, an important distinction between nursing and other professions must be made: nurses provide high-quality patient care by focusing on individual patient needs, expectations, and experiences in an environment that too often emphasizes costs and patient statistics. With this patient-centered focus, nursing is in an exceptionally good position to identify ways of improving quality of care.

Nursing must also document consumer perceptions of satisfaction with care delivered and perceptions of the quality of care received. The current philosophy in business is that quality is defined by the customer, not by the service provider. While health care is moving in this direction, there is still a long way to go. Nurses must embrace this philosophy, document aspects of patients' perceptions of nursing care, and become partners with patients in decision making. The outcome of this effort is likely to enhance nurses' important contributions to health care delivery.

Second, nurses have an opportunity to expand their share of the health care market by serving currently underserved populations. Although nurses already provide a great deal of the care in rural and inner-city areas, we must continue to expand these activities. Nursing must continue to provide care, and even expand the provision of care, to groups that lack access to primary care. It is these groups that experience many of the problems that have such profound effects on our society and on health care costs—lack of basic health care, lack of disease prevention, and violence. Nurses must also realize that many future opportunities will be outside of the hospital environment. Opportunities will exist in agencies and communities that bring the point of service closer to the consumer rather than closer to the provider.

Third, as a profession, nursing must continue to engage in and expand entrepreneurial activities. As the health care environment becomes more and more competitive, nurses will be in a better position to sell their services in the marketplace. So, too, may be other professionals who embrace this philosophy. As the resources available to pay for health care services become increasingly limited, it is likely that other professional groups competing for these resources will become increasingly savvy. Nurses must have the political, economic, and business skills to effectively market their product in this potentially volatile environment.

Fourth, nurses must employ computers and informatics to facilitate the provision of care to clients and to manage the delivery of health care. Computers can facilitate the development of databases, expedite the collection and retrieval of information, allow the integration of new knowledge, and hasten the analysis of large quantities of data to improve efficiency and productivity in health care delivery. Furthermore, informatics can improve diagnostic and consultation capabilities through the use of high-speed computer networks. It is imperative that nurses possess the requisite skills necessary to move forward in a computer-dependent environment.

Finally, nursing education must meet the challenge to better prepare students for the future. In addition to clinical training, nurses of the future will need a broad-based education that encompasses training in informatics, delivery models, economics, data analysis, and management. Future nursing leaders will need more intensive training in these and more diverse topics. A well-trained cadre of nurses will be needed to oversee patient care delivery in a variety of settings. Many health care organizations are restructuring so that all patient care services—including nursing—are provided through multidisciplinary, team efforts. Nurses must be prepared for leadership roles, not just in nursing but also in health care. Nurses in management roles will be called on to document efficiency and effectiveness in the modern health care organization. This requires the knowledge and ability to integrate clinical expertise with business information to oversee the delivery of care to patients.

KEY POINTS

- Many changes are occurring in nursing and health care today. Forces in our society affect access, quality, and cost issues; shape the health

care environment; and influence nursing and nursing care delivery.

- Total and per capita health care expenditures continue to rise. Without intervention, society will no longer be able to afford the care that technology and knowledge provide.

- An increasing number of people in our population have little or no access to affordable health care.

- Questions about health care cost and access lead to concerns about future quality of care.

- More and more care is being delivered on an outpatient basis; those who must be treated as inpatients require more complex and intensive care.

- Health care organizations are implementing new and innovative governance models, clinical ladders, and practice models to facilitate the efficient provision of patient care and to improve the quality of care delivered.

- Nursing can meet the challenges and opportunities that lie ahead by (1) documenting the contribution of nursing through patient outcomes, (2) expanding their share of the health care market by serving currently underserved populations, (3) employing computers and informatics to facilitate and manage the delivery of care, (4) engaging in and expanding entrepreneurial activities, and (5) educating nursing students to excel in a rapidly changing and complex health care environment.

CRITICAL THINKING EXERCISES

1. Considering the changing climate in health care, identify those issues that have changed the manner in which nursing care is provided.

2. Discuss how the changes in reimbursement over the past two decades have affected and will continue to affect the provision of nursing care.

3. Analyze how we can best allocate health care resources to meet the needs of the uninsured, or the most vulnerable populations in the United States.

4. Discuss the issues that managed care brings to health care, and how we as nurses can work with managed care organizations to improve quality, access, and cost-effectiveness of care.

5. Differentiate between shared governance, clinical ladders, and professional practice models as methods of structuring the nursing practice environment.

6. Forecast changes in health care delivery and the nursing profession in light of escalating costs, decreasing access, and concerns about quality of care.

7. Describe how nurses and the nursing profession might capitalize on opportunities presented by recent changes in health care delivery.

REFERENCES

Aiken, L. H., Havens, D. S., & Sloane, D. M. (2000). The magnet nursing services recognitions program: A comparison of successful applicants with reputational magnet hospitals. *American Journal of Nursing, 100*(3), 26–35.

Bednash, G. (2000). The decreasing supply of registered nurses: Inevitable future or call to action? *Journal of the American Medical Association, 283,* 2985–2987.

Berk, M. L., & Schur, C. L. (1998). Access to care: How much difference does Medicaid make? *Health Affairs, 17,* 169–179.

Block, L. E. (1997). Evolution, growth, and status of managed care in the United States. *Public Health Review, 25,* 193–244.

Brewer, C. S. (1996). The roller coaster supply of registered nurses: Lessons from the eighties. *Research in Nursing Health, 19,* 345–357.

Brown, S. A., & Grimes, D. E. (1993). Nurse practitioners and certified nurse midwives: A metaanalysis of studies on nurses in primary care roles. Washington, DC: American Nurses Association Publishing.

Buerhaus, P. I., Staiger, D. O., & Auerbach, D. I. (2000). Implications of an aging registered nurse workforce. *Journal of the American Medical Association, 283,* 2948–2954.

Chen, J., Radford, M. J., Wang, Y., Marciniak, T. A., & Krumholz, H. M. (1999). Do "America's best hospitals" perform better for acute myocardial infarction? *New England Journal of Medicine, 340,* 286–292.

Coalition on Health Care. (1998). How Americans perceive the health care system: A report on a national survey. *Health Care Finance, 23*(4), 12–20.

Congressional Budget Office. (1994, March). *Effects of managed care: An update.* Washington, DC: U.S. Government Printing Office.

Corley, M. C., Farley, B., Geddes, N., Goodloe, L., & Green, P. (1994). The clinical ladder: Impact on nurse satisfaction and turnover. *Journal of Nursing Administration, 24*(2), 42–48.

Creditor, M. C. (1993). Hazards of hospitalization of the elderly. *Annals of Internal Medicine, 118,* 219–223.

Cunningham, P. J., Kemper, P. (1998). Ability to obtain medical care for the uninsured: How much does it vary across communities? *Journal of the American Medical Association, 280,* 921–927.

Darman, R. (1991). Introductory statement: The problem of rising costs. Testimony before the Senate Finance Committee. Washington, DC: Executive Office of the President.

Dienemann, J., & Gessner, T. (1992). Restructuring nursing care delivery systems. *Nursing Economics, 10,* 253–258.

Folland, S., Goodman, A. C., & Stano, M. (1993). *The economics of health and health care.* New York: Macmillan.

Garber, A. M. (1996). To comfort always: The prospects of expanded social responsibility for long-term care. In V. Fuchs (Ed.), *Individual and social responsibility: Child care, education, medical care, and long-term care in America* (pp. 3–12). Chicago: University of Chicago Press.

Ginzberg, E. (1998). The changing US health care agenda. *Journal of the American Medical Association, 279,* 501–504.

Grindel, C. G., Peterson, K., Kinneman, M., & Turner, T. L. (1996). The practice environment project: A process for outcome evaluation. *Journal of Nursing Administration, 26*(5), 43–51.

Guild, S. D., Ledwin, R. W., Sanford, D. M., & Winter, T. (1994). Development of an innovative nursing care delivery system. *Journal of Nursing Administration, 24*(3), 23–29.

Hamrick, A. B., Whitworth, T. R., & Greenfield, A. S. (1993) Implementing a clinically focused advancement system: One institution's experience. *Journal of Nursing Administration, 23*(9), 20–28.

Health Care Financing Administration. (1999a). *1997 HCFA statistics.* Washington, DC: HCFA Press.

Health Care Financing Administration. (1999b). *Medicare enrollment trends, 1996–1998.* Washington, DC: HCFA Press.

Health Care Financing Administration. (2000). *1998 national health expenditures.* Washington, DC: HCFA Press.

Henry, B. (1992). Leadership, nurses, and patient satisfaction: A pilot study. *Nursing Administration Quarterly 16*(3), 72–74.

Inglehart, J. K. (1992). The American health care system: Managed care. *New England Journal of Medicine, 327,* 742–747.

Inglehart, J. K. (1999). The American health care system: Expenditures. *New England Journal of Medicine, 340,* 70–76.

Kuttner, R. (1999). The American health care system: Health insurance coverage. *New England Journal of Medicine, 340,* 163–168.

Lamm, R. (1997). Final report, April 1997, of the NLN Commission on a workforce for a restructured health care system. *Nursing and Health Care Perspectives,* 91–93.

Levit, K., Cowan, C., Lazenby, H., Sensenig, A., Mc-Donnell, P., Stiller, J., Martin, A., & the Health Accounts Team. (2000). Health spending in 1998: Signals of change. *Health Affairs, 19*(1), 124–132.

Levit, K. R., Lazenby, H. C., & Braden, B.R. (1998). National health spending trends in 1996. *Health Affairs, 17*(1), 35–51.

Litman, T. J. & Robins, L. S. (1997). *Health politics and policy* (3rd ed.). Albany, NY: Demar Publishers.

Mills, R.J. (2000). Current Population Reports, Washington, D.C.: U.S. Department of Commerce, Economics and Statistics Administration, U.S. Census Bureau.

Murray, M. (1993). Where are career ladders going in the 90s? *Nursing Management, 24*(6), 46–48.

Office of Technology Assessment. (1994, May). *Understanding estimates of national health expenditures under health reform.* Washington, DC: U.S. Government Printing Office.

Opperwall, B. C., Everett, L. N., Altaffer, A. B., Dietrich, J. A., Killen, M. B., Klien, R. M., Libcke, J. M., & Mitchell, M. A. (1991). ADVANCE—A clinical ladder program. *Nursing Management, 22*(5), 67–74.

Pear, R. (2000, June 20). A million parents lost Medicaid, study says. *New York Times,* p. A12.

Pew Health Professions Commission. (1995). *Critical challenges: Revitalizing the health professions for the twenty-first century.* San Fracisco: UCSF Center for the Health Professions.

Schultz, A. (1993). Evaluation of a clinical advancement system. *Journal of Nursing Administration 23*(2), 13–19.

Scott, J. G., Sochalski, J., & Aiken, L. 1999. Review of magnet hospital research. *Journal of Nursing Administration, 29*(1), 9–19.

Whetsell, G. W. (1999). The history and evolution of hospital payment systems: How did we get here? *Nursing Administrative Quarterly, 23*(4), 1–15.

Whitelaw, N. A., & Warden, G. L. (1999). Reexamining the delivery system as part of Medicare reform. *Health Affairs, 18*(1), 132–143.

PART II

Dimensions of Professional Nursing Practice

Concepts that extend across and influence the full range of nursing activities are referred to as dimensions. In this regard, nursing is a multidimensional discipline because it consists of political, economic, legal, and ethical influences, which have an impact on nursing care delivery and guide nursing practice.

The political dimension of nursing practice reflects the nurse's concern for, and response to, health policy legislation as it affects the health care of individuals, families, and communities. In addition, understanding the short-term and long-term implications of health policy is fundamental to taking a proactive position on issues that positively or adversely influence nursing and health care. The economic dimensions of nursing practice are grounded in the use of scarce resources, which ultimately affects payment for nursing services and the delivery of nursing care. An understanding of the relationship between the economic concepts of the supply of, demand for, and cost of health care services can help the nurse analyze health care delivery problems, pro-

pose solutions, and articulate the nursing role as the health care system is restructured. The legal dimension of nursing practice includes legal concepts, expectations, and consequences that surround the practice of nursing. While it is beyond the scope of this book to examine all of these areas in depth, an overview of the relationships that underlie the practice of nursing (including the nurse-state relationship, the nurse-employer relationship, and the nurse-patient relationship) is presented. As our population becomes more diverse, nurses provide care to clients from varied cultural backgrounds whose value systems may be quite unique. An overview of social and cultural influences and values and beliefs provides the basis on which to plan and implement individualized nursing care to clients from different cultural backgrounds. Finally, the ethical dimension of nursing practice that embraces both moral reasoning and ethical decision making can facilitate rational and intelligent decisions. These dimensions are further defined and explored in this section.

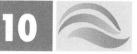
Health Policy and Planning

DEBRA C. WALLACE, PhD, RN

OBJECTIVES

At the completion of this chapter, the reader will be able to:

- Identify political, legislative, and economic factors impacting health policy.
- Describe the legislative and budget processes.
- Discuss the types of health programs mandated by federal health policy legislation.
- Examine health policies for their impact on nursing practice, education, and research.
- Delineate strategies for nurses to influence health policy and the implementation and regulation thereof.

PROFILE IN PRACTICE

Maureen Nalle, PhD, RN
Assistant Professor
University of Tennessee College of Nursing
Knoxville, Tennessee

My earliest years in professional nursing were spent in the military, as a member of the U.S. Army Nurse Corps. Beyond the demands of acquiring skills in the pediatric nursing specialty, socialization to the military lifestyle presented numerous challenges, not the least of which was understanding military protocol, procedure, and policy established by federal legislation.

During the course of a master's education at the University of Texas Health Science Center in San Antonio, I began to question who made the delivery, payment, and care decisions, and how those decisions affected professionals and consumers. My experiences as a clinical specialist in the private health care sector stimulated further interest in the area of health policy development. Doctoral studies in health promotion and health education included broader study of the social, economic, and political influences on health policy.

My participation in policy has been through active membership in the American Nurses Association and the Tennessee Nurses Association, where I serve on the board of directors, and on education and health policy committees that actively pursued legislative agendas.

As a maternal-child health professional, I have pursued advocacy roles to obtain adequate access to care for children and families. In 1996 I completed a health policy internship with the American Academy of Pediatrics, Department of Government Liaison in Washington, D.C. My current involvement is in community, state, and national maternal-child health initiatives. I also volunteer at the local homeless clinic and continue work with state leaders and fellow researchers to ensure competent and qualified child day-care workers.

As a faculty member, I promote student awareness and involvement in the policy process, including knowledge of current issues, participation in professional nursing organizations, and advocacy for clients. Instilling a belief in their own capacity for influencing nursing practice and health care is crucial to sustained participation. Preparing future professionals to contribute to the development and implementation of effective health policy is not only an obligation but also a privilege that reflects commitment to this important process.

Health policy is an area of concern for nurses at all levels of preparation, in all settings and specialties, and across all client groups. Health policy dictates delivery modalities, provider education, certification, provider qualifications, payment, the spectrum of services, and access to care. In addition to the policy itself, the rules and regulations concerning implementation of a policy directly impact nursing practice, education, administration, and research. Each nurse must have a working knowledge of health policy and regulation and how members of the largest health care profession can influence policy to increase the health and well-being of society.

Prior to the 20th century, health care was basically an individual or private sector responsibility. Many health care facilities were affiliated with religious and civic organizations and groups or educational institutions. Physicians had private office practices with out-of-pocket payment from clients. The federal government became involved in the regulation, provision, and financing of health care primarily during the early 1900s. Government involvement, scientific advances, and increased dollars associated with health care have resulted in the development of a health care industry that rivals the manufacturing and agriculture industries. This industry, including professional nursing, is affected by many political, economic, and social factors. Germane to the development, imple-mentation, and evaluation of health policy are politics, legislative and budget processes, regulation, leadership, and economics.

Politics

A variety of individuals, organizations, agencies, and state and federal processes are involved in developing health policy and the regulations for implementation. A citizen writes a congressman (or congresswoman) and argues that certain needs are not being met for technology-dependent children. An organization such as the American Association for Retired Persons writes, visits, and caucuses with congressmen on new and continuing needs of the elderly. Agencies such as the National Institutes of Health invite congressmen (or congresswomen) to attend and provide input in administrative hearings on priority setting, program development, and budgetary needs.

POLITICAL PARTIES

Three major political parties have been involved in legislation in the 1990s and early 2000s: the Republican National Committee (RNC), the Democratic National Committee (DNC), and the Reform Party. Political parties set forth the major issues of concern in the party platform during each presidential year convention. These platforms consist of "planks" that delineate the parties' philosophy and stand on issues. Platforms are a consensus of the convention delegates, but they also mirror the presidential candidate's stand and arguments to be used during the campaign. Platform issues, then, often become the agendas for state legislatures and the U.S. Congress. Many of the issues during the 20th century have been health related, such as gun control, abortion, Medicare, and AIDS. The most recent Republican and Democratic platforms can be obtained from the national offices or their web sites.

ORGANIZATIONS

In addition to the formal political parties, organizations are involved in the development of legislation. Two organizations with very close ties to the formal parties are the Grand Old Party Political Action Committee (GOPAC) and the Democratic Leadership Council. In fact, many congressional leaders are also members, leaders, and participants in these organizations, which highlight and disperse party philosophy, beliefs, and views on issues. Nonlegislative citizens also play a political role in health policy development and implementation through participation in and support of lay organizations and activities, such as Mothers Against Drunk Driving (MADD), the American Cancer Society, the March of Dimes, the National Organization of Women (NOW), and the National Rifle Association (NRA). Most professional organizations (e.g., American Medical Association [AMA], American Hospital Association [AHA], and American Nurses Association [ANA]) also develop legislative agendas, support political candidates, and employ lobbyists at state and federal levels.

Lay and professional organizations, whether or not associated with one political party, such as the American Association of Retired Persons (AARP), the NRA, the ANA, the National Home Care Association (NHCA), and the American Association of Health Plans (AAHP),

lobby legislators through grassroots activity, paid lobbyists, campaign support, and advertisements. Most health care professional organizations, including the ANA, have a paid lobbyist in each state capital and at least one in Washington, D.C. The proportion of membership dues not tax deductible because it goes to funding political and lobbying activities provides one indication of the cost and importance of these activities. The ANA uses approximately 22% of its dues for lobbying activities.

POLITICAL ACTION COMMITTEES

Political action committees (PACs) can be established solely or as a part of a formal organization to (1) raise, spend, and contribute money, (2) assist with campaigns, and (3) lobby on behalf of specific issues or persons. PACs initiate much of the legislative activity or inactivity on both the state and federal levels. For example, *Roe v. Wade*, which legalized abortion, has been a continued topic of discussion. The Christian Coalition and NOW pay for television advertisements, hold public rallies and demonstrations, distribute literature, and invite political and other famous figures to events supporting their positions. All of these activities, as well as financial support for politicians who have voted or will vote on further bills relating to this issue, make PACs increasingly powerful.

Often called *special interest groups*, PACs are representative of persons with specific needs that have been overlooked or not protected by society (AIDS, elders, homeless, poor children). PAC activity and contributions have changed how legislation is formed, what is passed, and the amount and type of appropriations approved. It is difficult for legislators to meet the needs of one special interest group and not another one because of the large number of citizens represented by these groups. As a result, there has been an increase in bills passed that either require additional federal monies, leave unfunded mandates, or require states to fund programs.

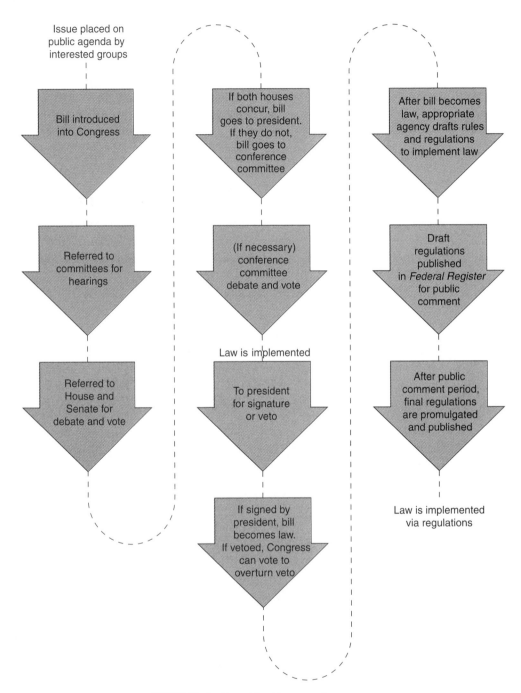

FIGURE 10-1 Formal health care policy process.

FINANCING

A recent concern has been access to legislators and the influence on legislation by PACs and financial contributors to campaigns. The Federal Elections Commission (FEC) regulates the type, amount, and reporting of such funds. State commissions handle those within state, county, and municipal governments. Each candidate, political party, and PAC is required to register and submit quarterly, monthly, or annual financial reports. However, the national party organizations (DNC, RNC, and so forth) have been required to report contributions only since 1991. This is traditionally referred to as "hard money." The documentation of "soft money" is minimal at best (FEC, 2000). *Soft money* is money given to the party, but for no specific purpose. It is often used to support campaign activities, but under a different guise. For example, instead of giving money to a senatorial campaign for travel to a state capital, the party supports a high school student workshop on a topic that invokes the candidate's position, thus averting the campaign finance rules constraining usage.

Campaign finance reports, as well as documentation of PACs, corporate, and other large contributors to each party and candidate, are required by the FEC and are available to the public (web site: www.fec.gov). The monies spent on media, travel, and food are extensive, especially at the congressional and presidential levels. One year prior to the 2000 election, the FEC reported that eight candidates for the presidency had raised $181 million (FEC, 2000). Presidential candidate George W. Bush raised $65 million in campaign funds before any state caucus or primary election had been held. In addition to funds raised by candidates, the government provides funds from the taxpayer-supported election fund. These monies are distributed to candidates after they raise a specified amount, but places a cap of $40 million dollars on what can be spent on primaries or precon-vention efforts for candidates who choose to accept these funds.

Legislative Process

A good explanation of how a bill proceeds through Congress is the recent revision of *How Our Laws Are Made* (U.S. House of Representatives, 1999). This document details the steps, processes, facilitators, and barriers to enacting legislation at the federal level from introduction through enrollment to the president (see Figure 10–1). House and Senate procedures are discussed, including leadership roles and responsibilities, committee assignment, readings on the chamber floor, and resolution between the two chambers. Many of the steps and processes, such as the house "hopper" and the system of bells and lights, originated in late 19th century. The *hopper* is the box where representatives initially place a piece of legislation they wish to be brought to the house for action. A *system of bells and lights* is placed throughout the capital building to notify representatives of the pending voting and other actions. Another major discussion in this document is how to "bury" or "kill" a bill, and how the majority party ideas prevail even in the most sacred workings of our democracy.

ADMINISTRATION AND COMMITTEES

In addition to the constitutionally mandated process and structure, each Congress establishes its own rules for administration and governance that affect how policies are made and which issues are considered. *Rules* include the number, type, and focus of committees where most of the legislative work takes place. In fact, committee chairmen, assigned because of seniority, develop the calendar of issues and legislation to be discussed. It has been true in the past, and will probably continue to be true, that bills brought forth for discussion and passage are not necessarily the purview of the particular committee. Rather, these issues may be germane to the ranking majority or minority leader for their constituents due to his or her personal beliefs and experience, or they may be related to financial support received from individuals, organizations, and corporations.

Committee structure is also determined for each Congress, with the exception of several mandated committees. The committee structure was fairly stable for the 30 years during which the Democrats controlled the House of Representatives and often the Senate. During that time, the Committee on Labor and Human Resources had primary responsibility for health care legislation and issues. With the new Republican majority in the House of Representatives in 1994 and that party's control over the Senate, committee structure was altered. Several committees were terminated, and the names and jurisdictions were changed throughout the 105th and 106th Congresses. A new Health, Education, Labor and Pensions Committee in the Senate was charged with primary health policy jurisdiction. However, many committees develop health-related bills and send forth authorizations and appropriations for those bills, such as the Agriculture Committee (nutrition) and the International Relations Committee (American Red Cross).

CONGRESSIONAL SESSIONS

Each Congress has two sessions for developing legislation. The 106th Congress began in January 1999 with the first session; the second session was held during 2000. Legislation that has passed through both houses, been resolved in conference committee, enrolled to the president, and signed become *public laws.* These laws are signified by the Congress in which they are passed as well as their chronological order of passage (e.g., PL 106–22). Financial allocations—more precisely, appropriations—are included in bills and usually include funding for 3–5 years. However, appropriations are dependent on the budget bills passed for each calendar year, and thus can be revised or repealed by subsequent congressional action.

CHAMBER RESPONSIBILITIES

A constitutional directive related to budgetary matters is that all bills, including an increase in federal income taxes, originate in the House of Representatives. Thus, the Senate cannot initiate an income tax increase, but it can increase spending limits and develop new programs that may result in the need for increased taxes. Either chamber can be the origin of bills that establish or increase taxes through other means, such as airport, gasoline, or Medicare taxes. The Ways and Means, Appropriations, and Finance Committees have input to the budget and review legislation originating in other committees that require new or continuing appropriations. Any legislation that includes appropriations, whether continuing or new, is required to be submitted by committees and subcommittees to those budget committees for calculation, inclusion in the fiscal year (FY) appropriations bills, and estimations of spending in the outlying years. On most occasions the budget committees change or alter the recommended allocations and refer these changes to the committee charged with a specific piece of legislation, as well as to the committee of primary responsibility for that specific area (e.g., health care, education, transportation).

The Senate has primary responsibility for approval of political appointments, such as judges, ambassadors, the surgeon general, cabinet members, and federal agency directors. In the 1990s the approval hearings were contentiously political and philosophical. Health-related issues such as sexual harassment, sex education, family planning, refugee support, and immigration laws served as litmus tests for appointee approval. Two other health issues, abortion and the death penalty, continue to be major points for discussion not only of health policy but also of the appointment of judges to state, appellate, and federal courts and the U.S. Supreme Court.

STATE ACTIVITIES

Most state legislatures also have two chambers, and leadership is similar to that of Congress, in that there is a Speaker of the House, Senate majority leader, and majority/minority whips to provide day-to-day administration of the legislative bodies. Chamber and committee leadership is determined by seniority, past party leadership, respective party caucuses, and persons who aspire to the party ideology and philosophy in setting legislative agendas. State legislatures also play a large role in the budgetary decisions and public services provided within the state. Many state constitutions require a balanced budget both submitted by the governor and approved by the legislature. Thus, even in states, outlying years of health programs and services can be in jeopardy through required annual appropriation decisions. Several states have instituted a lottery or specific types of gambling to increase revenues. For many states, this revenue is directly tied to education or specific health programs. Public health initiatives, such as adolescent tobacco use reduction, drunk driving prevention, and school health programs, are funded with these nonrecurring funds. Public education may also be supported by this type of fund. In that case, state-supported universities and public schools can be asked to increase enrollment, decrease faculty, or trim operations in order to stay within budget allocations. With the evolving shortage of educators, this type of situation threatens the quality and quantity of nursing education and thus nursing practice.

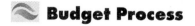 **Budget Process**

APPROPRIATION OF FUNDS

Appropriation bills are required to approve funding for running the federal government each fiscal year (October 1 to September 30). Bills, which represent spending by each cabinet department (e.g., Treasury, Labor, Commerce, Health and Human Services, Defense), require congressional approval and presidential signature no later than the beginning of each fiscal year. Near the end of each congressional session, all appropriation bills are combined into a general appropriation bill, which prior to 1997 was called the Omnibus Budget Reconciliation Act (OBRA). In 1998 and 1999 the titles were also focused on financial priorities, such as the Taxpayer Relief Act.

Through the president's proposed budget, with input from the administration's Office on Management and Budget (OMB), this process begins in Congress. After consideration of the proposed budget submitted by the White House, each chamber develops a budget resolution bill by April of each year. Additionally, all legislation under consideration that includes funding recommendations or appropriations is required to be submitted by committees to the Congressional Budget Office (CBO). The budget office reviews and calculates the actual costs to the federal government, as well as how a particular appropriation fits into the proposed budget or reconciliation bill. One of the problems with the revenue and expenditure estimates in the latter part of the 20th century was that there were three offices computing the figures: the CBO, the administration's OMB, and the General Accounting Office (GAO). These offices often came up with different estimates, depending on the estimates of inflation, economic growth, gross domestic product, and consumer price index numbers used. Thus, the final appropriations bill or reconciliation bill had several versions from the House and Senate, which the White House may or may not have supported. There was, of course, political influence on the computations and the final reconciliation appropriation bill.

Several times during the 1990s, these factors resulted in the lack of passage of a final reconciliation bill by the October 1 deadline. Rather, continuation appropriation bills were passed. In 1999, appropriations bills for cabinet departments became laws, and the continuation bill was not approved until the seventh vote. A *continuation bill* can be limited in effect until a specific date or until the replaced appropriation bill is enacted. This bill must be approved by regular processes, but it only allows legislative continuance of authorization and appropriations at the present level in order to keep the federal government running. Also, even though new authorizations may have been approved with funding, until the final appropriations reconciliation bill has passed Congress and is signed into law by the president, no changes can be made in programs, services, or funding. Thus, Congress completes the final reconciliation bill under political and legislative pressure. The federal budget bill often is achieved by "crisis" management in Congress. The lack of approval for a reconciliation bill caused the federal government to shut down on more than one occasion in the 1990s. This type of crisis management also allows special amendments to be added to the bills at the "midnight hour" in order for certain representatives and senators to agree to vote for the final bill. The deal-making and "pork barrel" special interest spending are added to what may have been appropriate legislation and allocations in an earlier version of a bill.

Emergency spending, or that not included in the fiscal year reconciliation bill, can be approved through supplemental appropriation bills. For example, after Hurricane Andrew in 1994 and Hurricane Floyd in 1999, special funds and Federal Emergency Management Agency (FEMA) increases were approved to provide disaster relief in Florida and North Carolina. Additional defense spending was allocated through supplemental bills for Desert Storm and the Bosnia crisis.

AUTHORIZATION OF PROGRAMS

Authorization bills (with funding requests) are required to establish or continue programs as well as to fund those mandates. The initial authorization is usually a separate bill named for the issue or program being established, such as the Older Americans Act, the Ryan White AIDS Act, or the Public Health Service Act. New governmental agencies may be initiated or established, as was the case with the Administration on Aging in 1965. Future authorization and reauthorization bills are required to make changes in governmental agencies, to expand programs, and to continue or alter funding levels. However, some authorization bills that are passed do not contain any funding levels. Rather, these bills are used to establish programs that are to be funded by governmental departments within present allocations or by individual states, or they are unfunded mandates. For example, the Brady Bill gun control legislation requires background checks on gun purchasers before a license is issued. The federal law contains no continuing funds; thus, states must provide funds or be in violation of the law, and as a result often suffer loss of government monies for law enforcement. Some authorization bills purposely contain no funding recommendations. On many occasions, these are political statements that legislators and political parties take credit for passing in the interest of a constituency or social need. However, the public is often unaware there is no funding to enact the legislation.

FISCAL CONSTRAINT

Several efforts were made during the 1980s and 1990s to mandate a balanced budget at the federal level. The Gramm-Rudman-Hollings law, which passed in 1985 (PL 99-177), required a gradual decrease in spending to result in a balanced budget by 1991. The Supreme Court subsequently found this law to be unconstitutional. During the 104th Congress, a major effort by the newly Republican-controlled House of Representatives was launched to pass an amendment to the U.S. Constitution to require a balanced federal budget. This attempt failed in Congress; thus, citizens did not vote on the constitutional amendment. However, Congress passed a Balanced Budget Act in 1997, which required a balance of expected revenues and expenditures by the federal government for the 1998 fiscal year. The next year, Congress passed the Taxpayer Relief Act of 1998 as the reconciliation bill that included additional child care exemptions and capital gains tax reform. In 1999, the reconciliation bill was the Taxpayer Refund and Relief Act. Although it passed both chambers of Congress, President Clinton vetoed the bill.

Appropriation or budget bills are required for the functioning of the federal government or other legislation, and thus "pet" or specialized programs are often attached to the budget bills in order to get them enacted. For example, several times during the 1980s the Nurse Education Act's appropriation bills were "tacked on" to the budget to ensure that they were passed during that fiscal year before Congress adjourned. Much of the time pork-barrel amendments are approved to gain the votes from specific congressmen. While the spending will benefit constituencies, the programs often are not federal mandates. Since many of these amendments are added at the midnight hour, much of the public is not aware of these expenditures until they have been approved. The president does not have line item veto and therefore must accept or veto each appropriation bill in its entirety to enact the fiscal year budget.

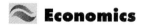 **Economics**

The federal budget for 1999 included 66% for mandatory spending. Approximately half ($786 billion) of the total budget is for entitlements, such as Social Security, Medicare, and Medicaid. Public dollars account for 46% of the $1.1 trillion national health expenditures (Health Care Financing Administration, 2000b). The president's proposed budget for FY 2001 has similar numbers (Office of Management and Budget, 2000). Also, a majority of the Department of Health and Human Services (DHHS) budget is for entitlement programs, which means that only a third or less of the amount appropriated by Congress for this department can be controlled. The National Institutes of Health (NIH), the Health Care Financing Administration (HCFA), and the Bureau of Health Professions (BHP) are included in the DHHS budget. Nursing leaders and others have continually worked to increase these budgets, and these efforts resulted in budget increases during 1999 and 2000. In FY 2000, HCFA appropriations totaled more than $320 billion, with federal Medicaid obligations totaling $112 billion (DeParle, 2000). The NIH FY 2000 budget was $18 billion and the National Institute of Nursing Research (NINR) non-AIDS budget was $82 million. The president's FY 2001 budget proposed $421 billion for DHHS, with increases in the State Children's Health Insurance Program, long-term care, Medicare preventive services, caregiver support, children's hospitals, and substance abuse. Increases in the NIH, NINR, and the Agency for Healthcare Research and Quality (AHRQ) research budgets are also included (Grady, 2000; Shalala, 2000).

In 1999, a federal surplus of $170 billion resulted from a thriving economy, a leaner governmental structure, and the Balanced Budget Act of 1997. However, when the Social Security Trust Fund "IOU" and national debt of over a trillion dollars is considered, it is questionable whether there is a surplus. The Social Security Trust Fund for several decades has been borrowed from each year to meet appropriations required to sustain the government and its other programs. Even when suggested in the late 1990s, there has been no "lock box" approach to stop this borrowing. Thus, the retirement income and Medicare programs that are funded by present workers' payroll taxes do not contain monies to fund those same workers when they reach age 65. The GAO estimates that the Social Security Trust Fund will be unable to meet its obligations starting in the year 2010. In fact, to continue funding Social Security and Medicare, double-digit increases in payroll taxes of 17% and 50%, respectively, would be required (Walker, 2000).

How to spend or save the surpluses resulted in continued disagreement in the 106th Congress second session. The major issues were whether to provide tax cuts, save Social Security, modify Medicare, or pay down the national debt. Debate continues over how a government with a large national debt and a large tax base can best serve its citizens, given the promises made to citizens regarding retirement and health insurance in old age.

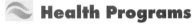 **Health Programs**

There are two main types of federal health care programs. *Discretionary programs* are those which are subject to annual appropriations by Congress and considered controllable budgetary items. These programs consist primarily of categorical health services, training, and research programs. Categorical health services are services for relatively narrowly defined categories of problems, such as programs for communicable diseases, family planning, and family planning services. An example of a training program is the Nurse Education Act, and an example of a research program is the National Institute of Nursing Research at the NIH.

Entitlements are those health care programs considered less controllable with respect to budgetary expense. Citizens are entitled to the benefits by law because of prespecified age, disability, or economic status. The federal government is obligated to pay these benefits regardless of the number of enrollees or the costs. The only major avenue to cut costs is by changing either the authorization or eligibility criteria through legislation. Costs cannot be limited by appropriating less money for expenditures. Social Security, veterans' compensation, and pensions are examples of income entitlement programs. Health care entitlement programs are Medicare,

Medicaid, and state Children's Health Insurance Programs. Much of the activity in the 105th and 106th Congresses was related to how to deal with the increasing costs for these entitlement programs, as well as to propose strategies for reforming the programs.

Implementation and Regulation

Multiple governmental agencies plan, implement, and evaluate health policy in the United States. The major agencies are headed by political appointment cabinet officials, directors, and administrators but are staffed by career civil servants. Congressional legislation and presidential executive orders and mandates can change auspices. The last major revisions occurred in 1996 after the Republican Congress and the Democratic vice president requested and mandated streamlining and reorganization of the government. The Balanced Budget Act of 1997 also mandated changes in the administration and implementation of federal programs. Prior to the 1990s there had been minimal change in most federal departments or regulatory oversight.

The DHHS is charged with protecting and ensuring the health of the nation and is headed by the Secretary of Health. Multiple agencies and divisions are included in the DHHS (Fig. 10–2) and several assistant secretaries are responsible for administrative aspects. The Surgeon General is an Assistant Secretary of Health and heads the Public Health Service. An Assistant Secretary for Aging heads the Administration on Aging and the Administration for Children and Families. Other agencies are headed by a commissioner (e.g., Food and Drug Administration) or director (e.g., NIH). Agencies include several sections or divisions. For example, there are 25 institutes and centers at NIH. In Atlanta and other regional offices, the Cen-

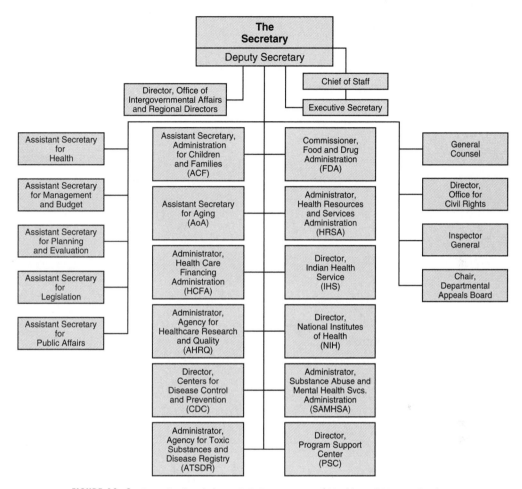

FIGURE 10–2 Organizational chart, U.S. Department of Health and Human Services.

ters for Disease Control and Prevention (CDC) houses 11 centers, institutes and offices, including the National Center for Health Statistics, the National Center for Chronic Disease Prevention and Health Promotion, and the National Center for Infectious Diseases (Centers for Disease Control, 2000). Most federal government agencies and states have civil rights, legal, public relations, and budget sections staffed by career employees. More recently, these agencies provide comprehensive web sites

for consumers and professionals to obtain program and contact information. Selected political, professional, and health-related agencies and organizations and their web sites are listed in Table 10–1.

Each agency has specific auspices or sponsorship, though not always consistent with the appropriation. The Department of Agriculture directs the commodity distribution program (e.g., nonfat dry milk, cheese products), the national school lunch program, farm programs, and food

TABLE 10-1 Selected Agencies and Organizations and Their Web Sites

Abbreviation	Organization or Agency	Web Address
AACN	American Association of Colleges of Nursing	www.aacn.nche.edu
AAHP	American Association of Health Plans	www.aahp.org
AEI	American Enterprise Institute	www.aei.org
AHRQ	Agency for Healthcare Research and Quality	www.ahrq.gov
AMA	American Medical Association	www.ama-assn.org
ANA	American Nurses Association	www.nursingworld.org
	Brookings Institute	www.brookings.org
BHP	Bureau of Health Professions	www.hrsa.dhhs.gov/bhpr
CBO	Congressional Budget Office	www.cbo.gov
CDC	Centers for Disease Control and Prevention	www.cdc.gov
DNC	Democratic National Committee	www.dnc.org
	Division of Nursing, Health Resources and Services Administration, Bureau of Health Professions	www.hrsa.dhhs.gov/bhpr/dn/dn.htm
FDA	Food and Drug Administration	www.fda.gov
FEC	Federal Elections Commission	www.fec.gov
FEMA	Federal Emergency Management Agency	www.fema.gov
GAO	General Accounting Office	www.gao.gov
GOPAC	Grand Old Party Political Action Committee	www.gopac.com
HCFA	Health Care Financing Administration	www.hcfa.gov
IOM	Institute of Medicine	www.iom.edu
NIA	National Institute on Aging	www.nia.nih.gov
NIAAA	National Institute on Alcohol Abuse and Alcoholism	www.niaaa.nih.gov
NIDA	National Institute on Drug Abuse	www.nida.nih.gov
NIH	National Institutes of Health	www.nih.gov
NIMH	National Institute of Mental Health	www.nimh.nih.gov
NINR	National Institute of Nursing Research	www.nih.gov/ninr
NLN	National League for Nursing	www.nln.org
OMB	Office of Management and Budget	www.financenet.gov/omb
OSHA	Occupational Safety and Health Administration	www.osha.gov
	Pew Charitable Trusts	www.pewtrusts.com
RNC	Republican National Committee	www.rnc.org
RWJ	Robert Wood Johnson Foundation	www.rwjf.org
USDHHS	United States Department of Health and Human Services	www.dhhs.gov
	United States House of Representatives	www.house.gov
	United States Senate	www.senate.gov
	W. K. Kellogg Foundation	www.wkkf.org

inspection. The HCFA directs Medicare, Medicaid, and Children's Health Insurance Programs, and the Department of Labor houses the Occupational Health and Safety Administration (OSHA). In addition to the federal levels, most states have similar agencies and auspices to manage public programs. For example, the Tennessee Department of Health houses the Bureau of TennCare to administer the Medicaid waiver program.

Whereas laws are written in broad language, the rules and regulations to implement these laws are written very specifically and often can be revised without changing the original law. Agencies are charged with implementation, financial oversight, legislative interpretation, and the development of regulation and rules governing their respective programs. Often agencies are required to interpret the purpose and intent of congressional or state legislation in order to implement such laws. The agency director's, staff's, and proponents' perceptions, political savvy, and experiences have an impact on this interpretation of the issue under consideration. Interpretations and changes in regulations can be related to the number and types of citizens served in a particular program, the increase or decrease in appropriations, the social or ethical values of directors and department head, and societal crises.

In some instances the auspices and appropriations are not consistent. The Department of Agriculture receives appropriations for the elder nutrition programs, but these are provided by the Administration on Aging through the state, regional, and local agencies. The Department of Labor has administrative responsibility for the Senior Community Service Employment Program, which is under the auspices of the Administration on Aging. The Bureau of Census collects vital data, but the National Center for Health Statistics and the Department of Labor analyze that data for developing policy and allocation decisions. Thus, some health-related policy legislation and appropriations require extra effort to determine the auspices, regulation, and

implementation, and whether there is duplication or omission.

As the health care industry evolves with new emphases, programs, and services, the governmental agencies must develop new strategies for evaluation of their implementation. Such evaluation for specific policies and their implementation has recently begun at the federal level. This evaluation of process, structure, and outcomes has become an emphasis, especially for the Social Security, Medicare, and Medicaid programs. Process and structure are often difficult to change in large bureaucratic organizations of state and federal government. An Annual Performance Plan required of agencies should assist in examining program and administrative efficiency. The recent emphasis on outcomes should lead to changes in process and structure in order to meet the objectives set forth. Two such health-related efforts are the *Healthy People 2010* (U.S. Department of Health and Human Services [USDHHS], 2000b) national objectives and the initiative to eliminate racial and ethnic disparities (USDHHS, 2000a).

Leadership

During the 20th century, several persons and organizations provided leadership to ensure the passage of major health policies and regulation. Surgeon Generals Everett Koop, Jocelyn Elders, and David Satcher strongly supported efforts to deal with chronic diseases, prevent and reduce health risks through education, and target efforts based on *Healthy People* national health objectives (USDHHS, 2000b). David Kessler, an FDA administrator, worked to protect consumers through regulation of nutritional and dietary supplements. He also argued for regulation of tobacco. The tobacco lawsuit settlement was reached, but not from the purview of the FDA. The lawsuit was brought by states' departments of justice suing for repayment of public dollars (Medicare and Medicaid) spent on providing health care to those with tobacco-related illnesses. The $360 billion settlement agreed to by the tobacco industry is to be paid over 25 years. Activities associated with the agreement were the termination of soliciting adolescent smokers, bans on tobacco advertisements within specific distances of schools, and further supplementation of education and prevention programs across the country. This is an example of the judicial branch of government playing a role in health policy and planning.

LEGISLATORS

Senators Edward Kennedy (D-MA), Barbara Mikulski (D-MD), Paul Simon (D-IL), and Nancy Kassenbaum (R-KS) led health-related legislative efforts during the 1980s, 1990s, and early 2000s in the U.S. Senate. In the House of Representatives, many efforts were led by Henry Waxman (D-WI), John Lewis, (D-GA), and Joseph Kennedy (D-MA). Foci for legislative efforts were programs for vulnerable populations such as children, elderly, and low-income persons, and appropriations for new and continuing programs. During 1999, Senator John Breaux (R-LA) and Senator Bill Frist (R-TN), a heart surgeon, headed the National Bipartisan Commission on the Future of Medicare, which sponsored the Medicare Preservation and Improvement Act of 1999. Although the bill did not pass Congress, the commission report is a major focal point for continued discussions of how to sustain Medicare. Additional health policy efforts in early 2000 were related to managed care (both private and public sector) and consumer rights regarding their health care coverage, personal information, and competency of providers. The issues of liability and welfare reform were led by the Republicans in the House of Representatives, and saving Social Security and Medicare were issues of Democrats and Republicans in both chambers. In fact, these latter issues were major campaign topics for candidates in the 2000 presidential election.

NURSES

Many nurses have provided leadership at the national level, to not only recognize nursing's contribution to health care but also to ensure quality and access to care. Former ANA presidents Virginia Trotter Betts and Beverly Malone were instrumental in setting Nursing's Agenda for Health Care Reform (American Nurses Association, 1991). These two nurses also assisted the ANA Council on Practice and various professional practice organizations to impact the passage of third-party reimbursement changes for advanced practice nurses, accreditation of home health agencies, and provision of childhood immunizations. Drs. Betts and Malone later were appointed Assistant Secretaries of Health at DHHS.

Debbie Gettis, a registered professional nurse, served as the AIDS advisor to President Clinton for 18 months. Because of the numerous intervention and outcomes studies she conducted while at the University of Pennsylvania and Case Western Reserve University, Dr. Dorothy Brooten, a nurse researcher, was elected to the Institute of Medicine, which advises Congress on health matters. Dr. Ada Sue Hinshaw was appointed the first director of the National Institute of Nursing Research. The present director, Dr. Patricia Grady, is a nurse who has a background in basic sciences, which she has used to develop collaborative agendas with other institutes in the areas of genetics, psychoneuroimmunology, chronic diseases, mental health, and aging. Nancy Bergstrom and Thelma Wells provided leadership in the development of the Agency for Health Care Policy and Research (AHCPR) guidelines for practice, and Nancy Fugate-Woods and Ora Strickland spearheaded a focus on women's health issues. Peter Buerhaus, an economist, and Linda Moody served as scientists at the national level to develop recommendations and projections for nursing workforce, staffing, and economic needs.

THINK TANKS, FOUNDATIONS, AND ORGANIZATIONS

Other sources of health policy and planning encompass private or public think tanks, philanthropic foundations, and policy centers. The Brookings Institute and the American Enterprise Institute support scholars in multiple fields to research, discuss, and evaluate social needs. Many of the needs are related to health, such as the environment, the welfare system, genetics, and individual versus states' rights. Also, the position papers on economics have often included costs in the health care arena and the aging of America. In addition to the think tanks, several foundations play a role in health policy and planning.

The Pew Charitable Trusts provide grants for health care demonstration and research activities and support studies of the health care industry. Recently, the Trusts supported the Pew Health Professions Commission to study the future needs of the health care system in the United States. Four reports have been issued (O'Neil, 1993; O'Neil & the Pew Health Professions Commission, 1998; Pew Health Professions Commission, 1995; Sugars, O'Neil, & Bader, 1991). These reports delineate the nature of health care work, the restructuring of health care professional regulation, the number and types of professionals needed, and the training and education of professionals. Much of the discussion is, by necessity, in the context of an evolving health care system with dynamics not yet known.

There are three major issues for nursing. First are the workforce needs, that is, what qualifications and the types of roles nurses will be required to fill. The American Association of Colleges of Nursing (AACN; 1999a, 1999b) and the ANA (1997) suggest, and the Pew report recommends, an increase in the number of RNs at the baccalaureate level and advanced practice nurses with master's level preparation.

A second issue is that of nurse educators with doctoral degrees to prepare nurses for the workforce needs. Although many doctoral programs have opened in the past two decades, the number of doctorally prepared nurse educators required for appropriate training and education of the projected workforce has not kept pace with market need. This lag is partially due to the large number of nurse faculty retiring in the early 2000s and partially due to the lack of incentives to stay in public rather than private sector positions.

A third issue is that of competency-based education and practice in which nurses demonstrate critical thinking, judgment and decision-making skills, and cultural competence, and engage in transdisciplinary practice. Curricular, regulation, and certification changes have been implemented. In the mid-1990s, the National League for Nursing Accreditation Commission (NLNAC) for baccalaureate and master's degree programs placed an increased emphasis on critical thinking and community-based care. The AACN (1996, 1998) put forth the essentials of baccalaureate and master's degree education, which include health care delivery, ethics, and competency-based education. The Commission on Collegiate Nursing Education (CCNE) and NLNAC, the professional accreditation bodies, required that undergraduate programs target their mission to local and regional health, rather than having a cookie cutter approach to curriculum. Master's programs were standardized for clinical and role competence, as well as mastery of the health care delivery system and economic knowledge and skills. This standardization has resulted in an increase in nurses with specialty certification. The American Association of Critical-Care Nurses (AACN), the Association for Women's Health, Obstetrical and Neonatal Nursing (AWHONN), and the Oncology Nursing Society (ONS) offered new certification for master's-prepared nurses.

Several other organizations have an impact on health policy and nursing. The Institute of Medicine (IOM), one of the National Academies of Science, advises Congress on health matters through position papers, expert witnesses, and recommendations for legislative initiation, approval, and funding. The IOM is often involved in discussions of and decisions for auspices and allocations for the Division of Nursing and nurse education acts in Congress. The American Public Health Association, the AMA, the ANA, and the American Dental Association all provide expert testimony to state and federal agencies and decision-making bodies on topics from product liability to school lunch programs, immunizations, disaster relief, and the cremation of deceased persons.

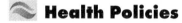

Health Policies

Health policies, or decisions regarding the health care system, are developed and implemented through several avenues. Congressional and state legislation, federal, state, and local rules and regulations for agencies, and appropriation decisions are methods to develop health policy. Some health policies are only legislation, while others are developed by multiple avenues. All of these avenues are impacted by public opinion, the economy, societal demographics, professional expertise, technology, and knowledge of health.

STATE NURSE PRACTICE ACTS

Legislation and related policies that directly affect nurses are the state practice acts (see Chapter 12). The nurse practice acts and corresponding rules and regulations define educational preparation and programs, eligibility for licensure, and the scope of practice. All states require passage of the NCLEX examination for RN licensure. Candidates for licensure must have graduated from a program approved by the state board of nursing, but the requirement for graduation from a nationally accredited school varies among states. Nursing practice in most states includes research, education, admin-

istration, counseling, and clinical practice or direct patient care.

Many national organizations also play a role in defining practice. The National Council of State Boards of Nursing develops the licensure examination for nurses. The American Nurses' Credentialing Center, as well as various national specialty organizations, determines eligibility, educational qualifications, experience, and examinations for national certification required in many states. This is especially true for advanced practice. In some states, an advanced practice nurse can practice without certification but cannot have prescriptive privileges unless national certification is obtained. In other states certification either is not required or is required for both.

State practice acts are statutes requiring legislative approval for establishment and amendment. In the past, the majority of changes occurred in the legislative arena. More recently, state boards of nursing have developed specific rules and regulations concerning practice that can be changed without legislative activity. This avoids the possibility of undesirable statute transpositions that might occur when "opening" the practice act for legislative revision. Additionally, the rules and regulations allow the nursing profession to articulate the practice, roles, and responsibilities of nurses, rather than others defining such.

HEALTH POLICIES 1900–1990

Three of the most influential health policies are the Social Security Act of 1935 and the amendments that established Medicare and Medicaid in 1965. Many of our national concerns with health and welfare have been addressed by amendments to these policies. Issues such as abortion, family planning, nutrition, and disability, as well as those related to vulnerable populations (chronically ill, mentally ill, elders, poor, and minorities), are included as major concerns and foci of programs and payments. These are also the largest programs in terms of population covered and dollars spent. With the aging of the population, technological and pharmaceutical advances, and changes in the racial-ethnic face of society, the original intent and expected costs of the programs have been far exceeded. A major issue today is how to continue these programs as a "safety net" with the means testing and entitlements that have been established.

Many bills and acts have been passed that directly and indirectly affect the health of society (Table 10-2). In the 1960s the Hill-Burton Act, which funded hospital construction, was a major focus. Legislation for payment to nurses was included in the Rural Health Clinics Act of 1977 and extended with the Omnibus Budget Reconciliation Act (OBRA) of 1989. In the 1970s and 1980s there was increased emphasis on disease prevention, risk reduction, and research on the leading causes of death (cardiovascular disease, cancer). The OBRA of 1982 established the diagnostic related groups (DRGs), which resulted in a prospective payment system for Medicare hospitalization. There was legislation regarding mental health, school lunch programs, disease research, and rural manpower. End-stage renal disease and disabil-

TABLE 10-2 Selected Policies Affecting Nursing and Health Care Before 1990

Year	Title	Content/Purpose
1935	Social Security Act	Established the Social Security Administration and pension income
1938	Food, Drug and Cosmetics Act	Provisions of safe and effective drugs through labeling; 1984 amendments applied to generic drugs
1941	Nurse Training Appropriations	To assist nursing schools in increasing enrollments and improving programs
1944	Public Health Service Act	Established the U.S. Public Health Service under one statute (Title 42, U.S. Code)
1964	Nurse Training Act	Initial federal act for professional nurse training
1965	Medicare (SSA amendment) Medicaid (SSA amendment)	Established health coverage for the elderly Established health coverage for the indigent
1965	Older Americans Act	Established the Administration on Aging, which provides a broad network of services to elders
1970	Title X Public Health Service Act	Established family planning grant programs aimed at low-income women
1973	Health Maintenance Organization Act	Established alternative to fee-for-service for government-subsidized employers
1982	Omnibus Budget Reconciliation Act (OBRA)	Added the prospective payment system (DRG) to Medicare hospital admission payment
1986	Protection and advocacy of individuals with Mental Health Illness Act	Established agencies to investigate and pursue legal action against abuse and neglect of persons with mental illness
1987	Nursing Home Reform Act (OBRA)	Standardized the types of services nursing homes must provide, quality, and patients' rights
1989	Amendments to Nursing Home Reform Act	Allowed NP/CNS to certify need for nursing homes
1989	OBRA	Medicaid direct payment for pediatric and family nurse practitioners

ity were added to Medicare eligibility. The 1987 OBRA (PL 101-203) changed Medicare payments to hospitals, changed health maintenance organization (HMO) requirements, and authorized nurse practitioners and clinical nurse specialists to certify patient needs for nursing home care.

HEALTH POLICIES 1990–2000

The 1990s were perhaps the most prolific decade for health policies and regulation for specific diseases, conditions, and vulnerable groups (Table 10–3). The Patient Self-Determination Act allowed persons to make decisions regard-

TABLE 10–3 Selected Policies Affecting Health and Nursing Passed in the 1990s

Year	Title and Number	Content
1990	Patient Self-Determination Act (PL 101-508)	Required all Medicare/Medicaid-paid health care institutions to provide/ask for advanced directives
1990	Occupational Safety and Health Act—amended (PL 101-552)	Describes general working conditions for health care workers, as well as statements for blood/body fluids, prevention of infectious disease, and biohazard waste
1990	Trauma Care Systems Planning and Development Act (PL 101-590)	Established guidelines for trauma care/services; replaced the 1973 EMS Act
1990	Americans With Disabilities Act (PL 101-336)	Prohibits discrimination in employment, transportation, accommodations, public services, and telecommunications for persons with disabilities
1992	Breast and Cervical Cancer Mortality Prevention Act (PL 101-354)	Provides grants to states for screening, referrals, educational programs to clients; training for professionals; quality assurance programs; research
1992	Mammography Quality Standards Act (PL 102-539)	Requires certification, accreditation, and inspection of centers, including equipment/technicians/records
1993	Family and Medical Leave Act (PL 103-3)	Establishes leave (job security) for persons caring for an ill child/family member, childbirth/adoption, or illness of employee; applicable to businesses with 50+ employees
1996	Welfare Reform Act (PL 104-93)	Adults limited to 5 years on welfare; must work within 2 years of starting on welfare
1996	Health Insurance Portability and Accountability Act (PL 104-191)	Provides for portability when changing jobs, limits preexisting conditions, requires congressional reports to evaluate the impact of the law
1996	Newborn's and Mother's Health Protection Act (PL 104-326)	Mandates medical decision for minimum 48-hour stay after delivery; provider includes midwife and NP
1997	Balanced Budget Act (PL 105-33)	Medicare direct payment to advanced practice nurses; Children's Health Insurance program; welfare-to-work
1998	Health Professions Education and Partnership Act (PL 105-392)	Consolidated health professions education and training, as well as minority health education and training; nursing education funding
1999	Healthcare Research and Quality Act (PL 106-129)	Changed name of AHCPR to AHRQ; mandates and funds quality and outcomes research

ing their own health care. The Ryan White Act was passed to deal with issues related to AIDS. New NIH guidelines for inclusion of women and children in research altered past trends, the use of past findings, and subsequent health policies. As the number of homeless persons increased, private and local public sectors had difficulty dealing with the costs and spectrum of services. The McKinney Homelessness Act established both funded and unfunded mandates. The Americans With Disabilities Act has impacted not only health care but also work environments and the justice system.

Policies and new regulations in the 1990s also impacted nurses and other health care workers. Parenting and caregiving concerns resulted in the Family and Medical Leave Act. OSHA guidelines were developed regarding "work-at-home" employees. Reauthorization of programs and allocations for older Americans, children, and indigent care each year also impact nursing and health care. The Health Professions Education Partnerships Act (HPEP) included the Nursing Education and Practice Improvement Act, which established the National Advisory Council on Nurse Education and Practice for studying workforce needs. A major purpose of the HPEP bill was to consolidate health profession education, training, recruitment of minorities, and rural placements. Family violence prevention, fetal alcohol syndrome, rural, children's, and Alzheimer's activities were included in the larger bill. Additionally, there were revisions in HCFA regulations during the latter part of 1998 and 1999 that changed payment, diagnostic capabilities, and reimbursement for advanced practice nurses as a result of federal legislation.

MANAGED CARE

Legislation of special interest is the Patient Bill of Rights or Managed Care Bill of Rights. Political and economic influences have, as of January 2001, resulted in a lack of legislative approval. A primary issue is that of accountability on the part of a managed care organization, which presently is absent and not included under most state insurance statutes. Since no federal legislation was passed, a presidential order was given and DHHS enacted regulations concerning consumer rights for Medicare and Medicaid beneficiaries. Medicare and Medicaid now have managed care options, with Medicaid ones being established through HCFA waivers to states in the early 1990s.

Although the issue of liability has not been clearly addressed, information concerning coverage and decisions regarding care have been established, and some states have passed similar legislation. The state policies primarily address the right to information concerning health coverage. For example, individuals have the right to notification of denial, changes in benefits, provider network, and network institutions such as hospitals and drugstores. Some bills provide the right to information, written and verbal, concerning the appeal or grievance processes and include a mechanism for arbitration over disputed denial of care.

The number of Americans on managed care plans increased steadily during the 1990s. In 1998, approximately 80% of Americans with employer-sponsored health insurance had managed care plans. Medicaid-managed care covers 16.5 million persons, or 54% of recipients; California and Tennessee have the largest number of recipients. Medicare beneficiaries originally had HMO options, beginning in 1997, but now have Medicare+Choice, which includes HMO, point-of-service (POS), and preferred provider organization (PPO) options. Six million persons (14%) are in managed care plans, which receive 18% of the payments (HCFA, 1999, 2000a).

Nursing and Health Policy

Health policy, regulations, allocations, and care impact nursing and are impacted by nursing in several ways. In addition to the leadership areas addressed in the previous section, nursing practice, education, and research are involved. The following sections address these areas.

PRACTICE

The new health care arena requires nursing administrators and staff to be aware of economic, communication, and ethical issues at a different level than previously encountered. This entails knowledge not only of budgets, but also of various health payment plans, the use of community resources, product evaluation, technology, and benchmarking against other like institutions, agencies, and practices. Consumers are also more educated and aware of their health needs and rights in today's world. Competency-based practice and a higher level of accountability are expected from society as a whole and consumers individually. Although the standard of care and types of services may be different according to a particular agency, setting, or location, a standard level of competency is required.

Standards provided by professional organizations, including the ANA's *Standards of Clinical Nursing Practice* (1998) and *Scope and Standards of Advanced Practice Registered Nursing* (1996), as well as specialty standards for practice, are a response to both societal and professional clarification of nursing. Identification of competencies, such as those provided for home care (Benefield, 1998) and continence care (Sampselle et al., 1997), will be required for all areas of practice. Effectiveness studies that support competent and quality practice also impact legislation. One of the early studies by Brooten and colleagues (1988, 1991) documented that follow-up care by master's-prepared nurses resulted in better health outcomes for mothers and children. Later, a similar research team found that a collaborative and coordinated discharge planning and advanced practice nurse (APN) follow-up for elders resulted in fewer hospital days and readmissions (Naylor & McCauley, 1999). Mundinger

(1999) and Mundinger et al. (2000) documented comparable patient satisfaction with care by nurse practitioners and physicians, and comparable or lower costs for care provided by nurse practitioners. These interventions indicate to legislators and the public that nursing contributes to better health outcomes, quality, and cost containment.

Self-development, continuing education, certification, and retooling will be required as the health care delivery system continues to evolve. This learning must be of a transdisciplinary nature, including language, client need, treatment, and evaluation of outcomes, quality, and access. While hospitals and clinics continue as major settings for acute medical care, long-term and other alternative care settings and delivery methods that assist clients to achieve health must be initiated and embraced. Case management for high-cost and high-risk clients can assist in meeting the need of specific populations (LoBianco et al., 1996). Homeless clinics, parish nursing and collaborative efforts with school systems are additional delivery methods that provide community-based care to vulnerable populations.

EDUCATION

Authorization for nursing education originated with the Nurse Training Act of 1964. Every 3 to 4 years the Nurse Education Act was reauthorized with appropriations. Between 1965 and 1971, more than $380 million was spent on nursing education for both students and institutions. Doctoral nursing students and nursing doctoral programs began receiving more emphasis and support during the mid-1970s. The 1980s and 1990s saw master's programs receiving larger allocations to provide tuition and stipends for preparation of nurse administrators, nurse practitioners, nurse midwives, and clinical nurse specialists. However, in the 1990s, with the onset of managed care and increased competition for health care dollars, the nursing education legislation was twice not acted on.

Passage of the Health Professions Education

Partnership Act in 1998 changed the tradition for several decades that nursing was the only health profession to retain a separate funding law. In previous decades, through political activism, nursing was able to gain support for education, even though no president had specifically funded nursing education in his proposed budgets. Congressional funding for nursing education has increased and expanded to include baccalaureate and multiple roles at the master's level, but enrollments have not increased to meet the projected needs in most areas of the country (AACN, 1999a). Many programs have increased ambulatory and community-based experiences, but most educational programs provide few experiences or courses in long-term care or a transdisciplinary health team approach. Rather, nursing students are having fewer opportunities for courses and experiences outside the nursing curriculum.

Accreditation of nursing programs was historically done by the National League for Nursing. Policies relative to accreditation came under scrutiny in the 1990s (see Chapter 2), and the National League for Nursing Accrediting Commission (NLNAC) was established as a free-standing entity. In 1999, the Council on Collegiate Nursing Education (CCNE), which evolved from the American Association of Colleges of Nursing, gained recognition from the Department of Education. How these changes will affect legislative authorization or appropriations is uncertain. It is certain that the Pew Report has had a major impact on congressional action and that nursing must seriously consider the recommendations: initiating new curricula, developing creative teaching methods, stimulating lifelong learning, establishing competency-based educational programs, and evaluating care delivered are necessary at all levels (Bellack & O'Neil, 2000). The AACN "essentials" documents for baccalaureate and master's education are excellent beginning guidelines, but these must be evaluated and revised as health care changes. Workforce and staffing studies, such as those being conducted by Dr. Barbara Mark and colleagues (Geddes, Salyer, & Mark, 1999),

the North Carolina Center for Nursing, and the AHRQ will become more germane to nurses at the local and state levels when nurses must lobby for increased scholarship funding, continued authorization of nursing programs, and reimbursement for advanced practice.

RESEARCH

The establishment of the National Institute of Nursing Research (NINR) at the NIH in 1993 and its reauthorization has affected nursing research most recently. NCNR was established in April 1986 with the purpose of providing a strong scientific base for nursing practice. Seven years later, on June 11, 1993, the NCNR became the NINR, the 17th institute of the NIH. NINR is an integral part of NIH, and the National Advisory Council participates in setting the agenda and budget for national health priorities. The program areas at NINR in the 1990s were consistent with the national priorities set by NIH and *Healthy People 2000/2010*. These areas included dealing with chronic illness and long-term care, health promotion and risk behaviors, reproductive and child health, and immune responses and oncology (National Institute of Nursing Research, 2000).

NINR also funds investigators who are not nurses, and nurses receive funding from institutes other than NINR. An interdisciplinary focus of projects is emphasized across program areas at many institutes, including the National Institute on Aging, National Institute of Mental Health, National Institute on Alcohol Abuse and Alcoholism, National Institute on Drug Abuse, and AHRQ. Agencies such as the CDC have funded nurse-directed studies on adolescent smokeless tobacco prevention (e.g., Stotts, 1997), and the Substance Abuse and Mental Health Services Administration has funded demonstration projects to prevent family violence in minority communities (e.g., duMont, 1999). Nurse scientists, such as Dr. Sally Weinrich, also have been invited to be investigators in the Human Genome project and other large interdisciplinary studies.

In addition to NIH, research directions have been guided by foundations such as the Robert Wood Johnson and W. K. Kellogg Foundations, which have funded many community and rural health initiatives. Findings from nursing investigations and experience have resulted in input to the development of practice guidelines. Nancy Bergstrom and her colleagues' work on decubitus ulcers and Jean Wyman and Thelma Wells's work on incontinence influenced the AHCPR practice guidelines for those health needs. These researchers also investigated the costs and effectiveness of interventions (Bergstrom et al., 1996, 1998; Jirovec, Wyman, & Wells, 1998; McClish et al., 1999). In addition, many of the early Ryan White AIDS programs and homeless shelters were nursing demonstration projects that have resulted in continued allocations and authorizations.

NINR, Sigma Theta Tau International, the four regional research societies, specialty organizations, Friends of NINR, and the National Nursing Research Roundtable meet annually to discuss and plan for the direction, implementation, and funding of nursing research. Regional and national conferences and the State of the Science Conference highlight nursing research findings that have an impact on health care delivery, costs, access, and outcomes. Congressional members and persons from local, state, and regional political and legislative arenas are invited to attend these meetings to discuss nursing and health care efforts and needs. Additional research activities include nursing fellowships and grants by the AHRQ, the Robert Wood Johnson Foundation, the W. K. Kellogg Foundation, and the Templeton Foundation. Nurses also fill positions as clinical researchers in medical centers across the country and conduct ongoing studies.

OUTCOMES AND QUALITY

Outcomes research is now required to determine the effectiveness and accountability of practice. There is much effort to defining what constitutes outcomes and how to measure them. Outcomes research is a priority in the area of health services research. A recent policy initiative was the enactment of the Healthcare Research and Quality Act of 1999, which changed the name of the Agency for Health Care Policy and Research (AHCPR) to AHRQ and provided additional funded mandates for quality and outcomes activities. This emphasis provides that research on outcomes and quality will be the foundation of future policy, regulation, and allocation decisions for health care.

National health indicators, *Healthy People 2010*, and the initiative to eliminate racial and ethnic disparities (USDHHS, 2000b) provide one set of outcomes and a measure of quality. Examining system outcomes is another avenue of research. These outcomes are those related to direct and indirect material and financial costs, length of stay, manpower, provider qualifications, and provider and payer satisfaction. Client outcomes such as consumer satisfaction, health status outcomes, adaptation, and function are another set of outcomes that require study. A final issue to be addressed is how outcomes and quality relate to and affect one another. This will be a specific area for nursing to address in future practice, education, and research efforts.

≋ Comment

As members of the largest group of health professionals, nurses can influence health care policy as individuals and as professionals. Consumers of health care, including nurses, desire affordable, accessible, and high-quality care. As professionals, nurses are obligated to ensure that the public has access to quality health care at controlled costs. Identifying and prioritizing client needs with sensitivity to culture and diversity, knowledge of treatments and interventions (both nursing and interdisciplinary) in one's area of practice, a focus on outcomes (client, system and provider), and ensuring safe, quality care in multiple environments are the basic requirements of professional nursing as we enter the 21st century.

Armed with information on how to influence health care policy, nurses serve as advocates for patients and become active participants in the formulation of effective health care policy. Organizational membership in regional, state or national organizations, and letter writing are two traditional activities for nurses involved in policy making. More focused involvement can be through collective actions as members of political action committees and political parties. Social, civic, professional, and lay organizations with interest in populations and concerns of interest also provide a mechanism by which nurses can influence legislation and allocation decisions. Another mechanism is to run for elected office or sit on boards, committees, councils, or commissions, especially those that make policy and funding decisions that affect health care. Consultation to elected officials, health agencies, foundations, educational institutions, and funding agencies provides opportunities to share expertise and communicate nursing needs and contributions.

Policy decisions regarding financial resources influence the type of nursing staff, the number of nurses, the amount and type of management and support services, and educational program and research funding—all of which affect the quality of nursing and health care. The settings and payment of care also affect access and the spectrum of services available. Using professional and personal knowledge, expertise, and experience, nurses can take action in research, practice, and education areas. Politics, legislation, and economics provide ample opportunity and challenge for nursing involvement. A major avenue to take advantage of these opportunities and meet the challenge of proving that access and quality health care for all can be achieved through involvement in the health policy arena.

KEY POINTS

● Health policy is influenced by many factors, including politics, economics, and personal and societal priorities.

● Legislation is a complex process that includes multiple players, takes time, and involves political and special interests.

● A large portion of the federal budget and expenditures is for health programs, specifically Medicare, Medicaid, and Social Security entitlements, which originally were a safety net for the most vulnerable.

● Federal and state legislation, as well as rules and regulations to implement policies, influence the availability, access, and spectrum of health care and nursing care.

● Managed care has not changed health care costs, but it has changed the way health care is delivered and to whom.

● An outcomes and quality focus is necessary for future nursing practice, education, and research.

● Nursing has influenced and been influenced by policy and allocation decisions.

● Nurses have a responsibility to participate in health policy and planning to ensure quality health care.

● Knowledge and involvement are key to influencing health policy.

CRITICAL THINKING EXERCISES

1. What are the major health care issues in your community, state, and region? Determine the outcomes desired. What are some solutions to these problems? How might you become involved in implementing these solutions?

2. Discuss how a practice, education, or research situation was directly affected by present health policy. What are the options for changing that policy? What are the barriers and facilitators to changing the policy?

3. Discuss how we should address entitlements with a health care provider, a health care economist or businessperson, and a client. Develop three strategies and share these with your state or national legislator and your professional organization.

4. What are your responsibilities to ensure access to quality, timely, appropriate, and cost-effective care?

REFERENCES

American Association of Colleges of Nursing. (1996). *The essentials of master's education for advanced practice nursing.* Washington, DC: Author.

American Association of Colleges of Nursing. (1998). *The essentials of baccalaureate education for professional nursing practice,* Washington, DC: Author.

American Association of Colleges of Nursing. (1999a, January). *Nursing school enrollments lag behind in rising demand for RNs, AACN survey shows* [On-line]. Available: http://www.aacn.nche.edu/Media/NewsReleases/enr198wb.htm

American Association of Colleges of Nursing. (1999b, April). *Faculty shortages intensify nation's nursing deficit* [On-line]. Available: http://www.aacn.nche.edu/Publications/issues/ib499wb.htm

American Nurses Association. (1991). *Nursing's agenda for health care reform.* Washington, DC: Author.

American Nurses Association. (1996). *Scope and standards of advanced practice registered nursing.* Washington, DC: Author.

American Nurses Association. (1997). *ANA response to the Pew Commission report* [On-line]. Available: http://www.nursingworld.org/readroom/pew.htm

American Nurses Association. (1998). *Standards of clinical nursing practice* (2nd Ed.). Washington, DC: Author.

Bellack, J. P., & O'Neil, E. H. (2000). Recreating nursing practice for a new century. *Health Professions Education, 21*(1), 14–21.

Benefield, L. E. (1998). Competencies of effective and efficient home care nurses. *Home Care Manager, 2*(3), 25–28.

Bergstrom, N., Braden, B., Kemp, M., Champagne, M., & Ruby, E. (1996). Multisite study of incidence of pressure ulcers and the relationship between risk level, demographic characteristics, diagnoses, and prescription of preventive interventions. *Journal of the American Geriatrics Society, 44,* 22–30.

Bergstrom, N., Braden, B., Kemp, M., Champagne, M., & Ruby, E. (1998). Predicting pressure ulcer risk: A multisite study of the predictive validity of the Braden Scale. *Nursing Research, 47,* 261–269.

Brooten, D., Brown, L. P., Munro, B. H., Cohen, S. M., Roncoli, M., & Hollingsworth, A. (1988). Early discharge and transitional care. *Image: Journal of Nursing Scholarship, 20,* 64–68.

Brooten, D., Gennaro, S., Knapp, H., Jovene, N., Brown, L., & York, R. (1991). Functions of the CNS in early discharge and home followup of very low birthweight infants. *Clinical Nurse Specialist, 5,* 196–201.

Centers for Disease Control and Prevention. (2000, June). *About CDC* [On-line]. Available: http://www.cdc.gov/aboutcdc.htm#cios

DeParle, N. A. (2000, February). *Statement by Nancy-Ann DeParle, Administrator, Health Care Financing Administration on fiscal year 2001 President's budget request to Subcommittee on Labor, Health and Human Services, Education, and Related Agencies of the Appropriations Committee, U.S. House of Representatives* [On-line]. Available: http://www.hhs.gov/progorg/asmb/budget/testify/b20000208b.html

duMont, P. (1999). *Family strengthening program.* Rockville, MD: Substance Abuse and Mental Health Services Administration.

Federal Elections Commission. (2000, February). *Campaign finance reports and data.* [On-line]. Available: http://www.fec.gov

Geddes, N., Salyer, J. & Mark, B. A. (1999). Nursing in the nineties: Managing the uncertainty. *Journal of Nursing Administration, 29*(5), 40–48.

Grady, P. A. (2000, March). *Statement by Dr. Patricia A. Grady, Director, National Institute of Nursing Research on fiscal year 2001 President's budget request for the National Institute of Nursing.* House Subcommittee on Labor-HHS-Education Appropriations, U.S. House of Representatives [On-line]. Available: http://www.nih.gov/ninr/3-2-2000statement.htm

Health Care Financing Administration. (1999, April). *National summary of Medicaid managed care programs and enrollment* [On-line]. Available: http://www.hcfa.gov/medicaid/trends98.htm

Health Care Financing Administration. (2000a, January). *National health expenditures 1998* [On-line]. Available: http://www.hcfa.gov/stats/nhe-oact/hilites.htm

Health Care Financing Administration. (2000b, January). *National health expenditures 1998–2008* [On-line]. Available: http://www.hcfa.gov/NHE-Proj/proj1998/hilites.htm

Jirovec, M. M., Wyman, J. F., & Wells, T. F. (1998). Addressing urinary incontinence with educational continence-care competencies. *Image: Journal of Nursing Scholarship, 30,* 375–378.

LoBianco, M. S., Mills, M. E., & Moore, H. W. (1996). A model for case management of high cost Medicaid users. *Nursing Economics, 14,* 303–307, 314.

McClish, D. K., Wyman, J. F., Sale, P. G., Camp, J., & Earle, B. (1999). Use and costs of incontinence pads in female study volunteers. *Journal of Wound, Ostomy and Continence Nursing, 26,* 207–13.

Mundinger, M. O. (1999). Can advanced practice nurses succeed in primary care market? *Nursing Economics, 17,* 7–14, 111.

Mundinger, M. O., Kane, R. L., Lenz, E. R., et al. (2000). Primary care outcomes in patients treated by nurse practitioners or physicians. *Journal of the American Medical Association, 283,* 59–68.

National Institute of Nursing Research. (2000, March). [On-line]. Available: http://www.nih.gov/ninr

Naylor, M. D., & McCauley, K. M. (1999). The effects of a discharge planning and home follow-up intervention on elders hospitalized with common medical and surgical cardiac conditions. *Journal of Cardiovascular Nursing, 14*(1), 44–54.

Office of Management and Budget. (2000, February). *FY2001 budget* [On-line]. Available: http://w3.access.gpo.gov/usbudget/index.html

O'Neil, E. H. (1993). *Health professions education for the future: Schools in service to the nation.* San Francisco: Pew Health Professions Commission.

O'Neil, E. H., & the Pew Health Professions Commission. (1998). *Recreating health professional practice for a new century.* San Francisco: Pew Health Professions Commission.

Pew Health Professions Commission (1995). *Critical challenges: Revitalizing the health professions for the 21st century.* San Francisco: UCSF Center for the Health Professions.

Sampselle, C. M., Burns, P. A., Dougherty, M. C., Newman, D. K., Thomas, K. K., & Wyman, J. F. (1997). Continence for women: Evidenced-based practice. *Journal of Obstetric, Gynecologic, and Neonatal Nursing, 26,* 375–389.

Shalala, D. E. (2000, March). *Testimony of the Honorable Donna Shalala, U.S. Secretary of Health and Human Services, before the Subcommittee on Labor, Health and Human Services, Education and Related Agencies, Committee on Appropriations, U.S. House of Representatives* [On-line]. Available: http://waisgate.hhs.gov/cgi-bin/

Stotts, R. C. (1997). *Preventing addiction to tobacco chewing (PATCH).* National Cancer Institute, 1 R01 CA76969-01.

Sugars, D. A., O'Neil, E. H. & Bader, J. D. (1991). *Health America: Practitioners for 2005.* Durham, NC: Pew Health Professions Commission.

U.S. Department of Health and Human Services. (2000a, January). *The initiative to eliminate racial and ethnic disparities in health* [On-line]. Available: http://raceandhealth.gov

U.S. Department of Health and Human Services. (2000b, March). *Healthy people 2010* [On-line]. Available: http://web.health.gov/healthypeople

U.S. House of Representatives. (1999, September). *How our laws are made* [On-line]. Available: http://thomas.loc.gov/home/holam.txt

Walker, D. M. (2000, February). *Medicare reform: Leading proposals lay groundwork, while design decisions lie ahead.* Testimony before the U.S. Senate Committee on Finance. GAO/T-HEHS/AIMD-00-103 [On-line]. Available: www.gao.gov

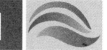

11

Economic Issues in Health Care

MATTIA J. GILMARTIN, PhD, RN

OBJECTIVES

At the completion of this chapter, the reader will be able to:

● Define the economic principles of supply, demand, and cost.
● Describe how the economic concepts of opportunity costs, price elasticity, complements and substitutes, competition, and marginal utility apply to the health care environment, and specifically to nursing.
● Define and differentiate the two methods of cost evaluation presented in this chapter.
● Discuss the interrelatedness of costs of care and quality of care.

PROFILE IN PRACTICE

Barbara A. Cross, MSN, CFNP
Nurse Practitioner
Elson Student Health Center
Charlottesville, Virginia

Economics is important for most college students and their families. At the university where I am employed, all students are required to have medical insurance. Depending on type of policy and the coverage it offers, students sometimes still find themselves faced with deciding whether to pay the copayment for medicines or eat or pay the rent. As a nurse in this setting, I often hear students expressing concern about the cost of medication and needing assistance in finding the best affordable, yet effective medication. The practitioners in our clinic will call on the pharmacist to assist us with this task. Our student health pharmacy offers students discounts on their prescriptions. For students whose insurance plan does not cover the drugs on the student health formulary, we call the neighborhood pharmacies

and compare prices to help the student find the best buys. Another way we have been able to assist students is by administering the first dose of the medication as a "now" dose in the clinic. This reduces the amount of medication the student has to purchase and thus reduces the cost. The pharmaceutical representatives have assisted us by keeping us supplied with samples of medications. At other times, instead of using the first choice of treatment for a condition, the second or third choice may be used if it is more affordable. So the challenge for us as practitioners in student health is to build a rapport with the students and provide an environment that allows them to share their concerns about their financial situations that can affect their health and treatment decisions.

The 1990s have been characterized as the economic era of health care service delivery (Brown, 1994; Johnson, 1994). In that decade, professional nurses and other health care providers saw a radical shift in the financing and organization of health care as a result of efforts to improve the economic effectiveness and efficiency of the U.S. health care system. Health economic concerns now permeate every aspect of nursing, and an understanding of basic economic issues has become essential not only to the nurse administrator, but also to the nurse educator, the nurse researcher, and the practicing clinician. In the current era, an understanding of economic principles is a fundamental and integral component of professional nursing practice. Because nurses are the largest professional group in the health care workforce, numbering approximately 2,558,874 in the United States (Health Resources and Services Administration, Bureau of Health Professions, 1996), their economic decision making has a direct effect on the financial performance of the organizations in which nursing practice occurs (Caroselli, 1996). Additionally, an understanding of economic principles and the tools of economic evaluation enables nurses to demonstrate the contributions of nursing practice to improving resource use in the production of health services.

Given the changing nature of the health care delivery environment and the emphasis on cost containment and resource efficiency in care delivery, health care providers must be able to incorporate economic principles into their administrative and clinical decision making. This chapter begins by introducing ten principles used in the study of economics and considers how these principles relate to health care and nursing. The interplay of economics and current health care issues such as the escalation of health care expenditures, problems of access to health care, the economic underpinnings of managed care, and the quality of care and technology use in the United States is then discussed. Two common cost evaluation methods

useful in demonstrating the economic effects of health care resource allocation decisions and skill development exercises are also presented.

Principles of Economics

Economics is the study of the distribution of resources across a population. Similarly, *health economics* is the study of the production and distribution of health care resources. The study of health economics is increasingly of interest and necessity not only to economists, health administrators, government policy formulators, and financiers of health care but also to providers of health care services (including physicians and nurses) and to consumers of health care.

Henderson (1999) identifies ten guiding principles, or concepts, necessary for the study of economics. Although economic theory is complex, it is guided by a relatively small set of principles. Henderson's ten principles are the following:

1. The principle of *scarcity and choice* addresses the problem of limited resources and the need to economize. There are not enough resources to meet all the desires of all the people, making rationing in some form unavoidable. We are forced to make choices among competing objectives—an inescapable result of scarcity.

2. The principle of *opportunity costs* recognizes that everything and everyone has alternatives. Time and resources used to satisfy one set of desires cannot be used to satisfy another set. The cost of any decision or action is measured in terms of the value placed on the opportunity forgone.

3. *Marginal analysis* is a way of thinking about the optimal use of resources. Decisionmakers weigh the trade-offs of a little more of one thing and a little less of another. In this decision-making mode, consideration is given to the benefits and costs of one more unit of a good or service.

4. *Self-interest* is a primary motivator of economic decision-makers. People respond to incentives and practice economizing behavior only when they as individuals can benefit from the behavior. In a just society, the pursuit of self-interest leads each individual to a course of action that promotes the general welfare of everyone in society.

5. *Markets and pricing* serve as the best way to allocate scarce resources. The market accomplishes this through a system of prices—everything has a price that a consumer is willing to pay for a good or service. Prices decrease if less is desired and increase if more is desired. The price mechanism enables a firm to gauge its output decisions in relation to consumer desires and buying behavior. When supply and demand are in balance the market is in equilibrium.

6. *Supply and demand* serve as the foundation for all economic analysis. Supply refers to the amount of a good or service available to consumers in the market. Demand refers to a consumer's willingness to purchase a particular good or service. Goods and services are allocated among competing uses by striking a balance (equilibrium) between the consumers' willingness to pay and the suppliers' willingness to produce goods and ration those goods via the pricing mechanism.

7. *Competition* forces those who own resources to use their resources to produce the highest possible satisfaction for society—consumers, producers, and investors. Competition stimulates efficiency in a market environment by rewarding the resource owners who do well in producing a good or service with the best combination of available resources and penalizing those who are inept or inefficient in resource allocation decisions.

8. *Efficiency* in economics measures how well resources are being used to promote social welfare. Inefficient outcomes waste resources, while the efficient use of resources enhances social welfare. Resource allocation is considered efficient when no one can be made better off without making someone else worse off. This equal-ized allocation state is known as the Pareto Optimum.

9. *Market failure* arises when the free market fails to promote the efficient use of resources by producing either more or less than the optimal level of output.

10. *Voluntary exchange* in a free market environment promotes economic efficiency and ensures that all mutually beneficial transactions occur. Every transaction will benefit both a consumer and a provider. The market system is grounded in the concept of consumer sovereignty—what is produced is determined by what people want and what they are able to buy. No one individual or group dictates what must be produced or purchased.

The ten principles listed above serve as a foundation for presenting a more detailed explanation of the dominant principles of supply, demand, costs, price elasticity, complements and substitutes, competition, and marginal utility as they relate to nursing practice and health care service delivery in the current market environment.

SUPPLY

The *supply* of health care refers to the availability of resources for delivery of health services. Resources include (1) health care facilities, (2) human resources, and (3) financing. Substantial changes have occurred within the last decade in relation to each type of resource.

Health Care Facilities. While hospitals continue to be the primary facility for delivery of health care, economic pressures have resulted in the closure of many traditional hospitals and the emergence of alternative delivery facilities such as ambulatory care centers and home health units (Stoline & Weiner, 1993). The second trend in the supply of health care services is the creation of integrated delivery systems, also known as integrated health systems (Shortell, Gilles, Devers, 1995). As a means to improve the efficiency of resource use, health care providers merge or form alliances to share resources (financial and human) to produce a spectrum of preventative, rehabilitative, and acute care services to meet population-based health needs. A third trend in the supply of health care services is stimulated by changes in the characteristics of patients requiring health care services. The production of patient care services outside the walls of the acute care hospital is related to declining patient length of stays for the acute care portion of service delivery. The "quicker-sicker" patient population is requiring greater quantities of home health services. Table 11–1 demonstrates actual changes in health care expenditures for selected services for the years 1994–1998. Note the large increase in home health care expenditures as compared with hospital care expenditures, and the changes in drug and nondurable supply spending.

Human Resources. Changes in the financing and organization of health care service delivery have a direct effect on the supply, education and training, and regulation of health care professionals. Box 11–1 illustrates a forecasting model to predict changes in the nursing workforce. Figure 11–1 shows another model.

In 1995 the Pew Health Care Commission and its Taskforce on Health Care Workforce Regulation issued a policy statement to revitalize the health professions to meet the changing market demands for integrated, population-based health care. The commission advocated the development of new skills and abilities for all health care professionals. Additionally, the commission recommended regulatory changes to control the supply and competence of the health professions to adjust the overall number and type of health care providers to meet the changing demand for health services.

The Pew Commission's recommendations for the nursing profession include:

1. Recognizing the value of multiple entry points to professional practice through educational preparation at the associate, baccalaureate, and master's levels to contribute different knowledge, skills, and abilities to the changing health care system.
2. Distinguishing between practice responsibilities at the different levels of educational preparation, with the associate degree being the entry level into hospital and nursing home practice, the baccalaureate degree as the entry to hospital-based care management and community-based practice, and the master's degree for specialty practice and independent practice as a primary care provider.
3. Reducing the number and size of basic nursing programs while expanding the number of master's-prepared nurse practitioners.
4. Recovering the clinical management role of nurses at all levels of professional practice (Pew Commission, 1995).

In response to the Pew Commission's recommendations for the nursing workforce, the American Nurses Association (ANA) voiced concern over the proposed regulatory mechanisms that weaken the profession's control over practice while expanding institutional control over the practice, competence, and regulation of professional practice. The ANA advocates the continuation of professional self-regulation through the setting of practice and ethical standards, certification, and other activities that ensure safe, high-quality services for the public (ANA, 1995).

Financing. Unlike many other markets where consumers pay directly for a product or service, consumers of health care predominantly purchase insurance, which in turn pays for the products and services, or they rely on subsidized insurance. It is the exception when the consumer of health care services pays directly for those services (especially hospitalization). The financing of health care is primarily provided by either private, commercial insurance companies

	Expenditures (in Billions)					Average Annual Growth (%)				
	1994	1995	1996	1997	1998	1994	1995	1996	1997	1998
National Health Care Expenditures	$947.7	$993.3	$1039.4	$1088.2	$1149.1	5.5	4.8	4.6	4.7	5.6
Hospital care	335.7	347.0	359.4	370.2	382.8	3.9	3.3	3.6	3	3.4
Physician services	193.0	201.9	208.5	217.8	229.5	3.8	4.6	3.3	4.5	5.4
Drugs and other medical non-durables	26.2	29.1	31.2	30.5	29.3	7	8.7	10.6	10.8	12.3
Home health care	81.5	88.6	98.0	108.6	121.9	14.1	11	7.1	-2.2	-4
Nursing home care	71.1	75.5	80.2	84.7	87.8	7	6.1	6.3	5.5	3.7

Note: Total expenditures for health care services have increased over time while the percentage of money invested (annual growth) in these services shows a pattern of decreasing over time. For example, overall expenditures in home health care services have increased each year, while the actual amount of money invested as a percentage of the previous year's expenditures has decreased over time. This reflects changes in overall spending patterns for health care services brought about by the Balanced Budget Amendment.
  From Health Care Financing Administration, Office of the Actuary, National Health Statistics Group [on-line]. Available: http://www.hcfa.gov/stats.

Box 11-1   Supply and Demand: Estimating the Nursing Workforce

In the current market environment the demand for nurses is in flux due to rapid changes in the organization of the health care delivery system. The supply of nurses available to the health care market is affected by five primary components: (1) predictions of the overall growth of the economy, (2) technology, delivery systems, and regulatory factors within the health care system, (3) economic factors influencing resource scarcity, (4) the availability of personnel in the health care sector, and (5) population factors driving the demand for health services. Historically the educational system, responsible for creating the nursing supply, and the health care delivery sector, which creates the demand for nursing services, have acted independently of one another. The uncertainty of the current marketplace along with opportunities for new nursing services requires the ability to accurately predict the need for appropriate nursing personnel to meet the emerging demand within the changing market environment.

Dumpe, Herman, and Young (1998) present the Forecasting Model of the Nursing Workforce to provide policymakers with information to make accurate decisions regarding the education and employment of nurses. The forecasting model is based on the theory of supply and demand and assumes that the demand for nurses and their services responds in a manner similar to the demand for any other good available in the marketplace. Additionally, the model is based on the assumption that it is possible to forecast the demand for nurses. The major economic concepts used in the forecasting model include supply factors, demand factors, the aggregate demand for nurses, the aggregate supply of nurses, contextual factors, market equilibrium, and the nursing workforce.

or by public entitlement programs, predominantly Medicare and Medicaid (Fig. 11-2). In 1991, 81% of all health care was financed by third parties (Letsch, 1993). The rising costs of health care are passed on in part to consumers, however, in the form of higher insurance premiums, deductibles, and copayments.

The financing of health care, whether by public or private third parties, changed dramatically in 1983 when Medicare introduced the prospective payment system. The former retrospective payment system allowed hospitals to recover their costs regardless of how excessive or efficient the costs and services were, and thus hospitals had no incentives to contain costs. In contrast, under the prospective payment system, payment rates are set before the provision of care and are based on diagnostic-related groups (DRGs). The hospital receives a fixed amount for an admission based on diagnosis and thus has the incentive to contain costs (conserve resources) (Dougherty, 1989).

The next major change in the financing of

health care services in an attempt to correct the excess and deprivation in the health care sector was managed care financing, introduced under the rubric of health care reform in the early 1990s (Enthoven & Kronick, 1991). Managed care uses the general economic principles of competition as a means to reduce costs and improve the efficiency of resources used in the production and delivery of health care services. Under this financing model, delivery organizations are paid a set amount per person in advance (prospectively) of the consumption of health care services. This prospective scheme provides the health care delivery organization with an incentive to reduce the cost of service to match the amount of prepaid resources received to deliver care to a defined group of patients. The economic mechanism of managed care is discussed in more detail in a later section.

The relationship of the supply of resources to produce a good or service and the demand for those goods or services by consumers forms the foundation of the market mechanism. Changes

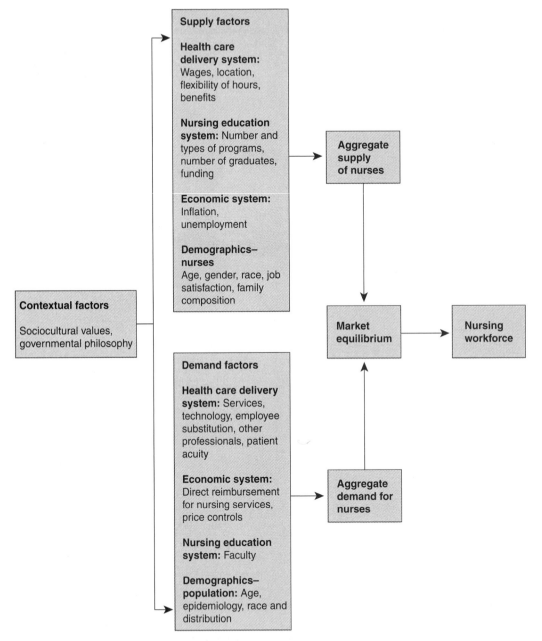

FIGURE 11-1 A model for forecasting the nursing workforce in a dynamic health care market. (Redrawn from Dumpe, M. L., Herman, J., & Young, S. W. (1998). Forecasting the nursing workforce in a dynamic health care market. *Nursing Economic$, 16*(4), 170. Reprinted with permission of the publisher, Jannetti Publications, Inc., Pitman, New Jersey.)

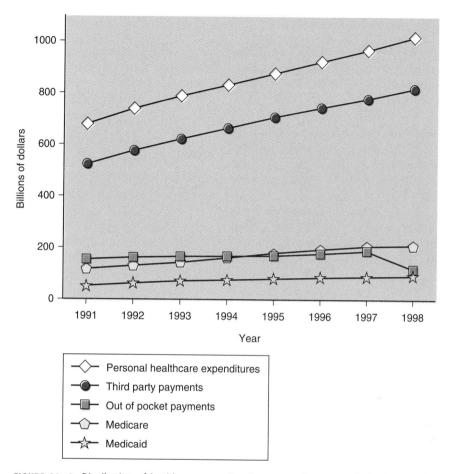

FIGURE 11–2 Distribution of health care spending by source of payment. Projections are for services delivered to individuals. (Data from Health Care Financing Administration, Office of the Actuary, National Health Statistics Group. (1999). [On-line]. Available: http://www.hcfa.gov/stats)

in the availability of health care facilities, health care providers, and funding for health care all affect the supply of health care services. Without available resources to provide services, the supply of health care is not able to meet the demand for health care.

DEMAND

Demand is the amount of a product or service that consumers are willing and able to purchase.

The concept of demand in relation to the health care market is somewhat difficult to understand. When a consumer purchases a dress or a car, it is the dress or the car that they want. In the health care market, a consumer purchases health care but really desires, with a few exceptions, health. Thus the demand for health care "is derived from the more basic demand for health" (Feldstein, 1983, p. 81). Consumers' purchase of health care is dependent on their perceptions of the impact of the care on their health (McMenamin, 1990). The decision to purchase health care is also dependent on the cost of the care to the consumer. Total consumer costs of health care include monetary costs (copayment, deductibles, insurance premiums, out-of-pocket expenses, and lost time and wages from work) and nonmonetary costs (risk, pain, inconvenience, etc.). The demand for health care depends on the willingness of consumers to purchase services after weighing the expected benefits of the care with the costs of the care. If consumers carry insurance, their direct out-of-pocket expenses for the care will be less than if they are uninsured (Feldstein, 1983). Therefore the insurance status of consumers impacts the costs of care (to the consumers) and thus their demand for care. This separation of consumers from the price of health care resulting from health insurance coverage (either private or public) has dramatically increased demand for health care services. However, since demand is based on willingness and ability to purchase, demand for health care does not necessarily correlate with need for health care.

Demand for health care services changes over time as societal demographics and morbidity patterns change. As the baby-boomers of the post-World War II era enter middle and old age in the coming decades, their demands for health care will contribute to the already expanding demands of an ever-growing elderly population. Cures for heart disease and cancer remain elusive, whereas the incidence of these diseases in the elderly remains significant. The AIDS epidemic has changed the types of health care services demanded and has led to the development of new treatments through research and development.

Demand for specific services is also influenced by the recommendations and decisions of health care providers (Feldstein, 1983). Because providers of care possess more knowledge regarding treatment options than consumers, the personal practice styles of providers, as well as how much information they share with consumers, can greatly impact the demand and con-

sumption of services (Rice & Labelle, 1989). Similarly, the risk of litigation by consumers can result in a "defensive practice" style by providers. Fear of litigation can lead to overprescription of (often unnecessary) diagnostic tests or therapeutic interventions and ultimately result in higher health care costs.

COST

Costs are resources required by the provider of services to produce health care products and services, as well as the amount a consumer pays to purchase the products and services. The costs to produce health care are the actual costs of inputs incurred for production, whereas the costs to purchase health care services are what the health care economy will bear (i.e., what the consumers and financiers are able and willing to pay). Thus costs are dependent on supply and demand. Costs may be monetary (pecuniary) or intangible (nonpecuniary). The pecuniary costs of care include salaries of health care providers, insurance premiums, the cost of supplies and equipment used during care, administrative overhead, pharmaceuticals, transportation, and lost salary of the consumer, as well as construction and maintenance costs and research. Nonpecuniary costs are those associated with the personal loss, pain, suffering, and other consequences associated with the consumption of health care services.

The costs of health care are affected by multiple factors, including the supply of services, the demand for services, and the use of medical technology. An increase in the input costs of providing a service increases health care expenditures while the quantity and quality remain constant. Efforts are focused on reducing health care expenditures through reducing the input costs of care without sacrificing the quantity and quality of services.

OPPORTUNITY COST

The resources consumed to produce or purchase a product or service are no longer available for the production or purchase of an alternative product or service. The value of the alternative product or service that is forgone is known as the *opportunity cost* (Pauly, 1993). The opportunity cost is therefore what is given up in order to obtain some good or service. A hospital that can afford to purchase only one of two diagnostic/therapeutic technologies must, in choosing one, give up known benefits of the other. The value of the forgone benefits (revenue generated, lives saved) is the opportunity cost. The concept of opportunity cost can also be applied to personal economic decision making. In the case of the associate degree–prepared nurse who decides to return to school full-time to pursue a baccalaureate degree, the opportunity cost of this career decision includes the lost earnings from not being in the workforce during the time it takes to complete the educational program.

PRICE ELASTICITY OF DEMAND

Price elasticity is the change in demand for a product or service in response to a given percentage change in its price. A situation where consumer demand for a good or service does not change due to a change in price is said to be inelastic. Demand is inelastic when a 1% change in price leads to a change in the quantity demanded that is less than 1%. Alternatively, a situation where the consumer demand for a good or service is relatively sensitive to a change in price that leads to a change in its demand is said to be elastic. Demand is elastic when a 1% change in price leads to a change in the quantity demanded that exceeds 1% (Henderson, 1999).

The price or cost that a person pays for health care is not only the monetary expense but also the person's inconvenience of waiting for and receiving services and the physical and psychological costs of care, including risk, pain, and discomfort. In deciding whether to purchase a health care service or procedure (e.g., an elective surgical procedure), an individual will weigh the expected benefits of the proce-

dure against the expected costs of the procedure (price in dollars, necessary time off work, anticipated pain, and complications). A change in the costs associated with the procedure, such as a less invasive technique that reduces price, length of stay, and associated pain, will influence the demand for that service. The degree of change (elasticity) of demand is dependent on the necessity of the product, the availability of alternative products (substitutes), and the percentage of income spent on the product (Cleland, 1990).

COMPLEMENTS AND SUBSTITUTES

Complements are products or services that are usually consumed jointly, such that an increase in the price of one decreases the demand for both. An example of complements in health care is intravenous fluids and tubing. If nursing services are complements to physician services, then an increase in the price of physician services will decrease demand for both physician and nursing services.

Substitutes, on the other hand, are goods or services that satisfy the same want or need, so that an increase in the price of one will increase the demand for the other. One example of substitutes in health care is two pharmaceuticals that have the same therapeutic effect. Another example is an obstetrician and a nurse midwife. If nursing services are substitutes for physician services, then an increase in the cost of physician services will increase the demand for nursing services.

In the physician arena there is an imbalance between generalists and specialists and a shortage of primary care physicians (Bocchino, 1993). This disparity between consumer demand and physician supply creates favorable opportunities for advanced practice nurses to practice in primary care capacities as physician substitutes. Nurses are making arguments for their use as substitutes for more expensive providers of care for services that they have been formally trained to provide. Similarly, delivery organizations, in an effort to reduce input costs, are incorporating the use of unlicensed personnel as substitutes for nurses for those activities that do not require licensure. Thus nurses are both substituting for some types of providers and being substituted for by other types of providers.

Physicians have traditionally held a monopolistic power as primary care providers, since regulations prevented others from "practicing medicine." As alternative providers of health care services demonstrate their ability to provide comparable services, regulations are being changed to allow these substitutes to enter the market and compete with physicians. Such changes in regulation have only come about since societal demands for more cost-effective providers have escalated while organized physician interests have lost political power.

With the use of advanced practice nurses as physician substitutes, competition between these two providers can occur on the basis of cost-effectiveness. Studies have demonstrated that the use of advanced practice nurses as primary care providers can reduce costs of outpatient care, including laboratory costs, per visit costs, per episode costs, and long-term management costs (Brown & Grimes, 1993; Schroeder, 1993; U.S. Congress, Office of Technology Assessment [OTA], 1986). Research studies have documented that nurse-managed care, when compared with physician-managed care, reduces the frequency of hospitalizations, reduces the acuity of those admitted, reduces the length of stay, reduces the cost of hospitalization, and has equivalent patient satisfaction ratings with service delivery (Michaels, 1992; Mundinger et al., 2000; Rogers, Riordan, & Swindle, 1991).

COMPETITION

In a perfectly competitive market, the market structure consists of numerous buyers and sellers each with no power over price, perfect information by all concerned, free entry and exit into the market, and a homogeneous product (Folland, Goodman, & Stano, 1993). The

health care market violates these assumptions of competition in several ways. First, providers of services are often so few that they possess monopoly power, and information asymmetry often exists between provider and consumer and between consumer and insurer. Second, barriers to entry into the health care field exist in the form of licensure and practice laws, and the services provided vary in type and quality. In addition, since most Americans rely predominantly on third-party reimbursement, consumers are insulated from the true costs of health care. Many consumers (whose insurance is paid by the government or by their employers) believe that health care does not cost them anything. Or consumers feel that they have already paid their share through insurance premiums and that they ought to get their money's worth (Stoline & Weiner, 1993). Thus consumers have no incentive to "shop around" for the best price. The separation of the consumer from costs has compromised the "ability of the marketplace to set prices that reflect societal value" (Letsch, 1993, p. 108).

The imperfections in the health care market lead to a situation called *market failure,* in which the buyers and sellers are unable to strike an equilibrium in supply and demand for goods and services and ultimately fail to produce a socially desirable level of output. In the health care delivery sector, supply-side drivers leading to market failure include the cost of care for hospital and physician services, access to care due to the prohibitive cost of health insurance, and medical outcomes and population health status in light of invested resources. Demand-side factors of market failure in health care relate to the third-party insurance mechanism, where the insurance company or government under the Medicare and Medicaid programs is the primary purchaser of health care services (Henderson, 1999). An effort to move the health care market to a more competitive market to correct the imbalance of supply and demand has been debated for the past decade and is discussed in more detail later.

MARGINAL UTILITY

Marginal utility is the extra utility (satisfaction, welfare, or well-being) gained from consuming one more unit of a good or service. In other words, it is the benefit obtained by purchasing more of a product (Folland, Goodman, & Stano, 1993). When the marginal utility of a product or service is low, the resources consumed by the purchase of the additional amount of that good or service is not used to its fullest potential. Thus the opportunity cost of purchasing one more unit of the good or service is high, since other goods or services that may have resulted in greater benefit or well-being were forgone. There are many examples in health care of use of resources for ser-

vices that have at best a questionable marginal utility. Many health care reformers argue that the resources consumed by high-cost, life-sustaining technologies could be better used for lower-cost, highly effective primary care services, such as immunizations.

For example, less than 5% of the total annual health care budget in the United States goes toward preventive health care services (Centers for Disease Control, 1992), despite the fact that approximately half of all deaths in the United States are attributed to lifestyle and behavior (McGinnis & Foege, 1993). The lack of resource commitment to primary care and wellness services results in higher-cost, reactive care for illness rather than proactive care for the promotion of health and prevention of illness. His-

---

Box 11-2 Methods to Evaluate Costs

The rising costs of health care necessitate the provision of more cost-effective ways to provide comparable services. In the current era, nurses must be able to demonstrate their accessibility, quality of services, and cost-effectiveness in order to validate existing and expanding roles, to broaden reimbursement policies for services that nurses are trained to render and are capable of providing, and to effectively complete with physicians and other providers of care. The two predominant methods of evaluating the economic costs of a service or program are cost-benefit analysis and cost-effectiveness analysis.

COST-BENEFIT ANALYSIS

Cost-benefit analysis is an analytical technique for evaluating the necessary resources and benefits of producing a particular project, program, or technique. Cost-benefit analysis requires assessment and evaluation of the costs and benefits of a program to determine if the benefits of a project outweigh its costs. In a cost-benefit analysis all costs and benefits undergo valuation and are stated in monetary terms. This process places a dollar amount on both monetary and nonmonetary costs and benefits so that a comparison can be made between competing projects or programs. In doing so, value or worth is assigned to nonmonetary aspects of the project's costs and benefits.

Cost-benefit analysis is a useful and powerful tool to justify the investment in nurse-managed services to managers responsible for resource allocation decisions. In this era of resource efficiency and service change, a critical skill for nurses across practice settings and role descriptions is the ability not only to speak the language of economics but also to demonstrate the unique value of nursing services in terms of cost, quality, and value. The widespread availability of personal computers and spreadsheet software makes cost-benefit analysis an accessible tool to a broad range of people. The calculations become effortless. Rather, quantification of the tangible and intangible costs is the difficulty of this method.
Box continued on following page

Box 11-2 **Methods to Evaluate Costs** *Continued*

The comparative nature of cost-benefit analysis is an attractive feature of this analytical technique, but in determining the "worthiness" of a project it is also a pitfall and a drawback. The major limitation of the application of cost-benefit analysis in health care scenarios is that the valuation of intangible costs such as pain or grief or premature loss of life not only varies from case to case, it also differs among analysts assigning the values. Specific criteria and arithmetic maneuvers have been suggested for determining the value of intangible costs and benefits, but they are controversial at best (Klarman, 1982; Pruitt & Jacox, 1991).

COST-EFFECTIVENESS ANALYSIS

Cost-effectiveness analysis is an analytical technique for comparing resource consumption between two or more alternatives that meet a particular objective (such as minimum quality of a product or production of a specific patient outcome). Cost-effectiveness analysis measures the costs involved with each alternative and determines the most cost-effective, or least costly (Kristein, 1983). In a cost-effectiveness analysis only monetary costs of inputs into each alternative are considered. Since the objective (or outcome) of the alternatives is assumed to be the same, the valuation of benefits is not considered (Folland, Goodman, & Stano, 1993). Thus cost-effectiveness analysis avoids making valuations while providing empirical evaluation of costs of alternative health care interventions.

An Example from the Field* The authors reported a cost-benefit analysis of an automated medication distribution system implemented on a 52-bed medical-surgical unit at Stanford University Hospital. Inefficiencies in medication storage and distribution and administration were becoming increasingly problematic as patient stays shortened and the volume of prescribed medications per patient increased. Nursing and pharmacy department costs were measured before and after the implementation of an automated point-of-service medication distribution system. Nursing costs associated with medication administration were tracked using extensive time and motion techniques. The researchers observed eight experienced unit nurses for an entire 8-hour shift over a 30-shift sampling period. Nursing costs related to medication administration were categorized into the distance traveled in feet to acquire patient medications, medication gathering time, and medication administration time. Pharmacy costs associated with stocking, auditing, and exchanging cart inventory were monitored and calculated.

Implementation of the automated point-of-service medication distribution system reduced nurses' time spent administering medication, as well as travel time between locations on the nursing unit to gather medications. An estimated cost savings of $33,547 for the nursing component of medication administration was attributed to the automated medication system. The cost savings captured in a reduction of the average travel distance freed nursing time for the performance of other interventions and activities. In terms of pharmacy costs, the automated medication system improved the capture of 182 medication doses per day, to produce a net increase in recovered medication costs of $66,430. The time gained by pharmacy personnel to check and restock the automated medication system was 40 minutes per day. Time saved from routine stocking activities by the pharmacy technicians was used to expand patient care services with the creation of an intravenous admixture service. Pharmacists' time was used to expand their patient monitoring role throughout the medical-surgical region.

* Modified from Wise, C. L., Bostrom, J., Crosier, J. A., White, S., & Caldwell, R. (1996). Cost-benefit analysis of an automated medication system. *Nursing Economic$, 14*(4), 224–231. Reprinted with permission of the publisher, Jannetti Publications, Inc., Pitman, New Jersey.

torically, nurses have served as health promotion/illness prevention advocates in the community, in outpatient settings, and even in acute care settings, educating patients about health promotion, illness prevention, and chronic disease management. In the early discourse on national health care reform efforts, American nurses advocated for increased resources for preventive services and for improved access to, and reimbursement of, nurse provider services (American Nurses Association [ANA], 1992).

The discussion so far has introduced the general economic principles and mechanisms that influence health care service delivery. The concepts of supply, demand, competition, complements and substitutes, marginal utility, cost, opportunity cost, and price elasticity illustrate the economic forces at play in the health care sector. The next part of the chapter draws on this foundation to examine the major economic issues and trends in health care that are shaping the discourse to improve economic efficiency within the sector (Box 11–2).

Health Care Costs and Access to Care in the 1990s

The widespread concern regarding the economic environment of the contemporary health care system is justified and results from problems of escalating health care costs and access to health services. The decade of the 1990s saw unprecedented change in the financing and organization of health care service in response to national expenditures for health care. The concern is not over the amount of money spent on health care but on the upward spiral of spending that seems to have no end. Aaron (1991) reports that the most frequently cited reasons for the escalation of health care spending include the expansion of the third-party payer system, an aging population, the explosion of

medical malpractice litigation, and the increased use of medical technology.

U.S. health care expenditures represent an increasing share of the gross domestic product (GDP), the combination of all goods and services produced in the domestic economy. In the health care sector, the percentage of expenditure is expressed as a ratio of total health spending to the overall value of the domestic economy. Projections in health care spending are based on data from estimates of per person income increases, the relative price of medical services, growth in consumer out-of-pocket share of spending, changes in enrollment in health maintenance organizations (HMOs) (as a surrogate for all changes associated with managed care), and control of public policy initiatives (Smith, Heffler, & Freeland, 1999).

In the United States, health care expenditures as a percentage of the GDP have grown at an unprecedented rate (Fig. 11–3), outpacing the growth of the entire domestic economy. The GDP grew 2.8% in 1991, whereas national health care expenditures increased by 11.4%, four times the rate of increase of the GDP (Letsch, 1993). The rate of growth of health care spending has exceeded the rate of growth of the overall economy over the past three decades. Health care expenditures in 1991 represented 13.2% of the GDP and totaled $751.8 billion. During 1993–1997, health care expenditures plateaued at 13.5% to 13.7% of the GDP. New predictions of national health expenditures are projected to total $2.2 trillion in 2008, growing at an average annual rate of 6.5% of GDP from their level in 1997 (Smith, Heffler, & Freeland, 1999).

The United States spends a larger percentage of its GDP on health care than do other industrialized nations (Fig. 11–4) Table 11–2 provides a comparison of health care spending patterns of the industrialized nations. Although it is helpful to compare U.S. health expenditures with those of other industrialized nations, these comparisons should be made with caution. Henderson (1999) points out that differences in

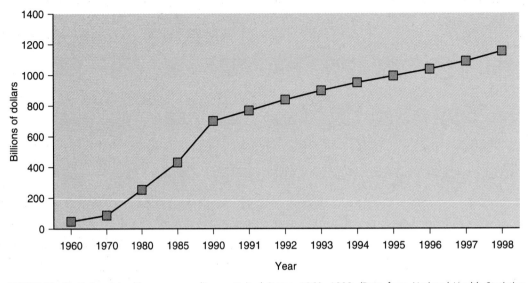

FIGURE 11-3 National health care expenditures, United States, 1960–1998. (Data from National Health Statistics Group, Office of the Actuary (1999). National health expenditures 1996. *Health Care Financing Review, 19*(1) (HCFA Publication No. 03400)).

population demographics, per capita income, disease incidences, and institutional features make direct comparisons difficult. Each country has built its health care system on a unique set of social values in terms of expectations for health care service and the investment as a society it is willing to make in the type of health care services produced. These compari-

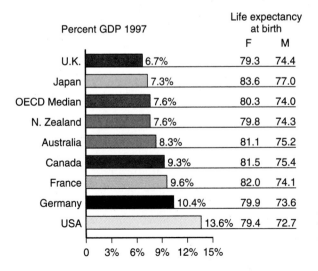

FIGURE 11-4 Comparison of health care expenditures and life expectancy for the industrialized nations. (Data from Organization for Economic Co-operation and Development. (1998). Health statistics [On-line]. Available: http://www.oedc.org)

TABLE 11-2 A Comparison of Key Health Care Statistics for the Industrialized Nations, 1995

	Canada	France	Germany	Japan	United Kingdom	United States
Population (millions)	29.6	58.1	81.7	125.5	58.6	263.1
GDP per capita (adjusted for currency parity, expressed in U.S. dollars)	$21,031	$19,393	$20,497	$21,795	$17,756	$26,438
Health care spending per capita	$2,049	$1,956	$2,134	$1,581	$1,246	$3,701
Health care spending as % of GDP	9.6%	9.8%	10.4%	7.2%	6.9%	14.2%

From *Health Economics and Policy,* 1st edition, by J. W. Henderson. ©1999. Reprinted with permission of South-Western College Publishing, a division of Thomson Learning. Figures are for 1995 and are based on Organization for Economic Cooperation and Development (OECD) data.

sons are made to demonstrate that countries all over the world are struggling with the common problem of controlling the growth of medical care spending. Although we can learn lessons from the social insurance models of health care financing used in the rest of the industrialized world, widespread reform of the U.S. health care system must fit our social value system.

Individual Americans are spending a greater percentage of their annual income on health services than in the past. Personal health care expenditures are third only to food and housing expenditures in household budgets (Folland, Goodman, & Stano, 1993). Personal health care expenditures have grown from $143 in 1960 to $346 in 1970, $1,064 in 1980, and $2,601 in 1990 (Letsch, 1993). The latest data reveal that personal health care expenditures reached an estimated $907.2 billion in 1996. The 275 million residents of the United States spent an average of $3,295 per person on personal health care in 1996. This figure is three times greater than the average per capita expenditure on health care in 1980 of $923 (Health Care Financing Administration [HCFA], 1999). By the year 2005, personal health care expenditures are projected to exceed $2.0 trillion, or 16.5% of the GDP. Long-term growth of personal health care expenditures reflects the combined effect of four major economic factors: economy-wide inflation, health care–specific in-

flation, population growth, and intensity of care (HCFA, 1999).

In addition to concern over the cost of health care, issues of access to health care are of equal importance. A rise in personal health care expenditures has caused an increase in the number of uninsured Americans (people who do not receive health coverage through their employer, do not purchase private insurance out-of-pocket, and do not qualify for Medicare or Medicaid) and an increase in the number of underinsured Americans. Many either do not get the health care they need or cannot pay for the costs of the health care they receive. The greatest financial barriers affecting access to health care services are poverty and uninsurance, while race, geographic location, and gender represent the greatest nonfinancial barriers in access to health care services (Addy, 1996).

The U.S. Census Bureau estimates that 44.3 million people in the United States, or 16.3% of the population, were without health insurance coverage during the entire 1998 calendar year. This figure represents a change in insurance status for approximately one million people from the previous year (Campbell, 1999). For those over 65 years of age, 1.1% of the population is uninsured. The widespread coverage of elderly Americans is due to the federally subsidized Medicare program. State-subsidized Medicaid benefits were extended to 14 million poor people in 1998, but 11.2 million poor people still had no health insurance, representing about 32.3% of all poor people (Campbell, 1999). Among the general population 18–64 years old, workers (both full- and part-time) were more likely to be insured than nonworkers, but among the poor, workers were less likely to be insured than nonworkers. About one-half, or 47.5%, of poor, full-time workers were uninsured in 1998 (Table 11–3). Figure 11–5 illustrates the percentage of educated people in the United States without health insurance in 1998.

MANAGED CARE AND MANAGED COMPETITION: THE ANSWER TO IMPROVED RESOURCE CONSUMPTION?

Issues of quality, access, and affordability of health care have fueled the most recent efforts of reform and change in the health care arena. Although national health care reform efforts failed in the early 1990s, the health care sector has seen unprecedented change in the financing and organization of care under the auspices of managed care. Over time, the term managed care has come to mean a variety of health care arrangements. In its broadest sense, managed care attempts to monitor and direct the use of health care services, thereby reducing health care costs. In the strictest sense, it refers to any health plan that directs its enrollees to a panel of physicians who have agreed to follow established guidelines to control the use of services and cost (Henderson, 1999). The intent of the managed care financing mechanism is to change the behavior of providers by placing controls on their side of the market.

The initial debate and impetus for reform of the U.S. health care system during the 1990s reflected concern over the spiraling cost of health care delivery. The various reform models for a competitive, market-based delivery model focus on providing incentives for delivery organizations to reduce the cost and improve the quality of care as a means to expand service to the over 40 million uninsured Americans. Health care reform efforts were put into motion to create a U.S. health system characterized by (1) guaranteed access for all persons, (2) a minimum standard of benefits for all, (3) a standard reporting form for patient care quality, (4) a choice of physician and hospital for the con-

TABLE 11–3 Health Insurance Coverage, 1998 (Numbers in Thousands)				
	All People		Poor People	
	No.	%	No.	%
Total	271,743	100.0	34,476	100.0
Total covered	227,462	83.7	23,325	67.7
Private	190,861	70.2	8,815	25.6
Employment-based	168,576	62.0	5,998	17.4
Government	66,087	24.3	17,199	49.9
Medicare	35,887	13.2	4,492	13.0
Medicaid	27,854	10.3	13,996	40.6
Military	8,747	3.2	664	1.9
Not covered	44,281	16.3	11,151	32.3

Note: The estimates by type of coverage are not mutually exclusive; people can be covered by more than one type of health insurance during the year.

From U.S. Census Bureau. (1999). Current population survey, March 1999. http://www.census.gov/ftp/pub

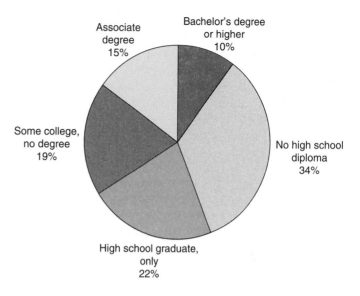

FIGURE 11–5 Percentage of U.S. population without health insurance, by educational level, 1998. (N = 199,731 persons age 18 or older.) (Data from U.S. Census Bureau. (1999). Current population survey, March 1999 [On-line]. Available: http://www.census.gov)

sumer, perhaps limited by choice of health coverage plan, (5) coverage not being denied because of preexisting health conditions, and (6) protecting existing standards of quality of care and, to the extent possible, improving them (Johnson, 1994).

In the original managed competition model proposed by Stanford economist Alain Enthoven (1988), costs are controlled through the market mechanisms of price competition. Multiple provider groups compete for contracts from consumers through bargaining pools composed of individuals and small business employers. Members of consumer groups pool their purchasing power, thus achieving economies of scale (bargaining power due to size, based on the principle of marginal cost) to get lower-priced coverage. Competition between provider groups should occur on the basis of each plan's prices, measures of quality of care, and level of enrollee satisfaction. Thus, consumers shop among the provider groups for the best deal. Theoretically, such competition would increase choice, drive costs down, and improve quality.

In Enthoven's original conception of man-

aged competition, eight techniques were advocated to stimulate effective resource use and exchange between the health insurance companies offering managed care plans to sponsored populations. These techniques include: (1) a system of accurate pricing, (2) standardized benefit packages, (3) an annual enrollment process managed by the sponsor (the consumer who purchases the plan—in this case, organizations that purchase health insurance on behalf of their employees), (4) assurance of continuity of coverage, (5) surveillance by sponsors, (6) quality assurance, (7) pro-competitive action by sponsors, and (8) sponsor management of subsidies (Enthoven, 1988).

Managed care and managed competition were introduced into the health care sector in an effort to stimulate competition and create an effective market mechanism to create a socially optimum use of resources to produce health care services. Managed care was offered to correct the occurrence of the imperfect market under the provider-driven fee-for-service delivery model. In the era of fee-for-service indemnity insurance, the primary factors that influenced economic decision making were technology, demographics, physician and hospital supply, and physician decision making (Etheredge, Jones, & Lewin, 1996). Instead of creating a socially optimum market, managed care and managed competition have created a new set of influences, which in turn have created a different type of market imperfection in the health care sector. Under managed care, the power between the health care provider, patient, and purchasing organization has been recast. System change under managed care is now influenced by (1) the purchasing power of buyers, (2) the role of price competition between payers (managed care organizations) and providers (health care delivery organizations and physicians), (3) the managed care industry and its practices, (4) the drive for market share among health plans, (5) the assumption of insurance risk in the selection of plan enrollees, (6) the effect of investment capital, and (7) new roles for employers and patients as decision makers influencing service delivery (Etheredge, Jones, & Lewin, 1996).

Since its introduction into the health care marketplace, managed care arrangements for employment-based health care coverage have accelerated at a swift pace. In a large-scale survey of employer-based health plans, Marquis & Long (1999) reported on the changes in employer-based health insurance purchasing patterns for the 1993–1997 time frame. Their findings confirmed the growth in managed care plans as the predominant type of employer-based health insurance. Additionally, they found that the managed competition mechanism was lacking in the purchasing of health benefits for employees. Namely, the changes in health plan enrollment patterns reflected employers' choices of types of plans to offer rather than voluntary selection among multiple options by employees.

The growth of the economically based system of health care service delivery has created a backlash among consumers and health care professionals. The backlash against the "socially immoral" practices of the managed care industry

focused attempts to preserve the quality of health care service delivery in the face of shrinking resources, to advocate consumer choice in selecting health care providers, and to protect professional decision making for the necessity of a given clinical service. While many consumers have benefited from more affordable and often expanded health care coverage, restrictions on choice of primary care physicians and access to specialty care, emergency care, and inpatient admissions have started a backlash that is beginning to resonate in state legislatures and Congress (Scott, 1997).

QUALITY OF CARE AND ECONOMICS

A cornerstone of change efforts focuses on improving the quality of health care service. In its economic sense, quality is the value gained from services for the amount of resources used in the production of those services. Concomitantly, health care quality can be defined as the degree to which health services for individuals and populations increase the likelihood of desired health outcomes and are consistent with current professional knowledge (Lohr, 1990). The idea that high-quality care equals high-cost care has emerged with the use of high-cost technologies. However, high cost does not always ensure high quality, and high quality does not have to come at a high cost. Consider the concept of marginal utility. There comes a point in the course of care when additional treatment will make little difference and will not improve the outcome. In fact, the quality of care may actually deteriorate by the continued input of services if the additional services have high risks of adverse effects (Davis et al., 1990).

In the current era of economic efficiency characterized by cost containment efforts, there are increased pressures and incentives to provide only those services that provide actual benefits to patients and to eliminate those services with marginal outcomes. From this economic force comes the need to determine the impact of care on the lives of patients. Such information regarding outcomes of care must become a propelling component in the decisions that affect resource allocation between competing services. To assess, evaluate, and document quality, data must be generated that provide indicators of quality of care. Outcomes research and technology assessment are attempting to move from evaluation of biometric measures (blood pressure, mortality) toward measurements of functioning, well-being, and quality of life in an effort to assess treatment effectiveness more comprehensively. The challenge of evaluating care is in balancing results from quality (assessment-of-outcomes) research with results from efficiency (assessment of cost-effectiveness) analysis. While the idea of incorporating cost research with quality research is logical (and necessary in the current economic environment), methodologies and data collection tools are relatively undeveloped and not standardized (Buerhaus, 1992). Nurses, already clinical experts in evaluating responses to care, must also become experts in quality and cost research as the field of outcomes research develops and grows.

Another component in improving the quality of health care service delivery follows the familiar "rule of rights"—"The right care to the right person at the right time by the right provider." The ANA's 1992 policy document, *Nursing's Agenda for Health Care Reform,* reflects nursing's professional value system by advocating universal access in response to the overwhelming number of Americans unable to enter the health care system. The inability to access care and the subsequent delay in treatment exacerbate health problems and escalate the costs of health care. The ANA advocates expanding professional nursing's roles and nurse-managed services to address the current unmet demand for health care services. Studies have shown that nurse practitioners enhance access to and the delivery of basic health care in a wide variety of geographic and practice settings, such as school-based clinics, long-term care facilities, correctional institutions, industrial health clinics, community health clinics, and community birthing centers, as well as in the more traditional settings of hospital ambulatory and inpatient departments and private practice offices (OTA, 1986; Safriet, 1992; Schroeder, 1993).

The Office of Technology Assessment's review of studies on care provided by nurse practitioners versus that provided by physicians found that nurse practitioners provide care equivalent to or superior to that provided by physicians in regard to assessment competency, patient compliance, resolution of acute problems, and improvement in patients' physical, emotional, and social functional status. Brown and Grimes's (1993) meta-analysis of 38 studies found that, compared with physicians, nurse practitioners provided more health promotion activities, scored higher on quality-of-care measures, achieved higher scores on resolution of pathological conditions and on functional status of their patients, and achieved higher scores on patient satisfaction and patient compliance. In addition, they found that patient knowledge was equivalent between patients of nurse practitioners and patients of physicians, and that nurse practitioners' patients experienced fewer hospitalizations. These studies also showed that care provided by nurse practitioners was more cost-effective than that provided by physicians (Brown & Grimes, 1993; Michaels, 1992; OTA, 1986; Rogers, Riordan, & Swindle, 1991). The role of the nurse practitioner as an accessible, cost-effective, and high-quality provider of primary care services has been validated, and nurse practitioners have demonstrated that quality does not have to be sacrificed to cost containment.

TECHNOLOGY

Health care technology has been cited as one of the significant drivers in the escalating costs of service delivery in the United States (Aaron, 1991). In its broadest sense, *technology* is any invention, innovation, or diffusion of knowledge that improves products or processes measured in terms of productivity or economic growth (Henderson, 1999). There are three types of technology available in the medical marketplace: nontechnology, halfway technology, and high technology (Thomas, 1974; Weisbrod, 1991). *Nontechnology* provides practitioners with the means of helping clients cope with illnesses that have no known cure. An example of nontechnology in health care is the use of mechanical ventilation for the client with respiratory failure from metastatic cancer. *Halfway technology* provides practitioners with the means of treating a client who has a particular disease by trying to postpone the effects of the disease process. An example of halfway technology is a total joint replacement for a client with degenerative bone disease. Lastly, *high technology* provides the practitioner with a treatment that either prevents or cures a particular disease or malady. The classic example of high technology in health care is immunization against a host of childhood diseases. The process of technological change from one stage to the next is dependent on the nature of the disease process, the state of scientific knowledge, and the amount of resources allocated to research and development (Henderson, 1999).

The expansion of health insurance since World War II has led to an interdependent relationship between health care technology and insurance and has dramatically impacted today's health care costs (Garber, 1994; Weisbrod, 1991). As individuals shifted the financing of services they received from themselves to insurance companies, individuals became removed from, and insensitive to, the actual costs of health care technologies. Because of the retrospective payment system, in which all services rendered were reimbursed, health care providers (namely, physicians and hospitals) had financial incentives to use any and all technologies available, regardless of cost. Research and development markets also had the financial incentives of reimbursement to continue to produce new health care technologies at any cost (Weisbrod,

1991). Consequently, there has been heightened and widespread patient and provider demand for greater technology (Callahan, 1990) and soaring health care expenditures.

In the current delivery environment the abundant development and use of low and halfway technologies has fueled the debate over the appropriateness of many disease-focused clinical interventions in improving health outcomes and overall health status. In today's health care market payers are increasingly willing to pay only for those technologies that are cost-effective and medically appropriate. The shifting focus of health care service and technological innovation toward health improvement and disease prevention provides the nursing profession with an opportunity to develop and demonstrate the effectiveness of nurse-specific interventions and service technologies.

Technology assessment and outcomes research are intended to help decision makers deal with the development, acquisition, and use of health care practices and technologies. The goal is to improve patient health, efficiency, and value. Technology assessment, as a form of policy research, evaluates the safety, effectiveness, and costs of technologies to provide the basis for clinical and social policies, including resource allocation. A comprehensive technology assessment encompasses four aspects of the technology: safety, efficacy-effectiveness, costs-benefits, and social impact (Pillar, Jacox, & Redman, 1990).

Technology assessment and outcomes research are time-consuming and costly. Traditional health care markets provide little incentive for the investment in the process. Under managed care, health care providers would be competing for contracts from consumers, since consumers would shop among the providers on the basis of reported price, quality indicators, and level of enrollee satisfaction. Providers would be accountable for quality and would stand to lose consumers if quality fell below the level of competitors. The managed competition approach provides an environment and the incentives for the generation of cost-effectiveness and quality outcomes data on health care technologies, since providers of care would compete on the basis of quality and cost.

Nursing practice, education, and administration are directly affected by the application of new medical and health care practices and technologies. However, there is little participation in technology research by nursing despite nursing's contribution to the implementation and assessment of technology in the clinical setting (Pillar, Jacox, & Redman, 1990). Nurses directly witness the individual as well as societal benefits and burdens that various practices and technologies bring and possess a wealth of clinical knowledge and expertise that could advance technology assessment. Nurses must become involved in multidisciplinary technology assessment and participate in the development of clinical practice guidelines as well as social policy regarding health care technologies (Box 11–3).

RATIONING HEALTH CARE TECHNOLOGY

The opportunity costs of health care, or the diversion of scarce and finite resources from other purposes (education, law enforcement, roads and highways, defense, etc.), generated largely by high-cost technology, are under scrutiny. Since demands for health care are insatiable, whereas resources are finite, and since society cannot afford to do everything that is now technically possible for every member of society, the need to explicitly ration health care resources has emerged. In the United States, many states have initiated legislation to enact a system of health care within their borders to provide incentives to control cost and create a more equal distribution of health resources for their citizens. One example of a state-based effort to ration health care services to reduce costs is the Oregon Health Plan.

Oregon's Basic Health Services Act has used a priority system incorporating outcomes of

---

Box 11–3 How to Read an Economic Analysis Paper

In the contemporary practice environment the allocation of limited resources in the production of health care services is a necessary component of clinical and policy decision making. As this chapter has illustrated, the economic cost of health care service delivery includes many tangible and intangible elements. A key skill for the professional nurse is the ability to critically analyze the quality of a study that reports the economic benefits of an intervention or new service. Greenhalgh (1997) presents a ten-question checklist that is useful in judging economic analyses of a health care service:

1. Is the economic analysis based on a study that answers a clearly defined clinical question about an economically important issue?
2. From whose viewpoint are the costs and benefits being considered?
3. Have the interventions being compared been shown to be clinically effective?
4. Are the interventions sensible and workable in the setting in which they are likely to be applied?
5. Which method of economic analysis was used, and was it appropriate?
6. How were costs and benefits measured?
7. Were incremental (one unit/one more individual) rather than absolute (overall) benefits considered?
8. Was the "here and now" given precedence over the distant future?
9. Was a sensitivity analysis performed?
10. Were "bottom-line" aggregate scores overused?

From Greenhalgh, T.: How to read a paper: Papers that tell you what things cost (economic analysis). *British Medical Journal, 315,* September 6, 1997, pp. 596–599.

treatment to establish a state Medicaid benefits package. The plan is based on the utilitarian principle of doing the greatest good for the greatest number of people. Therefore, high-cost technologies with marginal outcomes are not provided under the plan, whereas lower-cost, highly effective technologies are funded (Dougherty, 1991). Oregon has reduced growth in health care expenditures while delivering quality care by eliminating the use of technologies that have not been shown to be effective in changing health outcomes. The responsibility of prioritizing health services for inclusion or exclusion for coverage was placed on a Health Services commission. The commission is composed of five primary care physicians, a social worker, four consumers, and one public health nurse (Southard, 1992). As policymakers grapple with difficult resource allocation questions to improve the overall efficacy of health care service delivery, the inclusion of nursing expertise in the policy-making process can greatly impact not only resource allocation but also patient outcomes.

As a reference for comparative health system analysis on a national level, the United States often looks north, to the Canadian experience of state-funded National Health Insurance, as one possible solution to our health care crisis. Guaranteed access to care is one of the guiding principles of the Canadian health care system; other principles include universality, portability, comprehensiveness, and public administration of the plan on a nonprofit basis (Spence-Laschinger & McWilliam, 1992). The Canadian system, implemented in 1968 by the National Medicare Act, is a public insurance model, as opposed to a government-delivered services model such as exists in the United Kingdom. As in the United States, the Canadian system has economic constraints, and the majority of health care expenditures go to illness care in acute care settings. Canadian nurse advocates are calling for resource commitment to wellness and primary care services and for improved access to, and reimbursement of, nurse provider services (Spence-Laschinger & McWilliam, 1992).

Economics and the Future of Nursing

In 1992, Peter Buerhaus predicted several changes that nurses can anticipate as the provision of health care shifts to a more competitive marketplace:

- Intensifying pressure to provide nursing care in the least costly manner.
- Increased demand by licensed practical nurses, clinical pharmacists, physicians, and other economic competitors for regulations that either protect or expand their practice turfs, coupled with actions by employers to change both state nurse practice acts and institutional traditions that restrict them from achieving productivity gains and lowering labor-related costs.
- Developing opportunities to advance the value of nursing practice in all health care settings if the profession's research and management communities can successfully orchestrate a multifaceted quality assessment effort.
- Struggling to balance the tensions, costs, and benefits of pursuing a narrowly focused nursing quality assessment strategy with finding ways to integrate nursing's quality assessment concepts and methods into quality assessment systems and management initiatives that are controlled largely by non-nurses.
- Having to seriously consider what it is that purchasers and consumers want from nursing, and taking steps to satisfy these wants.

Nurses and the nursing profession face many significant opportunities and challenges in creating a new model of health care service delivery. The primary challenge of the economic era of health care service delivery is nursing's ability to reframe practice into an economic value equation to capture the cost, quality, and service of nursing care and knowledge-based technologies (Malloch & Porter-O'Grady, 1999). Eisler (1998) recommends a partnership economic model as a means of reframing the relational and technical essence of nursing practice. Partnership economics incorporates the best of capitalism, social responsibility, and the support for caring and ethical human relationships. The demonstration of the economic value of caring (Issel & Kahn, 1998) in the health service encounter provides a foundation to advance interventions that demonstrate the value (cost and quality) of nursing services to create a new reality of patient-centered health care delivery. Malloch & Porter-O'Grady (1999) provide a scenario to demonstrate the potential cost savings of health care service under the partnership economics model. They compare the costs of services for a patient with congestive heart failure (DRG 127) under the current fragmented,

event-based system of care delivery with services in an integrated, health management service scenario. In the economically conscious intervention scenario, the authors demonstrate that the attention to resource use, coordinated interventions, and patient involvement in service delivery can create a savings of $10,350 per patient for that DRG.

A knowledge of economics is no longer a luxury in contemporary nursing practice, it is a necessity. This chapter provides an overview of the many economic issues that are shaping the national discourse about health care service, its effect on our society, and, by extension, its effect on professional nursing practice. Professional nurses must have a basic understanding of economic forces and apply these principles within

TABLE 11–4 Web/Watch: Keeping Abreast of Economic Issues in Health Care

Web Site Description	Internet Address
National Institutes of Health Provides an overview of programs and activities of the federal government.	http://www.nih.gov
Health Economics Places to Go Provides links to sites related to health economics, policy, managed care and more.	http://www.medecon.de/hec.htm
National Center for Health Statistics The principal health statistics agency in the United States, its mission is to provide accurate, timely, and relevant statistics to inform policy and improve the health of the American people.	http://www.cdc.gov/nchswww/
RAND Corporation Not-for-profit institution dedicated to improving public policy through research. RAND conducts interdisciplinary health sciences research.	http://www.rand.org/organization/health
U.S. Census Bureau Provides statistics on population demographics and health insurance status.	http://www.census.gov/ftp/pub/hhes/www/hlthins.html
National Rural Health Association Dedicated to improving the health and health care of rural Americans through advocacy, communications, education, and research.	http://www.nrharural.org
Nursing World The official web site of the American Nurses Association. Provides access to the Online Journal of Issues in Nursing.	http://www.nursingworld.org
National Committee for Quality Assurance An independent not-for-profit organization that serves as the accrediting agency for the nation's managed care plans.	http://www.ncqa.org

Data from *Health Economics and Policy*, 1st edition, by J. W. Henderson. © 1999. Reprinted with permission of South-Western College Publishing a division of Thomson Learning. See also a web site maintained by J. Henderson at http://www.sw.college.com/bef/economics.html.

their practice environments if they are to participate in shaping a patient-centered, health-focused care delivery system. This chapter provides a foundation on which to build knowledge and skills to participate in the discourse of change. The Pew Commission (1995) identified lifelong learning as a characteristic of the health professional of the 21st century. Keeping abreast of changes in the dynamic health care economy is one way in which new knowledge shapes the practice environment and professional decision making. Journalistic accounts, professional publications, and Internet resources dedicated to the presentation and discussion of issues in health and nursing economics are widely available (Table 11–4). Professional nurses have the knowledge and expertise to create a socially just health care system. In the current era, nursing participation in decision-making activities will occur with the acquisition of new skills and the framing of nursing service within an economic context.

KEY POINTS

- Economics in health care represents the relationship among the supply, demand, and costs of health care.

- The supply of health care refers to the amount of health care facilities, personnel, and financing available to consumers. Supply levels are impacted by technological discoveries, costs for services, consumer demands, the level of competition in the marketplace, and the effect of government regulations.

- The demand for health care indicates what health care the consumer is willing to purchase. The demand level revolves around consumer needs and desires, the costs of health care, treatment selections ordered by health care providers, and general societal needs.

- The costs for health care reflect any financial expenditures contributed by providers or consumers to deliver and receive health care, as well as the intangible costs of receiving care. Factors influencing the cost of health care are numerous, ranging from consumer demands to advancements in medical technology to the status of the nation's economy.

- Economic concepts relevant to nursing practice include opportunity cost, elasticity, complements and substitutes, competition, and marginal utility. Nurses must be able to incorporate these economic concepts into their administrative as well as clinical decision-making processes.

- Cost-containment pressures require that nurse researchers be able to incorporate economic methodologies such as cost-effectiveness analysis and cost-benefit analysis into clinical and administrative research programs. Such economically as well as clinically based research can serve as the basis for policy decision making regarding regulatory reform, prioritization and rationing of health care technologies and services, and reimbursement for advanced practice nurses.

- Nurses can bring a unique perspective to the economic analysis of health care that can impact health care delivery systems, health policy, and, most important, patient care.

- The rising costs of health care necessitate the provision of more cost-effective ways to provide comparable services. Nurses must continue to demonstrate their accessibility, quality of services, and cost-effectiveness in order to validate existing and expanding roles, to broaden reimbursement policies for services that nurses are trained to render and are capable of providing, and to effectively compete with physicians and other providers of care.

CRITICAL THINKING EXERCISES

1. Discuss the economic concepts of supply, demand, and costs of health care as they relate to your nursing practice.

2. What are the implications for the nursing profession of the issues of:
   a. Access to health care
   b. Cost containment
   c. Quality of care

3. How can nurses in clinical practice become involved in decisions regarding the rationing of health care resources and services? How can nurses become involved in the formulation and evaluation of social policies regarding health care?

4. What suggestions do you have for restructuring the health care delivery system to address problems associated with access to care, cost, reimbursement, and quality of care?

5. Using Greenhalgh's criteria presented in Box 10–3, critique a paper presenting an economic analysis of a nurse-managed service or intervention.

6. In his book, *Not All of Us Are Saints: A Doctor's Journey With the Poor,* David Hilfiker, MD, tells a story of a homeless man and reveals an extreme example of the economic consequences of health care:

> After breaking his jaw several weeks earlier, Mr. McRae had gone to an emergency room, had his jaw wired shut to heal, and then been discharged back to the streets. Most likely, he had found it impossible to eat and drink enough to keep himself going, and so it was that the police found him severely dehydrated, unconscious, and close to death. [Subsequently,] Mr. McRae had been hospitalized for weeks at a cost of tens of thousands of dollars; attended to by teams of nurses, physicians, and social workers; and fed three carefully prepared meals a day. He was now about to be discharged to the streets, where he would sleep in a shelter, forage for food during the day, and wait in line in the evening in the hope of getting a bed for the night (Hilfiken, 1994, pp. 171–173).

What characteristics of our current health care system contributed to the outcome? What actions could have been taken, and by whom, to prevent the costly rehospitalization? What are some of the broader societal implications of this scenario?

REFERENCES

Aaron, H. J. (1991). *Serious and unstable condition: Financing America's health care.* Washington, DC: Brookings Institution.

Addy, J. A. (1996). Issues of access: What is going on in health care? *Nursing Economic$, 14,* 299–302.

American Nurses Association. (1992). *Nursing's agenda for health care reform.* Washington, DC: American Nurses Publishing.

American Nurses Association. (1995). ANA response to the Pew Commission Report [On-line]. Available: http://www.nursingworld.org

Bocchino, C. A. (1993). A new accountability in health care: Providers, insurers, and patients. *Nursing Economics, 11*(1), 44.

Brown, M. (1994). The economic era: Now to the real change [Commentary]. *Health Care Management Review, 19*(4), 73–82.

Brown, S. A., & Grimes, D. E. (1993). *Nurse practitioners and certified nurse-midwives: A meta-analysis of studies on nurses in primary care roles.* Washington, DC: American Nurses Publishing.

Buerhaus, P. I. (1992). Nursing competition and quality. In M. Johnson & J. McCloskey (Eds.), *The delivery of quality health care.* St. Louis: Mosby.

Callahan, D. (1990). *What kind of life: The limits of medical progress.* New York: Simon & Schuster.

Campbell, J. A. (1999). Health insurance coverage 1998. U.S. Census Bureau, Department of Commerce: Economics and Statistics Administration [On-line]. Available: http://www.census.gov

Caroselli, C. (1996). Economic awareness of nurses: Relationship to budgetary control. *Nursing Economic$, 14,* 292–298.

Centers for Disease Control. (1992). Estimated national spending on prevention—United States, 1988. *Morbidity and Mortality Weekly Report, 41,* 529–531.

Cleland, V. S. (1990). *The economics of nursing.* Norwalk, CT: Appleton & Lange.

Davis, K., Anderson, G. F., Rowland, D., & Steinberg, E. P. (1990). The impact of cost containment efforts on the quality of care. In *Health care cost containment* (pp. 200–217). Baltimore, MD: Johns Hopkins University Press.

Dougherty, C. J. (1989). Ethical perspectives on prospective payment. *Hastings Center Report, 19*(1), 5–11.

Dougherty, C. J. (1991). Setting health care priorities: Oregon's next step. *Hastings Center Report, 21*(3), 1–16.

Dumpe, M. L., Herman, J., & Young, S. W. (1998). Forecasting the nursing workforce in a dynamic health care market. *Nursing Economic$, 16*(4), 170.

Eisler, R. (1998). Partnership economics: Changing the rules of the game. Economic inventions that give value to caring work [On-line]. Available: http://www.partnershipway.org

Enthoven, A. (1988). Managed competition of alternative delivery systems. *Journal of Health Politics, Policy and Law, 13,* 305–335.

Enthoven, A., & Kronick, R. (1991). Universal insurance through incentives reform. *Journal of the American Medical Association, 265,* 2532–2536.

Etheredge, L., Jones, S. B., & Lewin, L. (1996). What is driving health system change? *Health Affairs, 51*(4), 93–104.

Feldstein, P. J. (1983). *Health care economics* (2nd ed.). New York: Wiley.

Folland, S., Goodman, A. C., & Stano, M. (1993). *The economics of health and health care*. New York: Macmillan.

Garber, A. M. (1994). Can technology assessment control health spending? *Health Affairs, 13*(3), 115–126.

Greenhalgh, T. (1997). How to read a paper: Papers that tell you what things cost (economic analyses). *British Medical Journal, 315*, 596–599.

Health Care Financing Administration (1999). Office of Actuary, National Health Statistics Group. *Health Care Financing Review, 19*(1) (HCFA Publication No. 03400). Available: http://www.cdc.gov/nchswww/data/hus98.pfd

Health Resources and Services Administration, Bureau of Health Professions. (1996). *Notes from the National Sample Survey of Registered Nurses*, March 1996 [On-line]. Available: http://www.158.72.83.3/bhpr/dn/survnote.htm

Henderson, J. (1999). *Health economics and policy*. Cincinnati, OH: South Western College Publishing.

Hilfiker, D. (1994). *Not all of us are saints: A doctor's journey with the poor*. New York: Hill & Wang.

Issel, L. M., & Kahn, D. (1998). The economic value of caring. *Health Care Management Review, 23*(4), 43–53.

Johnson, R. L. (1994). HCMR perspective: The economic era of health care. *Health Care Management Review, 19*(4), 64–73.

Klarman, H. E. (1982). Application of cost-benefit analysis to the health services and the special case of technological innovation. In R. D. Luke & J. C. Bauer (Eds.), *Issues in health economics*. Rockville, MD: Aspen.

Kristein, M. M. (1983). Using cost-effectiveness and cost/benefit analysis for health care policy making. In R. M. Scheffler & L. F. Rossiter (Eds.), *Advances in health economics and health services research*. Greenwich, CT: JAI Press.

Letsch, S. W. (1993). National health care spending in 1991. *Health Affairs, 12*(1), 94–110.

Lohr, K. N. (1990). *Medicine: A strategy for quality assurance*. Washington, DC: National Academy Press.

Malloch, K., & Porter-O'Grady, T. (1999). Partnership economics: Nursing's challenge in a quantum age. *Nursing Economic$, 17*, 299–307.

Marquis, M. S., & Long, S. H. (1999). Trends in managed care competition. *Health Affairs, 18*(6), 75–88.

McGinnis, J. M., & Foege, W. H. (1993). Actual causes of death in the United States. *Journal of the American Medical Association, 270*, 2207–2212.

McMenamin, P. (1990). What do economists think people want? *Health Affairs, 9*(4), 112–119.

Michaels, C. (1992). Carondelet St. Mary's nursing enterprise. *Nursing Clinics of North America, 27*(1), 77–85.

Mundinger, M. O., Kane, R. L., Lenz, E. R., Totten, A. M., Wei-Yann, T., Cleary, P. D., Friedewald, W. T., Sui, A. L., Shelanski, M. L. (2000). Primary care outcomes in patients treated by nurse practitioners or physicians. *Journal of the American Medical Association, 283*, 59–68.

Organization for Economic Co-operation and Development. (1998). *Health statistics*. [On-line]. Available: http://www.oedc.org

Pauly, M. V. (1993). U.S. health care costs: The untold true story. *Health Affairs, 12*, 152–159.

Personal health care expenditures: CY 1960–2005. (1998). *Health Care Financing Review, Medicare and Medicaid Statistical Supplement*, 20–21.

Pew Health Care Commission. (1995). *Critical challenges: Revitalizing the health professions for the twenty-first century* [On-line]. Available: http://www.futurehealth.ucsf.edu/summaries/challenges

Pillar, B., Jacox, A. K., & Redman, B. K. (1990). Technology, its assessment, and nursing. *Nursing Outlook, 38*(1), 16–19.

Pruitt, R. H., & Jacox, A. K. (1991). Looking above the bottom line: Decisions in economic evaluation. *Nursing Economics, 9*(2), 87–91.

Rice, T. H., & Labelle, R. J. (1989). Do physicians induce demand for medical services? *Journal of Health Politics, Policy and Law, 14*, 587–600.

Rogers, M., Riordan, J., & Swindle, D. (1991). Community-based nursing case management pays off. *Nursing Management, 22*(3), 30–34.

Safriet, B. J. (1992). Health care dollars and regulatory sense: The role of advanced practice nursing. *The Yale Journal on Regulation, 9*, 417–488.

Schroeder, C. (1993). Nursing response to the crisis of access, cost, and quality in health care. *Advances in Nursing Science, 16*(1), 1–20.

Scott, J. S. (1997). Who's sorry now? Managed care under seige. *Healthcare Financial Management, 51*(7), 28–30.

Shortell, S. M., Gilles, R. R., Devers, K. J. (1995). Reinventing the American hospital. *The Milbank Quarterly 73*(2), 131–160.

Smith, S., Heffler, S., & Freeland, M. (1999). The next decade of health spending: A new outlook. *Health Affairs, 18*(4), 86–95.

Sources of funding for health care services. (1998). *Health Care Financing Review, Medicare and Medicaid Statistical Supplement*, 22–23.

Southard, P. (1992). The Oregon Health Plan. *Journal of Emergency Nursing, 18*, 471–473.

Spence-Laschinger, H. K., & McWilliam, C. L. (1992). Health care in Canada: The presumption of care. *Nursing and Health Care, 13,* 204–207.

Stoline, A. M., & Weiner, J. P. (1993). *The new medical marketplace* (Rev. ed.). Baltimore, MD: Johns Hopkins University Press.

Thomas, L. (1974) *Lives of a cell.* New York: Bantam.

U.S. Congress, Office of Technology Assessment. (1986). *Nurse practitioners, physician assistants, and certified nurse midwives: A policy analysis* (Health Technology Case Study 37; Publication No. OTA-HCS-37). Washington, DC: U.S. Government Printing Office.

Weisbrod, B. A. (1991). The health care quadrilemma: An essay on technological change, insurance, quality of care, and cost containment. *Journal of Economic Literature, 29,* 523–552.

Wise, L. C., Bostrom, J., Crosier, J. A., White, S., & Caldwell, R. (1996). Cost-benefit analysis of an automated medication system. *Nursing Economic$, 14,* 224–231.

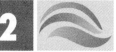

12

Legal Aspects of Nursing Practice

PATRICIA MCMULLEN, JD, MS, RN

OBJECTIVES

At the completion of this chapter, the reader will be able to:

● Describe the constitutional and administrative principles foundational to nursing practice.
● Analyze contract law and its effect on the nurse's employment relationships.
● Differentiate between torts of relevance to nursing practice.
● Discuss strategies the nurse can use to reduce legal exposure.

PROFILE IN PRACTICE

Elizabeth Frey, JD, RN
Jack H. Olender and Associates, P.C.
Washington, D.C.

As a nurse attorney in Washington, D.C., I handle medical malpractice cases on behalf of the plaintiff (the patient or injured party). I thoroughly enjoy handling these cases, for three primary reasons.

First, my goals as a practicing nurse were and are the same as my present goals. They are to be a patient advocate and to improve the quality of patient care. I believe that I am able to reach these goals as a lawyer practicing in the area of plaintiff medical malpractice.

Second, I believe that the patient who has been injured as the result of medical negligence is the underdog, if you will, and I prefer to represent those who are less fortunate. The patient generally does not have the amount of resources that physicians, hospitals, and insurance companies have, such as money, influence, and a good education. Other factors that place the plaintiff

at a comparative disadvantage in these cases include tort reform and the difficulty and cost involved in finding a qualified physician who is willing to review records and be an expert witness (which usually means testifying against a fellow physician). And, of course, the plaintiff has the burden of proof.

Third, I believe it is one of the best areas of law in terms of utilizing a nursing background. Most of my time is spent investigating cases prior to the filing of a lawsuit, and then, after suit is filed, performing discovery in which a nursing background is invaluable. As with any case, you must know and understand the facts and applicable law. To obtain the facts in a medical malpractice case, it is necessary to acquire the client's medical records, review them, and know and understand his or her condition as well as the care and treatment that he or she received. When the client contacts you because of an unfavorable outcome, you need to determine whether that negative outcome is a risk or consequence that occurred in the absence of negligence or whether it was the result of medical negligence. To do this, you must research the medical literature and determine what kind of medical experts are needed to render the necessary opinions. Then you must contact and retain the required experts. Where I have found my nursing background most helpful is in discussing cases with expert witnesses and in deposing physicians and other health care providers. You must have a good knowledge and understanding of medicine to handle such cases, and my nursing background has been invaluable in this regard. In fact, almost every medical malpractice law firm (plaintiff and defense) that I am familiar with has at least one nurse attorney.

Nurses confront legal principles on a daily basis. Legal concepts, legal expectations, and legal consequences surround the practice of nursing. An informed and safe nurse must be aware of the effect these legal principles have on nursing practice to reduce exposure to adverse legal consequences.

Law is defined as the sum total of man-made rules and regulations designed to assist people to order their society, organize their affairs, and settle their problems. *Statutory law* is established through the legislative process and expands each time Congress or state legislatures pass new legislation. *Common law* is decisional and expands each time a judge makes a legal decision.

The function of law is to create and interpret legal relationships. *Public law* defines and interprets relationships between individuals and the government. The major categories of public law are constitutional law, administrative law, and criminal law. *Private law* defines and interprets the relationship between individuals and includes contract law and tort law.

These areas of law have an effect on the practice of nursing. The clients' and nurses' constitutional rights and remedies are defined by *constitutional law*. *Administrative law* determines the licensing and regulation of nursing practice, as well as areas such as collective bargaining. *Criminal law* usually involves the nurse as a witness. However, it can also involve the nurse as a defendant who is accused of a crimi-

nal offense. *Contract law* identifies the common types of employer-employee relationships and determines the risks and protections inherent in each type of relationship. *Tort law* is concerned with the reparation of wrongs or injuries inflicted by one person on another. It defines the legal liability for the practice of nursing and identifies the elements that are essential for each tort. This chapter describes the interaction between law and nursing in three major areas: administrative law, employment law, and civil (or tort) law.

Administrative Law in Nursing

Nurses become aware of their board of nursing (the "board") and state nurse practice acts (NPAs) when they finish school and seek to acquire a license, if not before. Nurses are licensed under state NPAs. *Nurse practice acts* establish entry requirements into the profession, set definitions of nursing practice, and establish guidelines for professional discipline when a nurse fails to obey state laws or becomes incompetent. For most nurses, licensing will be their only direct contact with the board; however, many will find themselves tangentially involved with the board through some level of conflict about the definition of nursing. Few nurses will have direct contact with the board's disciplinary unit.

The power of the state to license nurses and other health care professionals originates in the U.S. Constitution (*Dent v. West Virginia*, 1889). The Tenth Amendment allows the states to enact legislation that is not preempted or prohibited by federal law. All states have a "police power" to enact legislation to protect the health, safety, and welfare of their citizens. Each state constitution has a health and welfare clause allowing it to pass such legislation.

LICENSING

Licensing is an exercise of the state's police power that is employed by the legislature to protect the health, safety, and welfare of its citizens. Through state licensing statutes, the nursing profession controls entry into the profession, the discipline of colleagues, and the nursing activities of nonnurses. Nurses themselves implement these controls because they are best qualified by their specialized knowledge to evaluate and oversee nursing practice.

Regulations controlling the licensing and practice of nursing have been enacted by all of the states, the District of Columbia, and the U.S. territories. National guidelines exist and serve as useful references for nurses in proposing and implementing state laws. For example, the American Nurses Association, the American Association of Colleges of Nursing, the National Organization of Nurse Practitioner Faculties, and other professional groups promulgate definitions and standards of nursing education and practice that are often incorporated into state NPAs. These NPAs are implemented through a state agency called the health professions board, nursing board, or a similar title. Rules and regulations promulgated by the board give meaning to the NPA.

The most visible function of NPAs is the control over entry of new members into the nursing profession. Nursing and other professions have been criticized for entry requirements that discriminate against minorities and the poor and discourage diversity. Thus, nursing

boards must continually examine their criteria for admission to the profession for bias. Some licensure questions facing the nursing profession include the following: Is licensing perhaps too restrictive by limiting entry into the profession? Do the tests and criteria used really identify the individuals who are good nurses, or do they shut out good nurses who are different from a homogenized stereotype? Does licensing protect the public, or does it really protect nursing professionals by eliminating competition? Should there be national licensure for nurses so that they could easily practice across state boundaries?

CONTROL OVER PRACTICE

The power to control entry and the power to discipline licensed and unlicensed practitioners give the profession an ability to exert control on the nursing market. Nurses are granted a privileged place in the occupational hierarchy, but it is a position challenged both by the public and by other professionals who fear the surrender of power. Nurses control the quality and standards of nursing care in the state because they control the disciplinary process of nurses through the NPAs. Thus, as in many other professions, NPAs leave public consumers of nursing care dependent to a large degree on members of the profession to control access to nursing services and maintain the quality of nursing care. The result is that nurses have the duty to advocate for patients not only at the bedside, but also before the licensing board for high-quality care from competent licensed practitioners. The ability of nurses to meet this great responsibility is challenged by members of the public who fear competing professional incentives. There has also been an argument that this is too much power to give any profession, since professionals are reluctant to discipline their own colleagues.

This power is also challenged by other professionals, from physicians to wound care specialists and lay midwives, who are afraid that nursing's scope of practice will compete with their own professional and financial incentives. NPAs permit nurses to function under a broad definition of nursing while restricting the practice of non-nursing personnel who might otherwise deliver many services provided by nurses.

Enforcement of the prohibition against the unauthorized practice of nursing is exemplified by the practice of lay midwifery. In many states, lay midwives have been absorbed into an area of nursing practice rather than being established as a separate profession. Practicing lay midwives who are not registered by the board of nursing may be served with cease-and-desist orders. Boards may also file criminal charges for misrepresentation against lay midwives with the local office of the state's attorney (*People of the State of Illinois v. Margaret Jihan*, 1989). Some boards have administrative fining powers for "unlicensed practitioners," which they can impose on lay midwives. These powers are invoked regardless of client satisfaction and often in spite of great public protest. Boards argue that a threat to the public safety and welfare is inherent whenever there is unlicensed practice, regardless of the specific fact situation. Similar processes have prevented nursing from taking over functions that have been absorbed into medical specialties.

Jurisdictions may overlap with other professions that perform some of the same functions as nursing. For example, the expanded role of the nurse has resulted in clashes with physicians at the regulatory level (*Sermchief v. Gonzalez*, 1983). While nursing boards have moved to limit the practice of unlicensed lay midwives, medical organizations have moved to limit the practice of several types of advanced practice nurses.

The above arguments illustrate the restrictive nature of licensing by limiting entry and practice. Is licensing too restrictive, or is licensing really too permissive by granting "blanket" licenses? Does licensing today permit nurses to practice beyond their actual competence? It is likely that no one nurse can competently perform all services that nurses are licensed to deliver. Although most nurses practice only in a limited field (e.g., surgery, obstetrics, oncology), a nursing license permits a nurse to practice in all areas of nursing. In addition, after initial licensure, there is little or no demonstration of performance competency. Initial credentials do not guarantee competency into the indefinite future. For this reason, some states and health care agencies are requiring mandatory continuing education or advanced certification as an indicator of ongoing competency.

EXTERNAL REGULATION OF NURSING PRACTICE

Policymakers debate how to regulate professional practice. Other external forces, such as health care legislation, managed care models, and financing of health care, also affect how nursing is practiced. Although it failed to pass in 1994, the Clinton Health Security Act (HSA) reflects prominent policy concerns. The HSA incorporated state law credentialing requirements for health care professions. Section 1161 provided for the override of state laws that restrict the practice of any class of health professions beyond what is justified by the skills and training of such professions. Section 3071(e) established funding for a program for advanced practice nurses and physicians assistants. Legislative proposals such as the HSA put nurses on notice that federal trends and federal laws are likely to have more impact on licensing in the future than in the past. Currently, all professional self-regulation is under attack. Consumers often do not perceive the professions as being the best ones to protect consumer interests.

If licensing is seen as a barrier to developing a free market in health care and a contributor to rising costs, it may be redefined in terms of a cost-to-performance ratio. An example of this principle is found in Title V of the HSA, which required periodic evaluation of actual performance of specific functions of licensed professionals. Licensing is supposed to protect the public from incompetence. Does a blanket license, covering practice over a broad range of specialties, accomplish that purpose? Further, do requalification tests scrutinize actual competence? These issues have yet to be resolved.

DISCIPLINARY AND ADMINISTRATIVE PROCEDURES

A board of nursing practice usually has both regulatory and adjudicatory power (Fig. 12–1). The *regulatory power* authorizes the board to develop rules and regulations for nursing licensure, nursing education, and nursing practice. The *adjudicatory power* authorizes the board to investigate, hear, and decide complaints that involve violations of the act and of the rules and regulations promulgated by the board. As mandated by the NPA, the board must ensure that a licensed nurse continues to practice within the standard of care, behaves professionally and ethically, and obeys all state laws. The NPA contains or incorporates a number of grounds to achieve this. The disciplinary action is on the license of the nurse, and that license may be suspended or revoked.

Boards are state administrative agencies. Their delegated powers are to protect the public from unfit nurses. It is important to understand the responsibility of state boards to protect the safety of the public. Boards can only limit or deny a nursing license. They cannot incarcerate a nurse, nor can they require a nurse to compensate a patient for damages, financial or otherwise. Most board actions cannot be used in a lawsuit against a nurse. If an injured patient does seek monetary damages, he or she must file a civil lawsuit against the nurse. If a party thinks a nurse has acted criminally, that party must contact the state's attorney's office.

A professional license is property protected by the U.S. Constitution. This means that it cannot be limited or taken away without "due process." Each state has an *Administrative Procedure Act* that guides state agencies in their dealings in order to guarantee this due process right. Each state agency has its own regulations that describe how the agency implements the law. These regulations can vary greatly from state to state, and even among professional boards within a state. A board of nursing in one state may hear all arguments concerning nursing issues. The board in a neighboring state may delegate this to an administrative law judge or a hearing officer. Within a state, a board of nursing may hear its own cases, whereas another professional board in the same state may have its cases heard by an outside hearing officer.

Due process requires a right to be heard, and it also includes "notice." A licensed nurse has a

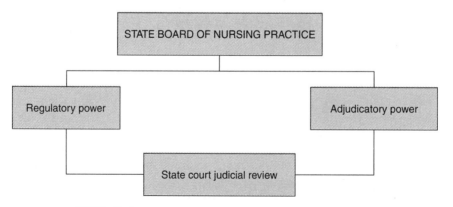

FIGURE 12–1 Enforcement of state law by the board of nursing.

duty to be aware of the state's NPA. The NPA is notice to nurses in that state about the grounds for which they may lose their license to practice. Further notice comes when a nurse receives a charging document. This paper advises the nurse that the board has probable cause to believe that the nurse is violating the NPA. It has to be specific enough to give the nurse notice about what any defense could be and about the time and place of the hearing.

Due process further requires that a nurse have the right to appeal any decision made by the board that seems improper. This appeal is usually to the state civil courts. In some states, the nurse may reargue the facts of the case, but in many states appeal is limited to such issues as whether the board had a right to hear the case and whether the board gave the nurse proper "due process" rights.

Although there are commonalities among all NPAs, each state has its own unique legislation. The nurse who moves from one state to another should obtain a copy of the new state's NPA. A convenient time to do this is during the process of applying for a license. The differences in state NPAs can be significant. For example, one state may impose no legal duty on a nurse to report the incompetence of a physician. In the next state, the nurse may find that failure to report such a physician can result in the loss of the nurse's license. The nurse needs to be familiar with the local NPA's requirements to obtain a license, boundaries and definitions of the practice, areas of discipline on the practice, and procedures in place to protect the nurse when the license is challenged by the board.

THE AMERICANS WITH DISABILITIES ACT

On July 26, 1990, the Federal government enacted the *Americans With Disabilities Act* (ADA). The ADA prohibits discrimination based on disability in employment, programs and services offered by state and local governments, goods and services delivered by private companies, and in commercial facilities. This is a federal law, and, like the constitutional right to due process, it applies to all states' boards. (The government's web site on the ADA can be found at http://www.usdoj.gov/crt/ada/ada-hom1.htm.)

Formerly, disabled nurses could be handled by the boards the same as any other nurse. Now, disabled nurses, such as those with a drug dependence who are *in treatment,* those with a handicap, and those with a mental illness, are granted special confidentiality. This is meant to encourage nurses to seek treatment, to report nurses who need treatment, and to ensure that the disabled are not the object of discrimination. Some boards have responded to this mandate by creating their own internal methods to comply with the ADA, such as a rehabilitation committee. Others have made arrangements with external groups, such as rehabilitation services that are provided privately or by a professional organization. A nurse in treatment for a protected disability does not have a public record connected with that disability.

The ADA also requires the board to make any special arrangements to facilitate access to practice by nurses. Examples are special communication services for the sensory impaired and handicapped access to the site of examinations or hearings.

Nursing and Employment Law

Most nurses work as employees rather than as independent practitioners. Nurse employees deal daily with the tension of being professionally independent and responsible for their actions in practice, while being simultaneously constrained by the standards and requirements of their employer. How can nurses' voices be heard and valued in creating work environments that promote the delivery of high-quality care? What avenues of redress do nurses have if they experience employee-management problems, such as hospital downsizing or cross-training of nonprofessionals to carry out nursing functions under their supervision? How can nurses tell whether they are employees or part of management for bargaining purposes?

CONTRACT LAW

Nurses who are employed work under some form of contract. A *contract* is a promissory agreement between two or more parties that creates (or modifies or destroys) a legal relationship (Prosser, 1984). A contract can be either in writing or in spoken language with specific terms, in which case it is called an *express contract*. A contract can also be based solely on the conduct of the parties. These contracts are referred to as *implied contracts.*

An enforceable contract must first be for the performance of legal goods or services. A nurse cannot contract to practice medicine, for example. Second, the parties must have legal capability to make the contract. This means, for example, that they must all have the mental ability to understand their actions and all be old enough to make a legal agreement. Third, all parties at the time of the contract must agree to do something, and they must agree on what that something is. Finally, there must be "consideration" (i.e., some kind of trade in which each party gets something from the contract). In a typical nurse employment situation, the employer receives nursing services, and the employee receives financial reimbursement.

All states have a *statute of frauds* that limits the enforcement of some contracts that are not written. These vary and are usually not significant to a nurse employee situation. It is obvious, however, that a nurse who wants to prove the specific terms of a contract will have difficulty with an oral contract.

Of more significance is the state *parole evidence rule*. This rule provides that if oral agreements are made that are different from the written contract, the courts will not allow them to add to or change the written contract. It will be difficult for a nurse to overcome a written contract (though it can be done), for example, by showing fraud or duress by the employer. When nurses agree to an employment position, they should be familiar with their employment contracts, should get them in writing, and should not rely on oral agreements that are not part of that written contract.

What about the role of the contract when the nurse is being terminated from employment or wants to leave that employment? A contract can be legally terminated when it has been completely performed, its terms have been met, both parties agree to a change, it becomes impossible (e.g., through the death of a party or the destruction of the subject matter), or both parties agree to annul the contract. A contract can also be terminated by a *breach*, which means that one of the parties fails to meet the terms of the agreement. When that happens, the other party can sue in civil court for any damages. For instance, an employee could sue for lost wages, and an employer could sue for lost profits. A nurse employee in a private setting could also file a grievance with the National Labor Relations Board. Of utmost importance for nurses is that most employment contracts are not individual contracts but are "at will." The next section clarifies this concept.

EMPLOYMENT AT WILL

Employment at will means that the employee has the right to quit employment anytime for any reason, or "at will." The employer has the parallel right to terminate the employee anytime for any reason, also at will.

The law of *Employment at Will* considers the employee and employer to have equal power, an assumption that nurse employees know does not reflect employee-employer realities. For this reason, it is a harsh legal doctrine. An example is an employee who is terminated for reasons that are against the public good, such as for joining a union or serving on a jury. Courts have found ways to restrict this doctrine, but they are limited to (1) public policy, (2) implied contract, and (3) good faith. Employees terminated against an implied contract are those who can show that this contract included hospital procedural manuals and personnel handbooks, employer's conduct or policy, or sometimes oral promises. An informed nurse employee must be familiar with such manuals and handbooks, document any oral promises, and get them in writing as soon as possible. What else can nurses do to enhance their protection as employees?

LABOR LAW

Approximately 20% of nurses employed in hospital settings are currently represented by unions (McMullen & Campbell-Philipsen, 1994). This means that they have formed a collective bargaining unit and can bargain with the employer as a group, in good faith, to make an agreement regarding similar interests in wages, hours, and working conditions. Collective bargaining agreements contain grievance procedures guaranteed to all employees. Furthermore, they usually contain a clause protecting the nurse employee from discharge except for "good cause." Nurses who work in a unionized facility cannot bargain individually with the employer. The employer must bargain with the union, which must represent all employees, whether or not they join the union (McMullen & Campbell-Philipsen, 1994).

Nurse employees can enforce employment agreements under the *National Labor Relations Act* (NLRA), enacted on July 5, 1935 (29 U.S.C. 141–178). The provisions of the NLRA are enforced through the National Labor Relations Board (NLRB) and various federal courts. The NLRB is a federal agency charged with implementing the NLRA, in much the same way that the nursing board implements the NPA. Its protections apply in all states.

Only nurses who are employees can participate in collective bargaining with the union. The NLRA also has a special provision allowing "professionals" to bargain collectively. In the past, many nurses who supervised health care workers, such as nursing assistants, were able to participate in collective bargaining under the "professional exemption." Nurse supervisors, however, were, and still are, excluded from collective bargaining participation and protection. In May 1994, the Supreme Court narrowed the NLRA coverage of professional nurses. In a split decision, the Court found that nurses who supervised others in a nursing home were part of management because such activities were "in the interest of the employer" (*NLRB v. Health Care and Retirement Corporation of America*, 1994). It is important to note that subsequent NLRB cases have determined that many types of nurses do not fall into the supervisory category and are eligible to participate in collective bargaining. In the case of *Providence Hospital and Alaska Nurses' Association* (1996), the NLRB determined that charge nurses, neurological outpatient rehabilitation nurses, and on-call home health leaders did not exercise "independent judgement in directing employees" and were, therefore, able to engage in collective bargaining. Despite this ruling, the full scope of the Supreme Court's decision in *NLRB v. Health Care and Retirement Corporation of America* is not yet clear; however, every nurse has to ask whether supervision of other employees might be interpreted as "management," thereby depriving the nurse of the right to bargain collectively and its protections.

GOVERNMENT EMPLOYEES

The NLRA applies only to privately employed nurses. Federal employees, such as nurses who work for the Veterans Administration, are covered under the *Civil Service Reform Act* of 1978. The employment rights of state employees are governed by each state's public employee statutes.

≈ **Tort Law in Nursing**

Another area of the legal system of particular importance to nurses is that of tort law. *Torts* are private civil wrongs, as contrasted with *crimes,* which are wrongs committed against the state (McHale, Tingle, & Peysner, 1998; Scott, 1998). The plaintiff, or person filing the law suit, files a tort action to recover damages for personal injury or property damage occurring from negligent conduct or unintentional misconduct (Prosser, 1984). *Unintentional torts* are those where persons suffer harm or injury as a consequence of an unintended, wrongful act by another person. Negligence and the related legal concept of malpractice are examples of unintentional torts (Sharpe, 1999). Several types of torts are often encountered in legal actions against nurses. These include negligence, assault, battery, false imprisonment, lack of informed consent, and breach of confidentiality. A

brief discussion of each of these types of torts follows. Case examples of various torts are included in Box 12–1.

NEGLIGENCE AND MALPRACTICE

Negligence occurs when a person fails to act in a reasonable manner under a given set of circumstances (Prosser, 1984). For example, if a person drinks excessively at a party, drives down the highway, and injures another motorist, the injured motorist could file a tort suit for negligence. Driving a car under the influence of alcohol or drugs is not typically considered reasonable conduct. Consequently, in addition to possible criminal action by the state where the accident happened, a negligence lawsuit would probably also result.

Unreasonable conduct by a nurse or other professional is a specific type of negligence, one referred to as *malpractice.* The nurse has the legal duty to provide the patient with a reason-

---

Box 12–1 Examples of Recent Cases Involving Nurses

Cafiero v. NC Board of Nursing, 102 N.C.App. 610, 403 S.E.2d 582 (N.C.App. May 07, 1991). A board of nursing suspended a nurse's license after the board determined she had negligently applied a heart monitor which resulted in an infant receiving an electrical shock. The court upheld the suspension of the license.

Karney by Karney v. Arnott-Ogden Memorial Hospital, 251 A.D.2d 780, 674 N.Y.S.2d 449, 1998 N.Y. Slip Op. 05900 (N.Y.A.D. 3 Dept. Jun 11, 1998). Patient was admitted to labor and delivery for evaluation of possible preterm labor. Initial testing excluded preterm labor. However, over time, patient complained of worsening contractions. For several hours, nurse failed to notify physician of patient's continuing complaints. Patient delivered a preterm infant with initial low Apgar scores. Jury awarded family $13.7 million. This award was appealed.

Kovacs v. Kawakami, 1:93cv02576 (D.C. Dist Ct Dec 16, 1993). Physician refused to see deaf patient at the time of a scheduled appointment unless she brought a qualified interpreter. Patient filed suit against physician under the Americans with Disabilities Act.

Nowak v. High, 209 Ga.App. 536, 433 S.E.2d 602 (Ga.App. Jun 08, 1993), certiorari denied (Oct 12, 1993). Nurse permitted to testify as an expert regarding whether a physician negligently administered IM phenergan to a patient.

Wendland v. Sparks, 574 N.W.2d 327 (Iowa Feb 18, 1998). Nurses, physician, and hospital were sued when patient went into cardiac arrest and physician directed the nurses not to resuscitate the patient. The patient's family sued for "loss of chance."

able *standard of care*. This is usually referred to as "what the reasonably prudent nurse would do under the same or similar circumstances." In malpractice lawsuits, the issue is whether or not the conduct of the nurse is below the standard established by law for the protection of others or whether the care given by the nurse involves an unreasonable risk of causing damage to another (McHale, Tingle & Peysner, 1998; Sharpe, 1999). The courts, based on long-established legal precedent, usually place the responsibility on the injured patient of establishing that the nurse acted wrongly. Initially, it is assumed that the nurse is innocent of the malpractice charge. Consequently, the plaintiff has the responsibility of establishing that the nurse's conduct was unreasonable. To accomplish this, the plaintiff must provide evidence related to four elements:

1. *Duty.* A duty is a legal obligation toward the patient (Scott, 1998). In health care settings, this legal obligation is usually based on express or implied types of health care service contracts (Sharpe, 1999). For instance, in prepayment health care systems, such as health maintenance organizations (HMOs), there is usually a written (express) contract between the HMO and the patient. The patient, through a health insurance plan or personal payment, pays a set fee for health care. In exchange, the HMO agrees to render certain health care services in a reasonable manner.

In other circumstances, the duty element may be based on a nonwritten (implied) contract (Aiken & Catalano, 1994). For example, if the patient is seen in the emergency room and signs an admission sheet guaranteeing payment of a reasonable fee for all services in the emergency room, there is an implied contract that the services received will be reasonable. For purposes of establishing the element of duty in a malpractice case against a nurse, the question at issue is, "Did the nurse have a legal obligation toward the patient?"

2. *Breach of duty.* This element of negligence and malpractice considers whether the nurse's conduct violated his or her duty to the patient

(McHale, Tingle, & Peysner, 1998). To determine whether or not there was a breach of duty, the plaintiff must show that the nurse's conduct did not comply with reasonable standards of care rendered by an average, like-specialty provider under similar circumstances (Prosser, 1984). There are a number of methods used to determine whether the nurse's care was reasonable. Expert witness testimony, nursing texts, professional journals, standards developed by professional organizations, institutional procedures and protocols, and equipment guidelines developed by manufacturers can all be used to decide whether the nurse's care complied with reasonable care (Aiken & Catalano, 1994; McHale, Tingle, & Peysner, 1998; Prosser, 1984; Sharpe, 1999). Use of detailed documentation techniques, such as those specified in the documentation guidelines (Box 12–2, Charting Basics), will help the nurse to establish that the care delivered was reasonable.

3. *Causation.* This element really addresses two issues: whether the nurse's action or inaction caused the patient's injury and whether the patient's injury was foreseeable (Aiken & Catalano, 1994; Prosser, 1984). To determine whether the nurse's actions or inaction caused the injury to the patient, lawyers frequently use the "but for" test (Prosser, 1984), which asks, "But for the acts or inaction of the nurse, would the injury to the patient still have occurred?" If the answer to this question is yes, then the first causation consideration is satisfied. The second part of the causation element looks at whether or not the nurse could have reasonably anticipated that his or her conduct might lead to patient harm (Aiken & Catalano, 1994; Hoffman, 1991; Sharpe, 1999).

4. *Damage.* For a patient to recover from a nurse in a malpractice suit, he or she must have suffered some type of damage (i.e., injury or harm). For example, if the nurse gave the patient the wrong medication but the patient did not experience any adverse effects, the damage element would be missing and the malpractice suit would be unsuccessful.

Box 12-2 Charting Basics

Documentation is always the big stickler for nurses. Knowledge of a few basic rules can help you protect yourself in the event of a lawsuit. And these rules can really help you communicate what great nursing care you deliver. Let's examine some tips that should prove helpful:

- *Never alter or falsify a record.* You will lose all of your credibility if it is discovered that you altered or falsified a record.
- *If you make an error, draw one line through it and explain why (e.g., wrong chart). Never use correction fluid or a sticker over an error.* You want others to clearly see what you have changed so that you maintain your credibility and your client goals.
- *Know and adhere to your agency's policies and guidelines.* Policies and guidelines help convey what the expectations are in your facility. They are frequently evaluated in lawsuits to determine whether what the nurse did or did not do complies with reasonable standards of care. Consequently, the policies and guidelines need to delineate what the reasonable expectations are. But they should not be so stringent that they cannot reasonably be accomplished.
- *Document in clear and chronological order.* If you need to go back, chart a "late note." If there is a lengthy delay in charting, explain why. It's important to keep orderly records. Remember always to date and time all notations. Nurses often leave blank spaces in the chart so that others can come back and make additions. However, blank spaces leave room for a sanitized record. It's a good idea to avoid gaps in charting. Incidentally, no one expects you to prolong a code to make a timely nursing entry. If you code a patient at 0900 and your adrenaline finally becomes manageable at 1100, just make a late entry note. This will make perfect sense to attorneys, judges, and other health team members.
- *Record accurate and complete information.* If there is an abnormality, chart your appropriate actions. Complete information is that data that another member of the health care team would need to reasonably care for that particular patient. If you fill your charting with irrelevant details, other providers will have a hard time locating the important facts. Part of your nursing role is to separate the critical information from the filler.

     If you identify a patient abnormality, don't forget to chart your appropriate nursing actions. Remember to record what the physician's response to your concerns was. An unsatisfactory response (or no response) from a physician warrants a call to your nursing superior.
- *State objective, factual information. Avoid conclusive statements like "well," "good," "fine," and "normal."*
- *Sign your legal name and title.* Always make your charting legible. A plaintiff's attorney can have a field day with illegible charting. If there is any way black could be interpreted as white, it will be.
- *Keep records in a safe and confidential manner.* Institutions and professionals are charged with the responsibility of maintaining a patient's privacy.
- *One last tip: Unusual circumstances warrant an incident report. But do not refer to the incident report in your notes.* Incident reports are designed to improve the quality of care rendered in an institution. They are not designed to communicate the needs of a particular patient. Generally, incident reports are not discoverable during a lawsuit. After all, courts want to promote quality care in institutions. However, if you refer to the incident report in your patient's chart, a little known legal doctrine may be applied. That doctrine is the doctrine of incorporation by reference. Under this doctrine, the incident report becomes part of the patient's record and not just the institution's quality assurance program, and is consequently discoverable.

Modified from McMullen, P., & Philipsen, N. (1993a). Charting basics 101. *Nursing Connections, 6*(3), 62–64. Washington Hospital Center, Washington, DC.

If sufficient evidence is established concerning all four of these elements and the defendant does not provide an adequate defense, the plaintiff can recover damages for *pecuniary* (monetary) and *nonpecuniary* (pain and suffering) injuries (Scott, 1998). The defendant nurse usually tries to ward off an adverse verdict by producing evidence that the nursing care was reasonable, that the patient's conduct contributed to the injury, that the time for filing the lawsuit (stature of limitations) has expired, or that he or she is immune from the lawsuit (Prosser, 1984). If, however, a defendant nurse is called to give testimony in a legal action, the strategies for giving oral testimony presented in Box 12–3 could prove very useful.

ASSAULT AND BATTERY

An *assault* is a deliberate act wherein one person threatens to harm another person without his or her consent and has the ability to carry out the threat (Prosser, 1984). A *battery* is an unconsented touching, even if the touching may be of benefit to the patient (Prosser, 1984). For example, a lawsuit for assault could result when a nurse threatens to medicate a competent person against his or her will. Battery would occur when the nurse actually administers the medication to the unwilling, competent patient.

In some circumstances, such as restraint situations, the law allows providers to touch patients without their consent. However, special circumstances and safeguards must be adhered to in order to excuse the battery. Initially, courts will look at whether the battery was needed to protect the patient, health care team members, or the property of others, such as those circumstances where the patient threatens to set a fire in an emergency room. Next, courts will examine whether restraining the patient was the least intrusive method to control the patient. For example, could the patient have been placed in a quiet room rather than being placed in a restraint? Finally, courts typically in-

---

Box 12–3 Giving Oral Testimony

- Bring your own attorney with you to review any records, for depositions or trials, to answer interrogatories, or for other legal requests if you are a party to a lawsuit.
- Never go to a deposition or a trial after working an off-shift; your brain will be mush!
- Thoroughly prepare for your testimony.
- Bring a recent, thoroughly updated copy of your résumé or curriculum vitae with you to the deposition or trial.
- During your testimony, always tell the truth.
- Dress professionally for your trial or deposition.
- If you are asked a question that is lengthy or convoluted, ask that it be restated and then rephrase it in your own words.
- Do not testify as to the medical standard of care.
- If you become fatigued during your testimony, ask for a brief break.
- Try to remain calm throughout the testimony.
- If asked whether a source is "authoritative" or a "classic," you will almost always answer no.
- Maintain eye contact during your testimony.
- Do not waive your signature.

Modified from McMullen, P., & Pepper, J. (1992). Surviving the legal hot seat. *Nursing Connections, 5*(2), 33–36. Washington Hospital Center, Washington, DC.

quire as to whether the health care team regularly reassessed the need to continue using the restraint. If the health care team can demonstrate that it has complied with these requirements, an unconsented touching will be excused. Consequently, nurses need to be sure that they provide detailed documentation to indicate that (1) the patient was a threat to self, others, or the property of others; (2) the restraint was the least intrusive means to control the patient; (3) there was regular reassessment of the need to continue the restraint; and (4) the restraint was discontinued as soon as practicable. It is also important to note that many hospitals and clinical facilities have specific procedures and protocols dealing with the application of restraints. Every nurse needs to be familiar with applicable agency policies.

INFORMED CONSENT

Informed consent lawsuits focus on whether or not the patient was given enough information before a treatment in order to make an informed, intelligent decision. In these types of cases, the focus will be on whether the patient was given adequate information concerning the nature of the proposed treatment, material risks, benefits of the proposed treatment, alternative therapies, and potential consequences if the patient decides against the treatment. In other words, did the patient get enough information so that he or she was the ultimate decision maker when a decision was made to pursue or abandon the proposed treatment?

In many states lack of informed consent is a separate tort action. In other states the plaintiff files a battery action alleging that the failure to give adequate treatment information constituted an unconsented touching.

It is important to note that there are a few pertinent exceptions to the doctrine of informed consent. An emergency situation is one example of an informed consent exception. If a patient was admitted to an emergency department with a severe hemorrhaging abdominal injury that required the immediate removal of his spleen, there could be an exception to the normal explanation of the splenectomy procedure and informed consent. Furthermore, not all patients desire information about a proposed treatment or procedure. In these situations, patients can waive their consent. Finally, some courts have allowed a provider to avoid full disclosure to a patient if disclosure of information might lead to further harm to the patient. This type of exception to informed consent is known as *therapeutic privilege*. For example, if the provider thought a patient's knowledge of terminal cancer would lead the patient to commit suicide, the provider might exert therapeutic privilege and not reveal the cancer to the patient.

Typically, the consent procedure rests in the hands of the physician who will be performing the treatment, and the nurse serves as a witness. When the nurse signs the "witness" portion of the consent form, he or she is attesting that the signature on the consent form is the patient's. If the nurse witnesses the physician giving the pertinent information regarding the treatment or procedure, the nurse may want to place "consent procedure witnessed" below his or her signature. If a lawsuit later develops concerning whether the provider gave the patient information concerning the procedure or treatment, the "consent procedure witnessed" statement can furnish powerful evidence that the patient did receive adequate information.

Today's advanced practice nurses often perform procedures and treatments that require consent, such as suturing, obstetrical care, and prescription of medications. In these circumstances, the advanced practice nurse must ensure that the patient has enough information to make an informed decision with respect to a proposed treatment.

Even if the patient does not sign a consent form expressly consenting to a proposed treatment or procedure, courts sometimes find that the patient gave implied consent to the treatment or procedure by coming to the health care facility and submitting to the treatment or procedure.

FALSE IMPRISONMENT

False imprisonment occurs when a person is unlawfully confined within a fixed area. The confined person must be aware of the confinement or harmed as a result of the confinement. To prevail in a false imprisonment action, the patient must prove that he or she was physically restrained or restrained by threat or intimidation and that he or she did not consent to the restraint (Prosser, 1984). False imprisonment suits may involve situations wherein a patient was kept in a mental health facility against his or her will and without a judicial order, or a restraint device was applied to a patient against his or her will.

The laws on false imprisonment vary from state to state. Most states allow some degree of patient confinement if the patient poses a serious threat of harm to self, others, or the property of others. In deciding whether a valid confinement occurred, judges and juries often look at the reasonableness of the decision to confine the patient, how long the patient was confined, whether the need for the confinement was regularly reassessed, and whether the least restrictive methods for detention of the patient were employed.

BREACH OF CONFIDENTIALITY

Confidentiality is the duty of health care providers to protect the secrecy of a patient's information, no matter how it is obtained (McMullen & Philipsen, 1993b). Until recently, patients had few legal remedies when the privacy of their medical records was breached. Today, state and federal laws provide patients with legal remedies to compensate them for confidentiality breaches.

Several cases demonstrate why there are valid concerns about medical record confidentiality.

In *Doe v. Roe* (1993), a flight attendant asked her treating physician not to reveal her HIV status to her insurer or her employer. The physician verbally promised not to reveal her HIV status. Several months later, the flight attendant found that her entire chart, complete with HIV information, had been forwarded to her employer. The attendant recovered damages against the physician for his breach of confidentiality and for breaching his expressed oral promise not to disclose her HIV status. Breach-of-confidentiality lawsuits have resulted wherein psychiatric, drug, and alcohol treatment information was released.

Typically, there is a very strict level of confidentiality for patients receiving drug or alcohol abuse treatment. Providers are usually prohibited from even disclosing information on whether a certain person is a patient. If a member of a health care team discloses confidential information, there may be federal statute violations (*Code of Federal Regulations*). In addition, state laws may exist that dictate who has authority to control access to medical records of patients who are incapacitated, incompetent, minors, or deceased. Information concerning these types of special situations is available through the state's attorney's office and through the employer's legal counsel.

~ Comment

A basic understanding of the impact of legal principles on nursing practice is essential to safe and effective performance as a nurse. It is also important to understand the role of the state board of nursing in the control and regulation of nursing practice. A thorough knowledge of employment rights and responsibilities when nurses enter into employment contracts can make nurses better negotiators. Knowledge of tort law is mandatory, not only to prevent being sued, but also to serve as both a professional and patient care advocate.

KEY POINTS

- The power of the state to license nurses is derived from the Constitution.
- Licensing of health professionals is intended to protect the health, safety, and welfare of the public.
- Nurse practice acts define the practice of nursing, identify the scope of nursing practice, set the requirements for licensure, and provide guidelines for disciplinary action.
- A nurse who is charged with a violation of a state's nurse practice act has a right to due process in the investigation, hearing, and decision of the charge.
- The *Americans With Disabilities Act* grants special confidentiality to nurses who are in treatment for protected disabilities.
- Nurses work under a contract, which is an express or implied agreement with an employer that creates a legal relationship.
- A collective bargaining agreement establishes a contractual relationship between the union and the employer.
- Torts are private civil wrongs, in contrast to crimes, which are wrongs against the state.
- Negligence occurs when a person fails to act in a reasonable manner.
- Malpractice occurs when the conduct of a nurse or other professional is below the established standard.
- Assault is a threat to touch or harm another person.
- Battery is an unconsented touching, even if the touching is beneficial to the patient.
- The principle of informed consent requires that the patient be given enough information before treatment to make an informed, intelligent decision about whether to pursue or abandon treatment.
- False imprisonment occurs when a person is unlawfully confined within a fixed area.
- The health care provider is duty bound to keep information about a patient confidential, no matter how it was obtained.

CRITICAL THINKING EXERCISES

1. Review your state nurse practice act and delineate the definition and scope of nursing practice. Evaluate its relevance for today's health care environment.

2. Discuss the administrative and disciplinary functions of state boards of nursing.

3. How does the right of due process protect the nurse? How does it protect the public?

4. What must a plaintiff prove in order to recover damages in the following situation? An IV was left in place for 5 days, although the hospital policy specified 2 days. As a result, the patient sustained a thrombosis and inflammation at the site.

5. Discuss the concepts of employment law as they relate to your employment situation.

6. Apply knowledge of tort law to formulate risk reduction strategies that could protect the nurse against legal action.

REFERENCES

Aiken, T. D., & Catalano, J. T. (1994). *Legal, ethical and political issues in nursing.* Philadelphia: Davis.
Code of Federal Regulations, Title 42, Part 2.
Dent v. West Virginia, 129 U.S. 114, 9 S. Ct. 231, 32 L. Ed. 623 (1889).
Doe v. Roe, No. 0369 (N.Y. App. Div., 4th Jud. Dept. May 28, 1993).
Hoffman, A. C. (1991). Torts. In American College of Legal Medicine (Ed.), *Legal medicine: Legal dynamics of medical encounters* (2nd ed.). St. Louis: Mosby.
McHale, J., Tingle, J., & Peysner, J. (1998). *Law and nursing.* Woburn, MA: Butterworth-Heinemann Medical.
McMullen P., & Campbell-Philipsen, N.D. (1994). The end of collective bargaining for nurses? NLRB v. Health Care and Retirement Corp. *Nursing Policy Forum, 1*(1).
McMullen, P., & Pepper, J. (1992). Surviving the legal hot seat. *Nursing Connections, 5*(2), 33–36.
McMullen, P., & Philipsen, N. (1993a). Charting basics 101. *Nursing Connections, 6*(3), 62–64.
McMullen, P., & Philipsen, N. (1993b). Medical records: Promoting patient confidentiality. *Nursing Connections, 6*(4).
NLRB v. Health Care and Retirement Corporation of America, 114 S.C.1778, 18 L.Ed. 586, 6 U.S.L.W. 4371, 146 L.R.R.M. (B.N.A.) 31, 18 Lab.Cas. 11,090 (May 3, 1994).

People of the State of Illinois v. Margaret Jihan, 537 N.E.2d 751m 127 Ill.2d 379, 130 Ill. Dec. 422 (1989).

Prosser, W. (1984). *Handbook of the law of torts* (4th ed.). St. Paul, MN: West.

Providence Hospital and Alaska Nurses' Association, 320 NLRB No. 49 (Jan. 3, 1996).

Sermchief v. Gonzalez, 660 S.W.2d 683 (Mo. 1983).

Scott, R. W. (1998). *Health care malpractice: A primer on legal issues for professions.* New York: McGraw-Hill.

Sharpe, C. C. (1999). *Nursing malpractice.* Westport, CT: Auburn House/Greenwood.

Web Sites of Interest

National Institutes of Health, Institute of Medicine Report on Medical Errors—To Err is Human: Building a Safer Health System. (2000). Washington, DC: National Academy Press. Available: http://www.nap.edu/books/0309068371/html. This publication is a recent report by the Institute of Medicine, which estimates that up to 98,000 people in the United States die each year as a result of medical errors. The report examined primarily hospital-based errors. Common errors and suggested solutions are addressed.

National Labor Relations Board. (2000, November). Available: http://www.nlrb.gov. Facts about the NLRB, labor law, weekly summaries, press releases, rules and regulations, and decisions are all available on this free government web site. Information is available in Spanish as well as in English.

Nurses Protection Group and Allied Health Providers. Available: http://www.npg.com. This free web site provides a weekly update of nursing malpractice cases and valuable information on malpractice/liability questions. Malpractice insurance information is also available.

U.S. Department of Justice Americans With Disabilities Act Home Page. (2000, October). Washington DC Available: http://www.usdoj.gov/crt/ada/adahom1.htm. The ADA Home Page gives valuable information on the history of the ADA, provisions of the Act, enforcement considerations, settlement information, technical assistance, new or proposed regulations, and ADA mediation information.

Versuslaw. (2000). Redmond, WA. Available:http://www.versuslaw.com. *Versuslaw* is a legal search engine. Cases from all states and the federal government are available. There is a modest fee for use of Versuslaw.

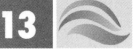

13

Ethical Dimensions of Nursing and Health Care

SARA T. FRY, PhD, RN, FAAN

OBJECTIVES

At the completion of this chapter, the reader will be able to:

- Describe how the subject matters of ethics and the methods of ethics are used to investigate morality.
- Apply a representative framework to analyze ethical conflicts in nursing practice.
- Comprehend how personal values and beliefs, professional moral standards, moral concepts of nursing, and ethical principles influence the nurse's ethical decisions and actions in providing patient care.

PROFILE IN PRACTICE

Terran Sims, RN, MS
Clinician 4
University of Virginia Health Systems
Charlottesville, Virginia

I became interested in ethics and ethical issues years ago when I was working in nephrology. At that time the number of dialysis units was limited and we had to decide who would be getting dialysis. There are similar issues now regarding the scarcity of organs for transplants. Because of my interest in ethics I took courses in biomedical ethics and received a master's degree with a specialty in this area. For the past several years I have been part of an interdisciplinary ethics consult service. This group provides 24-hour-a-day consultation for clinicians faced with ethical issues or dilemmas. The service includes physicians, social workers, nurses, clergy, geneticists, and others.

The major types of situations we deal with most often involve some type of communication problem. It may be that the patient has expressed certain wishes to some family members but not to all family members or the health care team. This can create difficulties in treatment planning. Since we are a tertiary care hospital in a rural area we often have family members trying to be involved in the treatment decisions of a loved one while being many miles away. They are often not aware that the patient's condition and wishes have changed, and this can cause a problem.

We also are asked to consult in situations where the competency of someone to sign a consent form is in doubt. We have learned that there is no overall guideline for a given patient. For example, some patients might be able to understand the ramifications of a simple medication instruction and be competent to consent to a simple procedure. However, this same patient may not be competent to sign a consent form for a complex oncology regimen.

I believe the field of biomedical ethics is always changing and becoming more complex, as is the constantly changing health care environment. There are many technological advances at the same time that we are being encouraged to control costs. Developing an expertise in ethics has expanded my role as a nurse clinician and provides daily challenges.

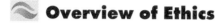 Overview of Ethics

The term *ethics* has several meanings. The term is sometimes used to refer to the practices or beliefs of a particular group of individuals, as in Christian ethics, physician ethics, or nursing ethics. *Ethics* also refers to the expected standards and behavior of a group as described in the group's code of professional conduct. Nurses and physicians are expected to maintain certain standards of ethical conduct as described by their professional codes of ethics (i.e., the American Nurses Association's *Code for Nurses* [1985] and the American Medical Association's *Principles of Medical Ethics* [1986]. The term *ethics* is also used to refer to a philosophical mode of inquiry that helps us understand the moral dimensions of human conduct. In this sense, ethics is an activity, a particular method of investigation, that one undertakes to respond to particular types of questions about human behavior.

Throughout this chapter, the term ethics will be used in all of the senses described above. "Ethics" will refer to the moral practices and beliefs of professionals who work together in the delivery of health care, the particular moral standards of a single group of professionals (nurses, physicians, and others), as well as a mode of inquiry based on certain principles. Ethics as a mode of inquiry helps us understand the moral dimensions of human conduct. To engage in or to *do* ethics is to undertake a particular method of investigation into matters of human concern (Fry, 1986).

Subject Matters of Ethics

Ethics has several subject matters or areas of inquiry (Fig. 13–1). *Descriptive ethics* investigates the phenomena of morality and then describes and explains the phenomena in order to construct a theory of human nature that responds to ethical questions. Those who investigate the moral reasoning patterns, moral judgments, and clinical decisions of nurse subjects are usually engaged in descriptive ethics. For example, Corley (1998) describes the ethical dimensions of nurse-physician relations in critical care units.

Normative ethics is an area of inquiry that investigates standards or criteria for right or wrong conduct. It usually begins with the question, "What ought I to do?" and examines various ethical principles, rules, or standards of right or wrong commonly associated with moral behavior. The moral weight of the perceived duties and obligations in human interaction is assessed, and theories about moral human conduct are often used to support one ethical judgment or action over another. Some common moral theories used in normative ethics are utilitarianism, natural law, formalism, and pragmatism.

Metaethics is a secondary level of inquiry that examines the nature of ethical inquiry itself. It gives us theories *about* ethics rather than theories *for* ethical conduct. Typical metaethical investigations consider the connections between human conduct and morality, the connections between ethical beliefs (values) and the facts of

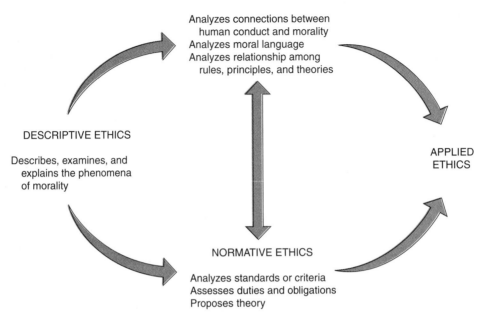

FIGURE 13-1   The subject matters of ethics.

the real world, and the relationships among ethical theories, principles, rules, and human conduct. Inquiry about the moral language of nursing (e.g., advocacy, accountability, cooperation, caring) falls within the area of metaethics as well.

The subject matters of ethics are closely related. One might start by engaging in descriptive ethics to describe moral phenomena (such as the protection of patients from harm), then engage in normative ethics to argue for the moral accountability of the nurse in patient care, and then engage in metaethics to explicate the meaning of accountability within a particular patient care situation. Sometimes it is not possible to engage in normative ethics without prior knowledge from metaethics, and vice versa. Both normative ethics and metaethics depend on descriptive ethics for the moral phenomena of human conduct. All three subject matters of ethics are particularly helpful in understanding the nature of the increasingly diffi-

cult ethical problems experienced by health professionals in the last decade.

VALUES

A *value* is a worthwhile or desirable standard or quality. Values can easily be identified in the everyday life experiences of any person. They can be expressed in language, in behaviors, or in standards of conduct that a person endorses or tries to maintain (Omery, 1989). Values are organized into a system that has meaning to the individual. This system of values represents the individual's set of beliefs about what he or she believes to be true. Some values are more important than others and are prioritized higher in an individual's value system. This hierarchy is usually fairly stable over time, but other values can and do replace higher values as a result of life experiences and an individual's reassessment of his or her values.

Once part of the person's value system, any

value can have motivational power and guide that person's choices. Unfortunately, individuals are often unaware of the values that motivate their choices and decisions.

Personal values are beliefs and attitudes held by an individual that form a basis for behavior and how each of us experiences life. For example, one nurse may personally value both cleanliness and honesty. These values are important to the nurse and either facilitate or prevent making certain judgments and carrying out specific actions. Personal values systems vary widely from person to person. One can never assume that another's personal value system is similar to one's own.

Each nurse has a personal value system influenced by upbringing, religious and political beliefs, culture, education, and life experiences. Identifying the personal values in one's value system through introspection and self-reflection is the first step in making ethical decisions. The second step is understanding what values are important to other individuals and the reasons why they are important. Each person prioritizes his or her values differently, based on his or her belief system and hierarchy of values. Someone else's value system is equally as valid as one's own value system.

Cultural values are values that are indigenous to a culture or people. They often influence our beliefs about health, illness, and what is morally required behavior in providing health care. Some cultures, typified by Western culture, value individual choice more than obedience to authority. Some cultures, such as some Asian cultures, value the elderly in the community more than other cultures. One culture may value health-promoting behaviors such as physical exercise more than another culture does. One's culture reinforces personal values.

Since nursing is practiced in many different cultural systems, any discussion of ethics must consider the values expressed by the culture of the population cared for and how those values relate to proposed nursing interventions. Many cultural values stem from religious beliefs and

may be acted out unconsciously by individuals. These values are deeply embedded in the background and experience of the person and cannot be called into question without questioning that person's very self-concept.

Professional values are general attributes prized by a professional group. Professional values in nursing are those promoted by the professional code of ethics and the practice standards of nursing. Nurses learn about professional values both from formal instruction and from informal observation of practicing nurses, and gradually incorporate professional values into their personal value system (Fry, 1994).

Some traditional professional values of nursing are based on preferences or taste: cleanliness, efficiency, organization, to name a few. Other professional values are based on moral norms: honesty, competence, compassion, and the like. Some of the professional values in nursing have a rich historical background founded on "nursing etiquette" (Box 13–1).

VALUES CONFLICTS

Values can easily conflict with one another and with individual rights and professional duties. Personal values may conflict with professional values, which in turn might conflict with cultural values. The nurse's value of providing good for the patient might conflict with her value of honoring the patient's choices or his right to make such choices. The nurse's value of giving safe medication dosages might conflict with the patient's value of relief from pain and the perceived professional duty to relieve suffering. The elderly patient's value of personal liberty or being able to get out of bed whenever he wants might conflict with the institution's value of patient safety, achieved by raising the side rails on the bed of every elderly patient at night. In each of these situations, the nurse must first identify the values involved, the value of relevant rights and duties, and where a conflict between values, rights, and duties is occurring. Then the nurse must make a decision

Box 13–1 Historical Note: Early Nursing Ethics and Etiquette

Early interpretations of nursing ethics tend to be associated with the image of the nurse as a chaste, good woman in service to others and as an obedient, dutiful servant. Florence Nightingale's good nurse was committed to the ideal of doing what was right. She was disciplined by moral training and could be relied on to do her duty in service to others.

This view of the good nurse as a good woman pervaded early textbooks on nursing ethics. In addition to being physically and morally strong, the nurse was required to be dignified, cultured, courteous, well-educated, and a reserved woman of good breeding. Moral virtue, moral duty, and service to others were thus established as important foundations on which later interpretations of nursing ethics would be built.

At first, the practice of nursing ethics was virtually indistinguishable from nursing etiquette and the performance of duty. Nursing etiquette included forms of polite behavior such as neatness, punctuality, courtesy, and quiet attendance on the physician. The nurse demonstrated her acceptance of her duties by following rules of etiquette, and by being loyal and obedient to the physician (Robb, 1921).

Some important distinctions were made between etiquette and ethics. Nurses learned proper ward etiquette in order to promote professional harmony in patient care—such etiquette became the foundation for all other nursing behaviors. Ethics, however, was taught to promote moral excellence and technical competence on the part of the nurse. Ethics was viewed as a science, the knowledge of which would enable the nurse to carry out prescribed duties with moral skill and technical perfection.

based on which values are most important. When moral values, rights, and duties are involved, resolving values conflicts becomes a complex ethical decision-making process (Fry, 1994).

Corley (1998) describes value conflicts between nurses and physicians when, for example, the nurses believe that the use of some technologies is unnecessarily prolonging a patient suffering whereas the physician views the treatment as a way to improve the patient's condition.

Moral Concepts in Nursing Practice

Advocacy, accountability, cooperation, and caring are moral concepts that comprise part of the foundation for nursing ethics. These concepts seem to enjoy a special place of honor among nursing standards and statements over the years.

Advocacy is the active support of an impor-

tant cause and a fundamental value of professional nursing (Hamric, 2000). It is sometimes used in a legal context to refer to the defense of basic human rights on behalf of those who cannot speak for themselves. For example, many institutions employ patient advocates who are expected to defend and speak for patients who cannot, by virtue of hospitalization or diminished autonomy as a result of illness, voice their own concerns or choices or assert their rights. The role of the advocate is to assert the patient's choices or desires on the patient's behalf, in the same way that a lawyer presents the case of her client, pleads for an interpretation of the case, and defends her client's rights.

There are several interpretations of the advocacy concept. One interpretation, the rights protection model, views the nurse as the defender of patient rights against an impersonal health care system. The nurse informs the patient of his or her rights, makes sure that the patient understands these rights, reports infringements of these rights, and is expected to prevent further violations of rights.

A second interpretation, the values-based decision model, views the nurse as the person who helps the patient discuss his or her needs, interests, and choices consistent with values, lifestyle, or personal plan of action. The nurse does not impose decisions or values on the patient but helps the patient explore the benefits and disbenefits of available options in order to make decisions most consistent with the patient's beliefs and values.

A third interpretation, the *respect-for-persons model,* views the patient as possessing certain human characteristics that require our respect. The patient's human dignity is respected and advocated regardless of whether or not the patient is self-determining or autonomous. As advocate, the nurse keeps the basic human values of the patient foremost among his or her

considerations and acts to protect the patient's human dignity, privacy, and choices (when applicable). When the patient is not self-determining, the nurse advocates the patient's welfare as defined by the patient while the patient was self-determining or as defined by the patient's surrogate decision maker. When no other person defines the welfare of the patient, the nurse promotes the best interests of the patient to the best of the nurse's nursing ability. In this role, the nurse assumes responsibility for the manner in which the patient's human dignity and other significant human values have been protected during the patient's illness and is accountable to society and other members of the nursing profession for how this important advocate role has been carried out.

This last model of advocacy seems to be consistent with the values in the ANA's *Code for Nurses* (Box 13–2). Indeed, the code describes

---

Box 13–2 American Nurses Association Code for Nurses

1. The nurse provides services with respect for human dignity and the uniqueness of the client, unrestricted by considerations of social or economic status, personal attributes, or the nature of health problems.
2. The nurse safeguards the client's right to privacy by judiciously protecting information of a confidential nature.
3. The nurse acts to safeguard the client and the public when health care and safety are affected by the incompetent, unethical, or illegal practice of any person.
4. The nurse assumes responsibility and accountability for individual nursing judgments and actions.
5. The nurse maintains competence in nursing.
6. The nurse exercises informed judgment and uses individual competence and qualifications as criteria in seeking consultation, accepting responsibilities, and delegating nursing activities to others.
7. The nurse participates in activities that contribute to the ongoing development of the profession's body of knowledge.
8. The nurse participates in the profession's efforts to implement and improve standards of nursing.
9. The nurse participates in the profession's efforts to establish and maintain conditions of employment conducive to high-quality nursing care.
10. The nurse participates in the profession's effort to protect the public from misinformation and misrepresentation and to maintain the integrity of nursing.
11. The nurse collaborates with members of the health professions and other citizens in promoting community and national efforts to meet the health needs of the public.

From American Nurses Association. (1985). *Code for nurses with interpretive statements.* Kansas City, MO: Author.

advocacy as acting so as "to safeguard the client and the public when health care and safety are affected by incompetent, unethical, or illegal practice by any person" (ANA, 1985). This means that the advocate role of the nurse has important long-range implications for the quality of patient care and the role of the nurse in the health care system. It is an important role that cannot be underestimated in today's world. Benner, Hooper-Kyriakidis, and Stannard (1999) have studied and provided rich examples of nurses in the role of advocate.

The concept of *accountability* has two major attributes: answerability and responsibility (Fry, 1994). Accountability can be defined in terms of either of these attributes, but answerability is the one preferred in the ANA's *Code for Nurses.* The code defines accountability as answerability for how one has promoted, protected, and met the health needs of the patient. It means to justify or to "give an account" according to accepted moral standards or norms for choices and actions that the nurse has made and carried out. It involves a relationship between the nurse and other parties and is contractual. The nurse is a professional who enters into an agreement to perform services and who can be held accountable for performing them according to agreed-upon terms and standards of practice.

The terms of *legal accountability* are contained in licensing procedures and state nurse practice acts. The terms of *moral accountability* are contained in the ANA's *Code for Nurses* and other standards of nursing practice in the form of norms set by the members of the profession. In the *Code for Nurses,* it is noted that accountability means "providing an explanation or rationale for what has been done in the nursing role" (ANA, 1985, p. 8). It is a very important concept of professional nursing practice and should be emphasized in the educational process. It is a concept from which important values are derived and principles are frequently formulated. Along with advocacy, cooperation, and caring, accountability forms the conceptual framework for the moral dimensions of nursing

practice and helps sustain the tradition of nursing by providing both the practice of nursing and the social role of nursing with a necessary historical content.

Cooperation is a concept that includes *active participation* with others to obtain quality care for patients, *collaboration* in designing approaches to nursing care, and *reciprocity* with those with whom nurses professionally identify. It means to consider the values and goals of those with whom one works as one's own values and goals. The ANA's *Code for Nurses* (1985) indicates support for cooperation as a moral value by its statement, "The nurse collaborates with members of the health professions and other citizens . . . to meet the health needs of the public" (p. 3).

Cooperation fosters networks of mutual support and close working relationships. The concept of cooperation supports such nursing actions as working with others toward shared goals, keeping promises, making mutual concerns a priority, and sacrificing personal interests to the long-term maintenance of the professional relationship. All these actions express feelings traditionally valued by all human beings and support professional collaboration in designing patient care.

Nursing's historical documents and professional statements have often emphasized different aspects of professional cooperation. For example, Isabel Hampton Robb (1921), an early nurse leader and scholar in the United States, linked cooperation to a special loyalty shared by members of the professional group:

[The nurse] must remember that, for the time being, she is a member of a large family and its privacy and internal affairs should be as loyally guarded as those of her own home circle. The individuality of each member of the family should be respected; the shortcomings or mishaps of any nurse should never be made a topic of conversation outside, either to friends in the city or to doctors. . . . The principle of loyalty must be maintained, irrespective of personal feelings (p. 139).

The concept of cooperation has also been expressed as the power that enables professionals to work together. The writings of Florence Nightingale (Nutting & Dock, 1907) emphasize this aspect of cooperation in the following passage:

> The health of the unit is the health of the community. Unless you have the health of the unit there is no community health. Competition, or each man for himself, and the devil against us all, may be necessary, we are told, but it is the enemy of health. Combination is the antidote—combined interests, recreation, combination to secure the best air, the best food, and all that makes life useful, health, and happy, There is no such thing as independence. As far as we are successful, our success lies in combination (pp. 277–278).

Cooperation appears to form the basis of Nightingale's idea human "combination," maintaining and strengthening a community of nurses working toward a common goal. It does not mean that conflicts will not occur or that the good of patients should be sacrificed for the maintenance of the nurse's relationships with colleagues or with the employing institution. It does mean, however, that individual goals and interests might need to be ethically compromised in order to achieve organizational and policy changes that will improve the quality of patient care.

Cooperation is also an altruistic concept because it expresses the human bonds that grow from working together and spending time together. It can threaten patient care if one's relationships to members of the profession or co-workers become more important than quality of patient care. The appropriate role for cooperation, however, is the maintenance of working relationships and conditions that express obligations toward the patient and are mutually agreed upon. Cooperation can help unite nurses and other health care workers toward the shared goal of improved patient care. Along with advocacy and accountability, cooperation helps form a strong conceptual framework that enables nurses to meet the requirements of professional practice.

The ethical concept of *caring* is valued in the nurse-patient relationship, and caring behaviors are often considered fundamental to the nursing role. Leininger (1984), for example, argues that caring has a direct relationship to human health and that all cultures and communities practice caring behaviors which serve to reduce intercultural stresses and conflicts. Such behaviors also protect human survival.

Nurse caring is specifically directed toward the protection of the health and welfare of patients. To some, caring is defined as a moral obligation or duty in special relationships. This means that the nurse, for example, is obligated to promote the good of the patient, for nurse and patient share a relationship that is created by the patient's need for nursing care. Nurses are obligated to show caring behaviors toward those in need of health care because doing so promotes their good.

Caring can also be defined as a form of involvement with others that creates concern about how other individuals experience their world (Benner, Tanner, & Chesla, 1996). Caring therefore involves being there for the patient, respecting the patient, feeling with and for the patient, and closeness with the patient.

The degree to which caring behaviors can be implemented in nursing practice is influenced by several factors. Nurse-related factors include such things as individual beliefs, educational experiences about caring, feeling good about nursing work, and one's own experiences in caring for others or in being cared for. Patient-related factors include whether or not the patient is hard to care for or confirms the nurse's caring behaviors. Other factors that influence nurse caring include time to care, administrative support for caring behaviors, and the physical environment where care takes place.

Some nurses have expressed concern about the extent to which nurses are expected to care for patients. For example, too much caring may result in nurses becoming physically and emotionally drained, "burnout," and unresolved nurse stress. There is a potential personal cost to caring on the part of the nurse that has not been adequately understood or investigated. Yet caring behaviors on the part of the nurse continue to be expected and valued by the profession and the public because caring is universally considered fundamental to the nursing role where human health is concerned.

Ethical Principles

Ethical principles are action guides to moral decision making and are an important element in the formation of moral judgments in professional practice (Beauchamp & Childress, 1994). They generally assert that actions of a certain kind ought (or ought not) to be performed, and serve to justify the rules that are often applied to patient care and the context of professional practice. The ethical principles important in nursing practice are beneficence, justice, autonomy, veracity, fidelity, and the sanctity of human life (Fry & Veatch, 2000).

BENEFICENCE

The obligation to do good and to avoid doing harm is understood as the ethical principle of *beneficence*. Acting on this principle means to help others gain what is of benefit to them, to reduce the risk of harm to patients, and to provide positive benefits to patients in terms of goods or assets.

Applying the principle in nursing practice often poses difficult problems for the nurse. For example, it is uncertain whether or not the nurse is obliged to take into consideration all of the ways in which the patient might be benefited. The *Code for Nurses* seems to imply that the nurse should do this when it states that the "nurse's primary commitment is to the health, welfare, and safety of the client" (ANA, 1985, p. 6). This is a substantial obligation that if literally interpreted, would entail multiple obligations toward the patient, some of which may actually lie outside the expertise or competency of the nurse.

A second problem in applying the principle is deciding whether the obligation to provide benefit has greater priority over the obligation to avoid harm. Some ethicists claim that the duty to avoid harm is a stronger obligation in health care relationships than the obligation to benefit (Beauchamp & Childress, 1994; Ross, 1939). If this is the case in nursing practice, nurses could fulfill the obligation to avoid harm by simply doing nothing for patients. Yet we would hardly call doing nothing for patients acceptable nursing care. The avoidance of harm must be balanced by the provision of benefit, and acceptable ranges of both benefit and risks of harm need to be established.

A third problem in applying this principle in nursing practice concerns the limits of providing benefit to patients. At what point do benefits to other parties (one's own family, the employing institution, co-workers) take priority over the benefits to the patient? Is the nurse obliged to provide benefits rather broadly or simply to the identified patient? Nurses need to be very clear about the boundaries of their obligation to provide benefits and avoid harm in patient care.

JUSTICE

Once the boundaries of the obligation to benefit and avoid harm are determined, nurses should be concerned about how benefits and burdens ought to be distributed among patient populations (Fry & Veatch, 2000). In other words, the nurse must decide what is a just or fair allocation of resources among patients under his or her care.

The formal principle of *justice* states that equals should be treated equally and that those who are unequal should be treated differently according to their needs (Beauchamp & Childress, 1994). This means that those equal in health needs should receive the same amount of health care resources. When some people have greater health needs, a principle of justice allows that they should receive a greater amount of health resources. This type of allocation is just because it distributes health resources according to need in a fair manner. While it is not possible to provide equal amounts of health care goods and resources for everyone in the society, it is possible to provide for every person's equal access to health care resources. Once access is achieved, then resources are ethically allocated according to individual need. The focus on need allows for the just distribution of resources among patients and prohibits the distribution of resources for other reasons.

AUTONOMY

The principle of *autonomy* ensures that individuals are permitted personal liberty to determine their own actions according to plans that they have chosen (Fry & Veatch, 2000). To respect persons as autonomous individuals is to acknowledge their personal choices.

One of the problems that occurs in applying a principle of autonomy to nursing care is that people are autonomous in varying degrees. Patients cannot make choices about their care entirely free from internal and external constraints. Internal constraints on patient autonomy are mental ability, level of consciousness, age, and disease states. External constraints on patient autonomy are the hospital environment, nursing resources, information for making informed choices, and financial resources.

The principle of autonomy may also be difficult to apply in patient care when there is a strong conviction on the part of the nurse or other members of the health care team that respecting self-determined choice is not really in the best interests of the patient. In this type of situation, the nurse may need to consider the limits of individual patient autonomy and the criteria for justified paternalism on the part of

the nurse. *Paternalism* is defined as the overriding of patient choices or intentional actions in order to benefit them (Beauchamp & Childress, 1994). Although paternalism is seldom justified in the care of patients, there is reason to believe that some situations warrant overriding patient autonomy when the benefits to be realized are great and the harms that will be avoided are significant (Childress, 1982).

Heeding a principle of autonomy means that nurses should also respect a patient's choice to refuse treatments. The basic human right of all patients to refuse treatment was formally legislated by the Omnibus Budget Reconciliation Act of 1990. The Patient Self-Determination Act became effective December 1, 1991, and requires all health care institutions receiving Medicare or Medicaid funds to inform patients that they have the right to refuse medical and surgical care and the right to initiate a written *advance directive,* a written or oral statement by which a competent person makes known his or her treatment preferences and/or designates a surrogate decision maker in the event he or she should become unable to make medical decisions on his or her own behalf (Box 13–3). A meta-analysis conducted in 1996 (5 years after the act was passed) found that 15%–25% of people have discussed advance directives (Miles, Koepp, & Weber, 1996). The most common reasons for not having advance directives are apathy, procrastination, and discomfort with the topic. Home health care agencies and managed care organizations are required to make this information available, in writing, at the time the patient comes under an agency's care.

In some situations, the nurse may need to assess whether an advance directive is an accurate statement of what the patient wants, whether a patient has fully taken into account the consequences of a treatment decision before completing an advance directive, and whether a surrogate decision maker is inappropriately making decisions for a patient with intact decision-making capacity (Mezey et al., 1994).

Box 13-3 Requirements of the Patient Self-Determination Act

- Provide written information to adult patients about their rights to make medical decisions, including the right to accept or refuse treatment and the right to formulate advance directives.
- Document in each patient's record whether the patient has previously executed an advance directive.
- Implement written policies regarding the various types of advance directives.
- Ensure compliance with state laws regarding medical treatment decisions and advance directives.
- Refrain from discrimination against individuals regarding their treatment decisions via an advance directive.
- Provide education for staff and the community on issues and the law concerning advance directives.

From Omnibus Reconciliation Act of 1990, Sections 4206 & 4751, P. L. 101–508, Nov. 5, 1990.

VERACITY

The principle of *veracity* is defined as the obligation to tell the truth and to not lie or deceive others (Fry & Veatch, 2000). Truthfulness has long been regarded as fundamental to the existence of trust among individuals and has special significance in health care relationships.

Truthfulness is expected because it is part of the respect that we owe persons. Individuals have the right to be told the truth and to not be lied to or deceived. Truthfulness also supports the relationship of trust that exists in special relationships. Nurses are obliged to be truthful because to not do so will undermine the effectiveness of the nurse's role with the patient and may, in the long run, bring about undesirable consequences for future relationships with patients.

When patients are seriously ill, nurses may sometimes withhold information from the patient because they think that the patient may not really want to know the truth about their condition. Studies of terminally ill patients, however, have indicated that despite illness, patients want to know the full truth about their conditions. The *Code for Nurses* points out that "truth telling and the process of reaching informed choice underlie the exercise of self-determination, which is basic to respect for persons" (ANA, 1985, p. 2). This means that the nurse is obliged to respect and follow a principle of veracity in providing nursing care to patients.

SANCTITY OF HUMAN LIFE

The issue of taking human life arises in a number of patient care situations and especially in decisions to withhold or withdraw life-sustaining treatments. It can also occur in situations of assisted suicide and whenever patients are suffering from disease or illness. The principle of sanctity of human life is defined as the obligation to not infringe on the sacredness of human life, or the obligation to not take human life (Fry & Veatch, 2000).

The taking of human life may be contemplated by the nurse whenever a patient is suffering. Someone might consider assisting the patient's death as an act of mercy. They might feel that the patient would be better off dead (or family members would be better off if the patient was dead). However, every nurse should consider whether or not the nurse should relieve a patient's misery by hastening his or her death in some manner. Is this a role for the nurse? Are nurses expected to make these types of judgments, especially when the patient is no longer capable of making his or her own decisions or of carrying out such an action on his or her own? Is there a difference between assisting a patient's death for reasons of mercy and withholding or withdrawing treatments for reasons of medical futility? Both actions will surely hasten the death of the patient, although with the latter action the patient will continue to live a while longer. The ANA's position statement on active euthanasia (1994) addresses some of these questions (Box 13–4).

Some ethicists claim that the above questions can be answered by applying the principles already discussed. In other words, the principles of beneficence, justice, and autonomy already provide arguments that will support the sanctity-of-human-life principle on the part of the nurse. Yet each of these principles has been demonstrated to be insufficient for questions about assisted dying in patient care. A principle of the sanctity of human life is needed to justify nurses' ethical reasoning for these situations.

The *Code for Nurses* seems to address this issue when it states, "Nursing care is directed toward the prevention and relief of the suffering commonly associated with the dying process. The nurse may provide interventions to relieve symptoms in the dying client even when the interventions entail substantial risks of hastening death" (ANA, 1985, p. 4). Yet the *Code for Nurses* also prohibits assisting the death of a patient when it states, "Nurses are morally obligated to respect human existence and . . . therefore they must take all reasonable means to protect and preserve human life when there is hope of recovery or reasonable hope of benefit from life-prolonging treatment" (ANA, 1985, p. 2).

Is withholding nutrition and hydration from a patient assisting his death? This question is at the center of some of the most controversial patient care issues confronting nurses today. Several philosophers (Lynn & Childress, 1983; Paris & Fletcher, 1983) and some legal cases (In the Matter of Mary Hier, 1984; Cruzan, 1990) have come to the conclusion that nutrition and hydration can be withheld for the same reasons that other treatments are with-

---

Box 13–4   Excerpts from the ANA's Position Statement on Active Euthanasia

The American Nurses Association (ANA) believes that the nurse should not participate in active euthanasia because such an act is in direct violation of the *Code for Nurses with Interpretive Statements* (*Code for Nurses*), the ethical traditions and goals of the profession, and its covenant with society. Nurses have an obligation to provide timely, humane, comprehensive and compassionate end-of-life care.

Active euthanasia occurs when someone other than the patient commits an action with the intent to end the patient's life, for example, injecting a patient with a lethal dose. . . . Active euthanasia is distinguished from assisted suicide. In active euthanasia someone not only makes the means of death available, but serves as the direct agent of death.

Honoring the refusal of treatments that a patient does not desire, that are disproportionately burdensome to the patient, or that will not benefit the patient can be ethically and legally permitted. Within this context, withholding or withdrawing life-sustaining therapies or risking the hastening of death through treatments aimed at alleviating suffering and/or controlling symptoms are ethically acceptable and do not constitute active euthanasia. There is no ethical or legal distinction between withholding or withdrawing treatments, though the latter may create more emotional disturbance to the nurse and others involved.

From American Nurses Association. (1994). *Position statement: Active euthanasia.* Washington, DC: Author.

Box 13–5 Excerpts from the ANA's Position Statement on Forgoing Nutrition and Hydration

The American Nurses Association (ANA) believes that the decision to withhold nutrition and hydration should be made by the patient or surrogate with the health care team. The nurse continues to provide expert care to patients who are no longer receiving artificial nutrition and hydration.

Artificial nutrition and hydration should be distinguished from the provision of food and water. Food and water provided to patients by mouth is the usual means of providing nutrition to patients. There are, however, situations in which nutrition can only be provided by artificial means. The provision of nourishment and hydration by artificial means (i.e., through tubes inserted into the stomach, into a blood vessel) is qualitatively different from merely assisting with feeding.

Like all other interventions, artificially provided hydration and nutrition may or may not be justified. It should be instituted or forgone only after a process of reasoned decision making focused upon an assessment of benefits and burdens to the patient. . . . The burdens vary with the illness of the patient, the substances to be delivered, the mode of delivery, and the anticipated outcomes. Some difficulties arise when it is unclear whether food and fluid are more beneficial or harmful. Since they are essential for life, this uncertainty leads to questions about whether life, under certain circumstances, would be a greater harm than death. As in all interventions, the anticipated benefits must outweigh anticipated burdens for the intervention to be justified.

When artificial nutrition is forgone, the nurse continues to provide high quality care, minimizes its effects (through mouth care, skin care, ice chips) and promotes patient dignity. The nurse demonstrates caring by continuing to provide expert care; pain control, skin care, personal hygiene, privacy and compassionate touch.

A process for transferring care of a patient to another qualified nurse, when a decision to forgo nutrition and hydration conflicts with the nurse's own personal beliefs and values, should be instituted at each institution.

From American Nurses Association. (1992). *Position statement: Forgoing nutrition and hydration.* Washington, DC: Author.

---

held, as long as there is clear and convincing evidence that this would be the patient's wish. Others, however, have been reluctant to accept the withholding of nutrition and hydration even when the patient has formally requested that this be done. Some scholars, for example, have expressed concern that the provision of food and fluids is a basic caring function that should always be required in the care of patients (Callahan, 1983). One reason given for this view is that the provision of food and fluids is symbolic of our care for the hungry and thirsty among us. If patients in terminally ill states do not experience hunger and thirst, however, does this mean that food and water should not be administered? The difficult nature of these questions is obvious. The ANA's position statement on forgoing nutrition and hydration (1992) offers guidance to the practicing nurse (Box 13–5).

In situations of doubt, the nurse must resort to the weight and importance of the obligation to respect human life in nursing practice. A sanctity-for-human-life principle is needed because nurses may often be uncertain whether or not their actions will contribute to the patient's death and whether or not such actions are morally wrong. Assisting a patient's death by facilitating the patient's suicide or by acts of active euthanasia under any circumstances is simply not an option for the nurse.

FIDELITY

Fidelity is the obligation to remain faithful to one's commitments (Fry & Veatch, 2000). Commitments that usually fall within the scope of fidelity are obligations generic to the trust relationship between patient and nurse. These obligations are keeping promises, maintaining confidentiality, and caring.

Individuals expect that promises will be kept in human relationships. We also expect that promises will not be broken unless there is a good reason. The same expectations concern the obligation of confidentiality, which is one of the most basic ethical requirements of professional health care ethics. However, exceptions to both obligations can sometimes be made. For example, some individuals maintain that it is morally acceptable to break promises when the breaking of the promise produces more good than if the promise is kept. Confidences are often broken for the same reasons.

It is also argued that breaking promises and confidences is morally acceptable when the welfare of a third party is jeopardized by the keeping of the confidence or promise. In the *Code for Nurses,* it is stated that the obligation of confidentiality "is not absolute when innocent parties are in direct jeopardy" (ANA, 1985, p. 4). Some form of this reason is usually given when confidences or promises are broken in order to report child abuse, homicide threats, or the laboratory results of a serious communicable disease.

Others, however, argue against the breaking of confidences, in particular on the basis of benefit to other parties. They claim that keeping information confidential is a right independent of consequences to others. While there may be good moral reasons to break promises to provide benefit to others, it is not morally acceptable to break confidences for the same reason.

One way to understand the conceptual nature of the moral commitments surrounding confidentiality and promise keeping is to ground these obligations in an independent principle of fidelity. Thus, in order to maintain fidelity with the patient, nurses should carefully consider the information that should be kept confidential and when promise keeping is a legitimate expectation in the nurse-patient relationship. The duty to keep one's commitments thus becomes the focus of these obligations, and not just the keeping of promises or confidentiality.

The duty to care is also included in aspects of the principle of fidelity. In fact, caring is consistently mentioned as one of the most important components of nursing practice, especially the care of the terminally ill patient. Individualized caring, affective behaviors, comforting, and nursing competence have all been mentioned by nurses and patients as important to caring and feeling cared for.

In summary, making moral decisions and carrying out moral actions are strongly influenced by the extent to which nurses incorporate ethical principles in their actions and relationships with patients. How do the principles of ethics apply to patient care, and how do nurses resolve conflicts of values in patient care?

Application of Ethics to Nursing Practice

No one denies that ethical decision-making ability is a requirement of professional nursing practice. Evidence of this ability is generally regarded as a desirable outcome of nursing education. Indeed, the majority of educational programs in nursing in the United States offer some course content in ethics. The goal is to assist the student to integrate his or her personal values and beliefs, the professional code of ethics, moral concepts of nursing practice, and ethical principles into a decision-making framework for making moral decisions and taking moral action (Fig. 13–2).

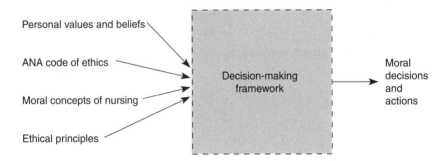

FIGURE 13–2 Essentials of moral decisions and actions in nursing practice.

≋ Decision-Making Frameworks

Are ethical decision-making frameworks really useful in nursing practice? If so, how does one choose such a framework? Ethicists recognize that there are many components and variables in decision making. No one decision-making method is appropriate or useful for everyone. However, ethical decision making can be enhanced by an orderly process of ethical analysis (Fry, 1994). Frameworks represent the process of analysis that one might make in making an ethical decision. They are useful in helping the decision maker examine (1) the values involved, (2) the context within which the decision will be made, and (3) the nature of the nurse's responsibilities in the situation. They do not provide a foolproof formula for arriving at the "right" decision. There is no recipe for ethical decision making in nursing practice. Each decision maker must supply his or her own values, cognitive ability, reasoning abilities, and moral intuitions to the process of arriving at an ethical decision. Frameworks for ethical decision making simply help the individual to analyze the value dimensions of a situation and utilize his or her abilities to arrive at an ethical decision.

Since ethical decision making is a cognitive and moral ability that can be taught in the educational process and learned by anyone with moral conscience, course content in ethics often includes ethical decision-making frameworks and their application in patient care situations. Used in conjunction with knowledge of the discipline of ethics, frameworks promote development of the abilities required for nursing practice.

The choice of a framework should be guided by the implicit values of the framework and their importance to the decision maker. Some frameworks clearly support the application of traditional theories of ethics and ethical principles to the patient care situation. Other frameworks help the nurse explore and analyze the context within which the value conflict has arisen and the views of the key parties to the decision. Nurses should not feel that one and only one framework works best in all situations.

The majority of ethical problems faced by the nurse are important but not necessarily complex. They are situations involving conflicts of values in fairly routine patient care situations. They become interesting and morally complex, however, when the values involved arise from strongly held cultural, religious, and moral beliefs. Because of the nature of values, a model of ethical decision making is offered here that can be used in conjunction with other models or used alone, depending on the situation.

A REPRESENTATIVE FRAMEWORK FOR CASE STUDY ANALYSIS

The following framework uses four questions to help the nurse, (1) understand the context within which the ethical problem has occurred,

(2) explore the significance of values central to the problem, (3) examine the meaning of the ethical problem to all parties involved, and (4) determine what should be done (Box 13–6).

1. *What is the story behind the values conflicts?*

By asking this question, the nurse begins to discover how the problem is defined by the parties experiencing the problem. The story needs to be told by each of the parties involved in terms of factual information (who did what) and in terms of the values of the parties involved (why the situation is seen as an ethical question), and the conflicts of values perceived by the parties involved. It is important to allow the story to be told in all its dimensions and through the eyes of all parties involved—the patient, the family members, the nurse, the physician, other health care workers, administrative official, and so forth. When the full story of the problem is known, the context within which the problem arose will be made explicit, and the various interpretations of the problem and the values of the parties involved will become clear. In this way, the value conflicts will be clarified. Ethical questions *always* involve conflicts between values.

2. *What is the significance of the values involved?*

In exploring the meaning of the values held by the parties involved, one gains insight into the nature of the values and their personal, religious, cultural, professional, and even political origins. Additional questions that might need to be asked include: What does it mean to "care" for this patient, and what are my nursing responsibilities to this patient? Are there any legal questions that might need to be explored by a legal representative? How do I, as a professional nurse, maintain my ethical integrity in this situation?

Exploring the significance of the values held by individuals in any situation is always very important. Ethical problems cannot be adequately resolved unless the value dimensions of the problem are known, respected, and considered in the decision-making process. This does not mean that all values will always be protected. In fact, in most conflicts the nurse plays a crucial role in assisting the involved parties to examine their values and the values of others so that the parties can begin to negotiate. In other words, the parties to the conflict will need to decide which values are most important to preserve and protect in this instance and which values might be of lesser importance. The goal of the professional nurse is to help the parties involved to respect each other's values and to help individuals prioritize their values and preserve the most important ones in the process of decision making. This can only be done when the significance of all values involved is known.

3. *What is the significance of the conflicts to the parties involved?*

In answering this question, the nurse learns how the parties involved related their values to the present situation. Values are never static. They are dynamic in that they change over time and in relation to significant human events and relationships. Situations of value conflicts likewise do not occur in a vacuum. They have a history and a necessary social, economic, and political content that make them significant or

---

Box 13–6   A Representative Framework for Case Study Analysis

1. What is the story behind the values conflicts?
2. What is the significance of the values involved?
3. What is the significance of the conflicts to the parties involved?
4. What should be done?

nonsignificant to the parties involved. The conflicts of values might lead to a decision that affects the quality of a person's life, how long he might live, the amount of guilt that other parties to the conflict might experience, the emotional and psychological stress that individuals might experience following the resolution of the conflict, and the nurse's professional demeanor.

The acknowledgment of conflicts of values might also lead to the formulation of policy that helps to resolve or prevent such value conflicts from occurring in the future. The nature of the value conflicts might have great signifi-

---

Box 13–7 Case Study: When the Duty to Be an Advocate Conflicts with the Duty to Contain Health Care Costs

Ramon Ortega, a 42-year-old farm laborer with a history of hypertension, had been experiencing headaches on an almost daily basis for 2 to 3 weeks. Disturbed by the persistent and severe nature of the headaches, he visited the state-supported health clinic serving his rural community. Ms. Tracey Anderson, the family nurse practitioner and sole staff of the clinic, listened as Mr. Ortega described his headaches. She then performed an initial examination, which revealed good general health with the exception of an elevated blood pressure of 190/108. Since Mr. Ortega had described some dizziness and visual disturbances during his headaches, Ms. Anderson also completed a neurological assessment. Everything seemed within normal limits except for Mr. Ortega's peripheral vision. Ms. Anderson's assessment demonstrated that he had some difficulty seeing objects in the visual field on his left side. Ms. Anderson realized that this disturbance was probably a manifestation of his present headache in combination with his known visual deficit. Since no other abnormalities were demonstrated, the possibility of a more serious problem seemed remote, in Ms. Anderson's judgment. Yet Mr. Ortega was very distressed by his headaches. He asked the nurse what he could do to prevent the headaches, or at least, what could be done to lessen the pain he was experiencing. Could she be sure no other problem was causing the headaches?

Several months earlier, Ms. Anderson would not have hesitated to refer Mr. Ortega to University Medical Center 110 miles away, for physician examination and a neurological evaluation of his headaches. She would have done this for no other reason than to relieve the patient of his worry and to confirm the absence of a more serious problem. She still believed that, on balance, the referral would be of some help. In recent weeks, however, the state agency that funds the rural health clinics had urged all health clinic personnel to be careful in referring patients for costly laboratory or evaluate testing with the added expense of clinic-sponsored transportation. There were decreased monies to support the personnel and services in rural health clinics since the agency had adopted a strict cost-containment program. In fact, the continued operation of the rural health clinics depended on how well individual clinics contained costs, even though they provided greatly needed services to populations like the low-income farm community in which Mr. Ortega lives.

Ms. Anderson had been cutting the operating costs of her clinic in every way she could, particularly in her judicious referral of patients to University Medical Center. But she could not overlook the fact that Mr. Ortega was distressed by his headaches, and there was always the possibility, albeit remote, that he was presenting with early signs of impending cerebrovascular disease, the effects of which could seriously affect him and his family. She was uncertain about what choice to make.

From Fry, S. T., & Veatch, R. M. (2000). *Case studies in nursing ethics* (2nd ed, p. 29). Jones and Bartlett Publishers, Sudbury, MA. www.jbpub.com. Reprinted with permission.

cance for health professionals who often must deal repeatedly with conflicts of values in the work environment.

4. *What should be done?*

By asking this question, the nurse explores all the ways in which the value conflicts might be resolved. Seldom is there a single "ethically correct" solution to a situation. In most cases, ethical decisions are reached based on the amount of information available at that time, the significance of the value dimensions, and the best judgment of the decision maker or the collective ethical stance of the group. Knowing a variety of possible ways in which the conflicts might be resolved gives the involved parties options to explore. These options should be explored in light of (1) the values held by the various parties, (2) outcomes that may occur, and (3) the moral rightness or wrongness of the various options. Some options might be ethically permissible (that is, they do not conflict with the professional code of ethics) but may not support the values of the key decision maker, other parties to the situation, or the community group consensus. Some options might not be ethically permissible although they might support important values. Some options might be ethically permissible for the patient, family members, or community group (i.e., consistent with their personal, cultural, and religious values) but not permissible for the nurse.

At some point, the key decision maker must choose a course of action based on his or her best judgment of what ought to be done. This decision is often very individual but is morally responsive in that it stems from a careful consideration of the context of the value conflicts, the values of all parties involved, the ethical relevance of these values, and the moral meaning of the situation to individuals involved. It is also a rational decision, based on a careful process of ethical reflection, and supported by the moral concepts of nursing and ethical principles.

Following the implementation of the choice or decision made, some assessment should be made about the outcome of the situation and the process that led to the decision. The nurse should always consider whether the process could have been improved and what implications, if any, the conflicts of values have for future patient cares situations.

To test your understanding of the above framework for case study analysis, use the framework in deciding what the nurse should do in the case study provided (Box 13–7).

Research on Nursing Ethics

The earliest record of a nursing ethics research project was Vaughan's study of the diaries of 95 student and graduate nurses who recorded the ethical problems they encountered in nursing practice over a 3-month period (1935). Vaughan's analysis identified a total of 2,265 moral problems, 67 problems of etiquette, and 110 questions about ethical behavior. The ethical problem the nurse subjects faced most often was the lack of cooperation between nurses and physicians, and between nurses in general. Vaughan concluded that the problem of lack of cooperation her subjects experienced signaled nurses' growing awareness of their responsibility to society and the role that they were playing in patient care.

Despite this early interest in descriptive ethics, nursing ethics research did not begin in earnest until the 1980s. Research efforts initially focused on the ethical reasoning abilities and ethical behaviors and judgments of practicing nurses (Crisham, 1981; Ketefian, 1981a, 1981b). Related studies focused on the moral reasoning levels of nursing students and nursing faculty (Munhall, 1980) and on patient values in relation to treatment choices (Gortner, 1984). More recently, studies have compared nurses' perceptions of moral problems in clinical practice with physicians' perceptions (Corley, 1998; Gamelspacher et al., 1986) and have analyzed nurses' beliefs about medical ethical decision making into objective and subjective value dimensions (Self, 1987).

These studies have focused on the ability of the nurse to make moral judgments, the hypothetical moral behavior of the nurse, nurses' perceptions of moral problems, or the value dimensions of nurses' and patients' beliefs about ethical decision making. The measurement tools and the procedures employed have been designed to evaluate the cognitive ability of nurses to perceive value dimensions or to make moral judgments. In most cases, study results have been interpreted according to theoretical structures outside the context of nursing. Kohlberg's stage theory of moral development has been the most frequently cited theoretical structure (Kohlberg, 1981), but bioethics theory (Beauchamp & Childress, 1994) and value theory (Self, 1979) have also been used.

During the 1980s and early 1990s, the focus of nursing ethics research shifted from a study of nurses' ethical perceptions and behaviors and how nursing ethics is taught to a study of how nurses make ethical decisions and plan patient care when confronted with complex moral issues. The use of nursing care resources by do-not-resuscitate (DNR) patients in medical intensive care units and the impact of the DNR order on nursing interventions have been studied (Lewandowski et al., 1985), while the identification of variables that are the best predictors of a DNR classification and the extent of nursing care required by the DNR patient have been examined in another research study (Tittle, Moody, & Becker, 1991). Other researchers have studied how nurses perceive their roles in the implementation of the Patient Self-Determination Act and how prepared nurses are to undertake this role in patient care (Silverman, Fry, & Armiger, (1994). More recently, changes in health care delivery have prompted researchers to study the types of ethical issues that nurses experience in practice, how disturbed they are by the issues, and the resources they use to resolve ethical issues (Fry, Riley, & Currier, 1999) (Box 13–8).

Observations that can be made about the current state of the art in nursing ethics research are the following:

1. Values, value changes, moral judgment, and levels of moral reasoning among nurses or nurse students have not been adequately correlated with formal educational ethics content in nursing curricula. It is also not evident that the formal teaching of ethics affects the development of moral judgment in practicing nurses or that the development of moral judgment and increased levels of moral reasoning among nurses has any effect on the performance of nursing functions or patient care outcomes. These are all areas for further study. We tend to think that ethics is an important component in the nursing curriculum and that the ability to recognize values, make moral decisions, and be accountable for decisions is important to the quality of nursing care. Yet we do not really know what type of ethics content is truly effective in the education of nurses. Nor do we know to what extent the effective teaching of ethics influences the ability of the nurse to give more competent patient care. Is the morally accountable nurse a more competent nurse?

2. The use of theoretical frameworks to interpret study results should be carefully evaluated. Since nursing is largely practiced by women, theoretical structures should include the process of ethical decision making by women as well as by men. Kohlberg's theory, derived from cognitive psychology and based on studies of male children, has been strongly challenged for its lack of relevance to the moral development and ethical reasoning of women (Gilligan, 1982; Noddings, 1984). Furthermore, researchers should use structures that can account for the nature and process of ethical decisions made by nurses in contrast to those of other health care workers, such as physicians.

3. The evaluation of nursing research on ethics needs to address the subject matters of ethics rather than typical subject matters of nursing. Units of analysis such as nurse, patient,

Box 13-8   A Clinical Nursing Ethics Research Study*

The purpose of this study was to identify the ethical issues experienced by registered nurses (RNs) in their practices and how frequently these issues occurred.

The population for the study was RNs practicing in six states in the northeast region of the United States. Systematic random sampling was used during 1997–1998 to select a 5% sample ($n = 8,536$) of the total population ($n = 159,183$).

A survey tool was developed, piloted, and satisfactorily tested for the psychometric properties of the 35-item ethical issues scale (EIS) in a survey of 521 nurses (internal consistency reliabilities of the three subscales of the EIS ranged from .77 to .83). Two mailings, each consisting of a cover letter, the six-page questionnaire, and a self-addressed and stamped return envelope, were sent to the sample.

Two thousand four hundred and eight (2,408) survey questionnaires were returned (return rate = 29%), and analysis was performed on 2,090 usable questionnaires. The typical nurse participant in the survey was a 44-year-old woman with a college degree, employed full-time as a staff nurse and with 19 years of nursing experience, and in her present position an average of 7.6 years. The most frequently experienced ethical issues for the RN participants during the previous 12 months were (1) protecting patients' rights and human dignity, (2) respecting/not respecting informed consent for treatment, (3) providing care with possible risk to the nurse's health, (4) using/not using physical or chemical restraints in patient care, and (5) staffing patterns that limited patient access to nursing care. The most disturbing ethical issues selected by the subjects were (1) staffing patterns that limited patient access to nursing care, (2) prolonging the living/dying process with inappropriate measures, (3) not considering the quality of a patient's life, (4) implementing managed care policies that threatened quality of care, and (5) working with unethical/incompetent/impaired colleagues. Over 30% of the RN participants reported that they experienced ethical issues in their practices one to four times per week or daily.

The findings from this study indicate that significant numbers of RNs in New England have frequently experienced ethical issues in their practices during the last 12 months. Indeed, almost one-third of the RNs experienced ethical issues almost daily. The issue they were most disturbed about (staffing patterns that limited patient access to nursing care) was also selected as one of the more frequently experienced ethical issues in practice.

This study provides data-based information about ethical issues that RNs experience in the workplace. However, further research is needed to determine the extent to which the workplace, as a contextual variable, influences how RNs experience ethical issues. The majority of the RN participants had completed their basic nursing education nearly 20 years ago, which suggests a need to learn new ways to address emerging ethical issues in the workplace. Appropriate education programs in the workplace to address the ethical issues RNs experience may therefore be necessary to assist nurses to practice ethically and ensure that patients' rights are protected.

* This study was conducted in collaboration with the Nursing Ethics Network.
From Fry, S. T. (1999). Ethical issues experienced by registered nurses: Their frequency and level of disturbance [Abstract]. In *Better health through nursing research: State of the Science Congress.* Washington, DC: American Academy of Nursing.

and the environment reflect traditional paradigms of nursing inquiry, but they tell us nothing about the discipline of ethics or the state of ethical inquiry in nursing. Ethical inquiry in nursing should be reviewed and evaluated according to the subject matters of ethics: descriptive ethics, normative ethics, and metaethics. We should also be encouraging nurse researchers to pursue research on ethics within these classifications.

4. The particular roles of nurses in ethical decisions that affect patients are not very clear. Nurses' abilities to recognize moral values, make ethical decisions, and support patients' or family members' decisions are believed to be very important to the quality of patient care. However, little is known about the types of ethical decisions made by nurses and how they affect patient outcomes. Nursing ethics research should attend to this lack of information.

KEY POINTS

- The moral concepts of advocacy, accountability, cooperation, and caring have important moral dimensions and compose part of the conceptual framework for nurses' ethical decision-making.

- The ethical principles of beneficence, justice, autonomy, veracity, the sanctity of human life, and fidelity are action guides to moral nurse actions but often conflict with one another or with other significant human values. It is important for nurses to use an ethical decision-making framework in patient care situations.

- Many ethical decision-making frameworks are available in the nursing literature. They provide a systematic approach to the ethical analysis of values conflicts and questions of what should be done in the nursing role.

- Descriptive ethics research is at a very early stage of development in nursing, and few good metaethical studies of nursing's moral concepts have been conducted.

- Normative ethics is also at a very early stage of development as a form of inquiry in nursing.

- Nurses should become familiar with the methods of ethics, the use of ethical decision-making frameworks, and the current state of nursing ethics research so that they can effectively contribute to the growth of ethical inquiry within nursing.

CRITICAL THINKING EXERCISES

1. To what extent should one's personal code of ethics, integrated with religious beliefs and cultural values, influence moral decision making in nursing practice?

2. If a terminally ill patient under your care asked you to help them end their life or assist them in dying, what would you do? Why?

3. Some ethicists have argued that there is nothing morally unique to nursing practice, that is, the same moral issues and questions arise in all health professionals' practices. Do you agree or disagree with this statement? Why?

4. The term "applied ethics" means the application of ethical theory, principles, and reasoning to a realm of practice. How do you apply ethics to your own area of nursing practice?

REFERENCES

American Medical Association, Judicial Council. (1986). *Current opinions of the Council on Ethical and Judicial Affairs of the American Medical Association—1986: Including the principles of medical ethics and rules of the Council on Ethical and Judicial Affairs.* Chicago: American Medical Association.

American Nurses Association, (1985). *Code for nurses with interpretive statements.* Kansas City, MO: Author.

American Nurses Association. (1992). *Position statement: Forgoing nutrition and hydration.* Washington, DC: Author.

American Nurses Association. (1994). *Position statement: Active euthanasia.* Washington, DC: Author.

Beauchamp, T. L., & Childress, J. F. (1994). *Principles of biomedical ethics* (4th ed.). New York: Oxford University Press.

Benner, P., Hooper-Kyriakidis, P., Stannard, D. (1999). *Clinical wisdom and interventions in critical care.* Philadelphia: Saunders.

Benner, P., Tanner, C., Chesla, J. (1996). *Expertise in nursing practice.* New York: Springer.

Callahan, D. (1983). On feeding the dying. *Hastings Center Report, 13*(5), 22.

Childress, J. F. (1982). *Paternalism in health care.* New York: Oxford University Press.

Corley, M. C. (1998). Ethical dimensions of nurse-physician relations in critical care. *Ethics for Nursing Practice, 33*(2), 325–337.

Crisham, P. (1981). Measuring moral judgment in nursing dilemmas. *Nursing Research, 30,* 104–110.

Cruzan v. Director, Missouri Department of Health, 110 S. Ct. 2841 (1990).

Fry, S. T. (1986). Ethical inquiry in nursing: The definition and methods of biomedical ethics. *Perioperative Nursing Quarterly, 2,* 1–8.

Fry, S. T. (1994). *Ethics in nursing practice: A guide to ethical decision making.* Geneva, Switzerland: International Council of Nurses.

Fry, S. T. Riley, J., & Currier, S. (1999). Ethical issues experienced by registered nurses: Their frequencies and levels of disturbance. In [abstract] *Proceedings: State of the Science Congress,* Sept. 15–19, 1999, Washington, DC.

Fry, S. T., & Veatch, R. M. (2000). *Case studies in nursing ethics* (2nd ed.). Boston: Jones & Bartlett.

Gamelspacher, G. P., et al. (1986). Perceptions of ethical problems by nurses and doctors. *Archives of Internal Medicine, 146,* 577–578.

Gilligan, C. (1982). *In a different voice: Psychological theory and women's development.* Cambridge, MA: Harvard University Press.

Gortner, S. R., et al. (1984). Appraisal of values in the choice of treatment. *Nursing Research, 33,* 319–324.

Hamric, A. (2000). What is happening to advocacy? *Nursing Outlook, 48*(3), 103–104.

In the Matter of Mary Hier, 464 N.E. 2d 959 (Mass. Ct. App. 1984).

Ketefian, S. (1981a). Critical thinking, educational preparation, and development of moral judgment among selected groups of practicing nurses. *Nursing Research, 30,* 104–110.

Ketefian, S. (1981b). Moral reasoning and moral behavior among selected groups of practicing nurses. *Nursing Research, 30,* 171–176.

Kohlberg, L. (1981). *The philosophy of moral development: Essays on moral development* (Vol. 1). New York: Harper & Row.

Leininger, M. M. (1984). Care, the essence of nursing and health. In *Care: The essence of nursing and health* (pp. 3–15). Detroit: Wayne State University Press.

Lewandowski, W., Daly, B., McClish, D. K., Juknialis, B. W., & Youngner, S. J. (1985). Treatment and care of "do not resuscitate" patients in a medical intensive care unit. *Heart and Lung, 14*(2), 175–181.

Lynn, J., & Childress, J. F. (1983). Must patients always be given food and water? *The Hastings Center Report, 13*(5), 17–21.

Mezey, M., Evans, L., Golub, Z., Murphy, E., & White, G. (1994). The Patient Self Determination Act: Sources of concern for nurses, *Nursing Outlook, 42*(1), 57–61.

Miles, S. H., Koepp, R., & Weber, E. P. (1996). Advance end-of-life treatment planning. *Archives Internal Medicine, 156,* 1062–1068.

Munhall, P. (1980). Moral reasoning levels of nursing students and faculty in a baccalaureate nursing program. *Image, 12,* 57–61.

Noddings, N. (1984). *Caring: A feminine approach to ethics and moral education.* Berkeley, CA: University of California Press.

Nutting, A., & Dock, L. L. (1907). *A history of nursing* (Vol. II). New York: Putnam's Sons.

Omery, A. (1989). Values, moral reasoning, and ethics. *Nursing Clinics of North America, 24*(2), 488–508.

Paris, J. J., & Fletcher, A. B. (1983). Infant Doe regulations and the absolute requirement to use nourishment and fluids for the dying infant. *Law, Medicine, and Health Care, 11*(5), 210–213.

Pellegrino, E. (1985). The caring ethic: The relation of physician to patient. In A. H. Bishop & J. R. Scudder (Eds.), *Caring, curing, coping: Nurse, physician, patient relationships,* pp. 8–30. Birmingham, AL: University of Alabama Press.

Prescott, P. A., Dennis, K. E., & Jacox, A. K. (1987). Clinical decision making of staff nurses. *Image, 19,* 56–62.

Robb, I. H. (1921). *Nursing ethics: For hospital and private use.* Cleveland: Loeckert.

Ross, W. D. (1939) *The right and the good.* London: Oxford University Press.

Self, D.J. (1979). Philosophical foundations of various approaches to medical ethical decision making. *Theoretical Medicine, 8,* 86–95.

Self, D. J. (1987). A study of the foundations of ethical decision making of nurses. *Theoretical Medicine, 8,* 86–95.

Silverman, H. J., Fry, S. T., & Armiger, N. (1994). Initial perspectives on implementation of Patient Self-Determination Act. *Journal of Clinical Ethics, 5*(1), 30–37.

Tittle, M. B., Moody, L., & Becker, M. P. (1991). Preliminary development of two predictive models for DNR patients in intensive care. *Image, 23*(3), 140–144.

Vaughan, R. H. (1935). *The actual incidence of moral problems in nursing: A preliminary study in empirical ethics.* Unpublished doctoral dissertation, Catholic University of America, Washington, DC.

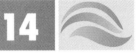

14

Social and Cultural Dimensions of Health and Health Care

KATHRYN HOPKINS KAVANAGH, PhD, RN

OBJECTIVES

At the completion of this chapter, the reader will be able to:

- Understand the ways in which cultural and lifestyle differences between nurses and clients affect nursing care.
- Describe the influence of cultural values and social norms on health, health care, and nursing.
- Discuss how a balance of sensitivity, knowledge, skills, and meaningful encounters allows nurses to manage diversity effectively.
- Identify strategies for culturally acceptable nursing assessment, communication, and intervention.

PROFILE IN PRACTICE: NURSING STUDENTS WITHOUT BORDERS

Bridget Kuczkowski, undergraduate student
University of Virginia School of Nursing
Charlottesville, Virginia

Rosalind de Lisser, BSN, RN
University of Virginia Health System
Charlottesville, Virginia

Teri Woodard, BSN, RN
Clinician II, University of Virginia Health System
Charlottesville, Virginia

Matthew Walden, undergraduate student
University of Virginia School of Nursing
Charlottesville, Virginia

Established in 1999, Nursing Students Without Borders (NSWB) is a student-run organization at the University of Virginia School of Nursing. The founding members sought to organize the concept of global community service into a health care program that has a sustainable impact on underserved communities. While expanding the perspectives and experiences of nursing students, the mission of NSWB is to launch health education initiatives, outline a network to access health care resources within the community, and distribute material donations.

The UVA chapter of NSWB is currently focused on educating San Sebastian, El Salvador, and its surrounding *cantones,* or rural communities. The region, home to 15,000 people, still suffers from the economic and developmental devastation incurred during a 12-year civil war that ended in 1992. Over the next 3 years NSWB has an education campaign in the San Sebastian schools that concentrates on first aid, hygiene, nutrition, and reproductive health. Other objectives for the co-op include independent research studies for the NSWB students, providing contemporary medical information and supplies to the town clinic and midwives, holding advanced first aid courses for the Red Cross volunteers, and training them to continue the educational drive.

The experience of teaching reproductive health in a different culture, specifically that of San Sebastian, El Salvador, was a valuable lesson, as nursing students were confronted with the existence of their personal and societal biases. Health care providers often inadvertently attempt to implement their own belief systems while attending to the needs of a patient. when the NSWB students arrived, the local school principals and the village physician cited a lack of knowledge about reproductive health as well as no existing channel to discuss the issue. Initially, lesson plans were drafted based on reports of families consisting of 4 to 13 children, soaring rates of adolescent pregnancy, and the prevalence of sexually transmitted infections. Having no prior contact with the community and its social practices, the curriculum preparers addressed the issues based on perceptions of their presentation in the United States. It was impossible to predict the degree of religious, cultural, and organizational influence on reproductive health practices in San Sebastian. Even less predictable was how the society would react to the introduction of the taboo topic of sexual and reproductive health.

In order to provide education on a controversial topic, it was crucial to observe and identify societal norms, weigh the findings with the realism that the entire community is not homogenous, and, finally, create a means for a diplomatic delivery of information. After their arrival, the students became cognizant of the cultural atmosphere in San Sebastian as well as their own intrinsic biases concerning reproductive health in the developing world. The students had to design an intervention that would permit the delivery of clinical knowledge while filtering out partiality. The purpose of the education initiatives was not to impose widespread solutions, such as small families are preferable to large ones or a specific age at which it is appropriate to have sex, but to introduce a knowledge base to the adolescents to consider within their cultural context. Being careful not to import biases, the students decided that the objective of the intervention was to be informed decision making. The intervention, reproductive health forums, fostered autonomous thought and informed discussion among the village adolescents about the balance between actions and their potential consequences. The talk, or *charla,* began with NSWB presenting objective information. The educational topics included family structure, pregnancy prevention, sexually transmitted infections, and AIDS. Following the educational segment was a question-and-answer session. After all the questions were addressed, the NSWB volunteers asked the adolescents how many siblings they had, and how many children they themselves wanted to have. The questions opened up discussions that illustrated different lines of reasoning about, and options for, reproductive health, all of which arguments were strengthened by the clinical information. The informality of the *charlas* fostered an open, educated dialogue and reflection on the positive and negative aspects of sexual activity. The *charlas* highlighted areas of the community's health concerns. A channel had finally been created; the adolescents conveyed what aspects of reproductive health they wanted more information on and discussed how they wished to interact within the sexual and social climate of their community.

The use of low-pressure *charlas* to address the difficult topics of sex, family planning, and infections was extremely effective. The adolescents were better able to understand their choices in making educated decisions regarding sexual activity and their future. For members of NSWB, the experience of teaching in San Sebastian, specifically the construction of an intervention to fit the cultural parameters of a community, resulted in the self-actualization of personal biases and cultural diversity. Having to give lessons in Spanish

and teach with minimal supplies prepared NSWB volunteers to work judiciously within the modern medical system and be able to improvise at a community site. From their experience mediating dialogues in San Sebastian, the students are better able to listen to patients as they communicate within their social context, and better able to draft interventions appropriate for a patient's lifestyle. As NSWB members practice in the clinical field, their depth of perception and awareness is evident in their problem-solving techniques, which focus on the bettering of the whole individual. In addition, skills such as adaptive teaching to involve both the patient and his or her support system, developing greater sensitivity to patient beliefs, and integrating nursing practice into diverse settings have directly enhanced their ability to provide care.

Nurses are increasingly being challenged to provide care to individuals and groups of people with diverse backgrounds, values, and expectations. This requires great flexibility on the part of the nurse because there is no single way to provide such care. The understanding of what constitutes "care" and "caring" varies widely, as does how the quality of care is evaluated. Nurses must be innovative in order to provide care that is recognized for its quality and is acceptable to members of diverse groups. This chapter is devoted to facilitating development of the sensitivity, knowledge, skills, and meaningful encounters that are essential to providing high-quality nursing care in a diverse and multicultural society.

CASE STUDY

Visiting

When Ellen began her clinical rotation on a large Indian reservation, her thinking revolved around what she could teach the community workers there. She spent days traveling many miles with various commu-

nity health representatives (CHRs). These were Indian men and women who had about 1 month's training (sometimes in addition to other training and student experiences). They then assumed roles as providers, visiting homes of other Indians, doing routine and basic care, and acting as liaisons between the Indian population and the biomedical system. Slowly Ellen realized how Lakota culture shaped the Indians' perceptions of health, illness, and their expectations for treatment and care. As the weeks went on and Ellen learned to be open to new ways of knowing and doing things, her interpretations changed, as her journal entries indicate:

Week 1: "The CHRs don't really do anything. They just go and drink coffee and sit down and visit."

Week 2: "I think they just visit because they don't know what else to do. They even talk about themselves there, and the problems their own kids are having. And they are all quiet a lot. Sometimes they hardly talk about the patient's problem."

Week 3: "You know, something happens when the CHRs visit, but I don't know what it is. I don't see how their visiting works, but I see that people appreciate it."

Week 4: "The patients do what the CHRs want them to do. Something goes on, but I don't get it—they never actually tell the patients what to do."

Week 5: "I still don't see how the visiting works when the CHRs don't do much instruction. They do other things—wash the quadriplegic man's long hair, dress decubiti, weigh babies, but mostly they visit. Somehow it works."

Week 6: "I've got it. Visiting is what the CHRs do. It is what is important and how they intervene. It is because of the visiting that the patients respond, not because of what the CHRs do when they visit."

Diversity and Health

Health and health care are influenced by culture, with its shared values and beliefs, and society, with its behavioral expectations, referred to as social norms. The theme of this chapter is diversity and its impact on nursing. Diversity is not defined here as ethnicity or race, as the term is often used in everyday language. Rather, diversity is defined broadly as differences that may be rooted in age, culture, health status, experience, gender, sexual orientation, racial or ethnic identity, or other aspects of sociocultural description and socioeconomic position (Kavanagh & Kennedy, 1992).

Effective interventions are founded on informed decisions, not chance happenings. In the management of diversity, "manage" is defined as affirmation and encouragement focused on development of full potential, not as manipulation to get compliance (Thomas, 1990). In assisting people with personal concerns and losses, nurses encounter patterns of similarities and differences that shape client care needs. Providing culturally appropriate care involves learning to balance sensitivity, knowledge, and skills to respectfully accommodate social and cultural, as well as biological, psychological, and spiritual, needs.

Why should nurses be concerned about diversity? Because groups and individuals interpret the world in ways that reflect how they view the world (i.e., from their perspectives and in the context of their own experience). What is considered normal or abnormal, caring or noncaring, appropriate or a waste of time or even offensive, depends on context. Health and illness are perceived in diverse ways, and there are many different expectations for appropriate care and treatment. Cultural values and social norms are major influences, and these often come from groups other than the Euro-American one most prevalent in nursing and health care in the United States.

The classic model of transcultural nursing relates the commonalities and differences among cultural worldviews that reflect various aspects of society to the diverse health systems (Fig. 14–1) (Leininger, 1991). This depiction of the many interrelated dimensions of culture and care is helpful for exploring important meanings and patterns of care. When working with clients who have cultural orientations that are different, in minor or major ways, from those of the nurse, these considerations are particularly significant.

Although Leininger's model of transcultural nursing provides valuable conceptual assistance, other tools may prove more helpful in actual nursing practice. Learning to recognize and use Diekelmann's inductively-derived "concernful practices" as they apply to specific groups of people provides an effective practice model (Kavanagh et al., 1999). What are the practices that are valued by individuals in the group? They reflect the values held by the groups encountered.

VALUES THAT SHAPE NURSING AND AMERICAN CULTURE

Nursing as a discipline reflects the generalized values of society, which in the United States is predominantly Eurocentric, middle class, Christian, and androcentric in view. Over time,

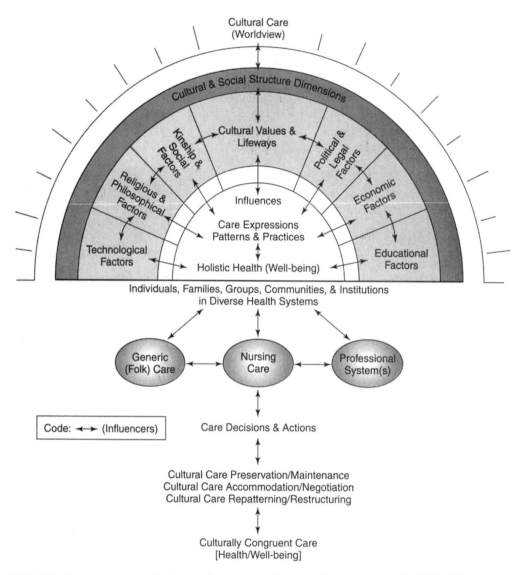

FIGURE 14-1 Leininger's model of transcultural nursing. (Redrawn from Leininger, M. (1991). *Culture care diversity and universality: A theory of nursing.* New York: National League for Nursing.)

American culture has generated social expectations that tend to minimize recognition of differences in both opportunity and experience. The American culture values personal freedom, independence, and individual achievement over the common good. The notion that everyone should be treated exactly the same is idealized. These themes fit well with the American values of action, productivity, materialism and consumerism, competition, and time as money

(DeVita & Armstrong, 1993). In combination, these predilections lead to routinizing health care for efficiency, resulting in a "one size fits all" model of treatment and care. Americans typically assume that problems can be fixed and should (and can) be done so economically and quickly.

Presumptions inherent in the American culture typically flow from this set of values. For example, it is presumed that each individual should be in control of his or her own destiny. Another presumption is that one's efforts should be rewarded, and if they are not rewarded, the efforts must not have been good enough. A further presumption is that people have the right and ability to control nature as much as possible (in contrast to living in harmony with it or being controlled by it in a fatalistic manner). Progress is defined in terms of technology and the future. Regarding health care, the presumption is that health care providers know more about clients' needs than clients do, although we are learning to listen to clients' desires and goals, and to recognize their beliefs, practices, and worldviews as resources. Because these ideals drive American society, they strongly influence its medical and health care systems. Yet values are merely abstract preferences, beliefs, and ideals that are inherently neither good nor bad. However, they should not be left unexamined or taken for granted because they strongly influence everyday life.

CRITICAL EXAMINATION OF VALUES

With nursing education comes an often unarticulated set of values and norms that must be made explicit and examined if nurses are to become informed and competent managers of diversity. Values require serious critique, not only because they strongly and subtly influence how society operates, but also because they empower better decisions about what aspects of society to accept, reject, ignore, or work to change. Some choices are in order. Nurses work in situations in which relatively firm and historically successful (at least from some points of view) sets of values are reflected throughout health care and in nursing. However, both humanity and the interactive rules are changing, and some of the values that predominate in society today do not fit well with the high-quality care that nurses strive to provide.

Much of the public is willing to accept the rules and directives of health care providers. They may complain about facilities and health plans, but overall, the medicalization of American society reflects a commitment to and investment in a nearly singular model of medical care. Even when consumers are told that they have rights and are expected to be involved in decision making about their own treatment and care (goals that are influenced by the values of individualism and independence), professional providers often continue to control the situation. However, today's consumer population is far more demographically and attitudinally diverse than it was in the past. Health care and nursing, reflecting society at large, are pressed to accommodate diverse values and beliefs. At present, health care is an aggregate of institutions built on a value system too inflexible to reflect its consumers' diverse needs.

VALUES THAT SHAPE WORLDVIEWS IN GENERAL

Despite the vast variability found among humans and within and between groups, we are all more alike than we are different. Every group and every individual must manage the same basic requirements of living to survive and to thrive. It is often helpful to visualize the basic, universal categories of values on a continuum. Ask yourself where you would place yourself along the continua of cultural values (Fig. 14–2) and how others' worldviews might differ from yours. Categories of values include orientations toward nature (including the supernatural), time, activity, relationships with other people, and the nature of humankind. Because

ORIENTATIONS TOWARD PERSON/NATURE RELATIONSHIPS

External forces   Living in   Mastery
control life _____   harmony _____   over
(fate)   with nature   nature

PREDOMINANT ORIENTATIONS TOWARD TIME

Past _____   Present _____   Future
                                   and immediate
                                   issues and concerns

PREDOMINANT ORIENTATIONS TOWARD ACTIVITY

Being   Individuals   Efforts to
is _____   must develop _____ develop will
enough   themselves   be rewarded

PREDOMINANT ORIENTATIONS TOWARD SOCIAL RELATIONS

There are   Ask others   All have
leaders, _____   how to solve _____ equal
and there are   problems   rights and
followers   control

Dependence   Interdependence   Independence
is okay _____   is valued _____   is best

THE NATURE OF HUMANKIND

People are   People are
basically good _____ basically evil
and can be   and can't be
trusted   trusted

FIGURE 14-2 Continua of cultural values. Ask yourself, "Where is ____ on each continuum?"

worldviews and value orientations are often taken for granted, they may be difficult to discern. The more you get to know yourself, your colleagues, and your clients, the more effective you will be at accurately recognizing your own and others' perspectives and their influence on relationships.

Health care professionals are increasingly aware of a need to consider their clients' views of the world. However, they may not be aware of the ways in which values influence the discipline of nursing, the expectations that common nursing practices communicate to others, or the influence of values in the formation of goals and priorities. The following example illustrates how values can influence clinical practice.

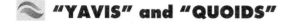 "YAVIS" and "QUOIDS"

Research going back to the 1960s indicates that even when the intent is to treat people fairly, implicit values may result in quite different outcomes. Members of some groups receive better care than others. Some people get less positive attention, have fewer choices and more pressure to conform to others' standards, or receive less vigorous treatment. Clients who exemplify the predominant values (reflected in the acronym YAVIS) often get more and quicker attention and better treatment than those clients characterized by the acronym QUOIDS (Kavanagh & Kennedy, 1992). The YAVIS are Young, Attractive, Verbal, Intelligent, and Successful (or at least potentially or apparently successful)—all traits that are highly valued in European-American culture. In contrast, QUOIDS might be Quiet, Ugly, Old, Indigent (poor), Dissimilar (in lifestyle, language, or worldview), or suspected of being Stupid. None of these characteristics bodes well in a youth-oriented, affluent, highly educated, technologically dependent, industrialized, and information-oriented society. Although someone carefully observing interactions in health care settings might quickly discern preferential patterns involving YAVIS and QUOIDS characteristics, those who work there are often oblivious to the biases that result when strong cultural values are not critically examined.

NURSING'S CHALLENGE

Decades ago, nursing moved beyond an emphasis on physical care into consideration of psychological factors. This shift provided a more comprehensive picture of the complex social realities experienced by people but still limited the focus of attention to individuals. Meanwhile, the presumption that one type of care fits everyone's needs, linked with a conviction that professionals' views are more valuable than clients' views, ignored the multifaceted contexts of ac-

tual experience. Despite empathy for its client populations, nursing's progress toward diversity management has focused on increasing tolerance rather than on appreciation and utilization of diversity. With the emphasis of much nursing care on technology, there is little evidence that nurses are thinking and practicing with real diversity-focused sensitivity, knowledge, or skill.

Contemporary American society is a composite of disparate populations. Nursing is in the position of providing care to diverse groups with diverse expectations, problems, and goals. Quite often, nursing's clients are people who are generally underserved. Today's nurses attend to both population-based and individual patterns and needs. In so doing, many realize that respectful encounter with topics such as race, ethnicity, religion, politics, and belief systems outside of biomedicine is essential to providing acceptable and effective care. Yet many nurses still practice with inherent belief that clients who disagree with them are simply wrong. Others acknowledge the diversity they encounter but are overwhelmed by its complexity. Yet being blind to the impact that diverse aspects of life have on actual experience creates obstacles to effective health care. On the other hand, integrating them into nursing care can result in high-quality and acceptable care that is rewarding to clients and nurses alike.

Even as nurses embrace both individuals and populations and engage in more sincerely holistic and negotiated models of care that include intuitive, subjective aspects of clients' realities (Kenney, 1995), those transformations occur more slowly than changes in society. However, the major concern is not catching up with increasing diversification. Rather, it is that nurses become competent and confident managers of diversity.

Relatively few nurses are prepared in nursing school to manage diversity effectively. The risk is that stereotypes, which by definition are incomplete and inflexible, may be reinforced. Another barrier to confronting diversity in nursing practice is the failure to critically examine the distribution of power. The discipline of nursing is remarkably ambivalent in its response to hierarchy. Nursing and nurses must scrutinize their attitudes toward strategies that promote true collaboration and participation in education, research, and practice. Sooner or later, nurses must learn to manage diversity humanely and effectively. The alternative is to be forced to change on others' terms.

Whether nursing acts or reacts, the trends are clear. U.S. society continues to diversify rapidly while the world becomes symbolically smaller. Increasingly, it is acknowledged that members of diverse groups have the right to their own lifestyles, values, and norms, including expectations for culture-specific care. In nursing, the ability to communicate and work interculturally and to understand culture-based care and caring practices is viewed as essential to providing high-quality, effective, and acceptable illness-alleviating and/or health-promoting care (Leininger, 1985, 1991).

CASE STUDY

Most nurses realize that stereotyping is risky. No one matches exactly those generalized descriptions of ethnic, racial, religious, gender, or other groups that we see on television or read about. On the other hand, many people are not aware of the extent of diversity *within* groups, and even within families. A recent example encountered in a Navajo health facility illustrates this. The Navajo traditionally try to avoid all discussion and involvement with death and dying. There is a fear that talking about dying may make it happen, and that being around someone who is dying may be unhealthy for those who are not. Consider this scenario. A woman in her 40s is dying of metastatic cancer. Her elderly mother, a very traditional woman who speaks only Navajo, is torn between wanting to be with her daughter in the hospital and wanting to avoid being near the dying woman. She sobs quietly just inside the room, but seems unable to approach the bed. The patient's father will not enter the hospital due to the many deaths that have occurred there over the years. It

seems there is little that the non-Navajo-speaking nurses can do, other than to be with the grieving parent and to replace the harsh paper towels she is using to blot her tears with softer tissues. These are significant interventions, but seem hardly adequate to the occasion. During his mother's final hours, the patient's son (who is in his 20s) arrives with his two small children. Unlike his grandmother, he is comfortable being with his mother, holding her hand and speaking to her, despite the lack of response he gets from her. The nurses, none of whom are or speak Navajo, are delighted to see the young man. They will assume that he will know how to comfort his obviously distraught grandmother. However, although he grew up within sight of his grandparents' home, the young man does not speak Navajo and his grandmother does not speak English. The dying woman represents the transitional generation who speaks both languages and lives—and dies—with one foot in each of the very different cultures.

PROTECTING AGAINST BIAS

There are more than 3,000 cultural groups, each of which interprets the world, including health and illness, somewhat differently. Combined with innumerable individual interpretations and experiences, it is obvious that no one can know everything about diversity. There are no reliable "how-to" manuals for nursing in a diverse society. It takes flexibility, willingness to learn, and ability to explore and understand multiple perspectives for nurses to provide acceptable care across significant cultural differences. To manage diversity well, nurses must be sensitive to both differences and commonalities, knowledgeable about expectable patterns of belief and behavior, and skillful at integrating their sensitivity and knowledge into appropriate assessment, communication, and intervention modalities. However, information about expectable patterns of behavior and their interpretation must always be tested against an individual's perception of a specific situation.

It is natural to have biases, to prefer some

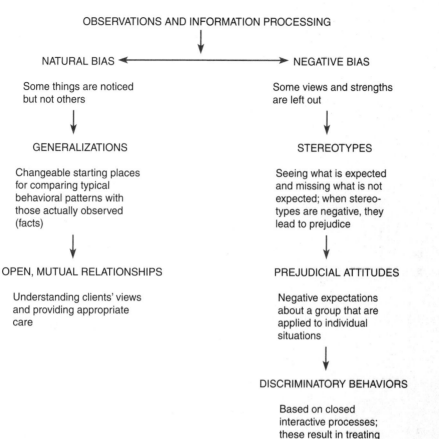

OBSERVATIONS AND INFORMATION PROCESSING

NATURAL BIAS ←————————————————→ NEGATIVE BIAS

Some things are noticed
but not others

Some views and strengths
are left out

GENERALIZATIONS

Changeable starting places
for comparing typical
behavioral patterns with
those actually observed
(facts)

STEREOTYPES

Seeing what is expected
and missing what is not
expected; when stereo-
types are negative, they
lead to prejudice

OPEN, MUTUAL RELATIONSHIPS

Understanding clients' views
and providing appropriate
care

PREJUDICIAL ATTITUDES

Negative expectations
about a group that are
applied to individual
situations

DISCRIMINATORY BEHAVIORS

Based on closed
interactive processes;
these result in treating
people unequally

FIGURE 14–3 Open versus closed information processing.

ideas, things, or behaviors and to find others less appealing. It is important to identify our biases, or they can distort the interpretation of the world around us. Objectivity does not imply a lack of bias; rather, it is the ability to avoid distortion of facts by personal or other preferences. Natural biases become negative when they are allowed to misrepresent and distort facts. People tend to see what they expect to see, and stereotypes hamper interpretation by supplying built-in blind spots. Communication ideally facilitates open, nonprejudicial relationships that can maximize understanding of clients' views and resources. A flowchart illustrating the outcomes of open and closed information processing is presented in Figure 14–3.

SOCIETY AND RESOURCES

American society does not always manage diversity well. Many people shy away from issues involving race, sex, or other aspects of life that, although important in everyday life, may be considered too personally or politically sensitive to discuss or even acknowledge. Despite the United States' image as a land of opportunity where effort is correlated with accomplishment and many people "get ahead" (although not always equitably so), American society is stratified. Resources are distributed through patterned social processes involving numerous interrelated factors. Among others, these factors include sex, education, income, occupation, religion, material possessions, health status, appearance, race, ethnicity, family name, residence, family composition, and landedness. The extent of influence of a given factor differs with time and circumstance. Despite civil rights to protect against discrimination, different opportunities are likely to be experienced by certain individuals and groups. Some examples are a single-parent versus a two-parent family, a wheelchair-bound worker versus his or her able-bodied peer, and a taxpayer who rents a home versus another who lives with a mortgage but, by "owning" property, qualifies for a more favorable tax return.

Social categories exist because some social criteria are weighted as more valuable than others. Classifying social worth is so much a part of everyday social life that it is often taken for granted. However, the outcome of social stratification is social inequality, which implies unequal life chances and opportunities. The long-term result of unexamined social processes may be unequal opportunity to achieve the basic resources of status, power, and wealth. In contrast to a middle-class individual with adequate health insurance, for example, an economically disadvantaged or socially disenfranchised person may not receive attention for a health problem until it seriously impedes his or her ability to function productively in society.

In the United States, the only industrialized country except South Africa without a national health care system, there is limited societal pressure to provide equitable care for all. Significant variation in mortality and morbidity rates is one outcome of unequal distribution of health care. American infant mortality rates are higher than those of most other industrialized countries and are particularly high among poor and nonwhite groups. Similarly, rates of premature deaths among nonwhite males below age 65 greatly exceed mortality rates for white males. These

statistics exemplify the costs of limited access to health care for large underserved populations.

THE "-ISMS"

Several interaction patterns that are grounded in bias, prejudicial in attitude, and discriminatory in their behavioral expression have acquired the label "-ism" because of their common word endings. Each -ism involves a tendency to judge others according to their match or lack of fit with a standard that is considered ideal or presumed to be "normal." Whatever the issue or level (personal or group), an -ism is centered on one's own judgment (Brislin, 1993). The three most powerful -isms in America are racism, sexism, and classism.

Racism and Ethnic Diversity. When America was originally envisioned as a cultural "melting pot," nearly all of its immigrants came from northern Europe, and most had Protestant origins. When members of culturally and racially different groups began to arrive in sizable numbers, the merged population experienced some painful, unassimilated lumps. The melting pot idea worked well only for those groups that would and could assume the values of the predominant population.

People did not blend in if they resisted giving up cultural values and traditions (i.e., they chose to keep their ethnic identities) or if they were physically "different." Race in American society has perpetuated a system of stratification based on skin color, hair texture, and other biological differences presumed to be significant. Many ethnic groups moved, with time, toward acculturation and assimilation. A few, such as the Amish and Hutterites, steadfastly maintained their specific cultures. People of color, however, experienced systematic barriers to "melting in," even if motivated to do so.

Advances in the physical and social sciences long ago redefined race as a social rather than a biological phenomenon, which left racist themes of inherent superiority and inferiority untenable. If the earth's more than 5.5 billion inhabitants were somehow mustered into a single line, starting with the darkest-skinned individual on one end and ending with the lightest-skinned individual on the other, that vast multitude could not be reliably sorted into races. Some are light and some are dark, but the great majority are some shade of brown. Skin color does not occur in discrete categories and cannot be used to predict ability.

Although ethnicity is a more viable tool than race for examining similarities and differences, the United States remains a society in which one's race influences everyday social experience. Race is one of the major issues to be dealt with if nurses are to manage diversity effectively. As with other -isms, failure to address the issue leaves important dimensions of health and health care unrecognized and potential resources unused.

Sexism and Gender Diversity. Sexism is one of the most obvious -isms, and one directly pertinent to nurses, whether male or female. As with other -isms, problems involving sexism cannot be completely resolved within the context of the health care system alone, for they reflect processes that permeate all of society. However, it is important to be aware of gender differences in opportunities to acquire status, power, and wealth. Similarly, it is important to be aware of the influence of those differences on health, access to health care, and adequacy of care, as well as on opportunities for professional career development in nursing.

In the United States, women earn significantly less money than men do for the same work and with the same level of preparation for that work. Single parents are typically women, a fact that reflects differences in gender-based rights and responsibilities, and their presence on the welfare rolls has greatly expanded. As more women assume roles as heads of households, bias toward the worth of women and their work is increasingly becoming apparent in under-valued, largely female occupations, such as nursing.

The manipulation of women's roles in society has not left men unaffected. As industrialization moved the locus of economic earning away from homes and farms and into factories and offices, men were removed from traditional familial involvement. While women, like children, were viewed as needing control and protection, Western men were deprived of equitable companionship and forced to assume stereotypically paternalistic roles. Characteristically stressed by expectations of achievement in the marketplace and estranged from emotional involvement at home, male roles only now are returning comfortably to the family. Society remains a long way from androgynous interchangeability of roles, however, as is illustrated by the relatively small proportion of men in nursing, although nurses comprise an otherwise educationally, ethnically, and experientially heterogeneous group. It should be kept in mind that sexism and gender issues are not limited to heterosexual populations. Advocacy of gay and lesbian providers and clients also requires sensitivity to, and knowledge of, social processes that are often overlooked by those unaware of their impact.

Classism. Class is defined as the ability to muster economic resources. It does not imply specific preferences, behaviors, or lifeways. Elitist attitudes often lead to assumptions that certain people are superior or inferior because of their social or economic status. The client who is poorly dressed, uses poor grammar, or otherwise "looks low class" may not be given the same treatment options offered to others whose appearance or behavior gives the impression of greater fiscal assets.

Class is related to health and health care in several ways. Universally, the greatest threat to positive health status is poverty. In the United States, although specific ethnic and racial groups are often stereotyped as having more or fewer health problems, it is really differences in socioeconomic status that are directly associated with health status (Fiscella et al., 2000). Race and ethnicity became confounded with class because of long-term inequality in the distribution of educational and occupational opportunities. Today there are significant class differences within racial and ethnic categories, and there is definite ethnic and racial variation within each socioeconomic class. The important points are to avoid stereotypic associations across categories and to recognize the impact that poverty has on access to, and eligibility for, care, priorities and coping patterns, relationships with health care providers, and overall health status. For example, people who live "hand to mouth" must be oriented toward present concerns and may not prioritize health practices that tend to pay off only in the future, such as immunizations, dietary restrictions, or even disease prevention strategies, such as those associated with reducing risk for HIV infection.

THE COSTS OF INEQUALITY

The desire to avoid confronting difficult issues often results in "colorblindness," "genderblindness," and similar phenomena. By pretending that everything is the same for everyone, societal patterns of differential treatment based on race or gender go unrecognized and are perpetuated. They are nonproductive because they deny variations in life experience that are both real and meaningful. It is painful to not have important characteristics recognized and acknowledged.

Overlooking or ignoring differences implies that specific experiences of individuals and groups are not important and that change is not necessary. Since many aspects of racism, sexism, and other systems of unequal opportunity (all those other -isms) are institutionalized in the social system, failure to recognize and change them both perpetuates and condones them. Effective and acceptable health care involves critical thinking and problem solving on all levels. Understanding social processes that underlie the perpetuation of social inequality empowers change by providers as well as consumers of health care.

AN EVER-CHANGING, DIVERSIFYING SOCIETY

The challenge of providing appropriate care becomes more manageable as we learn more about it, and more demanding as society continues to change. According to Census Bureau projections, before the middle of the 21st century the average U.S. resident will neither trace his or her heritage to Europe nor be what is commonly referred to as white. However, societal and cultural change does not occur readily or easily. It is predicted that the nation's crisis of values and ethics will deepen and racial and cultural tension will mount in response to pressures of intensified diversity. Creating and maintaining a sense of community is ever challenging. Although some people find these projections threatening and others find them hopeful, nursing at times seems to be stuck between fight and flight in dealing with such change.

Every nurse has encountered clients who seemed steadfastly resistant to every professional ministration. Some health care providers, out of a belief that they know what is best for clients, label a client's failure to respond as "noncompliance." This biased label deserves a closer look. In the beginning of this century, pressure to move toward the dominant value system was the norm; indeed, it was how one became "Americanized." Authority was granted to those in charge to control the attitudes and behaviors, as much as possible, of those who chose or were forced to use the institution's services. Other perspectives, including the client's, were marginalized, trivialized, or even overtly discredited. Times have changed. As the century closes, it is no longer acceptable to demand conformity to a single set of values and norms. Great social variation persists despite a homogenized culture that permeates nearly every household with standardized versions of fast foods, media event analysis, and consumer expectations. There is no longer a clear distinction between members of a provider group who set the goals and rules, and clients who must deny their own preferences to comply with the controlling group's expectations. As a society, we are moving toward a truer participatory democracy. In client care, democratic participation goes beyond a patient's bill of rights posted on the wall and soon forgotten.

WAYS OF UNDERSTANDING: EXPLANATORY MODELS

Since health, illness, and death are part of life, all people have conscious health-related needs. Knowledge about health and health care is not limited to professionals or professional ways of knowing. Every cultural group has at least one system of beliefs, diagnoses, treatments, and care to maximize control over distressing and life-threatening phenomena. How illness is defined, ideas about what caused it, and what is to be done about symptoms (when and by whom) are important concerns in every cultural system.

Explanatory models are the sets of explanations used to put ideas about the meaning, cause, process, and treatment of illness into familiar, workable frameworks. These models are used to understand health, health care, and illness within the context of complex cultural phenomena, including religion, economic situation, education, language, family and social organization, interaction patterns, ethnic orientation, and general perceptions of the world and self.

Biomedicine tends to view health problems as the consequence of trouble within the client or as resulting from interaction between the client and the natural world with its pathogens, environmental risks, and stressors. Members of social and cultural groups that do not use science as the basic explanation for everything often base their explanatory models within society (e.g., illness resulting from disharmonious social relations) or in supernatural belief systems (e.g.,

viewing disease as a punishment for sin or breaking a taboo).

Westernized definitions of health and illness are vague. There are numerous definitions of health, whereas illness is the culturally influenced individual experience of sickness. Biomedical science, in contrast, defines disease in objective terms of deviance from clinical norms or as the result of environmental insult. Mental health and mental illnesses are more difficult to delineate than physical status because of a lack of readily observable, discrete, and organic evidence. The result is reliance on assessment of behaviors rather than on definitive symptoms. Diagnoses involve the extent of social competence, which, to be valid, must be assessed against culture-specific criteria.

To members of many societies, concepts such as mental health have little or no meaning. One is either ill or not, and that distinction is based on somatic criteria that either allow or impede the ability to perform one's normal roles in society. A diagnosis and prognosis based on unobservable phenomena (as opposed to that obtained from laboratory or diagnostic tests) may seem absurd, and only impaired function motivates health care attention. Despite the predominance of biomedicine in the United States, popular (over-the-counter) and folk systems also proliferate and are widely used. Popular systems of health-related knowledge and resources are available through drug and health stores, in all forms of the media, and through information passed among personal acquaintances and networks. Folk or ethnomedical systems of beliefs and practices originate in traditional cultures and include healing rituals, herbal medicines, and systems of knowledge that reflect diverse cultural values and social norms. Within American society, professional biomedical systems, popular medicine (over-the-counter and nonprescription alternatives), and a variety of folk medical systems provide more varied services to consumers than many nurses imagine. Often more than one system is used at a time. Nurses can have powerful intermediary roles in negotiating the varied options.

INDIVIDUAL VERSUS GROUP IDENTITY

One assumption often taken for granted in nursing is that nurses care for individuals. It is important to realize that members of many societies do not perceive themselves first as individuals but as members of groups (typically, extended families). As an Asian nursing student explained it, she (an individual in Western eyes) is in her view a "small i"; her family is the "large I." Decisions are made by groups or by heads of groups for the good of the group. Individuals are first part of the whole family, and only secondly are they autonomous and separate persons. Therefore, although care may be appropriately individualized for each client, nurses must become more comfortable with perceiving clients in collective terms. Orientation to common units that are more than aggregates of individuals is traditional in some cultures.

It is similarly risky to assume that love is the idealized primary emotion in a relationship. Many cultural groups place far more value on respect and honor. Nor should nurses assume that biological relationships or formal ties such as marriage are the most significant ones. The individual who culturally is expected to make decisions is often a dominant male, regardless of who in the group is considered the focus of care or treatment. For example, community health nurses who try to encourage mothers to have their children immunized may have little impact unless the heads of households or community leaders are convinced of the value of inoculations.

CARE BARRIERS AND RESOURCES

There are numerous cultural and social phenomena that pose potential barriers in health care but also can serve as potential resources. Language, both verbal and nonverbal, is an obvious obstacle to, as well as a vehicle for, communication. Strong identities, such as with racial, ethnic, or gender groups, are reflected in attitudes, expectations, and practices related to health and care. Likewise, differences in ideas about relationships may encourage or discourage resource utilization (e.g., expectations of hierarchy or mutuality, independence or dependence, others who are perceived as different). Expectations of self-care or personal involvement in decision making may be perceived as an inappropriate imposition in some cultures. Many people view health professionals as experts who are expected to provide advice and direction. Furthermore, cultural expectations may be that illness results in a sick role that is characterized by dependence on others. For example, Rivera-Andino and Lopez (2000) describe how some Hispanic families believe it is their responsibility to shield family members from bad news or a poor prognosis.

CASE STUDY

Joy, a community health nurse (CHN), prepares to visit an elderly Native American woman who is characterized as "noncompliant" with her dialysis treatment and who consumes alcohol, and an elderly man who had been hospitalized with bronchitis. Joy has numerous other clients who could use home visits, but in the rural area in which they live, homes are difficult to locate and are miles apart, roads are often treacherous, and few people have phones for verifying availability. Each attempted visit involves the time of a translator as well as the CHN. Joy and the translator arrive at the home of the elderly woman. Mrs. Young was away having a healing ceremony. Joy interpreted this as a good sign; perhaps Mrs. Bird will return to dialysis after the ceremony. "What else can I do?" she said. "I can't leave her a note; she does not read English." She and the translator move on to the small home of the elderly man. They ask whether he is taking his medicine, and he shows them several bottles of pills, still full. They ask whether he has eaten breakfast. He describes bacon and eggs. But the unwashed dishes in the sink lack evidence, and the wood stove that serves both to heat the tiny dwelling and for cooking is not warm. "One order of Meals on Wheels coming up," quips Joy, "at least when they can get back there. But the pills? He knows I want him to take them. He says he has them for when he needs them. I will try to visit him more often and have others check on him, but I must respect his choices."

PROVIDING ACCEPTABLE AND CONGRUENT CARE

Given the diversity within society, its patterns of social interaction, and sundry cultural understandings of health and illness, it is not surprising that there is great variation in expectations for appropriate treatment and care. Overly simplified explanations of culture and health care can cause more problems than they solve. Nursing, like other health care disciplines, is learning to manage this diversity, which requires some substantive changes in care delivery systems.

To enhance health care, diversity must be understood in terms of the plasticity and flexibility of culture. This means avoiding stereotypes about people, being open to their many ways of understanding and adapting to the world, and allowing for a multidirectional flow of ideas. As barriers between health care professions are broken down, ideas also can flow creatively across disciplinary boundaries. Barriers between clients and care providers must also be broken down so that the sensitivity, knowledge, resources, and skills that both have can be incorporated into client care. In this multicultural view, boundaries are artificial and social identities are continuously renegotiated. Where cultures come together, there is creative ground (Kessler-Harris, 1992; Wali, 1992). Providers and clients can learn about and from each other and can negotiate appropriate goals, care strategies, and outcomes. The essential element is that respect be maintained by all involved so that mutual communication can be open to multiple perceptions.

NURSING'S UNIQUE POSITION

Nurses function as gatekeepers between clients and the health care system, and at times between clients' cultural backgrounds and American culture as it is reflected in health care. Nurses must therefore become comfortable with care meanings, patterns, and processes that allow flexibility in practice. Nursing has a unique opportunity to help other health care disciplines to negotiate their way in an ever-changing environment without a loss of collective identity and with a sense of the diversity that is inherently American. It takes a sense of the whole to appreciate the individual. Nursing's value of holism encourages awareness that each individual is like some others, like all others, and like no others. To be acceptable and appropriate, that individual's health care must follow the same pattern.

CULTURALLY CONGRUENT CARE

Care is the central, dominant, and unifying feature of nursing (Leininger, 1991). Providing care that is comprehensive must take into account culture-based factors related to systems of values and norms, technology, religion and philosophy, kinship and social relations, politics and law, economy, and education (Leininger, 1991). Language and environmental contexts are threads throughout those systems and further influence care patterns and expressions of individuals, families, groups, and societies. Nurses providing culturally congruent and culture-specific nursing care can intervene by preserving, accommodating, or repatterning (Leininger, 1988).

There are many strengths associated with traditional and popular (i.e., nonprofessional) systems of knowledge, care, and treatment. They are familiar and understandable to the client. Moreover, they are usually readily accessible, inexpensive, and noninvasive. Many clients find traditional healing systems more humanistic than scientific medicine and more sensitive to, and compatible with, their quality of life. Many health practices are harmless, some are useless, and others are harmful. Providing culturally congruent care involves being open to exploring the client's beliefs and practices, recognizing and reinforcing those that are positive and promoting change only in those that are known to be harmful. Cultural care preservation serves to maintain a state of health, aid recovery from illness, or assist with the dying process through reinforcement of traditional cultural values and lifeways that provide familiar, available, and nonthreatening resources.

Cultural care accommodation involves negotiation between professional and folk, biomedical, or nonscientific healing approaches. Rather than assuming that professional ways are better, interventions that are acceptable and relevant to clients can be negotiated using both the prescribed treatments of the biomedical system and the views and practices of the client's personal reference group. It is in this realm that most culturally acceptable nursing care takes place. For example, the nurse who wants to teach a special diet to a client can effectively do so by negotiating that diet within the client's normal framework of food practices, resources, and preferences.

Many cultural groups believe that all of life should be balanced: hot foods balanced with cold, hot illnesses treated with cold remedies, and so forth. This "hot-cold" theory does not relate to temperature but to meanings that are culturally ascribed to things and events. Dietary and treatment regimens can be "balanced" to fit the client's expectations as well as the professional's. The only requirement is that the nurse inquire about the client's beliefs and practices, treat the information with respect, and take the time to negotiate mutually acceptable plans and goals.

Cultural care restructuring or repatterning is the category in which most nursing care traditionally occurs. As change agents, nurses often act as culture-bearers, frequently discrediting alternative ways of doing things without understanding them. Occasionally it is essential to re-pattern behavior, as in cases of abuse or neglect. However, clients are generally more likely to value and follow nursing care that fits their ways of thinking.

COMMUNICATION

Communication is the core of much of nursing care. Clients always have a relationship with the problem as they see it, which may or may not be similar to professional assessment of the situation. Effective intervention requires the ability to understand the problem from both the insider's (client's) and the outsider's (nurse's) point of view (Kavanagh et al., 1999). One must learn what the client views as the problem, whom the client sees as being responsible for the problem, what the problem means to the client, and who the client thinks has control over the problem. It should be kept in mind that the influence of the nurse is less than the influence of the problem, unless the nurse's influence can be combined with that of the client to form a coalition. It is when the client and provider work together that they can problem solve.

As nurses move away from dependency on Eurocentric assumptions and references and become more sensitive to other ways of viewing the world, they become more comfortable learning about other explanatory models. Understanding various ways of thinking is important. Clients' beliefs about what causes problems are often directly related to what they view as solutions. A client who believes his illness resulted from a failure to pray or to go to church, for example, is likely to have little faith in medication as the resolution. Nurses interact well with clients and potential clients, so they are in an ideal position to explore over-the-counter and folk remedies that people use. When nurses work with a specific cultural group, it is useful to learn as much as possible about the folk illnesses and folk practices common to that group. While there is a large body of medical anthropological literature on such topics, the easiest way to access the information is to respectfully ask people about their beliefs and practices. When a sincere interest and nonjudgmental attitude accompany such questions, clients often openly share their perspectives. Recommended approaches for culturally appropriate care are presented in Box 14–1.

CULTURAL ASSESSMENT STRATEGIES

Cultural assessment in nursing involves systematic appraisal of values, beliefs, and practices to learn the context of client needs and to deter-

mine appropriate nursing interventions (Tripp-Reimer & Afifi, 1989). Such assessments are useful to identify general lifestyles and patterns that assist or interfere with nursing intervention or treatment regimens. There are several available assessment guides, as well as guides for interviewing. Categories for a basic cultural assessment are presented in Box 14–2.

All comprehensive assessment plans attend to value orientations, personal and family health histories, and social and cultural backgrounds. One cannot assume what beliefs, practices, or supports do or do not exist. Expected patterns must always be contrasted with actual, individ-

---

Box 14–1 Approaches Recommended for All Cultural Groups

- Provide a feeling of acceptance.
- Establish open communication.
- Present yourself with confidence. Introduce yourself. Shake hands if it is appropriate.
- Strive to gain your client's trust, but don't resent it if you don't get it.
- Understand what members of the cultural or subcultural group consider to be "caring," both attitudinally and behaviorally.
- Understand the relationship between your client and authority.
- Understand your client's desire to please you and his or her motivations to comply or not to comply.
- Anticipate diversity. Avoid stereotypes by sex, age, ethnicity, socioeconomic status, etc.
- Don't make assumptions about where people come from. Let them tell you.
- Understand the client's goals and expectations.
- Make your goals realistic.
- Emphasize positive points and strengths of health beliefs and practices.
- Show respect, especially for men, even if it is women or children you are interested in. Men are often decision makers about follow-up.
- Be prepared for the fact that children go everywhere with some cultural groups, as well as with poorer families, who may have few options. Include them.
- Know the traditional, health-related practices common to the group you are working with. Don't discredit them unless you *know* they are harmful.
- Know the folk illnesses and remedies common to the group you are working with.
- Try to make the clinic setting comfortable. Consider colors, music, atmosphere, scheduling expectations, pace, tone, seating arrangements, and so on.
- Whenever possible and appropriate, involve the leaders of the local group. Confidentiality is important, but the leaders know the problems and often can suggest acceptable interventions.
- Respect values, beliefs, rights, and practices. Some may conflict with your own or with your determination to make changes. But every group and individual wants respect above all else.
- Learn to appreciate the richness of diversity as an asset, rather than a hindrance, in your work.

Box 14-2 Categories for a Basic Cultural Assessment

* Ethnic origin, identity, affiliation, and values (ideas about health and illness, human nature, relation-ships between humankind and nature, time, activity, and interpersonal relationships); also relevant rites of passage, customs, art and symbols, and history
* Racial identity (ask, do not assume.)
* Place of birth; relocation and migration history
* Habits, customs, and beliefs associated with health, disease, illness, health maintenance, illness pre-vention, and health promotion; explanatory models; connections between health and religion
* Cultural sanctions and restrictions (what behaviors are encouraged or discouraged)
* Language and communication processes (verbal and nonverbal patterns; eye contact; touching; use of, and toleration for, silence; tempo; styles of questioning and persuasion; styles of decision making)
* Gender rules
* Healing beliefs and practices (relationships with folk, popular, and professional health systems; sym-bolism related to health and illness; what behaviors are considered normal or abnormal; care associ-ated with unusual or abnormal behavior; care associated with body fluids, body excretions, and body temperature; activities included in tending to one's body; substances and practices used in rituals; myths about health and taboos [substances and events to be avoided]; ideas and practices related to death, dying, and grief)
* Nutritional factors; food preferences, preparation, and consumption patterns (kinds of foods and amounts, schedules and rituals, eating environments, utensils and implements, taboos, changes with illness)
* Sleep routines, bedtime rituals, and environment (kinds of covering, sleepwear, comforting materials used, rules for sleeping and for awakening)
* Environmental resources and strains (the "fit" within the community)
* Economic status, resources, and living situation
* Educational history and background
* Occupational history and background
* Social network (types and amount of support available from family, other individuals and group resources; who and where kin and significant others are; what is expected and expectable of them; social interaction patterns)
* Self-identity/concept and sense of well-being
* Religious history, background, and beliefs
* Other spiritual beliefs and practices
* Usual response to stress and discomfort
* Meaning of care and caring (expectations, beliefs, and practices related to care; fit between nurse as provider and client as cultural seeker of health care, and between client and health system)

ual situations. It is often useful to explore local groups for information about an ethnic popula-tion in the area, and to solicit the assistance of the group leaders for problem solving and in-formation about acceptable interventions when it does not involve disclosure of individual cli-ents' circumstances.

In addition to cultural assessment, with its inclusive sociological and psychological dimen-sions, there must be consideration of biological and physiological norms for different groups. These include racial anatomical characteristics; growth and development patterns; variations in body systems; physiology of skin, hair, and mucous membranes; and diseases and illnesses common to the group.

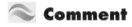

Comment

Diversity is here to stay. Both clients and health care professionals, reflecting the mosaic of society, continue to become more diverse. Failure to recognize diversity can be painful when what people value is not respectfully acknowledged and they are forced to comply with values and norms that are not their own. Every client has a right to culturally congruent care. Nursing is in a unique position to use its assessment, communication, and intervention skills to help delineate care appropriate and acceptable to specific clients. Competent management of diversity empowers all involved to work toward development of full potential.

KEY POINTS

- Cultural and social views of individuals and groups influence perceptions of health and health care.
- Diversity management uses affirmation and encouragement to move toward development of the client's full potential.
- Universal categories of values include orientation toward nature, time, activity, relationships with other people, and the nature of humankind.
- Open information processing can facilitate nurse-client relationships that maximize understanding of clients' views and resources.
- Nurses can protect against bias by recognizing and building on strengths found in diverse perspectives and experiences.
- Society has numerous built-in -isms that result in social inequities.
- The three most powerful -isms in America are racism, sexism, and classism.
- Explanatory models are used to understand health, health care, and illness within the context of complex cultural views and perceptions.

- Culturally congruent care must take into account culture-based factors related to systems of values and norms, technology, religion and philosophy, kinship and social relations, politics and law, economy, and education.
- Cultural assessment in nursing involves systematic appraisal of values, beliefs, and practices of the client.
- Nurses will either learn to manage diversity or be managed by it.

CRITICAL THINKING EXERCISES

1. What benefits are derived from understanding how cultural and lifestyle differences between nurses and clients affect nursing care?

2. Formulate strategies that nurses can use to effectively manage the influences of cultural values and social norms on health, health care, and nursing.

3. How could a nurse develop a balance of sensitivity, knowledge, and skills necessary to manage diversity effectively?

4. Discuss the effect on the client and the nurse when the nurse's perspective dominates the setting of goals and priorities, planning and intervention strategies, and assessment and evaluation criteria.

5. Discuss the effect on the client and the nurse when the client's perspective is used as the basis for setting goals and priorities, planning and intervention strategies, and assessment and evaluation criteria.

6. Describe an example of an -ism that you have observed in your professional experience. What measures were taken to reduce the effects of this bias on the individuals or groups involved? What measures could have been taken that were not?

7. In your experience, what strategies work well for the practice of culturally acceptable nursing assessment, communication, and intervention?

REFERENCES

Brislin, R. (1993). *Understanding culture's influence on behavior.* Fort Worth, TX: Harcourt Brace College.
DeVita, P. R., & Armstrong, J. D. (1993). *Distant mirrors: America as a foreign culture.* Belmont, CA: Wadsworth.

Fiscella, K., Franks, P., Gold, M. R., & Clancy, C.M. (2000). Inequality in quality: Addressing socioeconomic, racial, and ethnic disparities in health care. *Journal of the American Medical Association, 283,* 2579–2584.

Jackson, E. M. (1993). Whiting-out difference: Why U.S. nursing research fails black families. *Medical Anthropology Quarterly, 7,* 363–385.

Kavanagh, K. H., Absalom, K., Beil, W., & Schliessmann, L. (1999). Connecting and becoming culturally competent: A Lakota example. *Advances in Nursing Science, 21*(3), 9–31.

Kavanagh, K. H., & Kennedy, P. H. (1992). *Promoting cultural diversity: Strategies for health care professionals.* Beverly Hills, CA: Sage.

Kenney, J. W. (1995). Relevance of theoretical approaches in nursing practice. In P. J. Christensen & J. W. Kenney (Eds.), *Nursing process: Applications of conceptual models* (4th ed., pp. 3–23). St. Louis: Mosby.

Kessler-Harris, A. (1992, October 21). Multiculturalism can strengthen, not undermine, a common culture. *Chronicles of Higher Education,* pp. 83–87

Leininger, M. (1984). Transcultural interviewing and health assessment. In P. Pedersen, N. Sartorius, & A. J. Marsella (Eds.), *Mental health services: The cross-cultural context* (pp. 109–133). Beverly Hills, CA: Sage.

Leininger, M. (1985). Transcultural caring: A different way to help people. In P. Pedersen (Ed.), *Handbook of cross-cultural counseling and therapy* (pp. 107–115). Westport, CT: Greenwood Press.

Leininger, M. (1988). Leininger's theory of nursing: Cultural care diversity and universality. *Nursing Science Quarterly, 1,* 152–160.

Leininger, M. M. (1991). The theory of culture care diversity and universality. In M. M. Leininger (Ed.), *Culture care diversity and universality: A theory of nursing* (NLN Publication No. 15–2402, pp. 5–68). New York: National League for Nursing.

Pedersen, P. (Ed.). (1988). The three stages of multicultural development: Awareness, knowledge, and skill. In *A handbook for developing multicultural awareness* (pp. 3–18). Alexandria, VA: American Association for Counseling and Development.

Rivera-Andino, J., & Lopez, L. (2000). When culture complicates. *RN, 63*(7), 47–49.

Thomas, R. R. (1990, March–April). From affirmative action to affirming diversity. *Harvard Business Review,* pp. 107–117.

Tripp-Reimer, T., & Afifi, L.A. (1989). Cross-cultural perspectives on patient teaching. *Nusing Clinics of North America, 24,* 613–619.

Wali, A. (1992). *Multiculturalism: An anthropological perspective.* Report from the Institute for Philosophy and Public Policy (University of Maryland at College Park), *12*(1), 6–8.

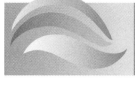

PART III

Themes in Professional Nursing Practice

Concepts common across all areas of professional nursing practice are referred to as themes. Of interest to nurses in a variety of practice settings, these themes serve as unifying threads for nursing practice. For example, regardless of the population being served or the setting, caring is an integral part of nursing. Health promotion and wellness are major thrusts in today's health care, and the effect of the environment on individual and community health is of paramount concern at local and national levels. Teaching is a fundamental nursing responsibility, whether the client is young or old, ill or well. Critical thinking and change challenge today's nurse to be flexible and creative to meet the ever-changing health care environment. Presented as a new chapter in the third edition, the evolving knowledge on the use of complementary and alternative therapies is presented as an introduction to this ever expanding field that has always been part of health care. Nursing research will continue to direct our patient care activities and promote improved treatment and care modalities. Finally, the impact of information technology on the planning and delivery of nursing care is a current theme that will become increasingly important in the future. These themes are discussed in this section.

15

Caring

JANET B. YOUNGER, PhD, NP, RN

OBJECTIVES

At the completion of this chapter, the reader will be able to:

- Understand the essential nature of care.
- Distinguish between human care and professional care.
- Understand care as a context for nursing intervention.
- Understand care as an intervention in itself.

PROFILE IN PRACTICE

Joy Buck, MSN, RN
Assistant Professor of Nursing
Shenandoah University
Winchester, Virginia

Like many nurses, I believe that caring is the heart of nursing. Nurses have been challenged, however, to come to a common definition of what it means to care and be caring. Nurse caring has been defined as a therapeutic process that facilitates mutual growth and health. Definitions of caring are founded on altruistic attitudes and behaviors and invoke thoughts of compassion, communication, continuity, and commitment—values that are common to nurses. Courage, another C word essential to nurse caring, is rarely included or discussed.

Caring is not easy. My early clinical experiences in acute care settings taught me many lessons about courage and caring. As a critical care and trauma nurse, having the courage to care meant advocating on behalf of patients and their families when their wishes were contrary to those of my peers and other care providers. Having the

courage to care meant ensuring the safety of patients and colleagues and challenging medical and nursing care that was substandard. Having the courage to care often meant having compassion and speaking the truth when it needed to be spoken, when no one else would. In my practice, having the courage to care has also meant bearing witness as patients and families experience devastating loss and pain.

My experiences in HIV/AIDS, hospice, and community nursing have provided me with the opportunity to confront my biases, my fears, and myself and to provide compassionate care to those in need regardless of the circumstances. I took care of my first two HIV/AIDS patients in 1983. We knew very little about AIDS then, especially in the rural setting where I practiced. Many health care providers were afraid; some even talked about leaving health care because of the fear. Although I was afraid, there was something about those first two patients that struck a chord within me. Those patients opened my eyes to the fact that although some of the fear of HIV was warranted, much of it was irrational. Those patients allowed me to see that although my fear was great, their fear and pain were greater. To me, caring meant that no one should have to go through what they were going through alone. Those two patients gave me the courage to spend the next 17 years in HIV care as a care provider, advocate, community educator, and prevention counselor.

I have learned many lessons about courage and caring from community-based HIV/AIDS and hospice nursing practice. For me and for many other nurses, the most challenging lesson has been to learn how to maintain the delicate balance between compassionate caring and appropriate separateness. Maintaining this balance in the context of community-based hospice nursing care requires the courage to be self-reflective and honest, and to ask "Whose needs are we really trying to meet, ours or others?" It also requires honesty in terms of personal strengths and limitations, and caring for colleagues and ourselves as we do those in need of nursing care.

Colleagues and students remind me every day of the courage it takes for nurses to care for others and ourselves. Regardless of the type of nursing practice, caring means having the courage to maintain the integrity of a professional nurse. It takes courage to take a leadership role in the ever changing health care system to ensure the health and safety of individuals, communities, and society.

In the past two decades, there has been an escalating interest in the concept of caring (Swanson, 1999). Care is a basic and necessary condition of life. Most animal species care for their young, and without this care the young would not survive. For example, some species of birds keep the same mate and same nest for life. They care for their eggs, they feed and protect their young, and the mates feed each other while nesting. These birds may fly thousands of miles to obtain food and then return to the same nest to care for the mate and the young. Most of this care is not only growth promoting but also is necessary for survival of the species.

In human beings maternal care normally begins before birth with the care a mother takes of herself during pregnancy and the care the father takes to provide for the addition to the family. Soon after birth, parental care takes the form of feeding, clothing, nurturing, socializing, and loving the child. Caring parents engage their infants in a watchful gaze that has been termed *en face* (Ainsworth et al., 1978). This means that the parent's attentiveness is manifested by canting her face in the same plane as the infant's and imitating the infant's expressions. Parental care is a great deal more than satisfying the physical and material needs of the infant. In fact, a startling scientific discovery of the 20th century was that infants in orphanages who had every physical and material need met but who did not have the consistent presence of parental care developed anaclitic depression and failed to thrive. Anaclitic depression is a severe loss of vitality of anaclitic origin, literally meaning "without care" (Spitz, 1946). If the absence of parental care is nearly absolute, even if physical needs are met, most children die. As a child grows, care is the most fundamental ingredient in the secure base provided by families that enables the child to develop. The certain knowledge of care enables exploration, experimenting, venturing out, developing and deploying talents, and developing a high level of self-reliance (Bowlby, 1969, 1979). Also of fundamental importance is that the care a growing person receives is a critical ingredient in that person's later ability to care for others and to form affectional bonds (Bowlby, 1979). Noddings (1984) grounds caring in the universal memory of being cared for. She traces one root of human caring to the longing to maintain, recapture, or enhance our most caring and tender moments. Noddings further claims that caring is the universal basis of morality.

The ability to care is developed throughout life. Erikson's (1982) theory of psychosocial development includes a stage of adult life that he calls generativity versus self-absorption. In this stage, care is the human strength that emerges from the struggle of the stage. Also, the principal mode of expressing generativity involves caring for future generations through family, work, community involvement, and similar pursuits. Erikson defines care as "the broadening concern for what has been generated by love, necessity, or accident—a concern that must consistently overcome the ambivalence adhering to irreversible obligation and the narrowness of self-concern" (p. 10). The stages in Erikson's theory are hierarchically related in a way that requires previous stages to be largely successful in their completion before success is likely at a later stage. This implies that a person who is developmentally capable of generative care would have previously acquired the developmental strengths of trust, autonomy, initiative, industry, identity, and intimacy and have these skills available to use in caring. Thus, care as Erikson describes it is not likely to occur in individuals who are immature in their own development.

It is no accident that health professionals refer to what they do in their practices as care. We as a nation are concerned about the availability of health *care*, We want insurance for dental *care*. and for medical *care*. Hospitals are places where people go to obtain nursing *care*. Other kinds of efforts are not typically referred to as care but as services. We obtain legal services and postal services. But suppose you see two advertisements and assume both to be true. One says they provide car services and the other says they provide car care. What would you assume to be the difference? Of central importance, then, is to understand what distinguishes care from services and professional care from human care.

What Is the Essence of Caring?

EARLIER DEFINITIONS

The word *care* comes from the Old English and Gothic word *kara,* which meant grief, lament, sorrow, or bed of sickness (Gaut, 1983). The *American Heritage Dictionary of the English Language* (third edition) defines care as

> a state of mind; a responsibility; mental suffering; an object of worry, attention, or solicitude; a caution in avoiding harm or danger; close attention; painstaking application; maintenance; watchful oversight; attentive assistance or treatment; to be concerned or interested; to have an attachment; the function of watching or guarding or overseeing; an organization, CARE (Cooperative for American Relief Everywhere); and feeling and exhibiting concern and empathy for others.

Marcel, an early existentialist philosopher, characterized a caring attitude in terms of "disposability, the readiness to bestow and spend oneself and make oneself available, and its contrary, indisposability." Those who are disposable recognize that they have a self to invest, to give. They do not identify themselves by their objects and possessions. They are present to the one who is cared for. Those who are indisposable, on the other hand, come across, even though physically present, as being absent, as being elsewhere. Marcel said, "When I am with someone who is indisposable, I am conscious of being with someone for whom I do not exist; I am thrown back on myself" (Blackham, 1959, p. 80).

PRESENT DEFINITION

Caring is a function of the whole person in which concern for the growth and well-being of another is expressed in an integrated application of the mind, body, and spirit toward maximizing positive outcomes in the one who is cared for. The expressions of caring, therefore, are quite broad and include, but are not limited to, the following: a feeling of compassion; an attitude of concern; a philosophy of commitment; a moral disposition in the situation; acts of doing for another; conscious attention to the monitoring, surveillance, and protection of well-being; the nurturance of growth; the courage of venturing into the experience of another and being fully present; and advocacy on behalf of another. Caring denotes a primary mode of being in the world and thus is fundamental to our understanding of human nature (Benner & Wrubel, 1989; Swanson, 1999). It may be expressed in a wide variety of activities, such as providing information, doing things, listening, helping, showing respect, and communicating (Warren, 1988). Leininger has identified 27 caring activities, which include helping, touching, nurturing, protecting, and supporting (Gaut, 1983). Leininger believes caring to be a universal phenomenon, although she notes that expressions, processes, and patterns vary among cultures (Leininger, 1988). Much of present writing in nursing theory suggests that caring is an essential component of nursing (e.g., Boykin & Schoenhofer, 1990; Watson, 1985). Swanson (1999), for example, describes nursing as informed caring for the well-being of others.

A more abstract form of care is existential care, which is compassion and care as a result of awareness of the common bonds of humanity, common fates, common experiences, and common feelings (Younger, 1995). Care may occur as a product of an individual relationship that has grown into rapport, but it does not always. Existential care does not require rapport with another, at least at first, but simply the acknowledgment of a shared human experience. This awareness enables us to care for another, not as a stranger but as another "I." Thus, as the philosopher Heidegger (1962) said, care is "a priori and primordial," no mere generalization but a real structure that appears in all (pp. 243–244). Swanson (1999) notes that when referring to the concept of caring, there is a need to be clear about whether the discourse is

about the capacity for caring, the concerns and commitments that underlie caring, conditions that inhibit or enhance caring, caring actions, or the consequences of caring.

CARE AS AN IDEAL

As a philosophical concept, care is an ideal, like truth, justice, or beauty. As an ideal, care can never be perfect or fully attained in human expression. Human beings are not capable of perfect care any more than we are capable of perfect truth, justice, or beauty. However, in striving for the ideal, we occasionally come close, and by so doing achieve something quite wonderful. A danger is in viewing such ideals concretely and expecting that they should be achievable and measured, and that those who fall short should be ashamed. A nurse who expected to care would likely feel guilty about moments of feeling selfish or about being unable to care for a particular patient. Another danger is to be too discouraged about the impossibility of perfection and fail to strive for that part of the ideal that might be achievable.

DIFFERENT MEANINGS OF THE WORD *CARE*

Not everyone who uses or hears the words care or caring means the same thing. Some may interpret it to mean only an emotional state and resent its use as devaluing the scientific and instrumental activities of nursing. Some others may use the expression "provide nursing care" to mean only performing technical skills. Again, this may be resented as denying the intellectual, humanistic, and existential component of nursing. Another use is to say "care" with an automaticity that lacks specific meaning, such as the phrase "nursing care plan." Still others see caring as a human trait and consider nurses' claim to caring as egocentric. This is particularly true of other health professionals. To be sure, any of the above interpretations falls far short of the meaning that is conveyed here. Given the possible confusion, it is usually a good idea to define the term before using it and assuming the same interpretation.

CARING IN NURSING

The expression of caring in nursing is well directed by Henderson's (1966) definition of nursing, which is "to do those things the patient would do unaided for himself if he had the necessary strength, will or knowledge; and to do this in such a way as to help him gain independence as rapidly as possible" (p. 15). The American Nurses Association (ANA) defines nursing as "the diagnosis and treatment of human responses to health and illness," which further guides the area of concern in nursing (ANA, 1980). Both of these definitions help us know what to care about. Thus, while there are aspects of caring in nursing that are specific to the purposes of nursing, the foundation of caring is common to human professions, to human beings, and indeed to most living beings.

PROFESSIONAL CARE

Human caring therefore is necessary for professional caring, but it is far from sufficient. Professional caring adds the additional defining characteristic of applying the knowledge of the discipline, including its art, science, theory, and practice, to the situation of concern. It requires acting in accordance with the standards of care, keeping abreast of current research, and sharing one's knowledge with colleagues. Professionals also evaluate their work and subject it to peer review to improve the quality. These actions increase the nurse's capability of effective caring. Without professional competence, it is not professional caring.

The professional relationship also requires acting in accordance with the ethical standards of the profession. Ethics of the caring relationship imply that a patient who entrusts his well-being and his private life to the hands of a professional will be dealt with responsibly. This responsibility means that the patient's privacy

will be maintained with confidentiality and that his/her well-being will be foremost in the professional's mind. It also means the nurse will refrain from meeting his or her personal needs through the relationship.

The separation of one's personal needs and well-being from the patient's or client's is called professional boundary. All professions have standards and regulations, in addition to ethics, that help define these boundaries. For nursing, the National Council of State Boards of Nursing (1996) has provided the following definition to assist in the interpretation of unprofessional conduct:

> Professional boundaries are the spaces between the nurse's power and the client's vulnerability. The power of the nurse comes from the professional position and the access to private knowledge about the client. Establishing boundaries allows the nurse to control this power differential and allows a safe connection to meet the client's needs (p. 2).

This definition is closely related to the understanding of caring presented in this chapter. It emphasizes the focus on the well-being of the patient and the importance of trust in the relationship. The National Council of State Boards of Nursing further provides the following definition of boundary violation that clarifies how boundary failures breach the trust:

> Boundary violations can result when there is a confusion between the needs of the nurse and those of the client. Such violations are characterized by excessive personal disclosure by the nurse, secrecy or even a reversal of roles. Boundary violations can cause delayed distress for the client, which may not be recognized or felt by the client until harmful consequences occur (p. 3).

Understanding professional boundaries and boundary violations distinguishes professional caring from other types of relationships. Thus, not all emotional involvement with another person constitutes caring. If the mother of a young child is overprotective and because of her own fearfulness prohibits the child from engaging in normal play activities which the child needs for development, that is not maternal care. These actions are more directed toward meeting the mother's needs for security. Although the mother may feel concern for the child, her actions do not promote the growth and well-being of the child, and therefore fall short of caring.

Sometimes a nurse becomes personally involved with a patient. The relationship becomes a friendship or even a romance. When this occurs, the relationship itself becomes more important to the nurse. When a nurse loses the ability to use professional knowledge fully for the well-being of that patient, the nurse's involvement is no longer considered professional care.

Sometimes the patient has an illness or condition that the nurse has also experienced. This experience can become a source of knowledge and skill, or it can be a personal experience that the nurse cannot get beyond. In such instances the nurse is actually absorbed in the continued care of himself or herself.

There are also times when a nurse may be unable to bear the pain or suffering of the patient. This may be manifested in one of two ways. In the first manifestation, the nurse may become quite detached and cease to engage the patient with the same watchful gaze, studied concern, or available presence. The patient becomes the object of some technical intervention that, regardless of how skillfully it is done, is not a product of the whole person of the nurse. In the second case, the nurse may give alcohol to an alcoholic or morphine to an addict, or tell patients that things will be fine when they are not. In these instances the nurse is so wrapped up in the patient's suffering that the focus on well-being is lost. In each of these cases the nurse is not engaged in professional care. It is a common, human mistake. It does not mean the nurse is incapable of caring, but needs to seek assistance in dealing with these feelings with other nurses, supervisors, or professional counselors. In all of these situations, recognition of the problem is often the most difficult step.

Caring as a Context for Intervention

Benner and Wrubel (1989) assert that caring is primary. Caring means being connected, and having that connection matter. It is the force that fuses thought, feeling, and action. It sets up what matters to a person; it also sets up what counts as stressful and what options are available for coping. Caring creates possibility and gives meaning. This is the first way in which caring is primary (Benner & Wrubel, 1989).

When patients feel cared for, it sets up the perception of a safe environment. The safety is like what the child experiences in an environment of parental care. It is predicated on the trust that someone more knowledgeable is monitoring the situation and will invariably act for well-being. This state is then accompanied by a lowering of vigilance, a sense of comfort, a willingness to explore, and a willingness to reveal more of the vulnerable self. It is helpful to contrast the sense one has when the environment is experienced as indifferent or dangerous. Nursing research has pursued the question of this contrast (Brown, 1986; Riemen, 1986; Swanson-Kauffman, 1986). Findings suggest that most people under those circumstances assume a guarded, defensive posture, and their stress level is much higher.

CARING AND ILLNESS

The experience of illness is very personal and, at the same time, universal. The personal experience is that illness always has a story. It is the story of a life interrupted. The nature of the interruption is very specifically related to the life itself. What plans have been changed? What meanings were assigned to whatever has been lost? What is the personal meaning of the reminder that life is vulnerable and time limited? To acknowledge the reality of pain and suffering means saying to oneself, "I may lose at any moment, through the play of circumstances over which I have no control, anything whatsoever that I possess, including those things which are so intimately mine that I consider them as being myself" (Weil, 1969, p. 287). This is true even when the illness is minor, but it is especially true when the illness produces a long-term or permanent change. Consider the trivial example of a person who has a flat tire en route to somewhere. Although the flat tire is trivial, the story of that journey to somewhere is epic. These stories of the journey are very personal, but in every illness there simultaneously exists an encounter with the universal. Caring involves learning the universal patterns of human fate. It is a voluntary involvement in the universality of pain, suffering, aloneness, fear, and a looming death. Caring also means involvement in the universal characteristic of constructing a life and restructuring meaning. Even a new mother is, in a day's time, interrupted from her old life and finds herself constructing a new life with a new person. This ceaseless activity of inventing, restructuring, and reinterpreting is universal, even though the outcomes are personal. For the nurse, it also means responding to a universal appeal that is made by one who suffers—that is, to care, the potential for which is in all.

Another type of activity that is not usually associated with the affective component of caring is careful monitoring. For example, a nurse in an intensive care unit spends much of the day monitoring information provided by machines. Is that caring? Certainly, the activity of very careful watching, like the mother's watching of her infant or the bird's watching its nest, is a component of the living prototypes of care. The fact that the patient may not talk is immaterial in answering the question. The full integration of the monitoring of information is a necessary element in order to call this professional care. The only issue that remains in answering the question is whether the nurse integrates this information with other kinds of information obtained from monitoring this patient as a whole person, and whether this nurse

acts as a whole person on behalf of the patient's well-being.

Caring is the force that takes the nurse into the patient's life while monitoring the patient's condition and selecting actions in an integrated goal-corrected movement toward well-being. Caring is the integrative force that organizes and binds together all of the resources of the nurse. Since nursing actions are really functional only when integrated, it is the context for nursing intervention.

The most demanding and deeply human aspect of caring is the expressive art of being fully present to another person (Davis, 1981). In the deepest sense, caring for the other is extending a human and humane presence to a fellow being—an action that reinforces caring. It transcends role obligations and acknowledges the vulnerable humanness of us all. To be present means to unconceal, to be aware of tone of voice, eye contact, affect, and body language—to be in tune with the patient's messages. The effect of this interaction is the reinforcement of self-esteem, the strengthening of spirit, and the healing and nurturing of the self. This is the ability to "convey by presence that my own fears and ego needs have been laid aside and I am yours." An act of human contact and concern provides the alienated with a human self-extension and, in itself, partially recreates the connection. Being present and available so that the patient's needs are responded to appropriately, so that "one's existence is acknowledged by another who cares" is confirmation (Drew, 1986; p. 40). The one who is caring sees the best self in the one who is cared for and works with this person to actualize that self (Noddings, 1984).

The suffering of another illuminates essential humanity under threat and is thus a profound call for the attention of the giver of care, a protector of humanity (Griffin, 1983). Since the nature of suffering is to call forth deep questioning of the truth of one's being and its meaning, care becomes a midwife of rebirth of a reconstructed life (Younger, 1995). Caring acknowledgment of patients' suffering legitimizes their experiences and gives them a feeling of personal integrity, wholeness, and value (Suchman & Matthews, 1988).

It is a frequent mistake to believe that people who do not speak of their caring do not care. This may be inaccurate, and a misjudgment of the true situation. In our society this misjudgment happens to men more often than to women, to physicians more often than to nurses, and to quiet nurses more often than to talkative ones. It is good to remember that caring may or may not be related to claims of caring. Furthermore, it may be demoralizing to one who cares to be accused of not caring. It has the effect of making the person feel misunderstood and alienated. Those conditions may then actually interfere with that person's ability to care or to receive support for caring, and thereby result in less care. Consider the situation of a nurse who believes that a mother who does not come often to see her hospitalized child does not care. If the nurse subsequently communicates that to the mother, is the mother more likely or less likely to feel supported in caring for the child?

CARE VERSUS CURE

Medicine is primarily concerned with the prevention, diagnosis, and treatment of disease. As such, it has sometimes been associated with cure in contrast to nursing, which has primarily been associated with care. Proposing that medicine is concerned with cure and nursing with care therefore may highlight some of the primary distinctions of the two disciplines. Would it be valid, though, to think that care is the province of nursing, and that cure belongs to medicine? Consider these questions. When a nurse debrides an ulcer, is that caring or curing? When a physician orders pain medication, what is that? Pain is a response to disease or trauma. The treatment of pain rarely cures the underlying problem. When a nurse practitioner orders acetaminophen for fever, is that medicine or

nursing? Fever is a response to disease and not the disease itself. Treating it does not cure the disease. Is a surgical procedure necessarily done for the purpose of cure? Each of these questions illustrates the ambiguity in trying to distinguish medicine and nursing by their caring or curing activities. More important, the distinction understates the wholeness of both physicians and nurses by suggesting each to be capable of using only part of the self.

Given the definition of caring presented in this chapter, caring would encompass curing if that possibility were present (Jecker & Self, 1991). Similarly, curing often involves altering the relationships between the disease process and the patient's natural defenses. Placing the patient in the best possible position to fight the disease or injury often involves acts of caring. Therefore, to believe that caring is confined to nursing and that curing is confined to medicine is unduly simplistic and unrealistically confining. Although the concepts of care and cure may be distinguished, in practice they are often well blended.

DEVELOPING MORE CARING ABILITY

Beginning nurses can develop their caring abilities in several ways. These involve strengthening the capacities of mind, body, and spirit, as well as increasing the ability to integrate these capacities. Everything nurses can discover or learn about the science of illness or its manifestations and about nursing interventions improves the ability to assess problems and understand what helps. Every technical skill that is perfected, whether it is the ability to give an injection with skill or to move a patient painlessly, contributes to care. The task of eliciting from the patient what is being experienced is tremendously complex. How do you get a patient to tell you how much pain, how much worry, how much knowledge he or she is experiencing? This is an artful combination of the questions asked and how they are asked, and there is never enough practice.

There is a type of knowledge of what it is like to be ill or to suffer or to be in pain that is not entirely intellectual and not entirely personal. Nurses may learn about this from listening to the experiences of their patients if they can listen without too much defensive avoidance. A lower level of exposure to that learning may be through artistic depictions of those experiences in literary works, artwork, and movies (Younger, 1990). Writers often draw on the very material that nurses encounter daily, and literary themes are often the same as the human themes that nurses need to recognize: endurance in the face of suffering, the quest for meaning, acceptance of loss. The depictions of suffering and illness are closer in their expression to the way patients describe their experiences than are descriptions found in textbooks. The human condition is expressed sensitively and articulately in literature, and the aesthetic appeal of these often calls forth compassion that is crucial to nursing. These literary works convey something complex in a more simple metaphorical form that can be grasped as a whole and understood. This is because they convey not only the facts, but also the context and meaning of the experience. The inexperienced nurse can risk entering into the vicarious experience of a story that would be beyond the professional level of experience. Also, performance is not required, so personal defenses may be relaxed, enabling the nurse to grow in knowledge, understanding, and compassion. Thus, literary works offer a way for nurses to gain maturity, understanding of human responses, and depth of compassion for others (Younger, 1990).

Another means of increasing one's ability to care is to use as professional models those nurses who demonstrate caring. Nurses who are not very knowledgeable or who have become so detached as to not know what their patients are experiencing may model behaviors that seem attractive because they are easier, but these behaviors will not result in professional care. However, an experienced nurse who is able to care may help by allowing a less experienced nurse to watch or to hear the stories of important experiences. Even more helpful is for the more experienced nurse to hear the problems of the novice and help with approaches and with encouragement. Much of caring requires some courage, so those individuals who encourage are very valuable colleagues.

Finally, nurses who wish to increase their ability to care for others must care for their own spirits (Lane, 1987). Lane tells us that we all desire to push back the horizons of our present life, aspiring to be something more, and that life is a journey on the road to somewhere. We are restless to know more, to love more, to create more, and to express a generosity within us that desires to give to the other, to make life better. Lane advises us to engage in inward turning to get in touch with the "wounded self" (Nouwen, 1972), which eventually helps us to be at home with ourselves, to be who we are, to accept the limitations life has imposed on us, and to go on.

CASE STUDIES
Examples of Caring

Each of the following clinical examples depicts certain aspects of caring. The situations differ, as does the form that caring takes.

EXAMPLE 1: The Neurointensive Care Unit

Ms. A is a nurse on the unit. Her patient is a young man with a gunshot wound to his head as a result of a shootout between two drug dealers. The patient has been unconscious since his admission. Ms. A is quite concerned about the well-being of her patient. She thinks about his possible recovery and wants to assist him in regaining his health and function. She does not condone his illegal activity, but that is not her concern in this situation. He is in need of nursing care. She is very knowledgeable about neuroanatomy and physiology and realizes that she must monitor every change in the patient's condition. She watches carefully all of the equipment that helps her assess the condition of his brain. She also uses all of her physical assessment skills to detect any complication that may arise. She assesses his level of consciousness at least every hour and talks to him in an attempt to penetrate his coma with some sense of life. He, however, cannot talk to her, nor is he at this moment aware of her care. Nonetheless, this is care. It is a product of her whole person on behalf of the patient's well-being.

EXAMPLE 2: The Oncology Unit

Mr. B, a nurse on the oncology unit, has been the primary nurse for his patient, a 53-year-old grandmother who has advanced cancer. She has been in pain and is aware that her prognosis is quite poor. While Mr. B is adjusting her IV line she says to him, "Are you a religious man, Mr. B?" Actually, Mr. B does not consider himself particularly religious, and furthermore he has a busy schedule this morning. He sighs inwordly at being called on to enter into this patient's suffering. This morning, at least, he would rather attend to other things. He is human and is not capable of perfect care. However, he is also an expert clinician in oncology, and he recognizes that it is not his religion that is at issue here; rather, the patient is seeking a human connection. He recognizes the pattern of the question and the way she asks it. He sits down on her bed, but not because he plans to stay a long time. This will not take very long. He wants to signal his intention to be fully present to her and to enter into her experience. Beginning truthfully, he says, "My own religion has its ups and downs—does yours provide you with some comfort now?" The question is gentle and not very demanding. The patient may choose to say a few more things about her religion and remain silent about other concerns. However, she may also choose to accept his gentle acknowledgment that there is really something here that is in need of comfort, and she may share this with him. In fact, she says, "I know that I have not much longer to live. I long to watch my grandchild grow a bit longer and offer more support to his parents. My comfort is in knowing that the Lord does things in His own good time and that He will provide for my children." He takes

her hand for a moment and says, "Your faith that the Lord will provide for your children seems a comfort to you now indeed." His answer is brief and tacitly accepting of everything she has said. He waits to see where she needs to go with this next. She pats his hand and says, "Well, you have others to take care of. Thank you so much."

EXAMPLE 3: The Nursing Student

Ms. C is a junior nursing student who is assigned to a 16-year-old girl who, because of a chronic illness that has worsened, is now in multisystem failure, including renal and hepatic shutdown. The patient wants to live, and the student perhaps identifies with this patient and recognizes that in a 16-year-old there is much living that can be lost. The student assesses the patient very carefully and spends nearly the whole night before her clinical experience researching what should be done for this patient. She arrives the next morning and presents her instructor with an excellent and exhaustive nursing care plan. The instructor looks at the care plan and then at the patient. From her experience she recognizes in this patient the unmistakable signs of impending death, and in this student she recognizes the lack of awareness of that reality. In the morning the student cares for the patient exhaustively. In the afternoon the patient dies. The instructor finds the student alone in an out-of-the-way corner of the unit. The student is maintaining a stiff upper lip and is nearly mute. The instructor talks to the student for a while, and the student says, "I should have done more." The instructor replies, "There was too much wrong. She couldn't be saved." The instructor begins to talk about the overwhelming problems of this patient and the unmistakable signs of impending death. The instructor then takes out a tissue to wipe the tears from her own eyes. The student says, "Nurses don't cry like this." The instructor replies, "Maybe not while things are happening and people need your help immediately, but after it is over we sometimes need a good cry." The student is then able to let go of her stiff upper lip and, in the safety of her instructor's acceptance, give way to her feelings.

In this situation the student is showing deep human care and excellent beginning professional care.

The instructor also shows human care and mature professional care. She also, as a professional, is creating more potential for care in this developing student. As she helps her develop professionally and learn to fuse her knowledge, humanness, and professionalism, she helps create a nurse more capable of care.

EXAMPLE 4: The Well-Child Clinic

Mr. D is a nurse practitioner in a well-child clinic in a neighborhood with much social and economic deprivation. His patient this morning is an 18-month-old boy and his mother. Mr. D is aware that this mother has had cultural experiences quite different from his own and that English is her second language and his only language. He thinks about that for a moment before entering the patient's room. He will do his best to understand, but this understanding can never be perfect. He is quite committed to fostering the health and growth of young people in this community. His knowledge of the normal growth and development of the child is excellent. Using that knowledge, he carefully assesses this child. The child, who was premature, is underweight; speech is nonexistent; the hematocrit is below normal; the immunizations are markedly behind; but most troublesome to him is the pattern of bruises with uneven levels of healing. He sits down and asks the mother, "How do you manage?" She says in broken English, "Life is very hard—three children, no money, no man—this boy bad." He asks a clinic helper who speaks her language fluently to help him talk to the mother. The mother denies abusing the child and indicates only normal punishment for misbehavior. Mr. D carefully considers the legal and ethical requirements of his situation. He must be an advocate for the child. He calls protective services. While waiting for them to come, he and the clinic helper talk at length to the mother about the normal behavior of children that age and their needs. Although momentarily he feels like shaking the mother, he listens to her and feels compassion for her while at the same time he is providing protection for the child. Thus he acts to promote the growth and well-being of both.

Each of these vignettes is an example of caring. All demonstrate a primary human quality finely honed by professional training and expressed humanly rather than perfectly. Each demonstrates some defining characteristic(s) of care. They depict nurses engaged with the whole of their professional knowledge, as well as their human spirits.

KEY POINTS

● Caring is a function of the whole person in which concern for the growth and well-being of another is expressed in an integrated application of the mind, body, and spirit of the one who is caring toward maximizing positive outcomes in the one who is cared for.

● Professional caring adds the defining characteristic of applying the knowledge of the discipline, including its art, science, theory, and practice, to the situation of concern and maintaining the fiduciary relationship. This is what distinguishes professional caring from basic human caring. Human caring, therefore, is necessary for professional caring, but it is far from sufficient.

● Definitions of nursing direct us in what to care about in professional practice.

● Caring as a context provides for the integration of activities of the mind, body, and spirit of the nurse on behalf of the well-being of the patient.

● Caring as an intervention is effective in giving patients a sense of personal integrity, wholeness, and value. In the suffering patient it helps to bear the burden.

● Caring as an activity integrates the information gained from monitoring the patient and activities on the patient's behalf into a constantly readjusted, goal-corrected intervention for the patient's well-being.

CRITICAL THINKING EXERCISES

1. Consider situations in which you have felt cared for. Analyze the situation. How did you know you were cared for? What was the effect of that care?

2. Consider situations in which you have been unable to care. Analyze the situation. What were barriers? What aspects of you as a whole person were affected?

3. What do you have to do to care for an individual who lives a life so adverse to your values as to create a conflict in you?

4. What is the difference between caring for someone you love, like your own child, and caring for someone you do not love, like a stranger?

5. Consider the example of a nurse who comes to work at 3:00 p.m. The assigned patient's chart reveals that a dressing, which is ordered once a shift, was done at 2:30 p.m. It is now 3:30; the nurse has time to do the dressing and considers doing it now. What does it mean in terms of caring to do it now?

6. Consider your development as a professional. What is missing from your full ability to provide professional care?

REFERENCES

Ainsworth, M. D. S., Blehar, M. C., Waters, E., & Wall, S. (1978). *Patterns of attachment*. Hillsdale, NJ: Erlbaum.

American Nurses Association. (1980). *Nursing: A social policy statement* (ANA Publication No. NP-63). Kansas City, MO: Author.

Benner, P., & Wrubel, J. (1989). *The primacy of caring*. Menlo Park, CA: Addison-Wesley.

Blackham, H. (1959). *Six existentialist thinkers*. New York: Harper & Row.

Bowlby, J. (1969). *Attachment and loss*. Vol. 1, *Attachment*. New York: Basic Books.

Bowlby, J. (1979). *The making and breaking of affectional bonds*. London: Tavistock Publications.

Boykin, A., & Schoenhofer, S. (1990). Caring in nursing: Analysis of extant theory. *Nursing Science Quarterly, 4*, 149–155.

Brown, L. (1986). The experience of care: Patient perspectives. *Topics in Clinical Nursing, 8*(2), 56–62.

Davis, M. (1981). Compassion, suffering, morality: Ethical dilemmas in caring. *Nursing Law and Ethics, 2*, 1.

Drew, N. (1986). Exclusion and confirmation: A phenomenology of patients' experiences with caregivers. *Image: Journal of Nursing Scholarship, 18*(2), 39–43.

Erikson, E. (1978). Life cycle. In J. Gardner (Ed.), *Readings in developmental psychology* (pp. 3–12). Boston: Little, Brown.

Erikson, E. (1982). *The life cycle completed*. New York: Norton.

Gaut, D. (1983). Development of a theoretically adequate description of caring. *Western Journal of Nursing Research, 5*, 311–324.

Griffin, A. P. (1983). A philosophical analysis of caring in nursing. *Journal of Advanced Nursing, 8*, 289–295.

Heidegger, M. (1962). *Being and time*. New York: Harper & Row.

Henderson, V. (1966). *The nature of nursing*. New York: Macmillan.

Jecker, N., & Self, D. (1991). Separating care and cure: An analysis of historical and contemporary images of nursing and medicine. *The Journal of Medicine and Philosophy, 16*, 285–306.

Lane, J. (1987). The care of the human spirit. *Journal of Professional Nursing*, 332–337.

Leininger, M. (1988). The phenomenon of caring: Importance, research questions and theoretical considerations. In M. Leininger (Ed.), *Caring: An essential human need*. Thorofare, NJ: Slack.

National Council of State Boards of Nursing. (1996). *Professional boundaries: A nurse's guide to the importance of appropriate professional boundaries*. Chicago: Author.

Noddings, N. (1984). *Caring: A feminine approach to ethics and moral education*. Los Angeles: University of California Press.

Nouwen, H. (1972). *The wounded healer*. New York: Doubleday.

Riemen, D. (1986). Noncaring and caring in the clinical setting: Patients' descriptions. *Topics in Clinical Nursing, 8*(2), 30–36.

Spitz, R. A. (1946). Anaclitic depression. *Psychoanalytic Study of the Child, 2*, 313–342.

Suchman, A., & Matthews, D. (1988). What makes the patient-doctor relationship therapeutic? Exploring the connexional dimension of medical care. *Annals of Internal Medicine, 108*, 125–130.

Swanson, K. (1993). Nursing as informed caring for the well-being of others. *Image: Journal of Nursing Scholarship, 25*, 352–357.

Swanson, K. (1999). What is known about caring in nursing science. In A. Henshaw, S. Feetham, & J. Shayer (Eds.), *Handbook of clinical nursing research*. Thousand Oaks, CA: Sage.

Swanson-Kauffman, K. (1986). Caring in the instance of unexpected early pregnancy loss. *Topics in Clinical Nursing, 8*(2), 37–46.

Warren, L. (1988). Review and synthesis of nine nursing studies on care and caring. *Journal of the New York State Nurses' Association, 19*(4), 17–21.

Watson, J. (1985). *Nursing: Human science and human care*. Norwalk, CT: Appleton-Century-Crofts.

Weil, S. (1969). Personality as affliction. In M. Lipman (Ed.), *Discovering philosophy*. Englewood Cliffs, NJ: Prentice Hall.

Younger, J. (1990). Literary works as a mode of knowing. *Image: Journal of Nursing Scholarship, 22*(1), 39–43.

Younger, J. (1995). Alienation of the sufferer. *Advances in Nursing Science, 17*(3), 53–72.

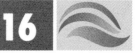

16

Health and Health Promotion

SANDRA P. THOMAS, PhD, RN, FAAN

OBJECTIVES

At the completion of this chapter, the reader will be able to:

- Compare and contrast several definitions and models of health.
- Compare and contrast several models of health behavior.
- Describe psychological, behavioral, and environmental factors related to wellness.
- Apply the Stages-of-Change model to a selected health behavior (smoking cessation).
- Apply the Health Belief Model to a selected health behavior (smoking cessation).
- Describe the use of evidence-based interventions to promote behavior change.
- Describe the goals of Healthy People 2010.
- Contrast several types of community-level health promotion programs.

PROFILE IN PRACTICE

Leslie El-Sayad, MSN, RN, FNP
Nurse Practitioner, Deer Lodge Medical Center
Deer Lodge, Tennessee

During my 13 years in primary care in rural eastern Tennessee, I have tried to avoid burnout and becoming jaded concerning my patients' motivations or lack thereof. But questions flit across my mind unbidden when patients make decisions that adversely affect their health. I think to myself, "Isn't it as plain as the nose on their face what they should do? Haven't I discussed that with them enough times?" Two principles have helped remind me to respect the patient's viewpoint on health.

1. *No one sets out deliberately to make a wrong decision.* This idea is based on one of nursing theorist Ernestine Wiedenbach's beliefs about the individual: Whatever the individual

does represents his or her best judgment at the moment of doing it. Given their immediate circumstances (and rural poor populations are more affected by immediate circumstances), past experiences, knowledge base, physical and mental state, and social or economic pressures at the time a decision is made, patients will make the best decision they are capable of making. Therefore, there is no looking back or chastising, only going forward with new knowledge. We cannot presume to know what is best for another person.

2. *Symptoms may have no meaning to a person unless there is a significant effect upon their life.* A person may have no wish to change any-

thing. A long lecture about the benefits of better health habits will not be helpful. People walk around with large tumors, constant dyspepsia, extreme dyspnea, or gnarled painful joints, but an ingrown toenail will bring them to the provider because they couldn't wear their boots. Risk factors do not have a one-to-one relationship to disease. They are risk factors, not guarantees of poor outcomes. Despite scientifically based predictions, patients will not buy into your suggested preventative measures if they see no gain.

It is difficult to promote health, but it's my job. Keeping the above principles in mind saves my sanity and helps me respect my patients' abilities on behalf of their health.

Ricky Jones is a 45-year-old long-distance truck driver who once used amphetamines heavily to help him stay awake while driving. He presently weighs 205 lb (height of 5′8″, medium frame) and expresses disgust with his weight and lack of physical fitness. After his annual physical examination, the nurse practitioner collaboratively sets initial goals of increasing Ricky's level of exercise and achieving a 10-lb weight loss. As Ricky departs, he wryly expresses a wish that amphetamines were still readily available so that he could diet more easily.

Many Americans share Ricky's longing for an easy way to lose weight or become fit. Millions of dollars are spent on books, tapes, pills, treadmills, and other exercise machines. But the outcomes Ricky seeks are not easy to achieve. Changing health behavior is difficult. Nurses, such as the family nurse practitioner profiled above, know how hard it is to motivate well people to undertake behaviors that lessen the likelihood of future illness. Some health professionals have a mistaken notion that the mere provision of didactic information will bring about health-promoting actions. But studies show that individuals are often aware of the risks associated with behaviors such as drinking and smoking; they modify their thinking about these risks so that they can continue the behaviors (Gerrard et al., 1996). Information is the solution only when ignorance is the problem. Health care providers need a more sophisticated understanding of the principles of behavior change. This chapter explores a variety of evidence-based interventions to change health behavior. But first, it is important to review ideas about health itself.

The Concept of Health

The concept of health is something of an enigma. Is it a state, a process, or a goal? Gadamer (1996) pointed out that health "is not something that is revealed through investigation but rather something that manifests itself precisely by virtue of escaping our attention." To the average layperson, it is *illness* that compels attention, a departure from taken-for-granted smooth functioning. Likewise, traditional medical and nursing curricula have prepared health professionals to care for the acutely ill. Many textbooks still place greater emphasis on morbidity and mortality than on health.

In contemporary nursing literature, authors assert that nursing has a mandate to promote *holistic health*. What does this mean? Unfortunately, some people think that holistic means "new age" or "alternative," something outside traditional beliefs or practices. Because the term holism is frequently misused, it may be useful to trace its origin. The word *holism* was first used on page 99 of a 1926 book by Jan Smuts, the first Prime Minister of South Africa and a lifelong student of biological evolution. Smuts rejected the mechanistic explanation of the world that was pervasive in his time. He saw physical matter and the mind as inseparable. And he believed that *holism*, a dynamic striving toward integration, was the ultimate principle of the universe. Not until the late 1950s and 1960s did these ideas begin to infiltrate the American health care delivery system. In medicine, Halbert Dunn began to speak of "high level wellness," the ultimate integration of body, mind, and spirit as an interdependent whole (1959, 1971). In nursing, Martha Rogers (1970) wrote about unitary human beings who are not reducible to parts or symptoms. She also emphasized the indivisible whole of person and environment.

Concurrent with the gradually shifting perspective of health professionals, a consumer wellness movement burgeoned, linked to the other human liberation movements of the 1960s and 1970s such as the civil rights and women's movements. Public dissatisfaction with paternalistic medical treatment and mystifying medical terms, along with a better educated, more affluent populace, contributed to a thirst for information about holistic therapies and self-care. Americans became preoccupied with self-care clinics, self-help groups, and the tantalizing potential of peak wellness and self-actualization. One prominent nursing theorist, Dorothea Orem, began to emphasize patients' self-care agency, recommending nursing intervention only when a self-care deficit is detected (1983). Education of the public for self-care became an important element of federal government policies and public health initiatives, such as the *Healthy People* initiative, first begun in 1979 and reformulated each succeeding decade. Motivated by escalating costs of care for sick workers, corporations began to demand that employees assume more responsibility for their health and provided them with exercise rooms, walking trails, and low-fat meal options in the employee cafeteria.

Models of Health

The actions of professionals are guided by their ideas about human beings and the meaning of the concept of health. For example, does health mean homeostasis or expanding consciousness? Smith (1983) has traced evolving conceptions of health across the centuries, categorizing them into four models (see Table 16–1).

CLINICAL MODEL

Listed first is the most narrow view of health, the *clinical model,* perhaps more readily recognizable to nurses as the "medical model." Health is simply the absence of disease or disability in this model. Upon examination of the physiochemical system of patient, the health care provider would declare "health" if no symptoms of any incipient illnesses were detected. Unfortunately, this narrow conceptualization of health is still dominant in many health care settings.

ROLE PERFORMANCE MODEL

The *role performance model* depicts health as the ability to fulfill one's customary social roles.

TABLE 16–1 **Models of Health**	
Model	Conception of Health
Clinical	Elimination of disease as identified through medical science
Role performance	Ability to perform social, occupational, and other roles
Adaptive	Ability to engage in effective interaction with environment
Eudaimonistic	Self-actualization of individual; optimal well-being

Data from Smith, J. (1983). *The idea of health: Implications for the nursing profession.* New York: Teachers College Press.

Thus, if a young mother is able to adequately carry out her child care activities, she would be deemed healthy. If she cannot perform these activities, she would be considered ill. The problem with this view of health is the distressful and stultifying nature of many people's occupational or familial roles. Scholars are now placing emphasis on the *quality* of experience in social roles, and the degree of *choice* about occupancy of these roles (Thomas, 1997a). Can individuals trapped in unsatisfying jobs or marriages achieve optimal health? What is the health impact of juggling *multiple roles* or experiencing *role conflict*? What if performance in one role (worker, for example) so dominates one's existence that performance in another role (parent) is compromised?

ADAPTIVE MODEL

Based largely on the ideas of Dubos (1965), the *adaptive model* emphasizes ability to flexibly adapt to ever-changing environments and challenges. Continuous readjustment to life's stressful demands is necessary. Healthy people are resilient and hardy. Disease is viewed as a failure of adaptation. While the adaptive model achieved popularity in nursing, as exemplified in the work of theorists such as Callista Roy (1970), there is a still broader conceptualization of health.

EUDAIMONISTIC MODEL

Drawn from the Greek philosophers and from the humanistic psychologist Abraham Maslow (1961), the *eudaimonistic model* depicts health as the complete development of the individual's potential, an exuberant well-being. Clearly, this model emphasizes human capacity for growth. Within nursing, theorist Margaret Newman (1978, 1994) has proposed that health is *expanding consciousness.*

Newer conceptualizations of health in the literature are consistent with Smith's adaptive and eudaimonistic models and Dunn's description of high-level wellness, mandating that today's health care providers must do more than address symptoms. Adopting a broader view of health has several implications for nursing practice: It becomes impossible to separate mind, body, and spirit. Moreover, the patient's embeddedness in family, friendships, culture, and the environment cannot be ignored. And there is greater recognition that the patient has power for healing within. The role of the nurse becomes that of *facilitator* of the patient's own innate capabilities for healing and growth. Skilled counseling becomes as important as technical competence.

Health Promotion and Disease Prevention

The terms health promotion and disease prevention, although used synonymously in the literature, actually have very different meanings. Flowing logically from adaptive or eudaimonistic views of health, *health promotion* refers to activities that protect good health and take people beyond their present level of wellness. By achieving lean and fit bodies and well-managed stress levels, individuals have a greater likelihood of achieving a high quality of life and reaching the goal of self-actualization. In contrast, *disease prevention* efforts are derived from the clinical model of health. Emphasis is frequently placed on avoidance, deprivation, or restraint. Behaviors are undertaken to prevent specific diseases. By limiting fat intake, one seeks to prevent obesity or cardiovascular disease. By refraining from smoking, one seeks to prevent pulmonary disease. Despite their distinctly different aims, health promotion and disease prevention may be viewed as complementary processes (Pender, 1996).

The importance of preventive efforts becomes obvious when we review statistics showing that men lose the equivalent of 11.5 well-years of life from morbidity, and women lose the equivalent of 15.6 well-years (Kaplan, Anderson, & Wingard, 1991). Mortality statistics likewise demonstrate the importance of lifestyle modifications to prevent premature death. The leading causes of death in the United States in the 1900s were infectious diseases such as typhoid and cholera. Subsequently, public health initiatives lengthened the American life span: vaccinations, fluoridation, improved maternal and child health, access to family planning, safer food and water, safer motor vehicle travel, and better occupational safety measures dramatically affected longevity and quality of life. By the 1950s, lifestyle became the primary cause of death. Presently, the chief causes of death (shown in Table 16–2), are strongly related to unhealthy behaviors such as smoking.

TABLE 16–2 Ten Leading Causes of Death in the United States, 1997

Males	Females
Whites	
Diseases of the heart	Diseases of the heart
Malignant neoplasms	Malignant neoplasms
Cerebrovascular diseases	Cerebrovascular diseases
Accidents/adverse effects	COPD and allied conditions
COPD and allied conditions	Pneumonia, influenza
Pneumonia, influenza	Accidents/adverse effects
Diabetes mellitus	Diabetes mellitus
Suicide	Alzheimer's disease
Chronic liver disease, cirrhosis	Nephritis, nephrosis
Nephritis, nephrosis	Septicemia
Blacks	
Diseases of the heart	Diseases of the heart
Malignant neoplasms	Malignant neoplasms
Accidents/adverse effects	Cerebrovascular diseases
Cerebrovascular diseases	Diabetes mellitus
Homicide/legal intervention	Accidents/adverse effects
HIV infection	Pneumonia, influenza
Diabetes mellitus	COPD and allied conditions
Pneumonia, influenza	HIV infection
COPD and allied conditions	Septicemia
Conditions originating in perinatal period	Nephritis, nephrosis
Hispanics	
Diseases of the heart	Diseases of the heart
Malignant neoplasms	Malignant neoplasms
Accidents/adverse effects	Cerebrovascular diseases
Homicide/legal intervention	Diabetes mellitus
Cerebrovascular diseases	Accidents/adverse effects
Diabetes mellitus	Pneumonia, influenza
Chronic liver disease, cirrhosis	COPD and allied conditions
HIV infection	Conditions originating perinatally
Pneumonia, influenza	Chronic liver disease, cirrhosis
Suicide	Congenital anomalies

From Hoyert, D. L., Kochanek, K. D., & Murphy, S. L. (1999). *Final death data for 1997. National vital statistics reports* (Vol. 47, No. 19). Hyattsville, MD: National Center for Health Statistics.

◠ Modification of Health Attitudes and Behavior

There is convincing empirical evidence that healthy lifestyles can significantly reduce mortality from cardiovascular diseases, cancer, obesity, diabetes, and human immunodeficiency virus/ acquired immunodeficiency syndrome (HIV/ AIDS). Therefore, the modification of health attitudes and behavior is one of the most important responsibilities of contemporary nurses. As shown in Figure 16–1, a comprehensive model of wellness includes interactive factors such as *psychological characteristics, health-promoting behaviors,* and aspects of the *environments* in which people live and work. Both attitudes and behaviors are modifiable by health care providers, as well as some (but not all) aspects of environments. In the sections that follow, we will examine a number of these modifiable factors. While *organismic variables,* such as genetic predispositions, certain personality characteristics (e.g., introversion versus extraversion), and demographic characteristics (age, income, gender, education, occupation, and race/

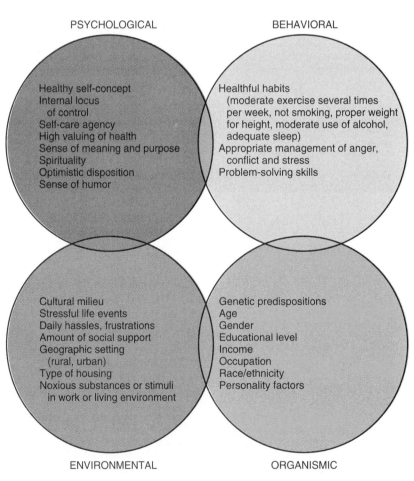

PSYCHOLOGICAL

Healthy self-concept
Internal locus
  of control
Self-care agency
High valuing of health
Sense of meaning and purpose
Spirituality
Optimistic disposition
Sense of humor

BEHAVIORAL

Healthful habits
  (moderate exercise several times
  per week, not smoking, proper weight
  for height, moderate use of alcohol,
  adequate sleep)
Appropriate management of anger,
  conflict and stress
Problem-solving skills

Cultural milieu
Stressful life events
Daily hassles, frustrations
Amount of social support
Geographic setting
  (rural, urban)
Type of housing
Noxious substances or stimuli
  in work or living environment

Genetic predispositions
Age
Gender
Educational level
Income
Occupation
Race/ethnicity
Personality factors

ENVIRONMENTAL

ORGANISMIC

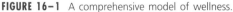

FIGURE 16–1 A comprehensive model of wellness.

ethnicity) are also important to consider in a comprehensive wellness model, most are not amenable to modification by health care providers.

PSYCHOLOGICAL ATTITUDES AND CHARACTERISTICS ASSOCIATED WITH WELLNESS

Self-Concept. Many theorists consider *healthy self-concept* (and closely related concepts such as self-acceptance or self-esteem) essential for wellness. It stands to reason that persons who feel better about themselves would be more inclined to enact self-care behaviors that promote good health. Abundant data demonstrate that self-destructive habits such as drug abuse are linked to lower self-worth or profound loathing of oneself. Some studies show that females are more concerned with self-concept and self-esteem issues than males (Thomas, Shoffner, & Groer, 1988). While experiences with parents, teachers, and peers all contribute to initial development of the self-concept, later life experiences offer opportunities to alter it. A client's negative evaluation of the self can be altered in an ongoing, supportive relationship with a nurse.

Locus of Control. *Locus of control* is a construct from Rotter's (1954) social learning theory. According to this theory, as individuals are exposed to reinforcements (rewards) for their behavior, they develop beliefs about their ability to control desired outcomes or rewards. Eventually most people have a stable general expectancy that reinforcements are contingent upon their own behavior (termed *internal locus of control*) or an expectancy that rewards are received on a purely random basis or dispensed by powerful others (*external locus of control*). This stable general expectancy has been given a variety of other names by researchers. For example, locus of control is subsumed in Kobasa's (1979) multidimensional *hardiness* construct and Antonovsky's (1984) *sense of coherence*. What does

locus of control have to do with wellness? Rotter's theory was modified for health by researchers such as Wallston (1989). Logically, individuals who have an internal locus of control are more likely to engage in positive health behaviors. They believe that the reinforcement (good health) is directly related to their own actions, not controlled by powerful others (such as doctors) or by the vicissitudes of fate. Although questionnaires are available to measure locus of control, a nurse can easily assess it by questions such as, "What do you think caused you to have this heart attack?" "Who do you think knows best what you really need?" "Do you normally follow instructions pretty well or do you prefer to work things out your own way?" Nursing interventions can be tailored accordingly. If the person has an internal locus of control, allow high participation in goal setting and selection of reinforcers. If the person has external locus of control, provide plenty of concrete guidance and support. For example, if the goal is weight loss, suggest involvement in a program with regular group meetings, such as Weight Watchers.

Self-Care Agency. *Self-care agency,* a term coined by nurse theorist Dorothea Orem (1983), refers to the *ability* to care for oneself, for which one must have knowledge, skills, understanding, and willingness. In working with a client, it is necessary to make an assessment of all of these. A parallel concept from social cognitive theory called *self-efficacy* (Bandura, 1986) has generated a sizable body of health psychology literature. According to Bandura's theory, when people perceive that they have efficacy to accomplish a specific behavior (for example, breast self-examination), they are predisposed to undertake the behavior. A recent study of older adults found that self-efficacy and outcome expectations significantly influenced exercise behavior (Resnick & Spellbring, 2000). Converging empirical evidence about the importance of self-care agency (and the analogous concept of self-efficacy) suggests that a nurse's first step in working with many clients is to enhance their belief in personal capability.

Values. *Values* are those elements that show how a person has decided to use his or her life. Values serve as a basis for decisions and choices. The nurse must assess the reinforcement value of health to an individual, in comparison with other life values such as pleasure, excitement, or social recognition. It is common for people to declare that they highly value health, although their behaviors contradict this declaration. A value system may contain conflicting values. For example, highly valuing achievement and financial prosperity may result in overwork and neglect of health. Assisting a patient to clarify conflicting values can be a useful intervention.

Sense of Purpose. Having a sense of meaning and purpose for one's life may be an important factor in individuals' responsiveness to health providers' instructions. *Purpose in life* includes having goals for the future and a sense of directedness. It is often helpful for a nurse to explore whether patients aim to follow a particular career trajectory, pursue an enjoyable hobby or avocation, or see their children and grandchildren grow and mature. In what way does each person aim to make a difference or leave a legacy? It makes sense that persons with clear goals may devote more effort to health maintenance, as most goals cannot be achieved without good health. There is empirical evidence that purpose in life is correlated with good health habits (Williams et al., 1991).

Spirituality. There is increasing recognition by health researchers and clinicians that spirituality is an integral component of holistic health/wellness. *Spirituality* is not synonymous with involvement in organized religion, but the sense of connection with a divine wisdom or higher power often motivates practices such as meditation, prayer, and church attendance. Studies have examined the relationship of spirituality with disease conditions (e.g., heart disease, cancer, mental illness) as well as health risk behav-

iors (e.g., smoking, drinking, using drugs) (Larson et al., 1998). Patients may be motivated to take health-promoting actions by a belief that the body is a temple for the spirit.

Optimism. Having an optimistic disposition is proving important to health, in studies conducted during the past two decades. Scheier and Carver (1985) assert that *optimism* is a stable personality characteristic with important implications for the manner in which people regulate their actions, particularly actions relevant to health. The construct of optimism includes tendencies to expect the best, look on the bright side, and anticipate good things in the future. The construct does not overlap with locus of control; one's expectations of favorable outcomes may be derived from perceptions of being lucky or blessed as well as from convictions of personal control. Higher levels of optimism have been associated with the likelihood of completing an alcohol treatment program (Strack, Carver, & Blaney, 1987) and with faster recovery of coronary bypass patients (Scheier & Carver, 1992).

Sense of Humor. While a *sense of humor* is a socially appealing trait, it also conveys health benefits. The physical effects of mirth have been compared to the effects of exercise. The efficiency of the respiratory system increases, and the cardiovascular and muscular systems relax (Kennedy, 1995). There is a correlation between humor and elevated endorphins, and laughter has been linked to higher levels of immunoglobulin A and lower levels of cortisol (Berk et al., 1989; Dillon, Minchoff, & Baker, 1985). Laughter is an excellent way to dispel stress and tension as well.

HEALTH BEHAVIORS ASSOCIATED WITH WELLNESS

Behaviors associated with wellness are listed in Figure 16–1. The first research about health behaviors was done in the 1950s by social psychologists who sought to explain the public's perplexingly low response to screening programs that were free or low-cost (Hochbaum, 1958). From this work, a model emerged that can be used to predict preventive health action. According to the Health Belief Model (HBM), an individual's perceptions of his or her *susceptibility* to a disease (and the *severity* of that disease), the perceived *benefits* of taking action, and *cues* to action (from media, health professionals, or family) contribute to the likelihood of taking preventive actions—provided that *barriers* are not too great (Becker et al., 1977). A decade of subsequent research with the HBM found barriers to be the most useful element of the model in predicting behavior such as physical exercise (Janz & Becker, 1984). Typical barriers are time, expense, and inconvenience.

In the 1980s, nurse researcher Nola Pender presented a model with similarities to the Health Belief Model but with greater emphasis on health-promoting behaviors. Based on research that tested Pender's Health Promotion Model, a revised version with fewer (10 rather than 13) determinants of behavior was proposed in 1996 (Fig. 16–2). Individual characteristics and experiences are theorized to impact perceptions of self-efficacy, benefits and barriers to action, and a variable called "activity-related affect," which refers to the feelings about the behavior in question. For example, is exercise fun or unpleasant? All of these factors, as well as interpersonal and situational influences, can influence commitment to a plan of action. Additionally, competing demands such as work responsibilities are taken into account in the prediction of health-promoting behavior, the outcome variable of the model. The model awaits empirical testing.

The interaction model of client health behavior (IMCHB) was developed by Cox (1982, 1986) to include the influence of the nurse-client interaction on health behaviors. As in the other models we have discussed, variables such as the client's motivation and previous health care experiences are included (here called *elements of client singularity*), and there are a number of health outcomes (such as *adherence*

to the recommended care regimen). The unique aspect of the IMCHB is the inclusion of factors such as the health professional's competence, information, and support. Research with this model has been reviewed by Carter and Kulbok (1995), who concluded that most studies have confirmed the proposed linkages among the model's variables. However, clearer definitions of some concepts were recommended.

Health Habits. Longitudinal studies have shown that several *health habits* are consistently correlated with better general health status and/or longevity. First reports of the well-known Alameda County study appeared in 1972. Seven practices were associated with health: never smoking, sleeping 7–8 hours nightly, using alcohol moderately, exercising regularly, maintaining proper weight, eating breakfast, and not eating between meals (Belloc & Breslow, 1972). In 1980, the relationship of these practices to mortality of the study participants was examined. Men following the seven practices had a mortality rate only 28% that of men following none to three practices; the comparable figure for women was 43% (Breslow & Enstrom, 1980). As the longitudinal study continued, five of the original seven health habits remained predictive of health status, but eating breakfast and refraining from eating between meals were not significant predictors (Wiley & Camacho, 1980).

Given that the benefits of healthful habits have been known for at least 20 years, the average American's adherence to recommended types and amount of exercise is discouraging. Even when an exercise program is started, the usual rate of dropout is 50% in the first 3 to 6 months (Pender, 1996). Many people have an aversion to exercise, mentally associating it with competitive sports or regimented calisthenics. Even as health club membership climbs—at least among the more affluent—too many Americans pay someone else to wash the car, use riding mowers to mow the lawn, and consider their treadmills as clothes racks. Nurses need to spread the word that it is not necessary

INDIVIDUAL
CHARACTERISTICS
AND EXPERIENCES

BEHAVIOR-SPECIFIC
COGNITIONS
AND AFFECT

BEHAVIORAL
OUTCOME

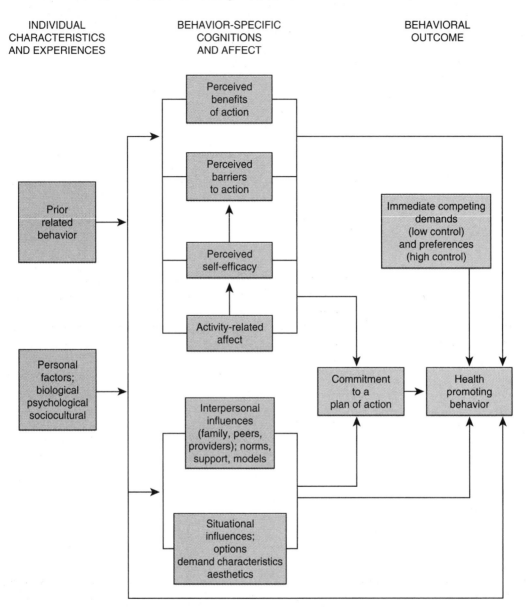

FIGURE 16-2 Pender's revised health promotion model. (From Pender, N. (1996.) *Health promotion in nursing practice* (3rd ed.). Reprinted by permission of Prentice-Hall, Inc., Upper Saddle River, NJ.)

to belong to a gym or use expensive equipment for regular physical workouts. Research shows that long-term adherence to an exercise program is more likely when the regimen is home-based rather than relying on participation in a group class at a gym (King et al., 1997). Nearly everyone can find a place to climb stairs or walk (shopping malls are a good alternative for those who live in unsafe neighborhoods). Soup cans can substitute for weights. Gardening, dancing, and biking are pleasurable as well as beneficial to the heart and muscle tone. Clients may be more motivated to exercise when informed of immediate benefits. For example, research shows that biking at a moderate rate for an hour reduces depression, anger, and confusion (Motl, cited in Kaplan, 1997). Studies also show that the greatest benefits in emotional state occur when people feel worst before they exercise (Gauvin, Rejeski, & Norris, 1996). Exercise can lift your spirits for as long as 2 to 4 hours (Kaplan, 1997).

One in three Americans is overweight, and American eating habits recently received a grade of C, based on the newest report about our food consumption from the U.S. Department of Agriculture (1997). Despite widespread media promotion of the food pyramid, we are nowhere near the recommended five to nine daily servings of fruits and vegetables. Our current intake of flour, grains, and beans is only two-thirds of what our grandparents consumed in 1910. Each of us consumes 150 lb of sweeteners (mostly sugar and corn syrup) per year, 25 lb more than in 1984. We drink twice as much carbonated soda as milk. And we still consume too much fat, 10 lb more per person than in 1970 (Liebman, 1997). Food is laden with emotional and social significance, complicating attempts at dietary modification.

According to the director-general of the World Health Organization, tobacco kills 4 million people annually; by 2030, it will kill 10 million per year (Brundtland, 1999). In the United States, public smoking has been discouraged by bans in offices, restaurants, and airports. Studies have shown that nurse-delivered smoking cessation counseling is effective (Hollis et al., 1993), and many Americans have kicked the habit. But smoking is on the rise among girls and women, with a concomitant increase in female lung cancer. Approximately 90% of new smokers are teenagers; 3,000 begin smoking every day (Lindell & Reinke, 1999). More adolescents are smoking today than at any time since the 1970s. Some 35% of high school stu-

dents smoke cigarettes, compared to 28% in 1991 (Centers for Disease Control and Prevention, 1996). Some youngsters have their first smoke in the sixth grade or earlier. These youngsters do not know they are exposed to more than 4,000 chemicals each time they light up, including arsenic and radioactive compounds such as polonium (Ruppert, 1999). Some of them have the mistaken belief that cigars, clove cigarettes, or chewing tobacco are healthy alternatives to cigarettes. The statistics on youth tobacco use are deeply disturbing, given the addictive potential of nicotine. Adolescent smoking is a powerful predictor of adult smoking (Chassin et al., 1996).

Approximately 70% of smokers do say they want to quit (Ruppert, 1999), but they cite many barriers to quitting: withdrawal symptoms, missing the companionship of cigarettes, less control of stress and moods, fear of weight gain, and lack of encouragement from family and friends. Some of the barriers can be dispelled by education. For example, new research shows that smoking does not relieve feelings of stress. In fact, it exacerbates stress (Parrott, 1999). Nevertheless, it is always a challenge to motivate a patient to stop smoking. James Prochaska and his research team have studied the stages of change in addictive behaviors (Prochaska, DiClemente, & Norcross, 1992). In working with a patient, it is helpful to use his model to assess the stage the patient is in. The Prochaska model is applied to smoking cessation in Table 16–3. Health professionals can promote client movement to subsequent stages by interventions that raise consciousness and increase self-efficacy. For example, adolescent girls who use smoking for weight control may be more inclined to consider cessation when they learn of its negative effects on the skin. Interventions to promote smoking cessation can be guided by the health belief model, as shown in Table 16–4. Lapses in abstinence are common, and clients must be encouraged to resume the strategies that initially helped them to quit. Successful quitters usually make several tries.

TABLE 16-3	Prochaska's Transtheoretical Model of Change Applied to Smoking Cessation
Stage 1: Precontemplation	Smokers do not see their smoking as a problem and do not intend to stop within the next 6 months.
Stage 2: Contemplation	Smokers see their smoking as a problem and think about quitting, but are not ready to change.
Stage 3: Preparation	Smokers intend to take action in the next month; some have made small changes, like cutting down on the number smoked or delaying the first smoke of the day.
Stage 4: Action	Smokers adopt a goal of smoking cessation and make an attempt to quit, involving overt behavior change and environmental modification.
Stage 5: Maintenance	Smokers work to prevent relapse and maintain abstinence.

Data from Prochaska, J. O., DiClemente, C. C., & Norcross, J. C. (1992). In search of how people change: Applications to addictive behaviors. *American Psychologist, 47,* 1102–1114.

Emotion Management. Appropriate management of *emotions* (particularly anger/hostility), interpersonal *conflict,* and *stress* has been recognized as essential to wellness for several decades, spurred by the research linking the angry, aggressively competitive Type A personality to coronary heart disease (Shoham et al., 1988). Anger is detrimental to health when it is too frequent, too intense, too prolonged, or managed ineffectively (i.e., by suppression, attacking another, or somatization). For example, suppressed anger is associated with higher blood pressure and eventual development of hypertension (Perini, Muller, & Buhler, 1991; Thomas, 1997b). Research by immunologists shows that intensely hostile interactions, such as arguments with a spouse, lower one's immunocompetence (Kiecolt-Glaser et al., 1993). The health-promoting way of managing anger is to wait until the initial physiological arousal abates, then discuss the anger-provoking incident with the provocateur or a confidant, and finally, take constructive action to resolve the problem. Persons who regularly discuss their anger in this way have lower blood pressure and better health (Thomas, 1997c). Health promotion efforts by

TABLE 16-4	Application of Health Belief Model in Interventions to Promote Smoking Cessation	
Factors	**Interventions**	
Perceived susceptibility	Teach about morbidity and mortality statistics of smokers versus nonsmokers.	
Perceived severity	Illustrate what happens to lungs and other organs when smoking; show pictures of diseased lungs, wrinkled skin.	
Perceived barriers	Identify barriers unique to the individual and counsel regarding common fears about weight gain, greater stress, and irritability.	
Perceived benefits	Identify benefits, such as more pleasant breath and body odor, increased energy, decreased cough, improved circulation, enhanced ability to taste, reduced risk of heart disease, stroke, and cancers of the mouth, throat, esophagus, lungs, bladder, cervix.	
Cues to action	Use telephone calls and postcard reminders. Provide pamphlets about cessation strategies. Organize support groups and buddy systems.	

nurses should include instruction about healthy anger management.

Problem Solving. *Problem-solving skills* must be taught to patients who do not know systematic strategies and techniques for enacting healthful habits or making changes in health behavior. For example, recovering alcoholics need to learn ways to slowly sip on nonalcoholic beverages at a party; dieters must practice polite refusal of foods at a family gathering. Middle school students may benefit from role-play of refusing illicit drugs at the skating rink. Individuals who lack assertiveness may need to rehearse firm requests for sex partners to use condoms. Assertiveness can also empower underserved groups to request needed community services or assistance from other members of the health care team. When giving exercise or diet prescriptions to patients, health care providers should ask what problems or barriers they envision; this will point the way to the skills they need to be taught.

Evidence-Based Interventions to Promote Behavior Change. Health professionals often use threats of future disease when urging behavior change. However, when people are frightened, they use denial to convince themselves that the threatening event (such as HIV/AIDS or cancer) is not likely to happen to them. Research shows that such threats of distant adverse outcomes are not as likely to be successful as motivational approaches that confer immediate benefits and rewards or reduce denial (Eitel & Friend, 1999). Even small changes may increase quality of life. Overweight women who lose as little as 5 lb handle everyday activities more easily and have fewer aches and pains (Fine et al., 1999).

A *health risk appraisal* (HRA) is a tool that can be used to provide clients with an estimate of biological age versus chronological age, an assessment of risk factors that may lead to health problems, and specific recommendations for behavioral changes that may lengthen their lives. A variety of computerized HRA instru-

ments are available, as well as paper-and-pencil versions of the tests. Some health risk appraisal tools are limited in scope, focusing only on a specific area, such as risk for coronary heart disease. Others assess broad areas, including the environment, education, stress, family history, and health behavior. These surveys are often administered during health fairs at community centers and shopping malls. A health risk appraisal instrument is best used in conjunction with laboratory tests (e.g., cholesterol, triglycerides) and the on-site measurement of some variables by professionals (e.g., blood pressure, triceps skin-fold thickness). Nurses should bear in mind that the accuracy of mortality predictions by health risk appraisals has been called into question. There could be adverse effects of informing persons that they have a shortened life expectancy (Weiss, 1984). Individuals who are given the results of their risk assessment along with a supportive educational process benefit more than persons who simply receive the test results.

The selection of incremental, achievable goals is also essential, as clients can be overwhelmed by the prospect of drastic changes, such as sweeping dietary modifications. Nurse practitioner Lynda Carpenito asks obese clients if they want to lose weight and, if the answer is affirmative, asks, "How much?" The client's goal becomes her goal. Then, with the client, two or three areas are chosen to work on (e.g., eating breakfast cereal each day, replacing bologna with low-fat/low-salt chicken or tuna) (Carpenito, 1998). Such an approach is far more likely to result in compliance than stringent calorie restriction. Clients should be taught that slow weight loss is preferable to rapid loss from fad diets (e.g., the low-carb diet), which can produce ketosis, gout, and other adverse consequences.

When health care providers write *prescriptions* for exercise or diet, adherence improves. In one recent randomized clinical trial, sedentary people either received verbal advice or written prescriptions (in addition to the verbal advice) about increasing physical activity. People in the group receiving written prescriptions were significantly more likely to increase their level of exercise (Swinburn et al., 1998). A strategy with proven effectiveness is *contracting*. The purpose of writing a contract is to arrange a favorable, positively reinforcing experience when the patient performs the desirable health behavior. Elements of a good contract are depicted in Table 16–5. A sample contract for weight loss appears in Figure 16–3.

Achieving an extra decade of life may be a significant motivator of healthful habits for some individuals. According to longitudinal studies of more than 360,000 patients, people who don't smoke and maintain low cholesterol (200 mg or below) and blood pressure (120/80 or less) can live up to 9½ years longer than those less careful about their health (Stamler et al., 1999). Death from cardiovascular disease, and from all other causes, was substantially reduced among adults with this desirable risk profile.

ENVIRONMENTAL FACTORS THAT AFFECT WELLNESS

Nurses must look beyond individual capabilities in our quest to help patients become healthier. The range of health-promoting choices available to individuals may be drastically limited by societal forces, structures, and policies (Butterfield, 1990). As depicted in Figure 16–1, numerous environmental factors affect wellness.

Culture. The cultural milieu in which a person develops and resides has a profound influence. In successful health promotion initiatives, the help of cultural insiders is solicited so that professionals can be aware of cultural norms and traditions before interventions are developed. Customs, laws, novels, films, television, and other cultural forces shape ideas about health and how to achieve it. It is culture that determines whether we think healthful body movement should take the form of tai chi or jogging, whether aging should involve accepting wrinkles or having face lifts. Culture can also convey conflicting messages. Paradoxically, Americans are saturated with media images of toned, sleek bodies, while fast-food restaurants beckon at every intersection. A visitor from another planet, confronted with our highly health-conscious but overweight, sedentary population, might conclude that most Americans have a death wish.

Environmental Influences. Many people are exposed to noxious substances or stimuli in the workplace. Asbestos, radiation, and toxic chemicals are just a few of the hazards workers en-

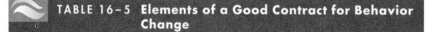

TABLE 16–5 Elements of a Good Contract for Behavior Change

- The behavior must be carefully selected and explicitly *described*.
- The behavior must be *measurable* (number of cigarettes smoked, minutes of exercise).
- A *data collection plan* must be developed (calendar, log, chart, graph, or diary).
- Client and nurse agree on the *goals* (short-term and long-term) and *time frame*.
- Client and nurse agree on the *reinforcers* (extrinsic and intrinsic).
- Reinforcers are specified for step-by-step *approximations* of the desired behavior.
- Client and nurse sign the *written contract*, and both keep a copy.
- Client and nurse evaluate *effectiveness* of the plan.
- The plan is *revised* as needed.

Desired outcome: Weight loss of 10 lb.
Long-term goal: To lose 2½ lb per week for 4 weeks.
Short-term goals: 1. Maintain 1,200 calorie/day diet.
                          2. Increase water consumption to eight glasses per day.
                          3. Avoid skipping meals.
                          4. Ride exercise machine:
                             Week 1: 15 minutes 3 times per week
                             Week 2: 20 minutes 3 times per week.
                             Week 3: 25 minutes 3 times per week.
                             Week 4: 30 minutes 3 times per week.
                          5. Weigh self on Monday mornings. Record weight on flow sheet.

Intrinsic rewards: Increased self-esteem and confidence.
                          Clothes fit better.
                          Improved physical fitness and appearance.

Extrinsic rewards: Upon successful completion of each day's regimen, a 20-minute bubble bath.
                          At end of each week, movie with a friend.
                          At end of contract, purchase of a new outfit.

Signature of nurse _____ Signature of patient _____ Date _____

FIGURE 16–3 Example of a health behavior change contract.

counter. Racist or sexist discrimination on the job may present a health hazard equivalent to (or even greater than) the factors that customarily receive more attention from researchers, such as excessive workplace noise or rotating shifts. Many Americans reside in substandard housing in neighborhoods where violence is commonplace. Many lack the security provided by a close-knit community of solicitous neighbors. They may have limited coping resources to withstand the daily bombardment of stressful events and hassles.

Stress. What happens when the environment bombards individuals with stressors? Researchers now know that *stress* is not simply a physiological reaction to environmental stimuli, as conceptualized by Selye (1956), but a psychological appraisal that the environmental demands exceed one's coping resources (Lazarus, 1991).

Early stress research focused on major life events such as foreclosure of a mortgage, bereavement, divorce, or job loss, demonstrating that an accumulation of such events could be detrimental to health (Holmes & Rahe, 1967). While these major life events are undoubtedly disruptive, minor daily hassles such as traffic jams and rude salespersons tax one's frustration tolerance as well (Kanner et al., 1981). Research on women has identified another type of stress, "vicarious stress," in which the misfortunes of loved ones add to a woman's psychological burden (Thomas & Donnellan, 1993). The added burden of worries about a friend's divorce or a grandson's illness may account for the consistency of research reports showing that women are more stressed than men across the life span (Davis, Matthews, & Twamley, 1999; Thomas, Shoffner, & Groer, 1988; Verbrugge, 1990). High stress can undermine enactment of health-promoting behavior. For example, during weeks with a high frequency of stressful events, people tend to exercise fewer days and for less time (Stetson et al., 1997).

Information about stress management is widely available, but the effectiveness of an individual's response to stressors depends on emotional well-being, physical status, personal history, and genetic vulnerabilities (Cohen & Herbert, 1996). One nurse researcher has proposed that individuals may emerge from stress states not demoralized and vulnerable, but healthier and stronger because they have mastered the challenges (Younger, 1991). However, health care providers must, once again, keep the environmental context in mind. Individuals in highly stressful environments may choose health-damaging behaviors to help them cope. One study showed that British working-class mothers smoked in full knowledge of the deleterious consequences because smoking was one of the few coping strategies available to them (Graham, 1984). Nearly one of every eight Americans lives in conditions of poverty, with an income below the federal poverty level (U.S. Public Health Service [USPHS], 1990). People living in poverty are not likely to perceive that they can master stress. In fact, when poverty is chronic and resources scant, individuals are likely to have pervasive powerlessness and a fatalistic outlook.

Social Support. Loving relationships with significant others may buffer or moderate stress. Connectedness to others is a central element in health throughout life. There is considerable empirical evidence that *social support* produces improved resistance to disease. Support from one's relatives and friends can include concrete material help, such as money and provision of information, as well as affirmation of self-worth and encouragement to maintain hope for a positive outcome of medical treatments. Extrafamilial support groups and health professionals can also play a vital role in encouraging exercise, smoking cessation, dieting, and other health-promoting actions. Stigmatized and marginalized client populations may lack a supportive network. Mobilizing social support can be an essential nursing intervention in such cases.

National Health Promotion Goals

Nurses' health promotion efforts must be undergirded and guided by an adequate understanding of U.S. public policy. The *Healthy People* documents published in 1979, 1990, and 2000 by the Public Health Service, U.S. Department of Health and Human Services, have focused on both individual and societal influences on health. These widely disseminated publications have drawn attention to health disparities among Americans and provided guidance to state and local planners of public health programs. Health promotion and disease prevention objectives are precisely stated and measurable. For example, a typical objective from *Healthy People 2000* was "increase to at least 50% the proportion of children and adolescents in 1st through 12th grade who participate in daily school physical education" (USPHS, 1990, p. 92). The precisely delineated objectives in the *Healthy People* documents have enabled measurement of the nation's progress.

The *Healthy People 2000 Review* showed considerable progress in reaching more than half of the nation's 300 objectives for the final decade of the 20th century (USPHS, 1999). For example, outbreaks of waterborne diseases and foodborne infections were reduced. Some objectives, such as the reduction of infant mortality, were only a slight fraction away from their targets. However, the report showed that movement was going in the *wrong* direction for one-fifth of the objectives. Notably, there has been little improvement in reducing the number of overweight individuals. As a corollary, the incidence, prevalence, complications, and mortality of diabetes are on the rise. Other disturbing trends include an increase in heavy drinking by high school seniors and increased deaths from falls and motor vehicle crashes (USPHS, 1999).

In *Healthy People 2010,* 467 objectives in 28 focus areas are proposed for the first decade of the new century. Many objectives focus on interventions to reduce illness, disability, and premature mortality, while others focus on strengthening public health services and improving dissemination of health-related information. As an example of the latter type of objective, comprehensive school health education is proposed for the prevention of adolescent violence, suicide, unintentional injury, and the use of tobacco, alcohol, and other drugs (USPHS, 2000). As in previous documents, each objective has a target for improvements to be achieved by the year 2010. Selected objectives and their targets are shown in Table 16–6.

Community Health Promotion

Increasingly, health professionals are collaborating with community leaders to design interventions such as youth activity programs, nutrition classes, school-based clinics, and health screenings. *Community health* is difficult to define, but it is more than the sum of the health states of individual members (Pender, 1996). Among the indicators of a community's health are communication patterns, ability to take organized action, level of social functioning (work and school attendance), proportion of individuals at the poverty level, crime rates, and traditional morbidity and mortality statistics. One type of community intervention has focused on improving the cardiovascular health status of entire communities. Examples include the Stanford Five City Project, the Pawtucket Heart Health

TABLE 16–6 Selected Examples of National Health Promotion Objectives as Identified in *Healthy People 2010*

Focus Area	Goal	Objective	Target
15. Injury and violence prevention	Reduce disabilities, injuries, and deaths due to unintentional injuries and violence	15-15. Reduce deaths caused by motor vehicle crashes	By 2010: 9 deaths per 100,000 (reduced from 15.8)
19. Nutrition and overweight	Promote health and reduce chronic disease associated with diet and weight	19-3c. Reduce the proportion of children and adolescents who are overweight or obese	By 2010: 5% overweight or obese children and adolescents ages 6–19 years (reduced from 11%)
25. Sexually transmitted diseases	Promote responsible sexual behaviors, strengthen community capacity, and increase access to quality services to prevent sexually transmitted diseases (STDs) and their complications	25-11. Increase the proportion of adolescents who abstain from sexual intercourse or use condoms if sexually active	By 2010: 95% of adolescents in grades 9–12 (increased from 85%)

Program, and the Minnesota Heart Health Program (National Heart, Lung, and Blood Institute, 1990). These programs attempt to reduce risk factors such as obesity, hypertension, smoking, sedentary lifestyles, and serum cholesterol levels. Community members become involved in media campaigns. Distinct programs are set up for different groups within the community. Points of contact with community residents include churches, stores, schools, and work sites. The results of these programs are varied. Benefits have been reduced tobacco use, lessened weight gain, lowered blood pressure, reduced cholesterol levels, and lowered coronary heart disease risks in general (Mittelmark et al., 1993; Salonen et al., 1989). In the Minnesota Heart Health Program, however, there were no differences in cholesterol levels, blood pressure, smoking, and exercise between communities that received health promotion interventions and communities that did not.

A second type of community program is the Healthy Cities initiatives, first developed in Canada and Europe. The first site in the United States, the Indiana Healthy Community Project, was developed by a nurse (Flynn, Rider, & Bailey, 1992). Rather than focusing on a predetermined health problem such as cardiovascular risk, the Healthy Cities initiatives address a broad range of concerns that are identified by community members, such as gang violence and job creation. Coalitions of community groups are formed to develop programming. The California Healthy Cities Project (1994) has initiated programs on environmental protection, healthy behavior, and economic development.

Both the Healthy Cities initiatives and the community-wide cardiovascular risk reduction programs are examples of aiming interventions at entire communities. Another type of programming considers members of a health maintenance organization (HMO) as a community. When managed care became a dominant form of health care delivery in the United States, there was great impetus to develop brief, low-cost interventions that could be delivered in natural settings, such as the primary care clinics visited by members of HMOs. Curry, Ludman, and Wagner (1996) developed a useful model for health behavior change in a managed care setting, specifically the Group Health Cooperative of Puget Sound in Seattle, which has 400,000 members. Interventions take place at multiple levels. At the level of the organization, activities include developing consensus on the health behavior targets, careful planning, and allocation of resources. At the practice level, roles are developed for all members of the practice team. At the individual level, client motivation and readiness to change are addressed. Also included in the model are client teaching (via group classes and self-help materials), telephone counseling, support, and follow-up.

This model was successfully implemented, first targeting tobacco use. At the individual level, the HMO offered a comprehensive stop-smoking program called Free and Clear. At the practice level, all primary care providers were given the protocol of the National Cancer Institute ("Ask, Advise, Assist, and Arrange"). Use of the protocol was encouraged through repeated workshops. Chart audits monitored provider implementation. Finally, at the organizational level decisions were made to provide coverage for both the Free and Clear program and nicotine replacement therapy. The HMO joined in community efforts to defeat a smoker's rights bill in the state legislature and to convince the *Seattle Times* to stop accepting tobacco advertisements. The result? Smoking prevalence among the HMO's adult members dropped from 25% to 17%. The model is presently being used for other targeted behavior changes such as cancer screening and diet modification (Curry et al., 1996).

Canadian researchers are studying the role of the family as an intermediary between community health promotion programs and subsequent changes in family members' risk behaviors. In the Quebec Heart Health Demonstration Project, four types of families (balanced, traditional, disconnected, and emotionally strained) were examined. Balanced families (characterized by a balance between focus on interior of the family and presence in the extrafamilial world) scored highest of the four types on valuing of health and were predicted to be more responsive to community health promotion programming (Fisher et al., 1998). Yet to be determined are ways to increase responsiveness of the more poorly functioning families. The greatest challenge of health promotion for the 21st century may be reaching the more vulnerable and disenfranchised members of our society and involving them in strategies to enhance and prolong their lives.

KEY POINTS

● Conceptualizing health more broadly than "the absence of disease" has significant implications for nursing practice.

● Health promotion and disease prevention have different foci, in that health promotion activities aim to take people beyond their present level of wellness, while disease prevention efforts are undertaken to prevent specific diseases.

● The major causes of death in the United States are related to lifestyle.

● A comprehensive model of wellness includes modifiable attitudinal and behavioral variables as well as environmental factors and nonmodifiable organismic characteristics.

● The Health Belief Model, Pender's Health Promotion Model, and Cox's Interaction Model of Client Health Behavior are useful in guiding health promotion research and practice.

● Prochaska's transtheoretical model can be used to assess client readiness to change health behavior.

● Motivational interventions are more likely to promote health behavior change than threats of future disease or distant adverse outcomes.

● Health care providers should make greater use of written prescriptions, contracting, and other evidence-based interventions.

● Nurses' health promotion efforts should be guided by national health promotion goals, such as those articulated in *Healthy People 2010*.

● Health promotion initiatives must target families and communities as well as individuals.

CRITICAL THINKING EXERCISES

1. Interview three persons regarding their definition of health. Compare their definition to the various theories and models presented in the chapter.

2. Assess your own health behavior, then select a behavior that you desire to change. It can be something that you wish to *increase* (e.g., aerobic exercise, meditation, flossing teeth), *decrease* (e.g., eating junk food), or *stop* (e.g., smoking, nail-biting). Develop a plan to change the behavior, then implement the plan for 1 month. Critically assess factors that facilitated or hindered achievement of your behavior change.

3. Select one detrimental health behavior, such as excessive drinking. Review the research literature regarding interventions to change this behavior. Identify gaps in this literature. For example, is it clear which interventions are most effective? Is there sufficient information about changing the behavior in women? In various ethnic and minority groups? In persons of diverse ages, sexual orientation, and socioeconomic status? Develop at least three questions for future research.

REFERENCES

Antonovsky, A. (1984). The sense of coherence as a determinant of health. In J. D. Matarazzo, S. M. Weiss, J. A. Herd, N.E. Miller, & S. M. Weiss (Eds.), *Behavioral health: A handbook of health enhancement and disease prevention* (pp. 114–129). New York: Wiley.

Bandura, A. (1986). *Social foundations of thought and action: A social cognitive theory.* Englewood Cliffs, NJ: Prentice-Hall.

Becker, M. H., Haefner, D. P., Kasl, S. V., Kirscht, J. P., Maiman, L. A., & Rosenstock, I. M. (1977). Selected psychosocial models and correlates of individual health-related behaviors. *Medical Care, 15* (5), 27–46.

Belloc, N. B., & Breslow, L. (1972). Relationship of physical health status and health practices. *Preventive Medicine, 1,* 409–421.

Berk, L., Tan, S., Fry, W., Napier, B., Lee, J., Hubbard, R., Lewis, J., & Eby, W. (1989). Neuroendocrine and stress hormone changes during mirthful laughter. *The American Journal of the Medical Sciences, 289,* 390–396.

Breslow, L., & Enstrom, J. E. (1980). Persistence of health habits and their relationship to mortality. *Preventive Medicine, 9,* 469–483.

Brundtland, G. H. (1999). The neglected epidemic. *American Journal of Nursing, 99*(11), 9.

Butterfield, P. G. (1990). Thinking upstream: Nurturing a conceptual understanding of the societal context of health behavior. *Advances in Nursing Science, 12*(2), 1–8.

California Healthy Cities Project (1994). *Connections, 6*(2), 1–5.

Carpenito, L. J. (1998). When clients teach me about noncompliance. *Nursing Forum, 33*(1), 3–4.

Carter, K. F., & Kulbok, P. A. (1995). Evaluation of the Interaction Model of Client Health Behavior through the first decade of research. *Advances in Nursing Science, 18* (1), 62–73.

Centers for Disease Control and Prevention. (1996). Tobacco use and usual source of cigarettes among high school students—United States, 1995. *Morbidity and Mortality Weekly Report, 45,* 413–418.

Chassin, L., Presson, C. C., Rose, J. S., & Sherman, S. J. (1996). The natural history of cigarette smoking from adolescence to adulthood: Demographic predictors of continuity and change. *Health Psychology, 15,* 478–484.

Cohen, S., & Herbert, T. B. (1996). Health psychology: Psychological factors and physical disease from the perspective of human psychoneuroimmunology. *Annual Review of Psychology, 47,* 113–142.

Cox, C. L. (1982). An interaction model of client health behavior: Theoretical prescription for nursing. *Advances in Nursing Science, 5*(1), 41–56.

Cox, C. L. (1986). The interaction model of client health behavior: Application to the study of community-based elders. *Advances in Nursing Science, 9*(1), 40–57.

Curry, S. J., Ludman, E., & Wagner, E. H. (1996, Summer). A model for health behavior change in managed care. *Outlook: Newsletter of the Society of Behavioral Medicine,* 5–6.

Davis, M. C., Matthews, K. A., & Twamley, E. W. (1999). Is life more difficult on Mars or Venus? A meta-analytic review of sex differences in major and minor life events. *Annals of Behavioral Medicine, 21*(1), 83–97.

Dillon, K., Minchoff, B., & Baker, K. (1985). Positive emotional states and enhancement of the immune system. *International Journal of Psychiatry in Medicine, 15*(1), 13–17.

Dubos, R. (1965). *Man adapting.* New Haven, CT: Yale University Press.

Dunn, H. (1959). High level wellness for man and society. *American Journal of Public Health, 49,* 88.

Dunn, H. (1971). *High level wellness.* Arlington, VA: Beatty.

Eitel, P., & Friend, R. (1999). Reducing denial and sexual risk behaviors in college students: Comparison of a cognitive and a motivational approach. *Annals of Behavioral Medicine, 21*(1), 12–19.

Fine, J. T., Colditz, G. A., Coakley, E. H., Moseley, G., Manson, J. E., Willett, W. C., & Kawachi, I. (1999). A prospective study of weight change and health-related quality of life in women. *Journal of the American Medical Association, 282,* 2136–2142.

Fisher, L., Soubhi, H., Mansi, O., Paradis, G., Gauvin, L., & Potvin, L. (1988). Family process in health research: Extending a family typology to a new cultural context. *Health Psychology, 17,* 358–366.

Flynn, B. C., Rider, M. S., & Bailey, W. W. (1992). Developing community leadership in healthy cities: The Indiana model. *Nursing Outlook, 49*(3), 121–126.

Gadamer, H. G. (1996). *The enigma of health: The art of healing in a scientific age* (F. Gaiger & N. Walker, Trans.). Stanford, CA: Stanford University Press.

Gauvin, L., Rejeski, W. J., & Norris, J. L. (1996). A naturalistic study of the impact of acute physical activity on feeling states and affect in women. *Health Psychology, 15,* 391–397.

Gerrard, M., Gibbons, F., Benthin, A., & Hessling, R. (1996). A longitudinal study of the reciprocal nature of risk behaviors and cognitions in adolescents: What you do shapes what you think, and vice versa. *Health Psychology, 15,* 344–354.

Graham, H. (1984). *Women, health, and family.* Brighton, England: Harvester Press.

Hochbaum, G. M. (1958). *Public participation in medical screening programs: A sociopsychological study.* U.S. Public Health Service Publication No. 572. Washington, DC: U.S. Department of Health and Human Services.

Hollis, J. F., Lichtenstein, E., Vogt, T. M., Stevens, V. J., & Biglan, A. (1993). Nurse-assisted counseling for smokers in primary care. *Annals of Internal Medicine, 118,* 521–525.

Holmes, T. H., & Rahe, R. H. (1967). The Social Readjustment Rating Scale. *Journal of Psychosomatic Research, 11,* 213–218.

Janz, N. K., & Becker, M. H. (1984). The health belief model: A decade later. *Health Education Quarterly, 11* (1), 1–47.

Kanner, A., Coyne, J., Schaefer, C., & Lazarus, R. (1981). Comparison of two modes of stress measurement: Daily hassles and uplifts versus major life events. *Journal of Behavioral Medicine, 4,* 1–39.

Kaplan, D. (1997). When less is more. *Psychology Today, 30*(3), 14.

Kaplan, R., Anderson, J., & Wingard, D. (1991). Gender differences in health-related quality of life. *Health Psychology, 10,* 86–93.

Kennedy, K. D. (1995). Invest in yourself: Have a laugh! Have a healthy laugh! *Nursing Forum, 30*(1), 25–30.

Kiecolt-Glaser, J., Malarkey, W., Chee, M. A., Newton, T., Cacioppo, J., Mao, H., & Glaser, R. (1993). Negative behavior during marital conflict is associated with immunological down-regulation. *Psychosomatic Medicine, 55,* 395–409.

King, A. C., Kiernan, M., Oman, R., Kraemer, H. C., Hull, M., & Ahn, D. (1997). Can we identify who will adhere to long-term physical activity? Signal detection methodology as a potential aid to clinical decision-making. *Health Psychology, 16,* 380–389.

Kobasa, S. C. (1979). Stressful life events, personality and health: An inquiry into hardiness. *Journal of Personality and Social Psychology, 37,* 1–11.

Larson, D. B., Swyers, J. P., & McCullough, M. E. (1998). *Scientific research on spirituality and health.* Rockville, MD: National Institute for Healthcare Research.

Lazarus, R. (1991). *Emotion and adaptation.* New York: Oxford University Press.

Liebman, B. (1997, April). The changing American diet. *Nutrition Action Healthletter,* 8–9.

Lindell, K., & Reinke, L. F. (1999, March/April). Nursing strategies for smoking cessation. *The American Nurse, 31,* A2–A6.

Maslow, A. (1961). Health as transcendence of environment. *Journal of Humanistic Psychology, 1,* 1–7.

Mittelmark, M. B., Hunt, M. K., Heath, G. W., & Schmid, T. L. (1993). Realistic outcomes: Lessons from community-based research and demonstration programs for the prevention of cardiovascular diseases. *Journal of Public Health Policy, 14,* 437–461.

Mullen, K. (1990). Religion and health: A review of the literature. *International Journal of Sociology and Social Policy, 10*(1), 85–96.

National Heart, Lung, and Blood Institute. (1990). *Three community programs change heart health across the nation* [Special edition]. Infomemo.

Newman, M. (1978). *Toward a theory of health.* Paper presented at Nurse Educator Conference, New York, NY.

Newman, M. (1994). *Health as expanding consciousness* (2nd ed.). New York: National League for Nursing Press.

Orem, D. E. (1983). The self-care deficit theory of nursing: A general theory. In I. W. Clements & F. B.

Roberts (Eds.), *Family health: A theoretical approach to nursing care* (pp. 205–217). New York: Wiley.

Parrott, A. C. (1999). Does cigarette smoking *cause* stress? *American Psychologist, 54,* 817–820.

Pender, N. (1996). *Health promotion in nursing practice* (3rd ed.). Stamford, CT: Appleton & Lange.

Perini, C., Muller, F., & Buhler, F. (1991). Suppressed aggression accelerates early development of essential hypertension. *Journal of Hypertension, 9,* 499–503.

Prochaska, J. O., DiClemente, C. C., & Norcross, J. C. (1992). In search of how people change: Applications to addictive behaviors. *American Psychologist, 47,* 1102–1114.

Resnick, B., & Spellbring, A. M. (2000). Understanding what motivates older adults to exercise. *Journal of Gerontological Nursing, 26*(3), 34–42.

Rogers, M. (1970). *An introduction to the theoretical basis of nursing.* Philadelphia: Davis.

Rotter, J.B. (1954). *Social learning and clinical psychology.* Englewood Cliffs, NJ: Prentice-Hall.

Roy, C. (1970). Adaptation: A conceptual framework for nursing. *Nursing Outlook, 18*(3), 42–45.

Ruppert, R. A. (1999). The last smoke. *American Journal of Nursing, 99*(11), 26–32.

Salonen, J. T., Tuomilehto, J., Nissinen, A., Kaplan, G. A., & Puska, P. (1989). Contribution of risk factor changes to the decline in coronary incidence during the North Karelia project: A within community analysis. *International Journal of Epidemiology, 18,* 595–601.

Scheier, M., & Carver, C. (1985). Optimism, coping, and health: Assessment and implications of generalized outcome expectancies. *Health Psychology, 4,* 219–247.

Scheier, M., & Carver, C. (1992). Effects of optimism on psychological and physical well-being: Theoretical overview and empirical update. *Cognitive Therapy and Research, 16,* 201–228.

Selye, H. (1956). *The stress of life.* New York: McGraw-Hill.

Shoham, Y., Ragland, D. R., Brand, R. J., & Syme, S. L. (1988). Type A behavior pattern and health status after 22 years of follow-up in the Western Collaborative Group Study. *American Journal of Epidemiology, 128,* 579–588.

Smith, J. (1983). *The idea of health: Implications for the nursing profession.* New York: Teachers College Press.

Smuts, J. (1926). *Holism and evolution.* New York: Macmillan.

Stamler, J., Stamler, R., Neaton, J. D., Wentworth, D., Daviglus, M. L., Garside, D., Dyer, A. R., Liu, K., & Greenland, P. (1999). Low risk-factor profile and long-term cardiovascular and noncardiovascular mortality and life expectancy: Findings for 5 large cohorts of young adult and middle-aged men and women.

Journal of the American Medical Association, 282, 2012–2018.

Stetson, B. A., Rahn, J. M., Dubbert, P. M., Wilner, B. I., & Mercury, M. G. (1997). Prospective evaluation of the effects of stress on exercise adherence in community-residing women. *Health Psychology, 16,* 515–520.

Strack, S., Carver, C., & Blaney, P. (1987). Predicting successful completion of an aftercare program following treatment for alcoholism: The role of dispositional optimism. *Journal of Personality and Social Psychology, 53,* 579–584.

Swinburn, B. A., Walter, L. G., Arroll, B., Tilyard, M. W., & Russell, D. G. (1998). The green prescription study: A randomized controlled trial of written exercise advice provided by general practitioners. *American Journal of Public Health, 88,* 288–291.

Thomas, S. P. (1997a). Distressing aspects of women's roles, vicarious stress, and health consequences. *Issues in Mental Health Nursing, 18,* 539–557.

Thomas, S. P. (1997b). Women's anger: Relationship of suppression to blood pressure. *Nursing Research, 46,* 324–330.

Thomas, S. P. (1997c). Angry? Let's talk about it! *Applied Nursing Research, 10*(2), 80–85.

Thomas, S. P., & Donnellan, M. M. (1993). Stress, role responsibilities, social support, and anger. In S. Thomas (Ed.), *Women and anger* (pp. 112–128). New York: Springer.

Thomas, S. P., Shoffner, D., & Groer, M. (1988). Adolescent stress factors: Implications for the nurse practitioner. *The Nurse Practitioner: The American Journal of Primary Health Care, 12*(6), 20–29.

U.S. Department of Agriculture. (1997). *Food consumption, prices, and expenditures.* Washington, DC: U.S. Department of Agriculture.

U.S. Public Health Service. (1979). *Healthy people: Surgeon General's report on health promotion and disease prevention.* Washington, DC: U.S. Department of Health and Human Services.

U.S. Public Health Service. (1990). *Healthy people 2000.* Washington, DC: U.S. Department of Health and Human Services.

U.S. Public Health Service. (1999). *Healthy people 2000 review 1998–99.* Washington, DC: U.S. Department of Health and Human Services.

U.S. Public Health Service. (2000). *Healthy people 2010.* Washington, DC: U.S. Department of Health and Human Services [On-line]. Available: http://web.health.gov/healthypeople

Verbrugge, L. (1990). The twain meet: Empirical explanations of sex differences in health and mortality. In M. Ory & H. Warner (Eds.), *Gender, health, and longevity* (pp. 159–199). New York: Springer.

Wallston, K. A. (1989). Assessment of control in health care settings. In A. Steptoe & A. Appels (Eds.), *Stress, personal control, and health* (pp. 85–106). New York: Wiley.

Weiss, S. M. (1984). Health hazard-health risk appraisals. In J. D. Matarazzo, S. M. Weiss, J. A. Herd, N. E. Miller, & S. M. Weiss (Eds.), *Behavioral health: A handbook of health enhancement and disease prevention* (pp. 275–294). New York: Wiley.

Wiley, J. A., & Camacho, T. C. (1980). Life-style and future health: Evidence from the Alameda County study. *Preventive Medicine, 9,* 1–21.

Williams, R. L., Thomas, S. P., Young, D. O., Jozwiak, J. J., & Hector, M. A. (1991). Development of a health habits scale. *Research in Nursing and Health, 14,* 145–153.

Younger, J. (1991). A theory of mastery. *Advances in Nursing Science, 14,* 76–89.

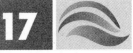

17

Complementary and Alternative Practices and Products: Components of Holistic Health Care

ANN GILL TAYLOR, EdD, RN, FAAN, VICTORIA MENZIES, EdM, MS, RN,
AND KATHLEEN BOYDEN, MSN, RN

OBJECTIVES

At the completion of this chapter, the reader should be able to:

- Identify complementary therapy as one component of an integrated health care system of the 21st century.
- Describe the frequency of use of complementary therapies in the United States.
- Discuss selected complementary therapies.
- Apply critical thinking to the application of complementary modalities in holistic health care.
- Cite considerations for the safe use of complementary therapies.
- Integrate the use of selected complementary therapies in nursing care.
- Develop a resource referral base for complementary therapy.

PROFILE IN PRACTICE

Victoria Menzies, RN, EdM, MSN
Doctoral Student
School of Nursing
University of Virginia
Charlottesville, Virginia

Graduating from a diploma school in Salina, Kansas, in 1969 and completing an MSN in psychiatric mental health nursing from the University of Virginia School of Nursing in Charlottesville, Virginia, in 2000 reveals part of my professional journey. My work experience began as an emergency department nurse. Then I became an ICU nurse, then a part-time private-duty nurse, and so gradually embarked on my current journey in complementary therapies. This part of my professional journey began the day I met a therapeutic touch practitioner in 1980. Twenty years later, I have practiced and taught a variety of complementary modalities. For 10 years, from 1987 to 1997, through private practice and a variety of courses, classes, workshops, and individual sessions in holistic lifestyle, I promoted complementary modalities, including a heart-healthy diet, the mind-body connection, meditation, therapeutic touch, and imagery techniques.

My experiences with a variety of imagery techniques along the way enhanced my skills and led to certification in interactive imagery modalities from the International Institute for Visualization Research and the Academy for Guided Imagery.

Additionally, the more I taught in adult education settings, participated in public speaking, and engaged in practice, the more I desired to become one of the researchers in complementary therapies whose work I was reading. This desire fostered my decision to pursue a PhD in nursing. Seeking a mentor who would support my interest in researching imagery as a nursing intervention led me to the University of Virginia, where my mentor/advisor is Ann Gill Taylor, EdD, RN, FAAN, founder and director of the Center for the Study of Complementary and Alternative Therapies. My professional goal is to blend teaching, research, and practice. Ultimately, I hope to contribute to the body of research literature on complementary and alternative practices and products.

A large percentage of persons worldwide are using complementary and alternative practices and products (CAPPs), also referred to as "complementary and alternative medicine" and "complementary and alternative therapies." However, these latter terms are not true descriptors in that the practices and products are not limited to medicine and the word "therapies" connotes "therapeutic," which has not been systematically documented through rigorous science for many of these practices and products. Despite some confusion in terminology, a significant percentage of the adult population in the United States (nearly 45% at the beginning of the new millennium) is trying a variety of these ancient and modern CAPPs to treat a variety of symptoms and conditions (Eisenberg, Kessler, Foster, et al., 1993; Eisenberg, Davis, Ettner, et al., 1998). These surveys indicate, too, that the American public is spending billions of dollars for CAPPs, most of which is not reimbursed by third-party payers.

In response to the increasing interest by the American people in the healing potential of CAPPs, in 1992 the federal government created

the Office of Alternative Medicine (elevated in 1999 to the National Center for Complementary and Alternative Medicine [NCCAM]). The mission of the NCCAM is to assure the American public, through rigorous research studies, that the widely used CAPPs do what the practitioners of these modalities and the manufacturers of these products claim. It is acknowledged today that anecdotes about the efficacy and effectiveness of practices for which there are not plausible explanations are insufficient, thereby giving importance to well-designed and well-executed research.

Practices and products categorized as complementary and alternative reflect a broad spectrum of modalities and beliefs. Consequently, what is defined as such varies, based on professional or occupational perspective. Among the early initiatives of the NCCAM was to identify broad categories of CAPPs as a first step toward classifying the more than 200 modalities, which are reported to have more than 10,000 uses. This categorization of CAPPs is shown in Table 17–1.

The term complementary medicine/therapies was introduced in the 1970s in the United

TABLE 17–1 Classification of Complementary and Alternative Practices and Products
Diet, nutrition, lifestyle changes
Mind/body control
Alternative systems of medical practice
Manual healing
Pharmacological and biological treatments
Bioelectromagnetic applications
Herbal medicine

Kingdom and refers to those practices and products that link the most appropriate therapies to the individual's physical, mental, emotional, and spiritual needs. In some cultures, "alternative" refers to those practices and products that are provided in place of conventional health care, many of which are outside the realm of accepted health care theory and practices in the United States.

Some nurse theorists and researchers believe that the terms "complementary," "unproven," "nontraditional," "unorthodox," and "alternative" are judgmental and in conflict with nurses' history and tradition of providing noninvasive, naturalistic therapies to the sick, in particular. Most nurses do not consider modalities such as those related to holistic health, caring, comfort, pain reduction or relief, and other symptom management as alternative to anything. Many of these practices, such as massage, are ones that nurses have provided over the years and are foundational to caring, compassionate, holistic nursing care. Some outside of nursing suggest that the definition of CAPPs is an evolving one that will change as more research-based evidence is made available and the field becomes better understood (Spencer, 1999).

Of importance to the practice of nursing and to nursing research are the phenomena of comfort; patient-centered, relationship-focused care; autonomy; and individual psychosocial differences. These phenomena have direct relationships to reasons persons seek out CAPPs (Box 17–1). Thus, learning about individual differences (including positive affect, negative affect, self-regulation, and coping styles) and the effects of these differences on the use of CAPPs is important to both practicing nurses and nurse researchers. Research has shown that the personality traits of individuals may facilitate the capacity to benefit from selected CAPPs (Owens, Taylor, & DeGood, 1999).

A few CAPPs have been studied sufficiently to provide conclusive evidence of effectiveness. For example, there are data to support a number of behavioral and relaxation practices used to treat pain and insomnia. However, data currently available are insufficient to show definitively that one practice or procedure is more effective than another for a given condition. Yet, because of psychosocial differences among persons, one procedure or product may be more suited than another for a given person National Institutes of Health [NIH], 1995).

Box 17–1 Reasons Persons Seek Out CAPPs

Complementary and alternative therapies foster:

- Sense of well-being
- Sense of control and self-efficacy
- Healing the person rather than curing the disease
- Partnership in which patient is active participant

Box 17–2 NCCAM Information Resources Available on CAPPs

NCCAM web site: http://nccam.nih.gov

NCCAM Clearinghouse

P. O. Box 8218

Silver Spring, MD 20907-8218

Tel.: 1-888-644-6226

   (toll-free, TTY/TDY, and fax-on-demand)

Fax: 1-301-495-4957

E-mail: nccamc@altmedinfo.org

The challenge today for health care professionals is to become informed about the indications for and contraindications to use of the myriad procedures and products that their patients are using, including the potential interactions of natural products with pharmaceuticals, foods, and lifestyles. A movement to offer some content about CAPPs in nursing, medicine, and pharmacy curricula is evident. However, at the National Conference on Medical and Nursing Education in Complementary Medicine held in June 1999 it became apparent that there is less agreement among faculty on the practical aspects of its integration. The NCCAM has recently focused on introducing CAPPs information into allopathic, osteopathic, nursing, dental, and pharmacy schools to capture the attention of young health professionals.

This chapter provides an overview of selected CAPPs to illustrate the diversity of practices and products the American public is using and to delineate the evidence-based information available. No attempt has been made to be exhaustive in this review of CAPPs. The discussion addresses some topics more than others, highlighting those CAPPs we judge to be more relevant to nursing practice than others. This sampling of CAPPs should contribute to nurses' desire to explore the field more extensively through the resources shown in Box 17–2.

Nutrition and Diet, Exercise, and Lifestyle Changes

Nutrition and diet, exercise, and lifestyle changes are not commonly thought of as CAPPs. However, the nursing profession has long recognized their benefits in a wide variety of health problems, including wound healing, reducing the effects of chronic illness, and improving overall health (Nightingale, 1859/1969; Whorton, 1999). In general, practices and products in this category are aimed at illness prevention and health promotion. The goals are to identify and treat risk factors or to support the healing and recovery process.

LIFESTYLE CHANGES

Healthy lifestyle choices contribute to one's well-being. Changes in lifestyle are intended to prevent disease and the development of illness. Lifestyle choices includes behavioral changes, dietary changes, exercise, and stress management. Some experts suggest that to be classified as a CAPP, a change in lifestyle must be based on a nontraditional system of medicine, applied in an unconventional way or used according to a non-Western approach. However, this distinction is unimportant. The point is that whatever these changes are called, as people integrate beneficial changes into their lives, the better they will manage their overall health (Jonas & Levin, 1999; McCamy & Presley, 1975; Orme-Johnson, 1997; Ornish et al., 1998).

EXERCISE

Sufficient exercise is essential to a healthy lifestyle. Historically, nurses have understood this, including Florence Nightingale, who pointed out the importance of exercise in improving and maintaining health (Nightingale, 1859/1969). Today, the health benefits of exercise for the immune system are well documented (Eliopoulos, 1999). Exercise is commonly prescribed by conventional and CAPP practitioners for health promotion and disease prevention. For example, in Ayurvedic medicine, which is based on a definition of health as a balance between mind, body, and soul, vigorous exercise and yoga stretching is encouraged to improve circulation, stimulate metabolism, and sharpen the mind (Goldberg, 1999). Conventional health care providers have prescribed integration of exercise according to the level of fitness and ability for many years. In chronic conditions such as type II diabetes mellitus, prostate disease, HIV/AIDS, osteoporosis, depression, and many others, research has suggested a beneficial effect of exercise on well-being (MacIntyre & Holzemer, 1997; McCarty, 1997; Moore & Blumenthal, 1998; Moyad, 1999).

DIET AND NUTRITION

Knowledge of disease prevention and health maintenance through nutrition continues to grow, but there is a paucity of funds and research to follow up promising initial results. For applications such as reversing chronic disease through nutritional intervention or determining levels of nutrients needed for optimal metabolic or immune function, there is typically a delay of several years or decades from initial results to widespread acceptance. For this reason, in 1994 the NCCAM identified "diet and nutrition in the prevention and treatment of chronic disease" as an important area of research (NIH, 1994).

The usual North American diet, high in animal fat and sugar, provides poor nutrition. The federal government's approach to dietary intervention, known as the Food Guide Pyramid, is intended to affect health through diet and nutrition by manipulating the typical diet so that foods with low nutritional value are eaten less and foods with more nutritional value are eaten more. However, this is only one approach to promoting health and preventing illness through dietary intervention. An array of alternative approaches, ranging from supplementation with vitamins and minerals to drastic dietary modification, either eliminating or adding certain types of foods or macronutrients to treat or prevent specific chronic diseases, represents a continuum of philosophies. The federal government's Food Guide Pyramid has been challenged by some in the medical profession, who believe that the recommendations fall far short of providing adequate nutrition and protection against cancer and cardiovascular disease (NIH, 1994; Ornish et al., 1998). The focus of the vast majority of these approaches is on eating more freshly prepared vegetables, fruits, whole grains, and legumes (NIH, 1994).

Specific vitamin, mineral, and food supplements added to the Western diet can have both preventative and therapeutic effects. In some cases, the prescribed amount of a supplement can exceed the recommended daily allowances (RDA). RDAs are defined as the average daily amounts of essential nutrients estimated, on the basis of available scientific knowledge, as adequate to meet the physiological needs of practically all healthy persons (Monsen, 1990). Many health advocates and practitioners believe that today's RDAs are not adequate for the daily stresses and environmental insults to which people are exposed (NIH, 1994), and that higher minimum levels must be ingested to ensure good immune functioning and maximum health status (Eliopoulos, 1999). The concepts of vitamin deficiency diseases and the RDAs have not kept pace with the growing understanding of the cellular and molecular functions of vitamins and other micronutrients. The distinction between nutritional and pharmacological doses of vitamins is meaningless, as high doses of micronutrients may be required to achieve normal metabolic processes in some people or in some conditions (Challem, 1999).

Several conditions have been identified to require more than the RDAs. For example, megadoses of folic acid are believed to prevent neural tube defects in newborns (Czeizel & Dudas, 1992), as well as to prevent complications in cardiovascular disease (Stampfer & Rimm, 1996).

The diet and nutrition category also includes food-elimination diets to modify hyperactivity disorders in children and the systemic symptoms associated with food allergies and food intolerance (Chez & Jonas, 1997). Alternative diets can also be a component of lifestyle programs to enhance wellness and minimize illness. Examples include vegetarianism, macrobiotics, and lifestyle-diet programs such as the Ornish Plan for reversing coronary heart disease and reducing cancer (Ornish et al., 1990, 1998). While we have learned much about diet and nutrition, the full extent of the effects of food additives, genetic engineering, soil depletion, pesticides, fungicides, and other crop sprays on the North American diet have yet to be studied.

NUTRITIONAL SUPPLEMENTS

The nutritional supplement industry is a multibillion-dollar industry in this country. This includes the use of foods, vitamins, and other nutritional supplements to promote health. Recently the U.S. Food and Drug Administration (FDA) issued a statement proposing guidelines to make claims for dietary supplements more informative, reliable, and uniform (U.S. Department of Health and Human Services

[USDHHS], 1998). The recommendations of experts such as Weil (1995), Murray (1996), and Graedon and Graedon (1999) can serve as reference.

Vitamin Supplements. There is a long history of vitamin and other nutritional supplements in the promotion of health and the prevention of disease. Today, evidence is mounting for the beneficial role of specific nutrients, including vitamins B_6, C, and E; beta-carotene and other carotenes; folic acid; calcium; and magnesium (NIH, 1994).

Vitamins and minerals are not harmful when consumed in the RDA (McEvoy, 1997; Reynolds, 1996); however, some supplements can cause serious adverse effects when taken in megadoses (Jonas & Levin, 1999). The adverse effects of many vitamin and mineral supplements are fully reviewed in Jonas and Levin (1999). The adverse effects of selected vitamins and minerals are shown in Table 17–2.

An association between vitamin and mineral supplementation and a decreased risk of cancer has long been suspected, but the data are not conclusive. Only modest evidence of the protective effects of nutritional supplementation with vitamins and minerals has been seen in numerous studies (Patterson et al., 1997). Multiple methodological problems in studies assessing the relationship between cancer risk and supplement use have been noted. Further rigorous studies are needed.

Shark Cartilage. Shark cartilage is categorized as a dietary supplement. Its use as a cancer treatment is based on the idea that sharks rarely get cancer due to special protective properties of the shark's cartilage (Jonas & Levin, 1999, p. 583).

Shark cartilage is thought to have antiangiogenic properties that may interrupt the blood flow to a tumor, thereby starving it of the nutrients needed for cell growth and proliferation (Spencer & Jacobs, 1999, p. 154). It may also protect cells against lesions by removing free

TABLE 17–2 Adverse Effects of Common Vitamins and Minerals	
Vitamin/Mineral	**Adverse Effect**
Vitamin A (retinol)	Skin changes, hair loss, bone and joint pain and tenderness, hepatotoxicity, neurological complaints, and psychiatric symptoms have been noted. Teratogenic effects are serious, including abnormalities of craniofacial, central nervous system, heart, neural tube, musculoskeletal, and urogenital systems.
Provitamin A (beta-carotene)	Generally considered to be safe; very few adverse effects have been recorded.
Vitamin D (cholecalciferol)	Can lead to hypercalcemia, manifested by nausea, vomiting, weakness, headache, bone pain, hypercalciuria, renal calcinosis, metastatic calcification, and hypertension.
Vitamin E (tocopherols)	Increases vitamin K requirements when taken in megadoses. Coagulopathy can occur in persons deficient in Vitamin K.
Provitamin B_3 (niacin = nicotinic acid)	Niacin is transformed into nicotinamide (vitamin B_3) by the liver. Niacin can produce flushing and hypertension headaches when taken in megadoses. Other adverse effects include pruritis, abdominal pain, diarrhea, peptic ulcer, skin rash, hepatotoxicity, hyperuricemia, hyperglycemia, and arrhythmias.
Vitamin B_6 (pyroxidine)	Can lead to severe peripheral sensory neuropathy and ataxia when given in large doses.
Vitamin B_{11} (folic acid)	Supplementation in very large doses can mask or precipitate the symptoms of vitamin B_{12} deficiency. For this reason, strict vegetarians should be advised of this risk.
Vitamin C (ascorbic acid)	Has not been associated with severe adverse reactions. Gastrointestinal symptoms, such as diarrhea and esophagitis, can occur in some persons. Also, there is a risk of developing renal calculi (oxalate stones) when taking vitamin C supplements.
Chromium	Associated with dichromate toxicity in persons using this supplement in herbal enema preparations. The adverse effects associated with toxicity include acute renal failure, gastrointestinal hemorrhage, and hepatocellular dysfunction.
Selenium	Can lead to toxicity, manifested by nausea, vomiting, abdominal cramps, watery diarrhea, nail changes, alopecia, dryness of hair, fatigue, irritability, and parasthesias, when given in large doses. This has been noted in persons using health food supplements containing megadoses of selenium.
Zinc	Associated with a risk of copper deficiency and anemia, as well as impaired immune response when taken in extremely large doses. A reduction in the lymphocyte stimulation response to phytohemagglutinin and chemotaxis and phagocytosis of bacteria by polymorphonuclear leukocytes are seen when zinc is taken in excessive doses.

radicals, which are essentially the short-lived forms of compounds with an unpaired electron in the outer shell. Because free radicals have an electron-seeking nature, they can be very destructive to electron-dense areas of cells, such as DNA and cell membranes (NIH, 1994). Shark cartilage is promoted as a poten-

tial treatment for malignant disease, despite the absence of conclusive evidence of efficacy (Boik, 1996; Markman, 1996). However, a large clinical trial being conducted at the M.D. Anderson Cancer Center, Houston, Texas, and at the Mayo Clinic in Rochester, Minnesota, with lung cancer patients may shed additional light on the efficacy of shark cartilage in cancer treatment.

The establishment of Dietary Supplements Research Centers by the NCCAM, with an emphasis on botanicals (medicinal plants), will advance the scientific base of knowledge about botanicals. The goals of these centers are to foster research across disciplines to identify health benefits and develop systematic evaluation of the safety and effectiveness of dietary supplements, in particular.

MIND-BODY PRACTICES

A burgeoning recognition of the undeniable alliance between mind and body exists (L. Dossey, 1999). Mind-body practices include any methods that individuals use to change their behavior or physiology to promote health and recovery from illness (Domar & Dreher, 1997). Since the days of Nightingale, nursing education has emphasized the interconnectedness between mind, body, and spirit. The specific goal of mind-body practices is to enhance the body's innate capacity for wellness and well-being by creating or restoring balance between the person's physiological and psychological characteristics and bodily functions (Chez & Jonas, 1997; Gordon, 1996; Purnell, 1999, May–July).

Mind-body practices, the least controversial and most widely used CAPPs, include meditation, imagery, biofeedback, hypnosis, various forms of yoga, t'ai chi, relaxation response therapies, music therapy, dance therapy, and prayer or spiritual practice (Chez & Jonas, 1997; Goldberg, 1999; Gordon, 1996; NIH, 1994; Purnell, 1999, May–July). The underlying philosophy of mind-body practices is that users are active partners rather than passive recipients in their health care (Goldberg, 1999).

Mind-body practices are used primarily with chronic conditions such as heart disease, depression, arthritis, cancer, and asthma and have been shown to be effective in treating hypertension, urinary and fecal incontinence, insomnia,

chronic pain, bulimia nervosa, and carpal tunnel syndrome (Castes et al., 1999; Garfinkel et al., 1998; Glavind, Mouritsen, & Lose, 1999; Gordon, 1996; Purnell, 1999; Sequeira, 1999). Mind-body practices have demonstrated clinical effectiveness in other conditions as well. These include relaxation response and hypnosis for the relief of chronic pain and insomnia, intercessory prayer on the outcome of patients admitted to a coronary care unit, and psychosocial support group sessions for extending the survival time of patients with metastatic breast cancer (Chez & Jonas, 1997; Goldberg, 1999; Gordon, 1996; Harris et al., 1999).

A basic premise in mind-body practices is that chronic stress and lack of balance contribute to illness and to a delay in recovery from illness (Goldberg, 1999). Although other professions have shifted emphasis from treating to teaching, from application to participation, thus making patient care a more fulfilling partnership, such has been the basic paradigm for nursing practice since its beginning.

MEDITATION

Meditation is a self-directed, cognitive practice through which an individual focuses attention on a specific thought or object to relax and calm the body, thus decreasing respiratory rate, heart rate, plasma cortisol, and blood pressure. Commonly the person concentrates on a single thought (harmony), physical activity (breathing), or sound (repeating a word or mantra, such as "one" or "peace") (Haskell et al., 1999; Purnell, 1999, May–July).

This cognitive practice can affect chronic pain, anxiety, depression, blood pressure, serum cholesterol and cortisol levels, and the frequency of seizures (Chez & Jonas, 1997; Diamond et al., 1999; Purnell, 1999, May–July; Taylor, 1999). Additionally, meditation can boost immune functioning, thus helping individuals who are immunocompromised (Diamond et al., 1999; Eliopoulos, 1999). Persons who meditate emerge from mental focusing with clearer minds, sharper thoughts, higher levels of mental function, and an improved sense of self-esteem (Benson, 1997; Eliopoulos, 1999).

IMAGERY

Imagery is defined as any thought representing a sensory quality and is hypothesized to be a means of communication between emotion, perception, and bodily change. Images may either precede or follow physiological changes, indicating that images have both a causative and a reactive role in relaxation. Some consider imagery to be the bridge between conscious processing of information and physiological change (B. M. Dossey, 1997; Haskell et al., 1999; Lubkin & Larsen, 1998).

Visualization is often used synonymously with imagery. This can be misleading, because *visualization* refers only to "seeing something in the mind's eye," that is, choosing images for a specific purpose. Imagery is the term reserved for those images that spontaneously occur from the unconscious, invoking and using the senses (Lubkin & Larsen, 1998; Payne, 1998). Visualization and imagery are internal experiences that may take place in the absence of any external stimulus and are accessed through thought and imaginal processes (Dossey, 1999; Payne, 1998).

Imagery is highly effective in reducing stress, heart rate, and blood pressure. Some persons with cancer have successfully used imagery to alleviate nausea, facilitate weight gain, and mobilize their immune systems. Also, geriatric patients have been shown to enhance their immunity through imagery (Ezra, 1999; Lubkin & Larsen, 1998; Milton, 1998; Purnell, 1999, May–July).

As with other forms of mind-body practices, imagery is not a substitute for other methods of pain control, but nurses can consider it an adjunctive treatment in comfort care (Esplen et al., 1998; Lubkin & Larsen, 1998). When used as distraction from pain, imagery increases pain tolerance; when used to produce relaxation, it decreases stress (Lubkin & Larsen, 1998).

Imagery has also been found to be effective in the treatment of bulimia nervosa (Esplen et al., 1998) and in helping individuals adjust to the demands of chronic illness (Stephens, 1999). Additionally, it has the potential to lower anxiety, facilitate wound healing, and reduce the feelings of helplessness, hopelessness, depression, and apathy associated with the grief process (Abrahm, 1998; Hatler, 1998; Stephens, 1999; Turkoski & Lance, 1996).

Evidence on imagery as a mind-body practice supports its use as a nursing intervention for redirecting physiological processes, stress and pain management, and health maintenance (Lubkin & Larsen, 1998). All forms of imagery are simple, cost-effective, and easy to use, yet mastering imagery techniques requires time and training (Goldberg, 1999; Lubkin & Larsen, 1999; Milton, 1998).

YOGA

Yoga is a traditional Indian culture and way of life that promotes a healthy body and a sound mind (McGrady & Horner, 1999; National Center for Complementary and Alternative Medicine [NCCAM], 2000; Ramaratnam & Sridharan, 1999). The term *yoga* means union (Eliopoulos, 1999; Goldberg, 1999; Haskell et al., 1999; Ramaratnam & Sridharan, 1999). As such it is a complex system of beliefs and practices that seeks to integrate and achieve a balance between the mind and the body. Yoga is a lifestyle that comprises dietary prescriptions, meditation, physical exercises, and release of energy (Lubkin & Larsen, 1998; McGrady & Horner, 1999; NCCAM, 2000).

Yoga practice reduces blood pressure and heart rate, facilitates pain relief, reduces anxiety levels and stress, increases circulation, and aids in digestive and respiratory problems (Eliopoulos, 1999; McGrady & Horner, 1999; NCCAM, 2000; Ramaratnam & Sridharan, 1999). Yoga and relaxation techniques are used to alleviate musculoskeletal symptoms, improve range of motion, and decrease tenderness and hand pain during activity in patients with osteoarthritis (Garfinkel et al., 1998). In addition, yoga is used as an adjunct in the treatment of mental disorders, asthma, and epilepsy (Ramaratnam & Sridharan, 1999).

Yoga and t'ai chi, as well as other forms of exercise, are recommended to lower blood glucose levels in individuals with diabetes mellitus (Eliopoulos, 1999). Yoga may also play a role in stroke prevention and, although there is little controlled research, patients with multiple sclerosis who practice yoga report symptom improvement (Diamond et al., 1999).

T'AI CHI CHUAN

T'ai chi chuan, described as a moving meditation (Lubkin & Larsen, 1998) and as *shadow boxing,* is a focused, deliberate set of meditative movements used to improve strength, balance, coordination, and concentration (Haskell et al., 1999; Peightel, Hardie, & Baron, 1999). Studies have shown improved cardiorespiratory function, lower blood pressure, reductions in heart rate, enhancement of mood, improved postural control in the elderly, stress reduction, and increased range of motion in patients with rheumatoid arthritis (Diamond et al., 1999; Haskell et al., 1999; Lubkin & Larsen, 1998; Peightel et al., 1999).

MUSIC THERAPY

Music is familiar, appealing, inexpensive, and low risk (Good, 1996; Milton, 1998), and can create an experience that increases a patient's level of physical, mental, and emotional comfort. Although Nightingale wrote about the effects of music on the sick, it was not until late in the 20th century that music and relaxation practices were recommended officially as adjunctive therapies in the management of acute pain (Acute Pain Management Guideline Panel, 1992). While the overall aim of music therapy is

to promote health and well-being (Ernst, Rand, & Stevinson, 1998; Milton, 1998), it is useful in the care of patients with Alzheimer's disease and other conditions (Kumar et al., 1999; McKinney, Tims, et al., 1997; Miluk-Kolasa & Matejek, 1996).

Music's effects are related to its various elements (tempo, pitch, harmony, melody, and rhythm), listener characteristics (age, language, culture, education, musical preferences), and means of delivery (headphones, speakers, open air). For example, reduced heart rate and blood pressure have been noted when the music played is familiar, desirable to the individual, and delivered through headphones (Schiedermayer, 1999, August).

When music is played, bodily rhythms begin to match the rhythm and tempo of the music (referred to as entrainment). The outcome of entrainment is that the bodily rhythms (heart rate, respiratory rate, brainwave patterns) synchronize with the beat or tempo of the music (Skaggs, 1999).

Music therapy provides individuals an opportunity to use their creativity and strength to cope with a psychological, physical, or emotional crisis and to maintain coherence (Aldridge, 1998). When integrated with conventional patient care, music plays a vital role in helping patients learn, regain, and maintain a healthy lifestyle (Mandel, 1996).

SPIRITUALITY AND PRAYER

Spirituality is often expressed as experiencing the presence of power, a force, or an energy. The word *spiritual* describes aspects of human behavior and experience that inspire devotion and direct behavior. In contrast is religion, a body of believers who share common beliefs, practices, and rituals. Those who are religious are generally spiritual (Krippner, 1995).

It is one's spiritual dimension that contributes to one's sense of wholeness and wellness. Changes in body image, comfort, mood, cognition, and interpersonal relationships related to illness can challenge a person's sense of self, life, and its meaning. Thus, recovery from illness is affected by one's spirituality (Waldfogel, 1997).

The link between spirituality and physical outcomes is evident when one engages in a repetitive prayer, word, sound, or phrase and specific physiological changes occur. These changes include decreased metabolism, heart rate, rate of breathing, and distinctive slower brain waves. The physiological state achieved represents the potential for an enhanced state of well-being.

Science has proved that prayer works (L. Dossey, 1993). There are more than 150 studies looking at the role of prayer, including whether prayer has a therapeutic effect on health in patients with AIDS and on those undergoing angioplasty (L. Dossey, 1999; Horrigan, 1999; Sicher et al., 1998). In two separate studies of the effect of remote, intercessory prayer on behalf of patients admitted to coronary care units, both studies showed statistically significant beneficial effects for the cardiology patients who received intercessory prayer (Byrd, 1988; Harris et al., 1999). Given that research supports spirituality as effective in health promotion and disease prevention, it is important that nursing curricula include opportunities for nurses to learn spiritual care skills needed to assist patients in gaining a perspective on life and its meaning.

The National Institutes of Health (NIH) has set aside funding for centers to conduct research that will seek to understand how one's beliefs, attitudes, values, and stress affect one's physical and mental health and how beliefs, values, and attitudes that affect health are developed, maintained or change. Outcomes from this research will be of particular interest to nurses.

Alternative Systems of Health Care

Many Americans think of mainstream biomedicine and health care as the world's standard; however, only 10% to 30% of health care is delivered by conventional practitioners (NIH, 1994). The remainder of care is provided by a range of practitioners, from one's self to organized health care systems such as traditional Oriental medicine, acupuncture, Ayurvedic medicine, homeopathic medicine, naturopathic medicine, and environmental medicine (NIH, 1994). Of these, homeopathy remains the most controversial, although it has the only officially established "alternative" drug production system regulated by the FDA (NIH, 1994). This section highlights homeopathy as a representative example of an alternative system of health care.

HOMEOPATHIC THERAPIES

Homeopathy is one of the most controversial yet widely used of the CAPPs (Jonas & Levin, 1999). It is based on the principle that "like causes like," which states that a substance that can cause negative symptoms when given to a healthy person can cure those same symptoms in someone who is sick (Belavite & Signorini, 1995). There are two main theoretical tenets: the principle of "similars" and the use of "dilutions" called "potencies" (Hahnemann, 1982). The principle of similars states that patients with particular signs and symptoms can be helped if given a drug that produces the same signs and symptoms in a healthy individual. The second principle states that remedies retain biological activity if they are repeatedly diluted and agitated or shaken between each dilution. These dilutions are said to produce effects even when diluted beyond Avogadro's number, in which no original molecules of the starting substance remain. How the solution "remembers" information from the original substance is speculative (Endler & Schulte, 1994).

Many scientists think that homeopathy violates natural laws (Sampson, 1995) and therefore any effect must be a placebo effect (Gotzsche, 1993; O'Keefe, 1986). Yet advocates claim that there are measurable and reproducible effects over placebo. For example, clinical trials show evidence of efficacy in the use of homeopathy for the treatment of hay fever, influenza, postoperative ileus, and pain from trauma (Kleijnen, Knipschild, & ter Riet, 1991; Reilly et al., 1994). Although evidence suggests that homeopathy can have an effect over placebo, there is a lack of independent replication of these study models (Linde & Jonas, 1999).

Today, homeopathic medicines are prescribed for a variety of physical, emotional, and psychological symptoms. The theory behind the practice of homeopathy is analogous to the use of allergy shots for severe allergies, or the use of a vaccine. Allergy injections contain a small dose of the allergen, resulting in an eventual tolerance to the allergen. Similarly, in a vaccine, trace amounts of a disease-causing pathogen are injected to aid in immunizing against disease (Eliopoulos, 1999). Homeopathy differs from allergy desensitization injections and vaccines in that vaccines and allergy injections do not become more effective by dilution as do homeopathic medicines.

In homeopathy, the goal is to match as closely as possible the effects of the remedy with the patient's symptoms. The more closely the remedy is matched with the patient's symptoms and complaints, the more effective the treatment. A well-known example is the use of belladonna to treat headache. Belladonna, a potent poison, can cause headache in its natural form, but when diluted according to homeopathic principles, it can relieve a headache (Eliopoulos, 1999).

Homeopathic remedies are sold in tablet, liquid, ointments, or granular form, often with sugar added. When patients use homeopathic remedies, they are advised to avoid caffeine, mint, and menthol products because these can act as an antidote to some remedies. Homeopathic remedies were legitimized by the United States Food, Drug and Cosmetic Act in 1938, over the strong objections of the medical community. Today, all homeopathic remedies are regulated by the FDA (Eliopolous, 1999).

MANUAL HEALING

Touch and gentle manipulation with the hands have been long used by nurses and other practitioners around the world. All manual healing modalities rely on the practitioner's hands as the primary means to assess (obtain the information through simple touch and palpation) and to treat the individual. The Chinese included touch in their diagnostic methods and massage in their healing practices centuries ago. Hippocrates discussed the benefits of therapeutic massage and directed his students in its uses, as well as in spinal manipulation, and Nightingale recruited nurses to comfort the sick and wounded through touch. Today, some perceive that health care practitioners have retreated too much from physical contact with patients, distanced in part by diagnostic equipment, time factors, and, in some instances, legal constraints.

Healing practices include both physical modalities and energy modalities. In this chapter, the focus is on massage and reflexology as examples of physical healing methods that use touch and pressure, and on therapeutic touch as an energy healing practice. These practices have more widespread use in professional nursing than other modalities in this category.

PHYSICAL MODALITIES

Massage. Massage therapy involves the manipulation of soft tissues of the body for the purpose of normalizing tissues and consists of a group of manual techniques that include applying fixed or movable pressure, holding, or causing movement of or to the body. Because touch is a form of communication, it also conveys caring. Nurses have long used components of massage to promote comfort and caring. However, the emphasis given to massage as an important element of patient care, particularly the back rub provided as a component of "bedtime (HS) care," began to receive less attention in practice in the decade of the 1960s with the emergence of technological innovations into patient care. Nonetheless, the benefits of massage remain important.

The most frequently recognized and described physiological effects of massage are increases in blood flow and lymph circulation, which aid in edema reduction and removal of inflammatory waste products, as well as improved delivery of oxygen and nutrients to the cell. Effects on the skeletal muscles include relaxation, relief of spasms and cramps, relief of myofascial pain, prevention or treatment of delayed muscle soreness, improved athletic performances (when massage is given before activity), and faster recovery from injury (when massage is applied following injury). The literature contains a significant number of studies on the positive effects of massage in patient populations ranging from persons with spinal cord injury, persons suffering tension headaches, patients with psychiatric illness, critically ill patients, and hospice patients to neonates, infants, and children. Many of these studies are integrated into the content of other excellent CAPP references (e.g., Spencer & Jacobs, 1999).

Reflexology. This physical modality is based on the principle that there are reflex areas in the feet and hands that correspond to all of the glands, organs, and parts of the body. Reflexology involves a unique method of applying pressure with the thumb and fingers to the specific points to achieve therapeutic benefits.

Popular belief holds that cultures have practiced some form of reflexology through the ages, with its roots in the ancient oriental art of pressure therapy or acupuncture. Reflexology is based on the theory that energy pathways exist throughout the body and that blockages of these pathways lead to energy loss, discomfort, or illness. Practitioners trained in reflexology apply pressure to each of the reflexes, thereby triggering a release of stress and tension in the area or body zone affected by the reflex as well

as an overall relaxation response. Persons on whom this procedure is performed typically express relief from tension and pain and report increased energy and a greater feeling of wellness than before experiencing the procedure. Needed, however, is research to support these anecdoctal reports.

ENERGY MODALITIES

Energy healing, sometimes referred to as "laying on of the hands," is among the oldest forms of healing. Worldwide, different peoples and cultures have developed such therapies using the person's energy or biofield. Some of the terms used to refer to the human biofield and the countries of origin include qi or chi (China), ki (Japan), prana (India), subtle energy (United States and United Kingdom), and life force (general usage term).

There is general consensus among practitioners who possess or develop the talents to perform biofield healing that the energy within the person's body also extends beyond the body for 6 to 8 inches or more. This extension of the human energy field beyond the body surface permits the practitioner to place the hands directly on the body or to work with the hands 2 to 4 inches above the body surface. Extension of the energy field external to the body tends to be variable and dependent on a person's general state of health, especially emotional state.

Although the human biofield is not a clearly defined phenomenon, and there is generally no accepted theory that accounts for it, current hypotheses to explain the biofield include the following:

- It is metaphysical and thus beyond the four dimensions of space and time, and is untestable.
- It creates an electromagnetic field effect.
- It reflects a currently undefined but potentially quantifiable field effect in physics.

Because there is not currently an explanatory model, and because explanations of the phenomena often mix concepts from physics and metaphysics, the range of perceptions among persons about the human biofield extends from "something near superstition" to science. However, practitioners of this healing modality believe that the biofield has a definable form, flux pattern, and polarities. They acknowledge that characterization of the biofield is far from complete and that determining its true nature is important to its further development among the healing arts.

Although there are ten major biofield therapies used in the United States, only therapeutic touch will be highlighted here. Table 17–3 lists characteristics of the major biofield therapies.

Therapeutic Touch. The contemporary technique that many nurses use that involves the human energy or biofield is therapeutic touch. Because this therapy is discussed in detail elsewhere in the nursing literature, including videotapes on the topic, here the authors simply provide an overview of this procedure and selected studies from the nursing literature.

First, the practitioner centers him- or herself and establishes the intention to attend to the person's unbalanced energy field. The practitioner may focus on a range of therapeutic intents, including, among others, stress relief, improvement in vitality, reduction of inflammation, and reduction in chronic or acute pain perception.

Next, the practitioner assesses the disturbances in the person's biofield, followed by a process of unruffling or smoothing the energy field through the use of his or her hands very near the physical body of the individual being treated. Through this process the practitioner is able to perceive the energy field of the recipient of the treatment. Final steps include reassessing the balance of the individual's biofield. Generally, treatment sessions range between 20 minutes to 1 hour for a successful application of therapeutic touch. The individual being treated generally is seated comfortably and clothed.

Despite a lack of a clear understanding of therapeutic touch, as well as other energy modalities as healing therapies, it has a long history of use with repeated references to it in the Eastern, European, and religious literature. Nurses in the United States have used therapeutic touch in clinical settings and, as with some other nursing interventions, long before nurse researchers began to conduct rigorous scientific studies to test its effects.

Nurse co-developer Kreiger and her students began a series of studies in the late 1970s and 1980s to test the effects of therapeutic touch in reducing patients' anxiety (Heidt, 1981; Quinn, 1984). In the 1990s additional studies reported on its efficacy in reducing anxiety in hospitalized children (Kramer, 1990), institutionalized elderly (Simington & Laing, 1993), and a high-anxiety population (Olson & Sneed, 1995).

Other ways in which therapeutic touch has been shown to be effective include a reduction in patients' reports of tension headaches (Keller & Bzdek, 1986), a reduction in patients' pain ratings after removal of molar teeth, and a reduction in musculoskeletal pain and anxiety (Lin & Taylor, 1999).

In contrast to the studies that reported positive findings are studies testing the efficacy of therapeutic touch in which positive results were not found (Meehan, 1993; Parkes, 1986). Factors contributing to the inconsistent study results include small sample size, lack of consistency in dependent variables assessed across the studies, and the brief duration of the therapeutic touch sessions.

Many opportunities exist for nurses to integrate selected manual and energy healing methods into their practices. Collaborative research is needed to obtain further evidence-based data on the physiological and neurological mechanisms associated with specific manual healing methods, as well as the range of clinical benefits that many of these modalities can offer.

TABLE 17-3 Summary Features of the Major Biofield (Human Energy) Therapies in the United States

Therapy	Year Originated	Developer	Theoretical Basis	Diagnostic Procedures	Certification	Placement of Hands	Mental Healing at a Distance	Therapeutic Intent
Healing science	1978	Barbara Brennan	Open system, incorporates chakras and psychic layers	High sense perception	Yes, after completion of advanced study	Both on and near the body	Yes	Treat the whole person and specific disorders
Healing touch	1981	American Holistic Nurses Association	Elements of therapeutic touch, healing science, and Brugh Joy's and other work	Tactile assessment	Yes	Both on and off the body	Yes	Whole person, specific disorders
Huna	Traditional Hawaiian		Involves mana (universal force) and aka (universal substance)	Various	No	Both on and near the body	Yes	Heal mind and body
Mari-el	1983	Ethel Lombardi	Vibrational energy is transmitted from a high source through the practitioner to the patient, affecting cellular memory and the endocrine system	Tactile assessment	No	Usually off the body	Yes	Heal and harmonize the life of the individual
Natural healing	1974	Rosalyn Bruyere	Operates on a belief in a universal principle of energy	Tactile assessment	Graduates are ordained	Not specified	No	Effect symptomatic relief, assist in proper use of energy
Qigong	Traditional Chinese		Qi flows through the body in meridians and other patterns; qi is delivered with great force by many practitioners called qigong masters	Varies with practitioners	Not usually	At the meridian points or at a short distance from the body	Yes	Healing of biological disorders

Table continued on following page

TABLE 17–3 Summary Features of the Major Biofield (Human Energy) Therapies in the United States *Continued*

Therapy	Year Originated	Developer	Theoretical Basis	Diagnostic Procedures	Certification	Placement of Hands	Mental Healing at a Distance	Therapeutic Intent
Reiki	Japan, 1800s; U.S.A., 1936	Mikao Usui (introduced by Hawayo Takata)	Spiritual energy with innate intelligence, channeled through the practitioner; the spiritual body is healed, it in turn is expected to heal the physical; uses rituals, symbols, spirit guides	Varies	Spiritual initiation (i.e., the power to heal is given after training)	A few standard hand placements (usually side by side, on the physical body)	Yes	
SHEN therapy*	1977	Richard Pavek	Biofield conforming to natural laws of physics, with a discernible flux pattern through the body	Conventional medical and psychotherapy instruments with questions designed to discover repressed emotional states	Yes, after internship; practitioners meet requirements of U.S. Department of Labor Occupational Code 076.264-640	Sequence of paired-hand placements, directly on the body, arranged according to flux patterns, usually with one on top and one underneath	No	Primarily emotional disorders and somatopsychic dysfunctions
Therapeutic touch	1972	Dora Kunz and Dolores Kreiger	Practitioner restores correct vibrational component to the patient's universal, unitary field	Tactile assessment	None	Generally near the body	Yes	Nonprescriptive healing of the whole person

* SHEN (Specific Human Energy Nexus) is a biofield method of treating the so-called psychosomatic and related disorders by releasing repressed and suppressed debilitating emotions directly from the body.

From National Institutes of Health. (1994). *Alternative medicine: Expanding medical horizons. A report to the National Institutes of Health on alternative medical systems and practices in the United States* (DHHS Publication No. NIH 94-066, pp. 137–138). Washington, DC: U.S. Government Printing Office.

Pharmacological and Biological CAPPs

APITHERAPY

Apitherapy, the therapeutic use of honey bee products such as bee pollen, royal jelly, honey, and bee venom, has been used since ancient times to promote health and healing. Bee pollen is used in natural remedies and food supplements. Royal jelly, which is produced by the bees of the hive to nourish the developing queens, is promoted as a youth-enhancing agent as well as a treatment for chronic arthritic conditions. Honey can also be used as an antibacterial for dressing wounds and burns and to promote healing. Perhaps the most controversial form of apitherapy is the use of bee venom, or "bee venom therapy" (BVT), for healing.

BVT has been used as an Oriental medicine for centuries. Subjects expose themselves to several stings per session to treat a variety of conditions, including rheumatoid arthritis, multiple sclerosis, irritable bowel syndrome, depression, and Bell's palsy. There are no published controlled human trials that show therapeutic effects in any of these conditions, and the biological activity of this therapy remains unknown. However, bee venom contains several proteins that have physiological effects. Mellitin, the most prevalent substance and one of the most potent anti-inflammatory agents known, may slow down the body's inflammatory response by inhibiting the amount of free radicals (electron-seeking compounds that are destructive to DNA and cell membranes) generated by the tissues. Some researchers suspect that bee venom works by stimulating the adrenal glands to release cortisol, one of the body's natural anti-inflammatory substances (Dietz, 1998).

Although earlier preliminary animal research results suggested that bee venom may have therapeutic effects (Chang & Bliven, 1979), reports of adverse effects are numerous and the effects may be severe, including localized swelling, itching, difficulty breathing and anaphylactic shock, eventually resulting in bronchospasm, laryngeal edema, respiratory failure, and possibly death (Wallace, 1994). The benefit to risk ratio of BVT must be carefully considered.

CHELATION THERAPY

The term *chelation* is derived from the Greek word *chele*, meaning to claw or to bind. Treatment with chelation consists of a series of intravenous infusions with ethylenediaminetetraacetic acid (EDTA), an amino acid complex (Jonas & Levin, 1999). EDTA hunts down harmful, positively charged metals and thus binds with these metals, to be excreted from the body through the kidneys (Jonas & Levin, 1999; Goldberg, 1999). The concept underlying chelation therapy is to restore adequate perfusion to all tissues of the body.

EDTA was first synthesized and used in chelation therapy to treat lead poisoning in 1930 (Goldberg, 1999). To date, chelation therapy has been safely administered to more than 500,000 patients in the United States to treat conditions ranging from lead poisoning to atherosclerosis and other chronic degenerative diseases such as arthritis, scleroderma, and lupus (Goldberg, 1999; Jonas & Levin, 1999).

Lack of evidence from clinical trials that chelation therapy affects any disease process has led to debate over both the safety and efficacy of this therapy. No recent studies document the efficacy of chelation therapy; however, in earlier studies 90% of all treated patients had marked or good improvement as a result of chelation therapy (Olszewer & Carter, 1989).

DMSO

Dimethyl sulfoxide (DMSO), a byproduct of the wood industry, is bacteriostatic and virostatic. It reduces the incidence of thrombus formation, has a tranquilizing effect, softens collagen due to its cross-linking effects, and is considered useful in treating scar tissue. DMSO has also been shown to cause differentiation in a number of human cancer cells in vitro (Boik, 1996).

Physicians in 125 countries, including Canada, Great Britain, Germany, and Japan, have prescribed DMSO for a variety of conditions since the 1960s, primarily for its anti-inflammatory effects, yet it has several other biological activities (Boik, 1996). For example, it is a potent solvent that carries molecules of low molecular weight across membranes, including the blood-brain barrier (Boik, 1996; Jacobs, 1996). It is widely used as a topical analgesic in burns, cuts, and sprains, with reports of pain reduction lasting up to 6 hours. As an antioxidant, DMSO is an effective anti-inflammatory agent in patients diagnosed with ulcerative colitis, rheumatoid arthritis, scleroderma, and interstitial cystitis (Boik, 1996; Jacobs, 1996).

The principal side effect of DMSO is an odd odor, similar to that of garlic, that emanates from the mouth shortly after use, even when the product is applied topically. Worldwide, some 11,000 articles document the medical and clinical implications of DMSO, yet in the United States, the FDA has approved it for use only as a preservative for transplant organs and for the treatment of interstitial cystitis.

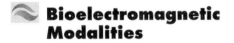

Bioelectromagnetic Modalities

The field of bioelectromagnetics explores interactions of static magnetic fields (SMFs) and dynamic electromagnetic fields (EMFs) with living tissue. Nurses are perhaps most knowledgeable about EMF exposures to which individuals are continuously subjected in their homes, in the workplace, and in public locations, such as near or under electric power lines. Though weak, these exposures can cause biological system changes. It has been hard until recently to get valid information about these effects, in part because the issue is highly politicized. While knowledge of the effects of both EMF and SMF on the cells, tissues, and body systems is impor-

tant for health promotion and prevention of adverse effects, in this chapter the focus is on SMFs. Little is known about the potential for efficacy and potential for adverse effects with exposure to varying doses of SMFs, yet American consumers spend more than $5 billion annually for SMF devices to treat a variety of symptoms.

From a historical perspective, SMFs have been used as potential therapeutic modalities for more than 4,000 years to treat a wide variety of ailments and conditions. Cleopatra supposedly wore a lodestone on her forehead while sleeping to prevent aging, and Tibetan monks put magnets on skulls to enhance their own minds during training. Widespread interest in the use of magnets in the United States was evident during the 18th century and into the early part of the 19th century, but then disappeared with the formalizaton of allopathic medicine. However, the focus on self-help strategies in the 1990s led to a resurgence of interest in the potential usefulness of magnets to enhance healing, particularly of bone fractures, lessening of the inflammatory process, and treatment of a wide variety of painful conditions.

For years, researchers in the field of bioelectromagnetic research have raised questions about what goes on and its significance in the cellular interactions (i.e., the magnetochemical concepts involved, the influence of varying magnetic field strengths and direction) to gain an understanding of the physical basis of magnetic field interactions with living cells and systems. Research has ranged from investigations of the underlying electromagnetic interaction mechanisms to the development of biomedical applications of external electromagnetic energy signals for use in clinical assessment, diagnosis, and therapy. In other words, bioelectromagnetic investigations can involve electromagnetic properties of biological matter, generation of endogenous electromagnetic fields by organisms, sensory perception of electromagnetic fields by organisms, and application of electromagnetic fields to alter, modify, or control biological function, and to induce therapeutic responses.

Exploration of SMF influences on biological systems is significant because intrinsic electromagnetic fields produced within the human body have critical functional roles. For example, there are the electrically excitable tissues that mediate neuronal and muscular activity through the production and release of bioelectrical and/or chemical signals. This activity occurs at the cellular and molecular levels to mediate essential activity, as in the case of cells generating and maintaining an electric field gradient across cell membranes. It is a possibility that the direction and strength of the magnetic field may actually be the cause of some bioelectromagnetic effects. Thus, it is important that clinicians, as well as researchers exploring this field, expand the conventional view that biological function results from biochemical interactions to include electromagnetic interactions as being fundamental to life processes (Walleczek, 1995).

Although the number of published studies testing the efficacy of SMF is small, preliminary findings from these studies and from case reports suggest potentially promising applications of static magnetic modalities in selected populations. Studies have demonstrated effectiveness in reducing neuropathic pain in various populations, including those with postpolio syndrome, fibromyalgia, low back pain, and knee pain (Vallbona, Hazlewood, & Jurida, 1997). A study of persons with fibromyalgia suggests that whole-body exposure to SMFs (sleeping on magnetic sleep pads for 6 months) reduces the report of pain associated with fibromyalgia and improves functional status in some persons (Alfano et al., 2000). In a review of magnetic therapy research conducted in Eastern European countries (Jerabek & Pawluk, 1998), clinical improvements were reported in patients suffering from rheumatoid arthritis, cervical osteoarthritis, and carpal tunnel syndrome.

Important questions concerning the mechanism whereby SMFs produce effects remain unanswered. Although the evidence of biological effects is greater for pulsed EMF stimulation than for SMF, there is emerging evidence that SMF may also have biological effects. For example, exposure to a quadripolar static magnetic field (four magnets with alternating polarity in a single plastic case) caused reversible blockade of the action potential firing and reduction of responses to the pain-producing substance capsaicin in cultured adult dorsal root ganglion cells (McLean et al., 1995). In laboratory studies, SMF altered cell immune parameters (Flipo et al., 1998) and significantly suppressed inflammatory processes (Weinberger, Nyska, & Giler, 1996). In other studies, researchers reported that levels of beta-endorphin increased 45% and serotonin levels increased 24% following an application of static magnets.

In summary, there is beginning evidence that there are beneficial effects of SMF on living systems. In clinical practice, SMF modalities may potentially offer economical and noninvasive therapy for pain and other symptom improvements in persons with fibromyalgia and other conditions for which conventional health care has treatment limitations.

Herbal Products

Herbs are used as therapeutic agents to maintain health and wellness and to treat illness (Mashour, Lin, & Frishman, 1998). Herbal preparations are the basis of some familiar drugs, such as salicin, the source of aspirin; digitoxin, from *Digitalis purpura;* ephedrine, from *Ephendra sinicia,* and the antihypertensive drug reserpine, from *Rauwolfia serpentina* (Mashour et al., 1998).

Consumers' use of herbs and medicinal plant products in the United States over the past two decades has skyrocketed. In 1997, 60 million Americans reported that they had used herbs in the previous year, accounting for $3.24 billion in sales (Miller, 1998), with sales projected to pass $5 billion in the year 2000. Researchers report that 70% of patients using herbal products do not reveal this to their primary care practitioners (Miller, 1998). While the general public usually views plant-based products as natural and lacking adverse effects, this notion can be dangerously misleading. In Europe, phytotherapy (herbal medicine) is an integral part of physicians' prescriptions, and they treat herbal products with the same clinical concern as they have for the synthetic counterparts of prescription medications (Eisenberg et al., 1998; Ernst, Rand, & Stevinson, 1998).

Under the 1994 Dietary Supplement Health and Education Act, herbal products are classified as dietary supplements and not drugs (USDHHS, 1995). Dietary supplements may bear claims that these products affect the structure or function of the body, but without FDA review, manufacturers cannot make a claim that these products can prevent, treat, cure, mitigate, or diagnose disease (USDHHS, 1998).

An estimated 15 million adults, 3 million of whom are age 65 or older, are at risk for potential adverse interactions involving prescription medications and herbs or high-dose vitamin supplements (Eisenberg et al., 1998). Four questions can guide clinician inquiries: (1) Is the selected preparation the best suited for the targeted symptoms? (2) What is the potential for drug-herb or herb-herb interactions? (3) What are the potential side effects of the herbal products? (4) What is the best way to educate the patient/consumer regarding these concerns?

Patients' growing interest in and use of herbal products has created the need for accurate information that is easily accessible to nurses, physicians, and pharmacists (Eisenberg et al., 1998; Ernst et al., 1998; Wong, Smith, & Boon, 1998). The paucity of scientific data on the 20,000 herbal products currently available on the market calls attention to the need for further research (Ernst et al., 1998; Mashour et al., 1998; Miller, 1998). Herbal reference are shown in Box 17–3.

ECHINACEA

Echinacea (*Echinacea angustifolia*, called the purple coneflower), is most often found in the Great Plains region of North America and is the most widely used medicinal plant of Native Americans, due to its healing and anti-inflammatory properties (Goldberg, 1999). Madaus, a German researcher, imported echinacea seeds to Germany and began conducting research on its immunostimulating properties. Today, echinacea is one of the most important over-the-counter remedies in Germany, where it is used for relieving symptoms of the common cold (Goldberg, 1999). Over 180 products are marketed in Germany, including extracts and fresh-squeezed juices from both the roots and the leaves of echinacea (Foster, 1991).

Echinacea is also popular in the United States. It is used as a stimulant to the immune system as well as for its antiviral effects (Jonas & Levin, 1999). The primary action of the plant on the immune system is through cell-mediated immunity (Luettig et al., 1989). Liquid echinacea preparations have been shown to have immune-stimulating activity, including increased lymphocytes, splenocytes, and phagocytes that ingest and destroy bacteria, protozoa, and cell debris (German Ministry of Health, 1989a).

Echinacea purpura, another species of echinacea, has distinct antiviral properties that make it a suitable herb for cold and flulike symptoms. It stimulates the individual's natural defense system, helping to fight off infection through direct means or through the production of interferon, a protein substance produced by the natural killer cells of the immune system (Jonas & Levin, 1999).

Recent research findings supported the use of echinacea in the early treatment of upper respiratory infection (URI) but offered little support for the prolonged use of the plant preparation to prevent URIs (Barrett, Vohmann, & Calabrese, 1999). It may have a role in prohylaxis by stimulating the cells responsible for nonspecific immunity, the first line of defense against virus-infected cells (Sun, Currier, & Miller, 1999). Clinical trials are needed to support use of the herb to prevent infection.

Box 17-3 Printed References and Web Sites Recommended for Herbal Products

FDA: A public domain search engine of the U.S. Food and Drug Administration.
http://www.fda.gov/fdahomepage.html
Using generalized search terms such as "herbal products" or refined search terms such as a single herb, e.g., ginseng, will provide multiple links to resources on herbal products.

Federation of American Societies for Experimental Biology (FASEB) is a membership organization of biomedical researchers. The goal of FASEB is to educate the public about the benefits of fundamental biomedical research. The website for their Office of Public Affairs includes a search engine. Online access to some journal articles is also available.
http://www.faseb.org/opa
Their membership includes the American Society for Pharmacology and Experimental Therapeutics as well as the American Society for Nutritional Sciences. A search of their web site, or inquiries to their Office of Public Affairs, offers resources for information on some herbal and medicinal plants geared to biomedical research.

The Herb Research Foundation (HRF) is a nonprofit research and education organization.
http://www.herbs.org/
Although a membership organization, there are multiple links to other search engines regarding herbal products.

WEBMD:
http://my.webmd.com/
This web site offers a search engine. Searching for "herbal products" provides multiple links to WEBMD-reviewed web sites

The American Herbal Pharmacopoeia Monograph Series (1997–2000). Santa Cruz, CA: American Herbal Pharmacopoeia.
http://www.herbal-alhp.org
The development of the American Herbal Pharmacopoeia (AHP) addresses significant deficiencies in the state of knowledge and quality control guidelines for herbal medicines in the United States. A privately owned web site, the editors of this monograph series provide an on-line sample copy of a monograph on St. John's Wort, or other herbal products, as well as the opportunity to acquire research materials on herbal products

University of Washington Medicinal Herb Garden:
Useful pictures of herbs
Cross-reference to MEDLINE abstracts
Resource appropriate to professional development
http://www.nnlm.nlm.nih.gov/pnr/uwmhg/

Modified from Winslow, L. C., & Kroll, D. J. (1998). Herbs as medicines. *Archives of Internal Medicine, 158,* 2192–2199.

Echinacea is well tolerated both topically and orally in adults and children. It is not recommended for those with progressive systemic disease states such as HIV, AIDS, tuberculosis, leukosis, collagenosis, multiple sclerosis, or other autoimmune disorders (German Ministry of Health, 1989b).

GARLIC

Garlic (*Allium sativum*), a bulbous herb, is considered a medicinal food and is useful for detoxification. Its applications include controlling dysentery, fighting parasites, lowering fever, and relieving abdominal cramping. Allicin, the chief component of this herb, is a strong antibacterial agent that is released when the bulbs are crushed.

Over 1,000 studies investigating garlic's physiological effects and its possible use in the treatment of infection, cancer, diabetes mellitus, hypertension, and hyperlipidemia have been published. Garlic's beneficial cardiovascular effects, including lowering lipid levels and its anticoagulant and antioxidant effects, are well documented (Bordia, 1981; Gibbs, 1996; Vorberg & Scneider, 1990; Warshafsky, Kamer, & Sivak, 1993).

One important adverse effect associated with garlic intake relates to bleeding when used concurrently with the anticoagulant warfarin (Coumadin). Elevated international normalized ratios (INR) and prothrombin times (PT) are reported when patients take these preparations concomitantly (Miller, 1998). Consequently, health care practitioners should routinely ask about the use of garlic when patients are taking other medications, particularly warfarin.

GINGER

Ginger (*Zingiber officinale*) has been widely used as both a spice and a medicine for centuries. The herb was used in China at least 2,500 years ago (Barrett, Kiefer, & Rabago, 1999). Ginger is an effective antiemetic and antispas-modic agent, particularly following gynecological surgery (Bone et al., 1990) and for morning sickness (Fisher-Rasmussen et al., 1990). However, the safety of this herb in pregnancy has not been evaluated through rigorous research (Fulder & Tenne, 1996).

Recent research suggests that ginger exhibits anti-tumor-promoting activity in experimental animal models (Surh, Lee, & Lee, 1998). Most recently, animal studies suggest a possible protective effect of ginger as an antilipidemic (Bhandari, Sharma, & Zafar, 1998). This has not been supported in research with humans.

Although the side effects of this herb are minimal, ginger may increase bleeding time (Petry, 1995). Therefore, ginger should be taken with caution when patients are taking anticoagulant medication (Miller, 1998).

GINKGO BILOBA

Ginkgo biloba is the top-selling herb in the United States, with sales near $140 million in 1998 (Brevoort, 1998). Extracts from the leaves of *Ginkgo biloba*, or maidenhair tree, are widely used to treat peripheral vascular disease or cerebral insufficiency (Ernst & Pittler, 2000). It improves cognitive function in persons diagnosed with Alzheimer's disease (Oken, Storzbach, & Kaye, 1998) and slows the loss of cognitive function in those with dementia (Brautigam et al., 1998; Ernst & Pittler, 2000; Jonas & Levin, 1999). *Ginkgo biloba* is superior to placebo when used to increase pain-free walking distance in persons with intermittent claudication (Ernst & Pittler, 2000; Pittler, 1999). This herb is also useful in the treatment of vertigo, tinnitus, headaches, and anxiety (Goldberg, 1999).

The pharmacology of *Ginkgo biloba* is only partially understood. It is an inhibitor of platelet-activating factor, which helps reduce aggregation and plays a role in reducing the bronchoconstriction that accompanies asthma. Ginkgo also stimulates the synthesis of serotonin receptors, which may explain the subjective improvement in mood among elders who have decreased serotonin receptors (Jonas & Levin, 1999).

Overall, *Ginkgo biloba* is relatively free of side effects. However, it should be used with caution in combination with other antiplatelet agents such as aspirin, garlic, ginger, ginseng, or warfarin (Coumadin) because the bleeding time can be prolonged (Graedon & Graedon, 1999; Jonas & Levin, 1999). Additionally, ginkgolic acids are potent contact allergens; therefore, allergic responses may occur. Additional information on this botanical product is expected from an NCCAM- and National Institute on Aging-sponsored 6-year study of *Ginkgo biloba* in 2,000 older people who are at risk for cognitive decline in memory. Researchers are comparing those older perons who take *Ginkgo biloba* with those taking a placebo.

GINSENG

The widespread use of ginseng is attributed to the multiplicity of its effects, even though wide variations exist among ginseng products (Ernst & Pittler, 2000; Jonas & Levin, 1999; Miller, 1998). Ginseng is effective in relieving menopausal symptoms except for hot flashes (Kronenberg, Murphy, & Wade, 1999). *Panax ginseng* is most often used as an adaptogen or tonic for increasing the body's resistance to stress and fatigue and to improve endurance Low, 1999, p. 363; Miller, 1998; Wong et al., 1998). Walking endurance in some persons with severe respiratory illness improves with ginseng use, and a lower fasting blood glucose level was associated with ginseng use in patients with type II diabetes mellitus.

Adverse effects attributed to ginseng preparations include hypertension, pressure headaches, dizziness, restlessness, anxiety, euphoria, vaginal bleeding, and mastalgia. Prolonged use has been associated with a *ginseng abuse syndrome,* which includes symptoms of hypertension, edema, morning diarrhea, skin eruptions, insomnia, depression, and amenorrhea (Des-

met, 1999, p. 119; Wong et al., 1998). Ginseng may potentiate the effect of monoamine oxidase inhibitors (MAOIs), stimulants (including caffeine), some psychiatric medications (including haloperidol), and sex hormones (Low, 1999, p. 363; Wong et al., 1998). Those with hormone-sensitive tumors should avoid its prolonged use (Low, 1999, p. 363). Because of the antiplatelet components of ginseng, concomitant use with warfarin (Coumadin), heparin, ginger, *Ginkgo biloba,* garlic, aspirin, and nonsteroidal anti-inflammatory drugs (NSAIDs) should be avoided. Also, women who are pregnant should avoid use of ginseng products until further studies bring resolution to potential teratogenic effects.

ST. JOHN'S WORT

St. John's wort (*Hypericum perforatum*) is widely promoted as a *natural* antidepressant (Cupp, 1999). It is popular in Germany, where physicians routinely prescribe herbal medicines to treat depression and anxiety. St. John's wort is superior to placebo in the treatment of mild to moderately severe depression (Chez & Jonas, 1997; Jonas & Levin, 1999; Klaus et al., 1996; Wong et al., 1998).

Some suggest the active ingredient in this herb is hypericin, a purported MAOI (Cupp, 1999). Others suggest the possibility that several active component groups, including the hypericins, synergistically influence various metabolic pathways involved in depression (Jonas & Levin, 1999).

St. John's wort extract inhibits serotonin, dopamine and norepinephrine reuptake in vitro. Consequently, when combined with other antidepressants, particularly serotonin selective reuptake inhibitors (SSRIs), hypericum has the potential to produce the serotonin syndrome (Cupp, 1999). Serotonin syndrome manifests as mild agitation and possible stomach cramping as a result of serotonin levels in the CNS rising too high too fast. More intense reactions can include severe agitation, panic attacks, hyperthermia, rigidity, delirium, coma, and death. Nurses should be attuned to the signs and symptoms of serotonin syndrome and recommend appropriate and immediate treatment of those who unknowingly combine this herbal product with another antidepressant regimen.

Other side effects of St. John's wort include phototoxicity, dry mouth, dizziness, confusion, gastrointestinal symptoms, allergic reactions, and fatigue (Cupp, 1999; Jonas & Levin, 1999). In addition to prescription antidepressant medications and tyramine-containing foods, the use of St. John's wort is also contraindicated in pregnancy, lactation, and exposure to strong sunlight (Jonas, 1999; Wong et al., 1998).

The safety and efficacy of St. John's wort are currently being investigated in a multisite clinical trial sponsored by the NCCAM and NIH.

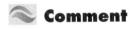 **Comment**

We began this chapter with an introduction to complementary and alternative procedures and products (CAPPs), estimates of consumer use, and a definition of what is meant by CAPPs, which will most likely continue to change as researchers complete rigorous scientific studies in this area. Although health consumers today are better able to take control of their health care outcomes, a large number of nurses and other health care professionals lack knowledge about CAPPs, thus creating a barrier to consumers achieving their goal. The evidence presented on selected categories of CAPPs shows that rigorous clinical studies are still needed to document treatment efficacy for many symptoms and conditions. Research monies are available for competitive research proposals through the NCCAM and cooperating institutes within the NIH. Consumer demand and pressure will continue to drive integration of selected CAPPs into the conventional health care system as well as prompt continued rigorous investigation in this field. These factors foster optimism and increase

the potential for additional evidence-based holistic care, facilitating the safe integration of selected CAPPs into health care in the 21st century.

KEY POINTS

- In 1992, Congress established the National Center for Complementary and Alternative Medicine (initially named the Office of Alternative Medicine) within the National Institutes of Health (NIH) to provide federal funding for rigorous research studies on CAPPs widely used by the American people.

- Definition(s) of what constitutes CAPPs will continue to evolve as more evidence-based data about this field become available through rigorous research and the treatments are subsequently integrated into the conventional health care system.

- A central objective of CAPPs is to improve the wellness state of persons through an emphasis on quality of life and its psychological, social, functional, and spiritual aspects.

- Increased consumption of a plant-based diet, selective dietary supplementation, and the use of mind-body practices, which are easily learned and carried out without supervision, show promise in health promotion and disease prevention.

- Important to nursing practice is nurses' knowledge about the many CAPPs resources available to guide patients seeking active partnerships in their care through the safe and responsible use of CAPPs.

- Momentum is evident in the movement to provide some level of instruction about CAPPs in the curricula of schools of nursing, medicine, dentistry, and pharmacy.

- Sufficient evidence-based data are available on many mind-body practices to support use of the modalities in a number of conditions, but insufficient data exist to indicate with confidence that one procedure or practice would be best for a given individual.

- Mind-body interventions often help individuals experience and express their illnesses in new, clearer ways.

- Mind-body practices provide patients the chance to be involved in their care, to make decisions about their health, to be touched emotionally, and to change psychologically through the process.

- The therapeutic potential of spirituality as well as religion is revealed through studies supporting significant benefits to both mental and physical health.

- Spirituality and its influence on healing in mental and physical health has been found to be of importance.

- The personality traits of individuals (i.e., positive or negative affect) may facilitate the capacity to benefit from selected CAPPs.

- Changes in the configuration of static magnetic fields can produce specific biological responses, and certain frequencies of magnetic fields have specific effects on body tissues.

- No generally accepted theory accounts for the effects of biofield (energy) therapies such as healing touch and therapeutic touch.

- Distinctions between curing and healing have been given little attention in conventional health care, but the distinction is important to patients with chronic illnesses who seek to integrate selected CAPPs into their care.

- Challenges to the clinician are to overcome perceived organizational, bureaucratic, and attitudinal barriers to the integration of those CAPPs for which there is demonstrated efficacy.

CRITICAL THINKING EXERCISES

1. Compare and contrast disease, pain and cure, and elements of the biomedical paradigm with suffering, care, and healing within the biopsychosocial paradigm that seems to fit the integration of CAPPs into health care.

2. Relate Florence Nightingale's 1859 ideas about environment, the use of the senses, clean air, nutritious food, spirituality, and nursing as a healing presence to practices that today are labeled CAPPs.

3. Talk with other nurses who have at least 20 years of experience in health care. Ask them to describe how many practices now referred to as CAPPs were at one time foundational to their practice of nursing.

4. What advice would you give to a patient with osteoarthritis who inquires about the use of herbal supplements for symptom management? Which herbal supplements could be used? What informational resources would you recommend?

5. Evaluate the patient history form used in your practice setting and examine its completeness for assessing and documenting the widespread use of CAPPs among Americans.

6. Mr. J comes into the emergency department complaining of frequent nosebleeds and blood in his urine and stool. His medical history reveals he has been taking Coumadin for several years after a heart valve replacement. He admits to taking a variety of herbal supplements for disease prevention and health promotion. Should the use of herbal preparations in this patient be of concern? Which herbal products should be avoided by patients taking Coumadin?

7. Discuss the major advantages of using spiritual care practices as a basis for patient care.

8. Recall a recent clinical scenario in which nothing seemed to go right for the patient and clinicians involved, and evaluate the situation from a spiritual care perspective. Describe how this situation might have been handled differently using spiritual care considerations.

9. A middle-aged woman who knows of your knowledge of the effects of SMF telephones you stating she has experienced two bone fractures within the last 6 months. She tells you her foot fracture is not healing well and asks for information about magnetic devices for use in promoting healing of the bone, and for recommendations for a reliable company from which to purchase magnets. How would you respond to this individual, given the state of knowledge and understanding of the efficacy and safety of SMF devices?

REFERENCES

Abrahm, J. L. (1998). Promoting symptom control in palliative care. *Seminars in Oncology Nursing, 14,* 95–109.

Acute Pain Management Guideline Panel. (1992). *Acute pain management: Operative or medical procedures and trauma. Clinical practice guideline* (AHCPR Publication No. 92-0032). Rockville, MD: Agency for Health Care Policy and Research, Public Health Service, U.S. Department of Health and Human Services.

Aldridge, D. (1998). Life as jazz: Hope, meaning, and music therapy in the treatment of life-threatening illness. *Advances in Mind-Body Medicine, 14*, 271–282.

Alfano, A. P., Taylor, A. G., Foresman, P. A., Dunkl, P. R., McConnell, G. G., Conaway, M. R., & Gillies, G. T. (2000). Static magnetic fields for treatment of fibromyalgia: A double-blind randomized controlled trial. Unpublished manuscript.

Ashar, B., & Vargo, E. (1996). Shark cartilage-induced hepatitis. *Annals of Internal Medicine, 125*, 780–781.

Astin, J. A. (1998). Why do patients use alternative medicine? *Journal of the American Medical Association, 279*, 1548–1553.

Barrett, B., Kiefer, D., & Rabago, D. (1999). Assessing the risks and benefits of herbal medicine: An overview of scientific evidence. *Alternative Therapies, 5*(4), 40–49.

Barrett, B., Vohmann, M., & Calabrese, C. (1999). Echinacea for upper respiratory infection. *Journal of Family Practice, 48*, 628–635.

Baum, A., Herberman, H., & Cohen, L. (1995). Managing stress and managing illness: Survival and quality of life in chronic disease. *Journal of Clinical Psychology in Medical Settings, 2*, 309–333.

Belavite, P., & Signorini, A. (1995). *A frontier in medical science.* Berkeley, CA: North Atlantic Books.

Benson, H. (1997). *Timeless healing: The power and biology of belief.* New York: Simon & Schuster.

Bhandari, U., Sharma, J. N., & Zafar, R. (1998). The protective action of ethanolic ginger *(Zingiber officinale)* extract in cholesterol fed rabbits. *Journal of Ethnopharmacology, 61*, 167–171.

Boik, J. (1996). *Cancer and natural medicine: A textbook of basic science and clinical research.* Princeton, MN: Oregon Medical Press.

Bone, M. E., Wilkinson, D. J., Young, J. R., McNeil, J., & Charlton, S. (1990). Ginger root—a new antiemetic. The effect of ginger root on postoperative nausea and vomiting after major gynaecological surgery. *Anaesthesia, 45*, 669–671.

Bordia, A. (1981). Effect of garlic on blood lipids in patients with coronary heart disease. *American Journal of Clinical Nutrition, 34*, 2100–2103.

Brautigam, M. R. H., Blommaert, F. A., Verleye, G., Castermans, J., Steur, J., & Kleijnen, J. (1998). Treatment of age-related memory complaints with ginkgo biloba extract: A randomized double blind placebo-controlled study. *Phytomedicine, 5*, 425–434.

Brevoort, P. (1998). The blooming U.S. botanical market: A new overview. *Herbalgram, 44*, 33–47.

Burton Goldberg Group (1999). *Alternative medicine: The definitive guide* (2nd ed.) Tiburon, CA: Future Medicine Publishing.

Bush, C. A. (1995). *Healing imagery and music: Pathways to the inner self.* Portland, OR: Rudra Press.

Byrd, R. C. (1988). Positive therapeutic effects of intercessory prayer in a coronary care unit population. *Southern Medical Journal, 81*, 826–829.

Castes, M., Hagel, I., Palenque, M., Canelones, P., Corao, A., & Lynch, N. R. (1999). Immunological changes associated with clinical improvement of asthmatic children subjected to psychosocial intervention. *Brain, Behavior, and Immunity, 13*(1), 1–13.

Challem, J. J. (1999). Toward a new definition of essential nutrients: Is it now time for a third "vitamin" paradigm? *Medical Hypotheses, 52*, 417–422.

Chang, Y. H., & Bliven, M. (1979). Antiarthritic effect of bee venom. *Agents and Actions, 9*, 205.

Chez, R. A., & Jonas, W. B. (1997). The challenge of complementary and alternative medicine. *American Journal of Obstetrics and Gynecology, 177*, 1156–1161.

Cupp, M. J. (1999). Herbal remedies: Adverse effects and drug interactions. *American Family Physician, 59*, 1239–1247.

Czeizel, A. E., & Dudas, I. (1992). Prevention of the first occurrence of neural-tube defects by periconceptual vitamin supplements. *New England Journal of Medicine, 327*, 1832–1835.

Desmet, P. A. (1999). The safety of herbal products. In W. B. Jonas & J. S. Levin (Eds.), *Essentials of complementary and alternative medicine* Philadelphia, Lippincott.

Diamond, B. J., Shiflett, S. C., Schoenberger, N. E., Nayak, S., Cotter, A. C., & Zeitlin, D. (1999). Complementary/alternative therapies in the treatment of neurologic disorders. In J. W. Spencer & J. J. Jacobs (Eds.), *Complementary/alternative medicine: An evidence-based approach* (pp. 170–207). St. Louis: Mosby.

Dietz, V. (1998). Honey bee venom in the treatment of arthritis. *Alternative Medicine Alert, 1*(2), 27.

Domar, A. D., & Dreher, H. (1997). *Healing mind, healthy woman.* New York: Henry Holt.

Dossey, B. M. (1997). *American Holistic Nurses Association core curriculum for holistic nursing.* Gaithersburg, MD: Aspen.

Dossey, L. (1993). *Healing words: The power of prayer and the practice of medicine.* New York: HarperCollins.

Dossey, L. (1999). *Reinventing medicine: Beyond mind-body to a new era of healing*. New York: HarperCollins.

Eisenberg, D. M., Kessler, R. C., Foster, C., Norlock, F. E., Calkins, D. R., & Delbanco, T. L. (1993). Unconventional medicine in the United States: Prevalence, costs, and patterns of use. *New England Journal of Medicine, 328,* 246–252.

Eisenberg, D. M., Davis, R. B., Ettner, S. L., Appel, S., Wilkey, S., Van Rompay, M., & Kessler, R. C. (1998). Trends in alternative medicine use in the United States, 1990–1997: Results of a follow-up national survey. *Journal of the American Medical Association, 280,* 1569–1575.

Eliopoulos, C. (1999). *Integrating conventional and alternative therapies: Holistic care for chronic conditions.* St. Louis: Mosby.

Endler, P. C. & Schulte, J. (1994). *Ultra high dilution: Physiology and physics.* Dordrecht: Kluwer.

Ernst, E., & Pittler, M. H. (2000). The efficacy of herbal drugs. In E. Ernst (Ed.), *Herbal medicine: A concise overview for professionals* (pp. 69–81). Oxford: Butterworth Heinemann.

Ernst, E., Rand, J. I., & Stevinson, C. (1998). Complementary therapies for depression: An overview. *Archives of General Psychiatry, 55,* 1026–1032.

Esplen, M. J., Garfinkel, P. E., Olmsted, M., Gallop, R. M., & Kennedy, S. (1998). A randomized controlled trial of guided imagery in bulimia nervosa. *Psychological Medicine, 28,* 1347–1357.

Ezra, S. (1999). Imagery. In C. C. Clark, R. J. Gordon, B. Harris, & C. O. Helvie (Eds.), *Encyclopedia of complementary health practice* (pp. 405–408). New York: Springer.

Fisher-Rasmussen, W., Kjaer, S. K., Dahl, C., & Asping, U. (1990). Ginger treatment of hyperemesis gravidarum. *European Journal of Obstetrics, Gynecology and Reproductive Biology, 38,* 19–24.

Flipo, D., Fournier, M., Benquet, C., Roux, P., Le Boulaire, C., Pinsky, C., La Bella, F. S., & Krzystyniak, K. (1998). Increased apoptosis, changes in intracellular Ca2+, and functional alterations in lymphocytes and macrophages after in vitro exposure to static magnetic field. *Journal of Toxicology and Environmental Health; 54*(1), 63–76.

Foster, S. (1991). *Echinacea: The purple coneflowers. Botanical Series,* No. 301. Austin, TX: American Botanical Council.

Fulder, S., & Tenne, M. (1996). Ginger as an antinausea remedy in pregnancy: The issue of safety. *HerbalGram, 38,* 47–50.

Garfinkel, M. S., Singhal, A., Katz, W. A., Allan, D. A., Reshetar, R., Schumacher, H. R. (1998). Yoga-based intervention for carpal tunnel syndrome: A randomized trial. *Journal of the American Medical Association, 280,* 1601–1603.

German Ministry of Health. (1989a). *Echinacea purpura leaf. German Commission E. Monograph for phytomedicines.* Bonn, Germany: German Ministry of Health.

German Ministry of Health. (1989b). *Echinacea purpura herb. German Commission E. Monograph for phytomedicines.* Bonn, Germany: German Ministry of Health.

Gibbs, W. W. (1996). Jungle medicine. *Scientific American, 275*(6), 20.

Glavind, K., Mouritsen, A. L., & Lose, G. (1999). Management of stress and urge urinary incontinence in women. *Acta Obstetrica et Gynecologica Scandinavia, 78*(2), 75–81.

Good, M. (1996). Effects of relaxation and music on postoperative pain: A review. *Journal of Advanced Nursing, 24,* 905–914.

Gordon, J. S. (1996). Alternative medicine and the family physician. *American Family Physician, 54,* 2205.

Gotzsche, P. (1993). Trials of homoeopathy. *Lancet, 341,* 1533.

Graedon, J., & Graedon, T. (1999). *The people's pharmacy guide to home and herbal remedies.* New York: St. Martin's Press.

Griffiths, P., & Livingstone, H. (1998). Treatment of encopresis by parent-mediated biofeedback in a child with corrected imperforate anus. *Behavioural and Cognitive Psychotherapy, 26,* 143–152.

Hahnemann, S. (1982). *Organon of medicine.* Los Angeles, CA: Tarcher.

Harris, W. S., Gowda, M., Kolb, J. W., Strychacz, C. P., Vacek, J. L., Jones, P. G., Forker, A., O'Keefe, J. H., & McCallister, B. D. (1999). A randomized, controlled trial of the effects of remote, intercessory prayer on outcomes in patients admitted to the coronary care unit. *Archives of Internal Medicine, 159,* 2273–2278.

Haskell, W. L., Luskin, F. M., Marvasti, F. F., Newell, K. A., DiNucci, E. M., & Hill, M. (1999). Complementary/alternative therapies in general medicine: Cardiovascular disease. In J. W. Spencer & J. J. Jacobs (Eds.), *Complementary/alternative medicine: An evidence-based approach* (pp. 90–106). St. Louis: Mosby.

Hatler, C. W. (1998). Using guided imagery in the emergency department. *Journal of Emergency Nursing, 24,* 518–522.

Heidt, P. (1981). Effect of therapeutic touch on anxiety level of hospitalized patients. *Nursing Research, 30*(1), 32–37.

Horrigan, B. (1999). "The mantra study project": Interview with Mitchell W. Krucoff. *Alternative Therapies in Health and Medicine, 5*(3), 74–82.

Jacobs, J. (1996). *Current status of DMSO* [On-line]. Available: http://www.dmso.org

Jerabek, J., & Pawluk, W. (1998). *Manetic therapy: The Eastern European research* [On-line]. W. Pawluk Publisher. Available: wpawluk@compuserve.com

Jonas, W. B., & Levin, J. S. (Eds.). (1999). *Essentials of complementary and alternative medicine.* Philadelphia: Lippincott–Williams & Wilkins.

Jourdain, R. (1997). *Music, the brain, and ecstasy: How music captures our imagination.* New York: William Morrow.

Keller, E., & Bzdek, V. M. (1986). Effects of therapeutic touch on tension headache pain. *Nursing Research, 35*(2), 101–106.

Klaus, L., Ramirez, G., Mulrow, C. D., Pauls, A., Weidenhammer, W., & Melchart, D. (1996). St. John's Wort for depression: An overview and meta-analysis of randomised clinical trials. *British Medical Journal, 313,* 253–258.

Kleijnen, J., Knipschild, P., & ter Riet, G. (1991). Clinical trials of homeopathy. *British Medical Journal, 302,* 316–323.

Knipschild, P., Kleijnen, J., & ter Riet, G. (1990). Belief in the efficacy of alternative medicine among general practitioners in the Netherlands. *Social Science Medicine, 31,* 625–626.

Kramer, N. A. (1990). Comparison of therapeutic touch and casual touch in stress reduction of hospitalized children. *Pediatric Nursing, 16,* 483–485.

Krippner, S. (1995). A cross-cultural comparison of four healing models. *Alternative Therapies in Health and Medicine, 1*(1), 21–29.

Kronenberg, F., Murphy, P. A., & Wade, C. (1999). Complementary/alternative therapies in select populations: Women. In J. W. Spencer & J. J. Jacobs (Eds.), *Complementary/alternative medicine: An evidence-based approach* (pp. 340–362). St. Louis: Mosby.

Kumar, A. M., Tims, F., Cruess, D. G., Mintzer, M. J., Ironson, G., Loewenstein, D., Cattan, R., Fenandex, J. B., Eisdorfer, C., & Kumar, M. (1999). Music therapy increases serum melatonin levels in patients with Alzheimer's disease. *Alternative Therapies, 5*(6), 49–57.

Lehrer, P. M. (1997). Health, homeostasis, and healing: Promises and paradoxes in the applied psychophysiology of asthma. *Biofeedback, 25*(2), 4–7.

Lin, Y., & Taylor, A. G. (1999). Effects of therapeutic touch in reducing pain and anxiety in an elderly population. *Journal of Integrative Medicine, 1*(4), 155–162.

Linde, K., & Jonas, W. W. (1999) Evaluating complementary and alternative medicine: The balance of rigor and relevance. In W. B. Jonas & J. S. Levin (Eds.) *Essentials of complementary and alternative medicine* (pp. 57–71). Philadelphia: Lippincott–Williams & Wilkins.

Low Dog, T. (1999) Phytomedicine. In W. B. Jonas & J. S. Levin (Eds.), *Essentials of complementary and alternative medicine* (pp 355–368). Philadelphia: Lippincott–Williams & Wilkins.

Lubkin, I. M., & Larsen, P. D. (1998). *Chronic illness: Impact and interventions* (4th ed.). Boston: Jones & Bartlett.

Luettig, B., Steinmuller, C., Gifford, G. E., Wagner, H., & Lohmann-Matthes, M. L. (1989). Macrophage activation by the polysaccharide arabinogalactan isolated from plant cell cultures of *Echinacea purpura. Journal of the National Cancer Institute, 81,* 669–675.

MacIntyre, R. C., & Holzemer, W. L. (1997). Complementary and alternative medicine and HIV/AIDS. Part II. Selected literature review. *Journal of the Association of Nurses in AIDS Care, 8*(2), 25–38.

Mandel, S. E. (1996). Music for wellness: Music therapy for stress management in a rehabilitation program. *Music Therapy Perspectives, 14*(1), 38–43.

Markman, M. (1996). Shark cartilage: The laetrile of the 1990s. *Cleveland Clinical Journal of Medicine, 63,* 179–180.

Mashour, N. H., Lin, G. I., & Frishman, W. H. (1998). Herbal medicine for the treatment of cardiovascular disease: Clinical considerations. *Archives of Internal Medicine, 158,* 2225–2234.

McCamy, J. C., & Presley, J. (1975). *Human life styling: Keeping whole in the 20th century.* New York: Harper Colophon Books.

McCarty, M. F. (1997). Exploiting complementary therapeutic strategies for the treatment of type II diabetes and prevention of its complications. *Medical Hypotheses, 49,* 143–152.

McEvoy, G. K. (1997). *AHFS Drug Information 97* (p. 2389). Bethesda, MD: American Society of Hospital Pharmacists.

McGrady, A., Graham, G. & Bailey, B. (1996). Biofeedback-assisted relaxation in insulin-dependent diabetes: A replication and extension study. *Annals of Behavioral Medicine, 18,* 185–189.

McGrady, A., & Horner, J. (1999). Role of mood in outcome of biofeedback assisted relaxation therapy in insulin dependent diabetes mellitus. *Applied Psychophysiology and Biofeedback, 24*(1), 79–88.

McKinney, C. H., Antoni, M. H., Kumar, M., Tims, F. C., & McCabe, P. M. (1997). Effects of guided imagery and music (gim) therapy on mood and cortisol in healthy adults. *Health Psychology, 16,* 390–400.

McKinney, C. H., Tims, F. C., Adarsh, M. K., & Mahendra, K. (1997). The effect of selected classical music and spontaneous imagery on plasma endorphin. *Journal of Behavioral Medicine, 20*(1), 85–99.

McLean, M. J., Holcomb, R. R., Wamil, A. W., & Pickett, J. D. (1995). Blockade of sensory neurons action potentials by static magnetic fields in the 10 mT range. *Bioelectromagnetics, 16,* 20–32.

Meehan, T. C. (1993). Therapeutic touch and postoperative pain: A Rogerian research study. *Nursing Science Quarterly, 6*(2), 69–78.

Merritt, S. (1996). *Mind, music and imagery*. Santa Rosa, CA: Aslan.

Miller, L. G. (1998). Herbal medicinals: Selected clinical considerations focusing on known or potential drug-herb interactions. *Archives of Internal Medicine, 158,* 2200–2211.

Milton, D. (1998). Alternative and complementary therapies: Integration into cancer care. *American Academy of Occupational Health Nursing Journal, 46,* 454–461.

Miluk-Kolasa, B., & Matejek, M. (1996). The effects of music listening on changes in selected physiological parameters in adult pre-surgical patients. *Journal of Music Therapy, 33,* 208–218.

Monsen, E. (1990). The 10th edition of the recommended dietary allowances: What's new in the 1989 RDAs? *Journal of the American Dietary Association, 89,* 1748.

Moore, K. A., & Blumenthal, J. A. (1998). Exercise training as an alternative treatment for depression among older adults. *Alternative Therapies in Health and Medicine, 4*(1), 48–56.

Moyad, M. A. (1999). Emphasizing and promoting overall health and nontraditional treatments after a prostate cancer. *Seminars in Urologic Oncology, 17,* 119–124.

Murray, M. (1996). *Encyclopedia of nutritional supplements*. Green Bay, WI: Impakt Communications.

National Center for Complementary and Alternative Medicine. (2000). *Mind-body control-fields of practice* [on-line]. Available: http://nccam.nih.gov/nccam/

National Institutes of Health. (1994). *Alternative medicine: Expanding medical horizons. A report to the National Institutes of Health on alternative medical systems and practices in the United States* (DHHS Publication No. NIH 94-066). Washington, DC: U.S. Government Printing Office.

National Institutes of Health. (1995, October 18). *NIH Technology Assessment Conference Statement: Integration of behavioral and relaxation approaches into the treatment of chronic pain and insomnia,* [on-line]. Washington, DC: Author. Available: http://text.nlm.nih.gov/nih/order.html

Nightingale, F. (1969). *Notes on nursing: What it is and what it is not*. New York: Dover Reprint. (Original work published 1859)

O'Keefe, D. (1986). Is homoeopathy a placebo response? *Lancet 29,* 1106–1107.

Oken, B. S., Storzbach, D. M., & Kaye, J. A. (1998). The efficacy of *Ginkgo biloba* on cognitive function in Alzheimer's disease. *Archives of Neurology, 55,* 1409–1415.

Olson, M., & Sneed, N. (1995). Anxiety and therapeutic touch. *Issues in Mental Health Nursing, 16,* 97–108.

Olszewer, E., & Carter, J. P. (1989). EDTA chelation therapy: A retrospective study of 2,870 patients. In E. M. Cranton (Ed.), *A textbook on EDTA chelation therapy* (pp. 197–211). New York: Human Sciences Press.

Orme-Johnson, D. W. (1997). An innovative approach to reducing medical care utilization and expenditures. *American Journal of Managed Care, 3,* 135–144.

Ornish, D., Brown, S. E., Scherwitz, L. W., Billings, J. H., Armstrong, W. T., Ports, T. A., McLanahan, S. M., Kirkeeide, R. L., Brand, R. J., & Gould, K. L. (1990). Can lifestyle changes reverse coronary heart disease? The Lifestyle Heart Trial. *Lancet, 336,* 129–133.

Ornish, D., Sherwitz, L.W., Billings, J. H., Gould, K. L., Merritt, T. A., Sparler, S., Armstrong, W. T., Ports, T. A., Kirkeeide, R. L., Hogeboom, C., & Brand, R. J. (1998). Intensive lifestyle changes for reversal of coronary heart disease. *Journal of the American Medical Association, 280,* 2001–2007.

Owens, J., Taylor, A. G., & DeGood, D. (1999). Complementary and alternative medicine and psychologic factors: Toward an individual differences model of complementary and alternative medicine use and outcomes. *The Journal of Alternative and Complementary Medicine, 5,* 329–541.

Parkes, B. (1986). Therapeutic touch as an intervention to reduce anxiety in elderly hospitalized patients. *Dissertation Abstracts International, 47,* 4775b (University Microfilms No. 13-31-462). Ann Arbor, MI: University Microfilms International.

Patterson, R. E., White, E., Kristal, A. R., Neuhouser, M. L., & Potter, J. D. (1997). Vitamin supplements and cancer risk: The epidemiologic evidence. *Cancer Causes and Control, 8,* 786–802.

Payne, R. A. (1998). *Relaxation techniques: A practical handbook for the health care professional* (3rd ed.). Edinburgh: Churchill Livingstone.

Peightel, J. A., Hardie, T. L., & Baron, D. A. (1999). Complementary/alternative therapies in the treatment of psychiatric illnesses. In J. W. Spencer & J. J. Jacobs (Eds.), *Complementary/alternative medicine: An evidence-based approach* (pp. 208–247). St. Louis: Mosby.

Petry, J. J. (1995). Garlic and postoperative bleeding. *Plastic and Reconstructive Surgery, 96,* 483–484.

Pittler, M. H. (1999). *Ginkgo biloba* extract increases pain-free walking distance. *Focus on Alternative and Complementary Therapies, 4*(4), 20–21.

Primack, A. (1999). *Complementary/alternative medicine: an evidence based approach*. St. Louis: Mosby.

Purnell, L. (1999, May-July). Complementary/alternative therapies: What are they? *DNA Reporter,* 7–9.

Quinn, J. (1984). Therapeutic touch as energy exchange: Testing the theory. *Advances in Nursing Science, 6*(2), 42–49.

Ramaratnam, S., & Sridharan, K. (1999). Yoga for epilepsy [review] [on-line]. *The Cochrane Database of Systematic Reviews, 4,* pp. 17+. Available: http://ovid.med.virginia.edu/

Reilly, D., Taylor, M. A., Beattie, N. G., Campbell, J. H., McSharry, C., Aitchison, T. C., Carter, R., & Stevenson, R. D. (1994). Is evidence for homoeopathy reproducible? *Lancet, 344,* 1601–1606.

Reynolds, J. E. F. (Ed.). (1996). *Martindale: The extra pharmacopoeia* (31st ed., pp. 1349–1396). London: Pharmaceutical Press.

Sampson, A. (1995). Homeopathy does not work. *Alternative Therapies, 1,* 48–52.

Schiedermayer, D. (1999, August). Music therapy for the relief of postoperative pain. *Alternative Medicine Alert,* 89–91.

Scott, V. (1996). A biofeedback approach to encopresis in Hirschsprung's disease. *Behavioural and Cognitive Psychotherapy, 24*(1), 83–90.

Sequeira, W. (1999). Yoga in treatment of carpal-tunnel syndrome. *Lancet, 353,* 689–690.

Shadick, N. (1999). Systemic drug therapy of osteoarthritis. In *American College of Rheumatology 1999 Annual Scientific Meeting: Conference summary index* [on-line]. Available: http://www.medscape.com/medscape/CNO/1999/ACR/

Sicher F., Targ E., Moore, D., & Smith, H. S. (1998). A randomized double-blind study of the effect of distant healing in a population with advanced AIDS: Report of a small scale study. *Western Journal of Medicine 169,* 356–363.

Simington, J. A., & Laing, G. P. (1993). Effects of therapeutic touch on anxiety in the institutionalized elderly. *Clinical Nursing Research, 2,* 438–450.

Skaggs, R. (1999). Music and imagery in healing. In C. Chambers Clark (Ed.), *Encyclopedia of complementary health practice* (pp. 430–432). New York: Springer. Inc.

Spencer, J. W. (1999). Essential issues in complementary/alternative medicine. In J. W. Spencer & J. J. Jacobs (Eds.), *Complementary/alternative medicine: An evidence-based approach* (pp. 3–36). St. Louis: Mosby.

Spencer, J. W., & Jacobs, J. J. (Eds.). (1999). *Complementary/alternative therapies in the treatment of pain.* St. Louis: Mosby.

Stampfer, M. J., & Rimm, E. B. (1996). Folate and cardiovascular disease: Why we need a trial now. *Journal of the American Medical Association, 275,* 1929–1930.

Stephens, R. (1999). Imagery as a means of coping. In J. F. Miller (Ed.), *Coping with chronic illness: Overcoming powerlessness* (3rd ed., pp. 467–480). Philadelphia: Davis.

Sun, L. Z., Currier, N. L., & Miller, S. C. (1999). The American coneflower: A prophylactic role involving nonspecific immunity. *Journal of Alternative and Complementary Medicine, 5,* 437–446.

Surh, Y. J., Lee, E, & Lee, J. M. (1998). Chemoprotective properties of some pungent ingredients present in red pepper and ginger. *Mutation Research, 402,* 259–267.

Taylor, A. G. (1999). Complementary/alternative therapies in the treatment of pain. In J. W. Spencer & J. J. Jacobs (Eds.), *Complementary/alternative medicine: An evidence-based approach* (pp. 282–339). St. Louis: Mosby.

Turkoski, B., & Lance, B. (1996). The use of guided imagery with anticipatory grief. *Home Health Care Nurse, 14,* 878–888.

Tyler, V. E. (1994). *Herbs of choice: The therapeutic use of phytomedicinals* (pp. 39–42). New York: Pharmaceutical Products Press.

U.S. Department of Health and Human Services. (1995, December 1). *Dietary Supplement Health and Education Act of 1994. U.S. Food and Drug Administration* [on-line]. Washington, DC: Author. Available: http://vm.cfsan.fda.gov/~dma/dietsupp.htm

U.S. Department of Health and Human Services. (1998). *FDA proposes rules to make claims for dietary supplements more informative, reliable and uniform* [press release, on-line]. Available: http://www.fda.gov

Upton, R. (2000). American herbal pharmacopoeia and therapeutic compendia: Analytical, quality control and therapeutic monographs. *The Journal of Alternative and Complementary Medicine, 6,* 95–96.

Vallbona C., Hazlewood, C. F., & Jurida, G. (1997). Response of pain to static magnetic fields in postpolio patients: A double-blind pilot. *Archives of Physical and Medical Rehabilitation, 78,* 1200–1203.

Vorberg, G., & Scneider, B. (1990). Therapy with garlic: Results of a placebo-controlled, double-blind study. *British Journal of Clinical Practice,* Suppl. 69, 7–11.

Waldfogel, S. (1997). Spirituality in medicine. *Primary Care, 24,* 963–976.

Wallace, J. F. (1994). Disorders caused by venoms, bites, and stings. In K. J. Isselbacher, E. Braunweld, et al. (Eds.), *Harrison's principles of internal medicine* (13th ed.). New York: McGraw-Hill.

Walleczek, J. (1995). Magnetokinetic effects on radical pairs: A paradigm for magnetic field interactions with biological systems at lower than thermal energy. In M. Blank (Ed.), *Electromagnetic fields: Biological interactions and mechanisms* (pp. 395–420). Washington, DC: American Chemical Society.

Warshafsky, S., Kamer, R. S., & Sivak, S. L. (1993). Effect of garlic on total serum cholesterol: A meta-analysis. *Annals of Internal Medicine, 119,* 599–605.

Weil, A. (1995). *Natural health, natural medicine.* Boston: Houghton Mifflin.

Weinberger, A., Nyska, A., & Giler, S. (1996). Treatment of experimental inflammatory synovitis with continuous magnetic field. *Israel Journal of Medical Science, 32,* 1197–1201.

Whorton, J. C. (1999). The history of complementary and alternative therapy. In W. B. Jonas & J. S. Levin (Eds.), *Essentials of complementary and alternative medicine* (pp. 16–30). Philadelphia: Lippincott–Williams & Wilkins.

Winslow, L. C., & Kroll, D. J. (1998). Herbs as medicines. *Archives of Internal Medicine, 158,* 2192–2199.

Wong, A. H. C., Smith, M., & Boon, H. S. (1998). Herbal remedies in psychiatric practice. *Archives of General Psychiatry, 55,* 1033–1044.

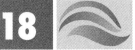

18

Challenges in Teaching and Learning

SARAH FARRELL, PhD, RN, AND JOAN L. CREASIA, PhD, RN

OBJECTIVES

At the completion of this chapter, the reader will be able to:

- Discuss the principles and practices of an effective teaching-learning experience.
- Compare and contrast major teaching-learning theories.
- Distinguish between child-centered and adult-centered teaching and learning.
- Design teaching-learning experiences for individuals and groups
- Discuss the role of information technology in teaching

PROFILE IN PRACTICE

Tami H. Wyatt, MSN, RN
Graduate Student
University of Virginia
School of Nursing
Charlottesville, Virginia

No one knows the importance of teaching in the nursing profession more than school nurses. In addition to caring for their patients, school nurses teach to promote wellness and prevent disease. Their task has become more challenging as many students today have special health needs. Due to rapid medical advancements in neonatal care, babies can survive serious illnesses that used to be fatal. However, some of these children enter the school system with developmental delays or chronic illnesses. School nurses also face a growing number of students with chronic diseases, including asthma and obesity,

most likely associated with environmental hazards and lifestyles.

The role of school health personnel is expanding at the same time that their methods must change. In this information age, consumers and health care providers rely on technology and the Internet for information. Nurses, therefore, must use instructional technology and the Internet to deliver effective instruction to consumers, families of consumers, and other health care personnel such as school staff.

Recognizing the new demands on school nurses, I focus my efforts on developing dynamic instruction to meet the special education needs of today's schoolchildren. To do this, I am active in national, state, and local school health initiatives.

I served as a member of the Southern Regional Educational Board School Health Guidelines Task Force to develop requirements for entry-level school nurses that included specific teaching-learning abilities. The task force promoted the following initiatives for school nurses:

- Develop community partnerships to provide resources and services to schoolage children.
- Teach and counsel students about health.
- Use technology to get up-to-date information and to expand teaching skills.

The task force learned that with national initiatives focusing on technology-rich education, state and local communities must follow suit.

Nurses working in schools often request creative educational methods, such as distance education and the Internet, to deliver education modules. To meet this need, I developed a web resource for children with asthma and their health care providers (http://faculty.virginia.edu/sfarrell/tami/asthma). I plan future web resources on obesity, nutrition, ADHD, and diabetes.

I also am developing an interactive storytelling program to teach children with asthma how to manage, treat, and cope with their asthma. The program will allow children to participate in an interactive story about a cartoon character with asthma and allow them to develop their own story based on personal experiences and feelings.

As a member of the local School Health Advisory Board, I have worked with community health leaders and health educators to develop Internet-based health education and multimedia programs in the areas of substance abuse, first aid, and natural disasters. I have also guided and instructed children in developing their own health-based multimedia.

To be creative with teaching and learning with schoolage children, we need to seek technology-rich and interactive learning environments. Many school nurses find themselves educating children about wellness and diseases. Their methods of teaching and learning will vary, but technology will continue to play a crucial role. Savvy health educators and nurses will learn to develop and deliver effective instruction through advanced instructional technology and the Internet.

The nurse's role with patients and families encourages, promotes, and frequently demands planned teaching-learning experiences. Most readers have probably encountered patient-teaching situations similar to the following:

- The mother of a 2-year-old newly diagnosed with juvenile diabetes needs to learn how to monitor her child's blood sugar and give his insulin injections.
- A 54-year-old African-American lawyer has just been diagnosed with hypertension. He needs information about the signs and symptoms of his disease, the side effects of medications, and the importance of diet and exercise in relation to this health problem.

- A hospice nurse visits a new patient at her daughter's home. The 32-year-old daughter wishes to be her mother's primary caregiver and needs to learn how to change her mother's colostomy bag.
- An 18-year-old girl who comes to the family planning clinic for birth control pills has little knowledge about safe sex. She is dating an abusive man with a history of intravenous drug use.

Few nurses have had formal preparation or coursework in teaching and learning. While nursing textbooks emphasize the teaching role of the nurse, most provide little information about the process of teaching and learning. Taylor (1994) notes that the nurse's role as teacher has assumed critical importance and that the nurse needs to be cognizant of changing content as well as new technologies.

This chapter presents the principles and practices of effective teaching-learning experiences, reviews some of the major teaching-learning theories, distinguishes between andragogy and pedagogy, presents research on teaching-learning styles, provides tips for designing successful teaching-learning experiences, reviews evaluation methods and discusses future uses of information technology in the teaching-learning arena.

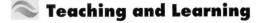 ## Teaching and Learning

Teaching is a set of planned, purposeful activities that assist the learner in acquiring new skills, knowledge, attitudes, or values. From the mid- to late 1900s, most teaching and training efforts stressed the process of teaching (i.e., writing instructor objectives and lesson plans) and focused little on learning (i.e., learner outcomes and performance).

Learning is defined as "the way in which individuals or groups acquire, interpret, organize, change, or assimilate a related cluster of information, skills, and feelings and construct meaning in their personal and shared family/work lives" (Marsick & Watkins, 1990, p. 4).

Cognitive psychologists, behavioral psychologists and experienced teachers all tend to believe that active learning is superior to passive learning. It has been said that lecturing is the least desirable method of teaching. In general, the following percentages tell a story. According to Dale (1969), we learn:

10% of what we read
20% of what we hear
30% of what we see
50% of what we see and hear
60% of what we write
70% of what we discuss
80% of what we experience
95% of what we teach

This suggests that the most effective way to learn something is to attempt to teach it to someone else. Because of the strong connection between the two, the teacher not only learns what is being taught, but quickly discovers what has not been learned. One strategy is to encourage the student or client to take some time to teach about the specific health topic to someone else—a roommate, a significant other, a stranger on the street.

Teaching is considered a formal function, whereas much of learning can be informal and incidental. Informal learning results from interactions with others through networking, coaching, and mentoring. Self-directed learning may also be termed informal learning. Incidental learning consists of learning from mistakes, assumptions, beliefs, attributions, and internalized meanings and is often a byproduct of another activity. Perhaps this is one reason why the most successful learning often takes place in groups, such as weight loss groups, grief support groups, and parenting groups, where clients help one another and the teacher is seen more as a guide or a facilitator.

TRANSFER OF LEARNING

The key to successful learning is determining how important the new learning is to the learner's ability to function effectively in his or her daily life and world. The more the learning environment resembles the actual environment where the learning will be applied, the more likely learning will be applied (Knowles, 1980). Learning transfer can be enhanced by focusing on behavior rather than knowledge, setting realistic expectations, and establishing rewards. Factors that inhibit transfer of learning include unclear expectations, poor timing, no ownership by the learner, isolated teaching, and limited opportunity for reinforcement or application (Kemerer, 1991).

MUTUALITY AND TRUST

The most successful teaching-learning experiences involve a process in which an interpersonal relationship of shared mutuality and trust is established between the teacher and the learner. In such a relationship, the nurse is viewed as the knowledge and information expert on health and the client is seen as the expert on the need for information, support, and related health behaviors within the particular context of his life. The accent is on the learner actively engaging, discovering, and taking responsibility for new ways of acting and problem solving. An example is a nurse assisting a new mother in the process of breast-feeding her newborn.

LEARNING IN THE INFORMATION AGE

With so much health care information now available on the Internet, the nurse's role as broker of information is more important than ever (Brennan & Friede, 2000). Patients now come to a clinic with information printed from a web site. As content experts, the nurse must be able to critically evaluate this web content in order to help the patient make informed choices. Internet health sites can be evaluated using a variety of evaluation schemes (Grassian, 1998; McGonigle, 1998). Box 18–1 lists McGonigle's five-step plan for evaluating websites.

Use of the Internet enhances the active learning of the patient and provides a vehicle for communication between the nurse as provider of services and the patient as informed receiver of services. Information technology includes the traditional and emerging methods of discovering, retrieving, and using information. Through technology, learning can become more interactive than other formal methods of teaching such as a lecture. The World Wide Web is a graphical version of the Internet that accommodates multimedia. The multimedia can include pictures, artwork, music, sounds, and other forms of visual and auditory illustrations. Effective teachers will use a variety of methods to enhance those who learn by different modalities. Examples of patient education web sites are listed in Box 18–2.

CHARACTERISTICS OF EFFECTIVE TEACHERS

Most of us teach the way we were taught, imitating the behaviors of the best teachers we have known and minimizing the worst behaviors of those teachers we did not like. To be an effective teacher, however, requires that we develop a sound educational theory and research base, learn the specifics of the teacher-learner roles, find new ways of interrelating, and continually explore new teaching methods. In addition, we must be able to critique our own performance and be willing to be critiqued by others (DeYoung, 1990).

Five characteristics are consistently attributed to excellent teachers in the college setting: (1) enthusiasm, (2) clarity, (3)preparation/organization of material, (4) ability to stimulate the learner, and (5) love of knowledge (Sherman et al., 1987). Although there are few studies that

---

Box 18–1 *Teaching and Learning with Information Technology: How to Evaluate Web Sites*

Step 1   Authority
Step 2   Timeliness and Continuity
Step 3   Purpose
Step 4   Content: Accuracy and Objectivity
Step 5   Structure and Access

From McGonigle, D. (1998). How to evaluate web sites. Available: http://www.hhdev.psu.edu/nurs/ojni/dm/V2N2.html

---

Box 18–2 Ten Top Sites for Patient Education

1. Kaiser   http://www.kaiserpermanente.org
2. Mayo Clinic   http://www.mayo.edu
3. McKesson   http://www.mckesson.com
4. Medtronic   http://www.medtronic.com
5. Amgen   http://www.amgen.com
6. Bristol-Myers Squibb   http://www.bms.com
7. Columbia HCA   http://www.medtropolis.com
8. Humana   http://www.humana.com
9. Johnson & Johnson   http://www.jnj.com
10. WebMD   http://www.webmd.com

Based on http://www/Webcriteria.com (downloaded March 27, 2000).

---

define and evaluate teaching effectiveness in nursing, categories such as availability to the learner, knowledge of subject, interpersonal style, teaching methods, teaching style, and evaluation methods have emerged (Reeve, 1994).

Emerging health and nursing research studies have begun to explore which instructional strategies work best with which populations. Peveler and others (1999) found that information leaflets positively affected adherence to drug treatment in primary care. On the other hand, Dixon-Woods (2000) found problems with relying on printed materials for patient education.

Wyatt (1999) argues that the educational programs most likely to succeed are those developed with a strategic plan based on theory of instruction, design, and learning, and the integration of the three. She describes a number of instructional strategies that empower the patient and integrates theories related to health promotion behaviors. While not specifically teaching learning theories, the models are helpful in understanding individual empowerment and motivation. These include the health belief model, self-efficacy, locus of control, cognitive dissonance theory, stages of readiness, and adult learning theory.

Teaching-Learning Theories

There is no shortage of theories on the teaching-learning process. Some theories focus on changes in the learner, whereas others describe the preferred teaching methods. Since no single approach to teaching and learning is effective for all clients, the nurse must draw from a variety of perspectives when designing teaching-learning experiences for the client. An overview of selected teaching-learning theories follows.

THEORIES OF LEARNING

Theories of learning can be divided into four major classifications: behaviorist, cognitive, humanistic, and empowerment.

Behaviorist Theories. The *behaviorists* believe that changed behavior (new learning) results from a stimulus and a conditioned response that requires reinforcement (a reward). Behaviorist theories include modeling or repeated practice of a new behavior until it is internalized (Bandura, 1971), stimulus substitution (Wolpe & Lazarus, 1966), operant conditioning (Skinner, 1953), and stimulus response (Pavlov, 1927), all of which positively or negatively shape or condition the learner. Another behaviorist theory is connectionism, or trial-and-error learning (Thorndike, 1913).

Teachers who subscribe to behaviorist theories will give learners feedback about their performance and reward movement toward the desired behavior. For example, "You've reached your long-term goal of a 20-pound weight loss this week. What tangible or intangible reward (other than food) are you going to give yourself? What is your plan for maintaining this weight over the next several months? How will you reward yourself then?" Table 18–1 summa-

rizes the learning principles and teaching applications relative to behaviorist theory.

Cognitive Theories. *Cognitive theory* is based on an internal change in the perception (information processing) of the individual. This change is neither obvious nor measurable and allows the individual to receive information from the environment in multiple ways. Cognitive theories include information processing, or moving from simple to complex skill (Gagne, 1974), field theory, in which the positive and negative forces for change are identified (Lewin, 1951), hierarchical structure, or identification of levels

---

TABLE 18–1 Learning Principles and Teaching Applications Relative to Behaviorist Theory

Major Theories and Theorists

Connectionism	E. L. Thorndike
Stimulus-response	I. Pavlov
Operant conditioning	B. F. Skinner
Stimulus substitution	J. Wolpe and A. Lazarus
Modeling	A. Bandura

Learning Principle	Teaching Application
Humans learn through trial and error.	Provide opportunity for problem solving.
Learning develops over time.	Provide adequate practice time; plan retesting or repeat demonstrations both immediately and at later intervals.
Given a stimulus, the learner responds.	Plan teaching strategies to trigger desired response; avoid unnecessary information that may detract from desired response.
Positive and negative feedback influence learning; positive feedback is remembered longer.	Reward learner for all correct behavior; praising positive behavior is better than punishing mistakes.
Learning is strengthened each time a positive response is received or a negative consequence is avoided.	Continue praise and positive reinforcement throughout the teaching transaction.
Learning occurs through linking behavior with associated response.	Proceed from simple to complex; provide information to show that learning is occurring.
Learning remains until other learning interferes with original learned response.	Assess prior experience with subject; some "unlearning" may be needed before new learning can take place.

TABLE 18-2   Learning Principles and Teaching Applications Relative to Cognitive Theory

Major Theories and Theorists	
Cognitive discovery	J. Piaget
Field theory	K. Lewin
Information processing theory	R. Gagne
Hierarchal structure	B. Bloom

Learning Principle	Teaching Application
Learning is based on a change in perception.	All learning cannot be readily observed; information must be internalized.
Perception is influenced by the senses.	Use multisensory teaching strategies; adjust environment to minimize distractions.
Perception is dependent on learning and is influenced by both internal and external variables.	Assess attitude toward learning, past experiences with similar situations, culture, maturity, developmental level, and physical ability before designing teaching plan.
Personal characteristics have an impact on how a cue is perceived.	Identify learning style and target it in the teaching process; develop a flexible approach.
Perceptions are selectively chosen to be focused on by the individual.	Focus learner on what is to be learned; provide support and guidance.

of learning (Bloom, 1956), and discovery learning, in which children progress through predictable stages of cognitive development (Piaget, 1954).

Teachers who use cognitive theories believe that when learners perceive a need to acquire new knowledge, skills, or attitudes, they will be motivated to learn. For example, alcoholics who become dedicated members of Alcoholics Anonymous following the loss of their job, family, and other social supports may have a high level of motivation to learn new behaviors. A summary of cognitive theory and applications is presented in Table 18-2.

Humanistic Theories. In *humanistic theory,* learning is self-motivated, self-directed, and self-evaluated. The teacher provides information and support to help learners increase their cognitive and affective functioning. Humanistic theories are the oldest classic theories and include an-

dragogy or adult-centered learning (Knowles, 1984), hierarchy of needs (Maslow, 1970), self-directed learning (Rogers, 1969), reality theory of self-awareness learning (Glasser, 1965), perceptual-existential theory or self-determined learning (Combs, 1965), and values clarification learning (Dewey, 1938).

Teachers who use humanistic theories will encourage learners to set their own goals and work toward them. For example, a nurse might ask a diabetic client, "When do you think you'll be ready to give your own insulin injection? What activities or steps would help you get ready to do this?" Table 18-3 summarizes teaching applications and learning principles relative to humanistic theories.

Empowerment Theories. These *motivated-based theories* suggest that the learner's motivation to practice health promotion is influenced by how strongly the individual feels empowered. According to the health belief model, individuals are motivated to change if they believe there may be serious risk or consequences. An instructional program applying the concepts of the health belief model provides motivation for change, focuses on behavior necessary to promote change, and provides a mechanism to promote patient empowerment (Wyatt, 1999). Parker et al. (1999) used an empowerment model in working with abused pregnant women to decrease the frequency and severity of subsequent violence.

PATTERNS OF KNOWING

Before the 1950s the apprenticeship model of education in nursing often produced graduate nurses who determined what was right and wrong in nursing practice by observing more experienced nurses, memorizing rules and facts about specific tasks, and seldom asking questions (Ashley, 1976; Reverby, 1987). In contrast, today's graduates face an increasingly complex and specialized practice that requires a rich theory base, critical thinking skills, and a value system for making ethical decisions (Oermann, 1994).

Several patterns of knowing have been identified in the nursing literature. They include: (1) ethics, the moral knowledge in nursing; (2) aesthetics, the art of nursing; (3) personal knowledge in nursing; and (4) empirics, the science of nursing (Carper, 1978). *Ethical knowledge* seeks credibility for providing care and focuses on matters of obligation or what ought to be done. *Aesthetic knowledge* is used to creatively structure, design, and implement nursing care. *Empirical* or scientific knowledge is based on objective evidence obtained by the senses, validated and verified by others, and used to describe or predict nursing actions and outcomes. *Personal knowledge* is a synthesis of knowing based on past experiences that is integrated into current situations. Chinn and Kramer (1995) built on Carper's work by developing the conceptualizations described in Table 18–4.

TABLE 18-3 Learning Principles and Teaching Applications Relative to Humanistic Theory	
Major Theories and Theorists	
Self-directed learning	C. Rogers
Hierarchy of needs	A. Maslow
Perceptual-existential theory	A. Combs
Values clarification	J. Dewey
Reality theory	W. Glasser
Andragogy	M. Knowles
Learning Principle	**Teaching Application**
Learning is self-initiated.	Promote self-directed learning.
Learner is an active participant in teaching-learning transaction.	Serve as a facilitator, mentor, and resource for learner to encourage active learning.
Learning should promote development of insight, judgment, values, and self-concept.	Avoid imposing own values and views on learner; support development of learner's self-concept.
Learning proceeds best if it is relevant to learner.	Expose learner to new, necessary information; pose relevant questions to encourage learner to seek answers.

TABLE 18–4 **Patterns of Knowing**			
Ethics	**Aesthetics**	**Empirics**	**Personal**
Valuing	Engaging	Describing	Opening
Clarifying	Intuiting	Explaining	Centering
Advocating	Envisioning	Predicting	Realizing

Modified from Chinn, P. L., & Kramer, M. K. (1995). *Theory and nursing* (4th ed.). St. Louis: Mosby.

ANDRAGOGY AND PEDAGOGY

Knowles (1980) described *andragogy* as the art and science of helping adults learn. The adult learner has a multitude of life experiences on which to build and is motivated by the desire for self-growth and self-direction. Characteristics of adult learners have implications for teaching methodology, as illustrated in Table 18–5.

Pedagogy is the art and science of teaching children. In contrast to andragogy, pedagogy is primarily initiated, planned, and facilitated by the teacher. The nurse's understanding of growth and development and age-appropriate expectations ensures a successful teaching-learning experience with children. For example, non-verbal communication, use of touch, and a soothing tone of voice can be effective teaching strategies with infants and very young children who have not yet developed language skills. The use of play, exploration, and observation with puppets have all proved to be useful teaching strategies with toddlers and preschoolers. Since schoolage children have a larger vocabulary and greater repertoire of problem-solving skills and abilities, they can learn better through formal teaching interactions, such as coloring, creating, handling objects, and asking questions. Finally, adolescents, who are struggling for their identity and are strongly influenced by their peers, challenge the teacher to respect their growing intelligence by designing more creative teaching-learning experiences. For example, the hazards of substance abuse can be communi-

TABLE 18–5 **Characteristics of Adult Learners and Implications for Teaching**	
Characteristics	**Implications**
Adults want to learn but do not always respond to traditional methods of teaching.	Diverse ways of learning, such as small project groups, teams, independent study, etc., need to be offered.
Life experiences influence how adults learn.	Learning can be enhanced by sharing these life experiences through use of discussion, role-playing, and case method.
Adults learn best if they can actively participate in learning.	If adults help to plan and conduct their own learning experiences, they will learn more than if they are passive recipients.
Identifying usefulness of the learning to the individual can enhance overall motivation of adult learner.	Learner must be involved in a mutual process of formulating learning objectives in which needs of learner, subject, institution, and society are taken into account.
Adults can be anxious about their ability to succeed.	Learning environment needs to be characterized by physical comfort, mutual trust, respect and helpfulness, freedom of expression, and acceptance of differences.
Adults enter learning experiences with different levels of learner readiness.	Learning will be more effective when programs are sequenced to allow for different levels of learner readiness.
Adults like to apply learning to more immediate life problems or situations.	Learning experiences organized around life problems will be more relevant than those organized around subject topics.

TABLE 18–6 Comparison of the Assumptions of Pedagogy and Andragogy

	Pedagogy	Andragogy
Self-concept	Dependence	Increasing self-directiveness
Experience	Needs to be built on	Learners are a rich resource for learning
Readiness	Biological development Social pressure	Developmental tasks of life roles
Time perspective	Postponed application	Immediate application
Orientation to learning	Subject centered	Problem centered

Modified from *The modern practice of adult education: From pedagogy to andragogy* by Malcolm Knowles. © 1988 by Cambridge. Used by permission.

cated to adolescents by posters displayed outside cafeterias or other popular gathering places.

Pedagogy requires different assumptions than does andragogy. While the life experiences of adults serve as a rich resource for learning, the life experiences of children are minimal. In addition, the child's orientation to learning is usually subject centered, whereas the adult's is problem centered. Table 18–6 compares the assumptions underlying pedagogy and andragogy.

The design of teaching-learning experiences necessarily differs for children and for adults. For example, the climate for pedagogy is more formal and authority oriented, whereas the climate for andragogy is more collaborative and informal. Learning objectives are usually formulated by the teacher in pedagogy while being mutually negotiated in andragogy. A comparison of pedagogy and andragogy design elements is shown in Table 18–7.

TABLE 18–7 Comparison of the Design Elements of Pedagogy and Andragogy

	Pedagogy	Andragogy
Climate	Authority oriented Formal Competitive	Mutual Collaborative/informal Respectful
Planning	By teacher	Mechanism for mutual planning
Diagnosis of needs	By teacher	Mutual self-diagnosis
Formulation of objectives	By teacher	Mutual negotiation
Design	Logic of the subject matter Content units	Sequenced in terms of readiness Problem units
Activities	Transmittal techniques	Experiential techniques (inquiry)
Evaluation	By teacher	Mutual rediagnosis of needs Mutual measurement of program

Modified from *The modern practice of adult education: From pedagogy to andragogy* by Malcolm Knowles. © 1988 by Cambridge. Used by permission.

LEARNING STYLES AND PREFERENCES

Few would argue that each of us learns in different ways. For example, some individuals prefer a lecture, others a group discussion, and still others problem solving a case study. A rich literature and research base exists on these individual differences in preferences and learning styles (Kolb, 1984). Learning styles are individual variations in the way people perceive, remember, and think, or distinctive ways of comprehending and using information. Two learning styles frequently used are Witkin's field dependence-independence model and Kolb's experiential learning theory model.

According to Witkin's model, the *field-dependent* individual perceives the whole but not the parts of a learning situation, whereas the *field-independent* person separates the background information from the whole. These differences are reflected in both the interpersonal characteristics and the learning behaviors of these individuals (Witkin, 1977). For example, field-dependent individuals learn in a global fashion, have a short attention span, view the teacher as a facilitator, and prefer the discussion method. Field-independent individuals, on the other hand, are analytical in their learning, focus on ideas and concepts, have long attention spans, view the teacher as an information giver, and prefer the lecture method.

Differences in learning styles also influence how teachers teach (Witkin, 1977). For example, field-independent teachers lecture, use questions to introduce topics, emphasize standards and principles, and provide both positive and negative feedback. Field-dependent teachers, on the other hand, design student-centered learning experiences, teach facts, use questions to check student learning after instruction, and link what is taught to life experience.

Mesoff (1979) identified differences in field-dependent and field-independent learning styles in research studies with groups. Field-dependent individuals were found to be participant observers, emphasized cooperation and collaboration,

facilitated group process, conformed to peer pressure, looked for feedback, and were motivated by the other group members. Field-independent individuals were shown to be active participants, tested out opinions and ideas, assumed group leadership (especially in a vacuum), were less affected by peer pressure and feedback, and were motivated by meeting challenges. Table 18–8 summarizes the differences in field-independent and field-dependent learners, teachers, and group members.

The Kolb model is based on experiential learning theory (ELT) developed from the works of Jung (1971), Dewey (1938), Lewin (1951), and Piaget (1970), all of whom emphasized both the process of learning, especially active participation, and the environmental influences on learning. Kolb's Learning Style Inventory (LSI) is designed to identify an individual's learning style preference as one of the following: (1) accommodator (active doer and risk taker), (2) assimilator (abstract conceptualizer and reflective observer), (3) converger (problem solver and decision maker), and (4) diverger (active doer and reflective observer). A sample of the LSI can be found in Kolb (1984) or on-line (Kolb, 2000).

Nursing Research on Learning Styles. A few studies have been conducted examining nurses' learning styles. Garity (1985) used Witkin's tool and found that head nurses had field-dependent learning styles, and Sherbinski (1994) used Kolb's tool and found that the predominant learning style of nurse anesthetist students was the assimilator style, which emphasizes reflective observation and abstract conceptualization. The assimilator learning style also was predominant in a study of diploma nursing students (Rakoczy & Money, 1995). In a sample of 93 home health aides, however, 56% were divergers and preferred instructional processes that presented materials or information in a concrete learning style (Colucciello, 1993). No studies were found that addressed client learning styles. In a critical review, Thompson and Crutchlow

TABLE 18–8 Comparison of Field-Dependent and Field-Independent Learners, Teachers, and Behavior in Groups

Field-Dependent Learning Style	Field-Independent Learning Style
Learners	
Global (wholes; gestalts)	Analytical (reflective; complex)
Relational	Idea or concept oriented
Short attention span (speed skater)	Long attention span (distance skater)
View teacher as facilitator	View teacher as information giver
Prefer discussion method	Prefer lecture method
Teachers	
Design student-centered learning experiences	Lecture
Teach facts	Emphasize standards and principles
Use questions to check student learning after instruction	Use questions to introduce topics
Link what's taught to life experience	Give both positive and negative feedback
Behavior in Groups	
Participant observers	Active participants
Emphasize cooperation, collaboration, and participation	Test out opinions, ideas, and hypotheses
Facilitate group process	Take on group leadership
Conform more to peer pressure	Less affected by peer pressure
Look for feedback	Less influenced by feedback
Motivated by group members	Motivated by meeting challenges

(1993) supported the use of Kolb's model and recommended that nurse researchers conduct studies investigating the influence of learning style on the learning environment.

～ The Teaching-Learning Plan

The steps in the teaching-learning plan parallel those of the nursing process and include assessing the learner, developing learner objectives, selecting teaching-learning strategies, implementing the teaching plan, and evaluating outcomes.

ASSESSING THE LEARNER

There are some key elements that should be explored when assessing the learning needs of clients. These include (1) knowledge level, (2) developmental characteristics (e,g., age, reading ability), (3) preferred sensory channel (i.e., auditory, kinesthetic, visual), (4) motivation or readiness to learn, (5) anxiety level, (6) health values, and (7) health status. An effective way to gather some of this information is through questioning. Characteristics of the learner can serve as enhancers or barriers to learning and influence the outcome of the teaching-learning experience (Table 18–9).

ASSESSING SPECIAL GROUPS

Clients who are from an unfamiliar culture or who are challenged in some way often have complex and unique learning needs. Assessing the special characteristics of these learners will aid in identifying learning needs and choosing teaching strategies that are appropriate and effective.

Cultural Considerations. Nurses caring for diverse populations must be culturally sensitive to the traditions, taboos, and values that facilitate or interfere with the teaching-learning process. For example, in the Asian population it is important to "save face," and these clients may not indicate a lack of understanding or may be uncomfortable answering questions about sexual functioning. Because Africans respect authority figures, they may be reluctant to ask questions about their care if the questions seem to challenge the caregiver.

When a learner from an unfamiliar culture is being assessed, a systematic appraisal of the client's beliefs, values, and health care practices is essential. Barriers to communication and preferred methods of learning must also be identified, since both may be culturally based. Several free web-based programs are available to assist in translating documents into different languages (e.g., http://www.babelfish.com). These programs are useful as a beginning step in translating teaching materials. However, all documents translated in this manner should be checked by a native speaker to ensure cultural congruency.

Challenged Populations. The reading ability of the client is a critical consideration when printed materials are used for teaching. It is important to carefully assess the client's reading level and ability to understand the written word if printed teaching materials are used. This assessment must respect the client's dignity, as many people are embarrassed by their reading difficulties. Statements about forgetting one's reading glasses often indicate an inability to read. This statement should be accepted as stated while the nurse offers to read the content to the client. When developing or selecting teaching materials, one must take care that the reading level is appropriate for the target audience. The reading level of printed materials can be determined by using most word processing programs.

Individuals who are visually or hearing impaired may require adapted educational materials. Reading materials in large print or audiotapes can be used with the visually impaired, and sign language or closed-captioned videos can be used with the hearing impaired. For those with a language barrier, an interpreter may be needed. Individuals who have impaired mobility may require adaptations in the teaching plan to accommodate their level of functioning.

DEVELOPING LEARNER OBJECTIVES

It is sometimes difficult for new teachers to develop concise and measurable learner objectives. The purposes of learner objectives are (1) to communicate what the learner is to know and do, (2) to guide in the selection and use of teaching materials, and (3) to evaluate whether the learner learned what the teacher tried to teach. For example, "Today we'll watch a video of patients giving their own insulin injections [media], tomorrow we'll practice drawing up insulin together [demonstration and return demonstration], and the next day you'll have

TABLE 18–9 Learner Characteristics That Influence Learning	
Enhancers	**Barriers**
Moderate anxiety	Fear
Trust in caregiver	Denial of health problem
Motivation	Fatigue
Perceived threat or seriousness of illness	Pain or physical discomfort
Health-oriented beliefs and practices	External demands (job, family, other responsibilities)

the opportunity to give your own insulin injection (evaluation)."

Bloom divided learning objectives into two categories: (1) cognitive (Bloom, 1956) and affective (Krathwohl, Bloom, & Masia, 1964). Cognitive objectives are concerned with the learner's mastery of different levels of cognition along a continuum from simple to complex: (1) knowledge, (2) comprehension, (3) application, (4) analysis, (5) synthesis, and (6) evaluation. Examples of cognitive objectives include the following:

- Lists correct signs and symptoms of health problem (knowledge).
- Describes relationship between exercise and weight loss (comprehension).
- Schedules 30 minutes of exercise three times weekly (application).
- Calculates amount of hidden fat in restaurant offerings before ordering (analysis).
- Prepares and cooks meals for self and family with more low-fat choices (synthesis).
- Revises exercise and dietary choices as needed (evaluation).

Affective objectives describe changes in the learner's interests, attitudes, appreciations, values, and emotional sets or biases. Levels of affective objectives include (1) receiving, (2) responding, (3) valuing, (4) organizing a value system, and (5) characterizing a value complex. Examples of affective objectives include the following:

- Accepts that present weight is unhealthy (receiving).
- Shows willingness to comply with health belief of increased exercise to decrease weight (responding).
- Desires to attain optimum weight (valuing).
- Forms judgment about the responsibility of the individual for maintaining optimum weight (conceptualization of a value).
- Revises health beliefs about weight, diet, and exercise as new information becomes available (value complex).

Much more has been written about cognitive objectives than about affective ones in the general educational and nursing literature. Present changes in society, the global economy, and health care would seem to indicate the need to pay as much, if not more, attention to the affective domain of learning.

SELECTING TEACHING-LEARNING STRATEGIES

Primary considerations in effective teaching and learning are setting the climate and selecting appropriate strategies. Some obvious ways to facilitate a climate conducive to learning include attention to room size, temperature, noise level, seating arrangements, and availability of supplies. The degree of formality or informality that sets the tone of the teaching-learning experience is also important. For example, teaching about dietary and activity recommendations to recovering stroke patients may involve a more formal and serious presentation. In contrast, a class for new parents on how to bathe the baby may be more informal and relaxed.

Cognitive capacity, psychosocial development, and physical maturation and abilities of the learner are important considerations when one is choosing a teaching strategy (Whitman et al., 1992). Selection of appropriate strategies is also influenced by cultural and environmental factors. Many individual strategies are available for designing effective teaching-learning situations.

Questioning Techniques. Teacher questioning that enhances critical thinking has a positive impact on meeting learner needs. Two types of questioning practices are important: phrasing the questions and probing the responses. Clearly phrased questions are stated simply, use words that are easily understood, focus on the content, and stress specific thinking skills. For example, "When you had your last asthma attack, were you near someone who was smoking?" Or, "How do you plan to increase your physical activity without jeopardizing your cardiac status?"

There are many ways to ask probing questions to clarify exactly what the client means, such as a more exact description of pain intensity. Additional ways include questions that increase awareness of potential motivations, refocusing the conversation when it begins to wander from the topic at hand, and asking about emotional reactions to the situation.

Demonstration. Frequently, a learning situation involves a demonstration in which a teacher shows an individual or group how to perform a particular task. To facilitate a demonstration, prepare the materials before the audience gathers and analyze the steps ahead of time. Additional tips include:

1. Start the class on time.
2. Arrange the group around you so that all can see.
3. Explain ahead of time what will happen and what to look for.
4. Demonstrate slowly and deliberately.
5. Explain each step.
6. Allow time for questions after each step.
7. Use humor to keep people alert.
8. End with a final summary and more questions.
9. Have the learners return the demonstration.

Group Discussion. A group discussion is a purposeful conversation and deliberation on a topic of mutual interest carried out under the guidance of the leader. Discussion enables participants to express opinions and to learn about topics of mutual interest. This technique provides maximum opportunity for the acceptance of personal responsibility for learning and sharing experiences and opinions with others. Focus groups are types of group discussions that have been used in research and to obtain information from the patient-consumer point of view.

Role-Playing. Selected members of a learning group spontaneously act out specific roles. This technique is used to bring participants into the closer experience of feeling and reacting to a problem. It promotes understanding of one's own and others' feelings and viewpoints. Types of role-playing include:

1. Drama: Helps participants gain insight into other people. (Plot, characters, and scenes are developed previously.)
2. *Exercise:* Larger, more complex, and prolonged version of role-playing in which groups are interacting.
3. *Psychodrama:* Directed primarily at the therapeutic treatment of individuals.
4. *Simulation games:* Learners act out their understanding and insight in handling "live" problems or "critical incidents" using gaming techniques.

Different media can also enhance teaching and learning. Questions to ask in choosing and using media, as well as their individual differences and special considerations, are summarized in Table 18–10.

EVALUATING THE TEACHING-LEARNING EXPERIENCE

Evaluation consists of determining the worth of a thing. It includes obtaining information for use in judging the worth of a program, product, procedure, or objective, or the potential utility of alternative approaches designed to attain specified objectives. In planning, designing, implementing, and validating teaching-learning experiences, knowledge of the theories and methods of evaluation is extremely important.

There are three evaluation methods that can be used concurrently in teaching and learning: formative, summative, and peer. *Formative evaluation* takes place while the teaching-learning experience is in progress. Its purpose is to identify needed changes in material, content, or teaching style in order to better meet overall program learning objectives. *Summative evaluation* occurs at the end of a teaching-learning episode and may focus on learner satisfaction, the level of learner performance, the incidence of occurrences related to the subject area (e.g., fewer episodes of hyperglycemia secondary to testing blood sugars more frequently), improved self-care skills documented through a home visit, or satisfaction with a lifestyle change (e.g., change in diet or exercise documented through a follow-up phone call). Information from summative evaluations is used to judge the value of the present teaching-learning experience compared with alternative methods or experiences.

Although learners are certainly important evaluators of teacher effectiveness, teachers should also be evaluated by peers, particularly if they

---

TABLE 18-10 Choosing and Using Audiovisual Materials

Assessment Questions:

1. Is the material accurate and current?
2. Is the age/learning level appropriate?
3. Is it interesting?
4. Is it the best available in the price range?
5. Is it an acceptable time length?

6. Is it worth the time and money?
7. Are the appearance and quality satisfactory?
8. Is it appropriate for the size audience?
9. Is the equipment available; can I operate it?
10. Is a different medium a better choice?

Media	Advantages	Considerations
Audiotapes	Useful for individuals and groups; involves auditory learners Economical, easy to prepare Can be used independently	Assess hearing with individuals, room size with groups Make backups or use good-quality tapes Review mechanics, check batteries or power
Books/pamphlets	Useful for individuals; involves visual sense Easy to use Allows client to self-pace	Assess reading ability and level of material Cost; must obtain permission to copy Texts go out of date rapidly
Computer programs	Allows self-pacing, multisensory involvement Sequential programs can be used by all learner levels Entertaining	Requires added time to learn computer use Equipment expensive Professional programming required
Films	Suitable for groups; involves sight, hearing Can stimulate emotions, build attitudes May be available from a public library Useful for compression of time and space	Does not permit self-pacing Difficult to produce Expensive to buy; allow time for order Requires darkness, special equipment
Flipchart/chalkboard	Suitable for groups; involves sight Allows step-by-step buildup Inexpensive	Bulky to transport Back to audience while writing Not reusable
Models/real objects	Useful for individuals/small groups Multisensory involvement Permits demonstration and practice	May not be easy to obtain Models costly Models often easily damaged
Posters/overheads	Useful for individuals/small groups; involves sight Easy to produce, inexpensive May be reused, easy to store	Requires viewing space and/or equipment Avoid crowding; consider color, size, and space For best appearance, have professionally done
Slides	Suitable for large groups Inexpensive, easy to produce/duplicate Easy to add/subtract material	Need partial darkness Test equipment, have extra light bulb Duplication of color slides expensive

---

Box 18-3 Sample Evaluation Questions

FORMATIVE EVALUATION OF A PARENTING CLASS

1. Things I know about my parenting are . . .
2. I learned these three things about my parenting from tonight's class . . .
3. I would like to know or ask about parenting . . .
4. If I were teaching a parent like me, I would . . .

SUMMATIVE EVALUATION OF A SERIES OF CLASSES ON PARENTING

1. What was the most effective part of the parenting classes for you?
2. Give one example of a new concept, fact, skill, or attitude you have added to your knowledge or experience.
3. How do you expect to apply this new knowledge to your parenting practices?
4. Explain briefly how you believe this knowledge will improve your parenting practices.

PEER EVALUATION OF A PARENTING CLASS

1. Emphasized major points of the teaching-learning presentation

    ____ Very well   ____ Well   ____ Satisfactorily   ____ Not very well

2. Selected appropriate content

    ____ Highly evident   ____ Evident   ____ Somewhat evident   ____ Little evidence

3. Able to ask and/or answer difficult questions

    ____ Very well   ____ Well   ____ Satisfactorily   ____ Not very well

4. Interacted effectively with learners

    ____ Very effective   ____ Effective   ____ Somewhat effective   ____ Not effective

---

are novices and are expected to grow and develop. *Peer evaluation* conducted by a colleague or an outside observer offers a different perspective on the effectiveness of the entire teaching-learning episode. An evaluation of this type calls for an experienced teacher who can evaluate against more sophisticated criteria, such as selection and organization of content, utilization of the literature, evidence of learning needs assessment, ability to ask or answer difficult questions, and quality of teaching style. Sample questions from each of these types of evaluations are provided in Box 18–3.

Technology in Teaching and Learning

Emerging information technology tools are having an impact on the teaching-learning process.

There is new terminology that corresponds to the tools being developed for both hardware (e.g., desk-based computers, laptops, video-phones) and the Internet. Asynchronous and synchronous methodologies provide a distinction between various programs that provide a teaching and learning environment using extant technology. *Synchronous* in this context refers to methods of teaching and learning that are coexistent. *Asynchronous* refers to acts of teaching and acts of learning that are not simultaneous, such as e-mail messages sent between a student and a teacher.

Synchronous learning includes the face-to-face lecture and discussion formats often used in all levels of education including colleges and universities. People are familiar with these methods. Initially, technology brought more asynchronous methods. These include e-mail, news groups, and document browsers with search engines. Newer technology brings back some of the preferences for synchronous styles. These synchronous tools include chat rooms, white boards, and interactive slide shows. Using the Internet, a teacher and a learner can be in a chat room in different parts of the world and simultaneously interact in a teaching-learning situation.

Technology is changing education at all levels. In the late 1990s children and adolescents were more digitally literate than older generations. These children will become adult consumers of health care and will be accustomed to teaching and learning experiences using technology and the Internet. They will be facile with electronic communication and chat rooms in ways that facilitate the efficiency of learning and correspond to their personal lifestyles.

The way nurses communicate as patient educators will change as well. The Pew Health Professions Commission (O'Neil & the Pew Health Professions Commission, 1998) developed 21 competencies for the 21st century related to education. This interdisciplinary group identified numerous recommendations for educational experiences in the classroom and clinical setting. In this recommendation, nurses will continually be lifelong learners as well as teachers and will need to adapt to the future technology in both roles.

Future Trends in Teaching and Learning

Technology is changing the way we teach. Future teaching-learning experiences will focus on information management, problem solving, and decision making rather than memorization. Nurses will have access to technology in devices that fit in the palm of their hand, to assist them with the explosion in knowledge (Simpson, 1999). Teaching methods will center on more experiential learning, such as interactive simulations on the Internet.

The knowledge explosion and emergence of major scientific developments mean that nurses

become continuous lifelong learners who emphasize how to think critically, how to accept the need to relearn, and how to deal with the constancy of change.

Teaching remains an important component of the professional nurse's role. To effectively implement the teaching role, a thorough understanding of the teaching-learning process is vital. Nurses must take into account variations in client health status, risk factors, cultural considerations, and a myriad of other factors to develop effective teaching-learning experiences. Adapting teaching and learning to new practice environments and changing health values of the nation will continue to challenge the profession.

KEY POINTS

- Behaviorist theories are based on the premise that learning occurs through a stimulus-response sequence, followed by consistent feedback.
- Cognitive theories propose that learning is related to an internal change in perception that is influenced by both internal and external variables.
- Humanistic theories state that learning is self-initiated and should promote the development of insight, judgment, values, and self-concept.
- Andragogy and pedagogy are based on different assumptions and design of the teaching-learning experience.
- Characteristics of adult learners influence the teaching-learning process.
- The field-dependence/field-independence model and the experiential learning model are two paradigms that focus on learning styles and preferences of the learner and teacher.
- The teaching-learning process parallels the steps of the nursing process, beginning with assessment, followed by planning, implementation, and evaluation.
- Assessment of the learner is multifaceted and includes demographic, psychosocial, cultural, physical, behavioral, and cognitive factors.

● Planning the teaching-learning experience focuses on developing learner objectives and selecting appropriate teaching-learning strategies.

● For successful implementation of the teaching plan, the environment must be conducive to learning,

● Evaluation of the teaching-learning experience includes the level of achievement of learner objectives and the effectiveness of the teacher.

● Among the future trends in teaching and learning are a reliance on information management, the development of critical thinking and problem-solving skills, and a focus on experiential learning for the continuous lifelong learner.

CRITICAL THINKING EXERCISES

1. Evaluate the effectiveness of the teaching-learning process in your own area of clinical practice. What are the typical activities of the teacher and the expected outcomes of the learner? What evaluation methods are used to determine whether learning objectives are achieved? What changes would you make in the teaching-learning process to improve its effectiveness?

2. Select a learning theory and health deviation of your choice (e.g., behavioral theory and diabetes). Develop learning objectives in the cognitive and affective domains. What teaching strategies would be effective in achieving those objectives with an adolescent client? With an older adult?

3. For each characteristic of the adult learner presented in Table 18–5 identify a specific strategy you would incorporate in the design of an effective teaching-learning situation.

4. Analyze teaching materials (care plans, pamphlets, audiovisuals) in use at your clinical facility for evidence of educational, gender, or cultural bias. Select two of these and describe the changes needed to make them culturally acceptable.

REFERENCES

Ashley, J. (1976). *Hospitals, paternalism, and the role of the nurse.* New York: Teachers College Press.

Bandura, A. (1971). Analysis of modeling processes. In A. Bandura (Ed.), *Psychological modeling.* Chicago: Aldine.

Bloom, B. (1956). *Taxonomy of educational objectives: Handbook I. Cognitive domain.* New York: David McKay.

Brennan, P. F, and Friede, A. (2000) Public health and consumer uses of health information: Education, research, policy, prevention and quality. In E. H. Shortliffe & L. E. Perreault (Eds.), *Medical informatics: Computer applications in health care and biomedicine.* New York: Springer.

Carper, B. (1978). Fundamental patterns of knowing in nursing. *Advances in Nursing Science, 1*(1), 13–23.

Chinn, P.L., & Kramer, M. K. (1995). *Theory and nursing* (4th ed.). St. Louis: Mosby.

Colucciello, M. (1993). Learning styles and instructional processes for home healthcare providers. *Home Healthcare Nurse, 11*(2), 43–50.

Combs. A. (1965). *The professional education of teachers.* Boston: Allyn & Bacon.

Dale, E. (1969). *The core of experience.* Indianapolis: Merrill.

Davis, T., & Murrell, P. (1993). *Turning teaching into learning: The role of student responsibility in the collegiate experience.* Washington, DC: George Washington University Press.

Dewey, J. (1938). *Experience and education* New York: Macmillan.

DeYoung S. (1990). *Teaching nursing.* Redwood City, CA: Addison Wesley.

Dixon-Woods, M. (2000). The production of printed consumer health information: order from chaos. *Health Education Journal, 59*(1), 108–115.

Garity, J. (1985). Learning styles: basis for effective teaching. *Nursing Educator, 10*(2), 12–16.

Gagne, R. (1974). *Essentials of learning for instruction.* Hinsdale, IL, Dryden.

Glasser, W. (1965). *Reality therapy.* New York: Harper & Row

Grassian, E. (1998) *Thinking critically about World Wide Web resources.* Los Angeles: UCLA College Library, Regents of the University of California.

Jung, C. (1971). *Psychological types.* Princeton, NJ: Princeton University Press.

Kemerer, R. (1991). *Understanding the application of learning.* In *New Directions for Adult and Continuing Education* (No. 49, pp. 67–80). San Francisco: Jossey-Bass.

Knowles, M. (1980). *The modern practice of adult education: From pedagogy to andragogy* (Rev. ed.). Chicago: Follett.

Knowles, M. (1984). *The adult learner: A neglected species* (3rd ed.). Houston: Gulf Publishing.

Kolb, D. (1984). *Experiential learning: Experience as the source of learning and development.* Englewood Cliffs, NJ: Prentice-Hall.

Kolb, D. (2000). *Learning Style Inventory* [on-line] http://trgmcber.haygroup.com/learning/lsius.htm

Krathwohl, D. R., Bloom, B. S., & Masia, B. B. (1964). *Taxonomy of educational objectives: Handbook II. Affective domain.* New York: David McKay.

Lewin, K. (1951). *Field theory in social science.* New York: Harper & Row.

Marsick, V., & Watkins, K. (1990). *Informal and incidental learning in the workplace.* New York: Routledge.

Maslow, A. (1970). *Motivation and personality.* New York: Harper & Row.

McGonigle, D. (1998). *How to evaluate web sites* [on-line]. Available: http://cac.psu.edu/~dxm12/siteval.html

Mesoff, B. (1979). *Cognitive style and interpersonal behavior: Implications for human relations training settings.* East Lansing, MI: National Center for Research on Teacher Learning. (ERIC Document Reproduction Service No. ED 185 442)

Oermann, M. (1994). Professional nursing education in the future. *Journal of Obstetrics, Gynecologic and Neo-Natal Nursing, 23*(2), 153–157.

O'Neil, E. N. & the Pew Health Professions Commission. (1998). *Recreating health professional practice for a new century.* San Francisco: Pew Health Professions Commission.

Parker, B., McFarlane, J., Soeken, K., Silva, C., & Reel, S. (1999). Testing an intervention to prevent further abuse to pregnant women. *Research in Nursing and Health, 22,* 59–66.

Pavlov, I. (1927). *Conditioned reflexes* (G.V. Anrep, Trans.). London: Oxford University Press.

Peveler, R., George, C., Kinmonth, A., Campbell, M., Thompson, C. (1999) Effect of antidepressant drug counselling and information leaflets on adherence to drug treatment in primary care: Randomised controlled trial. *British Medical Journal, 319,* 612–615.

Piaget, J. (1954). *The language and thought of the child* (3rd ed.). London: Routledge & Kegan Paul.

Piaget, J. (1970) *Genetic epistemology.* New York: Columbia University Press.

Rakoczy, M., & Money, S. (1995). Learning styles of nursing students: A 3-year cohort longitudinal study. *Journal of Professional Nursing, 11,* 170–174.

Reeve, M. (1994). Development of an instrument to measure effectiveness of clinical instructors. *Journal of Nursing Education, 33,* 15–20.

Reverby, S. (1987). *Ordered to care: The dilemma of American nursing, 1850–1945.* New York: Cambridge University Press.

Rogers, C. (1969). *Freedom to learn.* Columbus, OH: Merrill.

Sherbinski, L. (1994). Learning styles of nurse anesthetist students related to level in a master of science in nursing program. *Journal of the American Association of Nurse Anesthetists, 62*(1), 39–45.

Sherman, T., Armistead, L., Fowler, F., Barksdale, M., & Reif, G. (1987). The quest for excellence in university teaching. *Journal of Higher Education, 48,* 65–84.

Simpson, R. (1999). What does IT have in store for nursing? *Nursing Management,* October, 14–18.

Skinner, B. (1953). *Science and human behavior.* New York: Macmillan.

Taylor, C. M. (1994) *Essentials of psychiatric nursing.* St. Louis: Mosby.

Thompson, C., & Crutchlow, E. (1993). Learning style research: A critical review of the literature and implications for nursing education. *Journal of Professional Nursing, 9,* 34–40.

Thorndike, E. (1913). *The psychology of learning.* New York: Teachers College Press.

Whitman, N. I., Graham, B. A., Gleit, C. J., & Boyd, M. D. (1992). *Teaching in nursing practice* (2nd ed.). Norwalk, CT: Appleton & Lange.

Witkin, H. (1977). Field dependence and interpersonal behavior. *Psychological Bulletin, 84,* 661.

Witkin, H., Moore, C., Goodenough, D., & Cox, P. (1977). Field-dependent and field-independent cognitive styles and their educational implications. *Review of Educational Research, 47,* 1–64.

Wolpe, J., & Lazarus, A. (1966). *Behavior theory techniques: A guide to the treatment of neurosis.* Oxford: Pergamon Press.

Wyatt, T. H. (1999) Instructional technology and patient education: Assimilating theory into practice. *International Electronic Journal of Health Education, 2*(3):85–93.

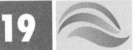

19

Critical Thinking

C. FAY RAINES, PhD, RN

OBJECTIVES

At the completion of this chapter, the reader will be able to:

- Define critical thinking.
- Identify the components and characteristics of critical thinking.
- Understand the relationship of critical thinking to problem solving and decision making.
- Compare and contrast critical thinking, clinical judgment, and the nursing process.
- Apply critical thinking in nursing practice situations.

PROFILE IN PRACTICE

Elizabeth R. Lenz, PhD, RN, FAAN
Anna C. Maxwell Professor of Nursing Research
Associate Dean for Research and Doctoral Studies
Columbia University School of Nursing
New York, New York

Critical thinking: it's recognizable when someone does it well and certainly evident when it is not happening. During the past 20 years we have talked increasingly about critical thinking in nursing, but that wasn't always the case. In the early 1960s, when I was entering the profession, serious efforts to change the "handmaiden" image of nursing were only just beginning. Clearly, if one's role is defined as handmaiden, rather than as colleague or independent decision maker, critical thinking is not particularly important, or even desirable. Rather, blind, noncritical obedience is the order of the day. As nursing has become more truly professional and nurses have func-

tioned with increasing autonomy in increasingly complex situations, critical thinking has become a most important and valued competency.

What elements converge to produce a good critical thinker? It seems to me that there are several requisites, not the least of which is intelligence. While a necessary condition, it is no guarantee that critical thinking will occur without both training and a nourishing environment. We assume that critical thinking is something that can be learned; hence we address it at all levels of nursing curricula.

Based on my experience, I believe that two essential types of learning provide the basis for critical thinking. The first is substantive. It is impossible to think truly critically about something you do not understand or about which you possess only partial information. Mastery of the theory and research findings that relate to the problem or issue to be addressed is critical, yet it is not something that nurses always take time to do. Unfortunately, we have been less successful than other professions, namely medicine, in socializing our practitioners to value learning as a career-long pursuit, yet pursuit of the most state-of-the-science information is an essential ingredient of critical thinking.

The second type of learning is about the process of critical thinking itself. The skills of raising questions, using logic, and comprehensively considering alternative perspectives, explanations, and courses of action can often best be learned experientially within a structure that encourages and, in fact mandates, that kind of thoughtful consideration. The model that comes to mind is the daily medical rounds in which physicians-in-training are challenged to present cases and to lay out their diagnostic reasoning clearly for others to critique. Equally valid as an environment for cultivating critical thinking is that found in many of the social sciences and humanities, where freewheeling debate and open challenge of ideas is encouraged. At first frightened by that kind of candor during my doctoral studies in sociology, I later came to value greatly the critical input of my peers. More of that kind of willingness to challenge each other's assumptions and ideas within an atmosphere of mutual respect would benefit our profession.

For me the groundwork for critical thinking was laid early in my education. Fortunately, the faculty responsible for the BSN program I attended were forward-thinking and highly committed to the emerging definition of nursing as a true profession, with the requisite obligation to base action on scientific knowledge and clear and logical thinking. Without labeling the goal as such, we were consistently encouraged, groomed,

and enabled to be critical thinkers. We were continually challenged by being asked to provide rationale for our decisions, to make explicit all of the alternative approaches and explanations we had considered and rejected, and to explain why. Not inconsequentially, the school was in a small liberal arts institution, where we were exposed on a daily basis to a wide range of points of view and disciplinary perspectives and assumptions. If anything, the nursing students were the "odd balls," whose pragmatism and goal-directedness seemed strange to the arts, sciences, and music majors. I wrestled more than once with how in the world assignments like dissecting the symbolism in *Moby-Dick* might be relevant to my career in nursing, but I now appreciate the mind-expanding contribution that such activities made to my ability to think critically.

The base hopefully having been laid during one's professional education, critical thinking depends not only on training, but also on an environment or context that enables, encourages, and rewards it. Regretfully, today's employment picture in nursing is typically one in which there is precious little time for contemplation. Downsizing, high proportions of nonprofessional personnel, high levels of acuity, and high productivity requirements may discourage critical thinking. That means every effort must be made to counter the tendency to let it slide, and to encourage, nurture, and reward it, even if that means bucking the tide and incurring some additional short-term costs.

The "community of scholars" type of environment to which top educational institutions aspire should, by definition, be conducive to critical thinking. Nevertheless, even in those settings, time and energy to engage in deliberation, to exchange ideas and to critique them openly are scarce, and the kind of culture that encourages such scholarly dialogue is relatively rare. When it is in place, it is wonderful! One of my most exciting opportunities to engage in intense and prolonged critical thinking was when a group of four colleagues and I were "freed up" from many of our routine responsibilities to plan a PhD program "from scratch." In weekly full-day sessions we argued, debated, challenged, cajoled, compromised, and created. We drew on what we knew substantively about nursing, science, philosophy, and the disciplines of our respective doctorates (none of which was in nursing). It was hard work, but invigorating. The ground rules were that no idea was to be belittled or rejected out of hand; all perspectives were heard and considered. Importantly, we were given time to think with minimal interruption and maximum flexibility; accordingly, the end product was excellent, and the process truly energizing! Such time away from the routine is rarely available in today's environment, but the model is certainly not without merit. Essential are a culture and a leadership that permit and encourage critique without recrimination.

In clinical settings, time to engage in deliberative critical thinking is even more difficult to attain. Rather, critical thinking seems to be expected to occur routinely without much cultivation. Benner's model of progression from novice to expert suggests that excellent clinical experience fosters critical thinking that eventually

becomes almost automatic and intuitive. However, I assert that the level of critical thinking that is displayed by clinical experts needs to be developed deliberately and strategically. The clinical environment in which I have seen critical thinking encouraged most effectively was one in which the expectations were explicit, it was measured routinely in the practice context, relevant learning and growth opportunities were provided, and it was taken into account in performance evaluation. In other words, the nursing leadership in that academic medical center truly valued critical thinking and was willing to assign it priority.

Nursing has reached the point in its evolution where a consistent and continuous pattern of critical thinking by its practitioners is a mandate—a sine qua non. The assurance that critical thinking will be truly woven into the fabric of our profession will depend on our ability to recruit and retain intelligent, interested, and committed nurses; to provide challenging educational opportunities that develop the requisite competencies; and to provide and sustain the kinds of environments in which critical thinking is valued and demanded.

A cornerstone of professional nursing practice is the ability to process information and make decisions. The demands of clients from diverse backgrounds with multiple health care needs, coupled with the demands of a complex health care system, require higher-order thinking that is not solely content based. It is essential that professional nurses think critically in order to process complex data and make intelligent decisions in planning, managing, and evaluating the health care of their clients. Similarly, critical thinking is essential if nurses are to make productive contributions toward establishing the future direction of health care. To become a critical thinker, a nurse must understand the

concept of critical thinking, identify the skills and internalize the dispositions of a critical thinker, and deliberately apply critical thinking principles to clinical situations.

The Concept of Critical Thinking

In recent years critical thinking has received considerable attention as an essential component of educational programs and of nursing practice. The underlying point of many of these discussions is that there is a need for higher-order thinking as the complexity of our world increases. Critical thinking accommodates this complexity as it is a nonlinear process based on reason, reflection, knowledge, and instinct derived from experience (Catalano, 2000).

DEFINING CRITICAL THINKING

Critical thinking, as a concept, has been examined and presented from a variety of perspectives. An early definition, proposed by Watson and Glaser (1964), described *critical thinking* as the combination of abilities needed to define a problem, recognize stated and unstated assumptions, formulate and select hypotheses, draw conclusions, and judge the validity of inferences. A less prescriptive definition was offered by Ennis (1989), who characterized critical thinking as "reasonable reflective thinking focused on deciding what to believe or do" (p. 4). Paul (1992) stated that critical thinking is a process of disciplined, self-directed rational thinking that "certifies what we know and makes clear wherein we are ignorant" (p. 47). Alfaro-LeFevre (1999) presented critical thinking as controlled, purposeful thinking which focuses on using well-reasoned strategies to achieve desired outcomes. *Critical thinking for nursing,* as described by Bandman and Bandman (1995), is "the rational examination of ideas, inferences, assumptions, principles, arguments, conclusions, issues, statements, beliefs, and actions" (p. 7) and includes the following functions:

- Discriminating among use and misuse of language
- Analyzing the meaning of terms
- Formulating nursing problems
- Analyzing arguments and issues into premises and conclusions
- Examining nursing assumptions
- Reporting data and clues accurately
- Making and checking inferences based on data
- Formulating and clarifying beliefs

- Verifying, corroborating, and justifying claims, beliefs, conclusions, decisions, and actions
- Giving relevant reasons for beliefs and conclusions
- Formulating and clarifying value judgments
- Seeking reasons, criteria, and principles that justify value judgments
- Evaluating the soundness of conclusions

Conclusions are drawn as a result of this reasoning process. In nursing practice, the desired outcome of this reasoning is effective action.

There are conflicting viewpoints as to whether critical thinking is subject-specific or generalizable (U.S. Department of Education, 1995). Meyers (1991) believes that before critical thinking skills can be developed, mastery of basic terms, concepts, and methodologies must occur. McPeck (1990) agrees, noting that only by immersion in the discipline can critical thinking skills be fully developed. He argues that being an effective critical thinker in one area does not mean that one will be an effective thinker in another area because knowledge and skills differ in various fields. Einstein, who was an expert critical thinker in physics but inept in other areas, is an example of this point. Ennis (1987), on the other hand, suggests that there are principles of critical thinking that bridge many disciplines and can transfer to new situations, although some familiarity with the subject matter is necessary.

The Delphi Report. An attempt to define critical thinking by consensus was begun in the late 1980s, and the results became known as *The Delphi Report.* The Delphi research project used an expert panel of theoreticians representing several disciplines from the United States and Canada to develop a conceptualization of critical thinking from a broad perspective (Facione, 1990). The resulting work described critical thinking in terms of cognitive skills and affective dispositions. The outcome was a definition of *critical thinking* as the process of purposeful, self-regulatory judgments: an interactive, reflective reasoning process (Facione & Facione, 1996). A critical thinker gives reasoned consideration to evidence, context, theories, methods, and criteria in order to form a purposeful judgment. At the same time, the critical thinker monitors, corrects, and improves the judgment. The Delphi project produced the following consensus definition from its panel of experts:

> We understand critical thinking (CT) to be purposeful, self-regulatory, judgment which results in interpretation, analysis, evaluation, and inference, as well as explanation of evidential, conceptual, methodological, criteriological, or contextual considerations upon which that judgment is based. . . . CT is essential as a tool of inquiry. As such, CT is a liberating force in education and a powerful resource in one's personal and civic life (American Philosophical Association, 1990).

The Delphi participants identified core critical thinking skills as interpretation, analysis, inference, evaluation, and explanation. These critical thinking cognitive skills and subskills are listed in Table 19–1.

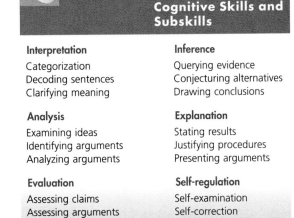

TABLE 19–1 Critical Thinking Cognitive Skills and Subskills

Interpretation
Categorization
Decoding sentences
Clarifying meaning

Analysis
Examining ideas
Identifying arguments
Analyzing arguments

Evaluation
Assessing claims
Assessing arguments

Inference
Querying evidence
Conjecturing alternatives
Drawing conclusions

Explanation
Stating results
Justifying procedures
Presenting arguments

Self-regulation
Self-examination
Self-correction

SUMMARY OF DEFINITIONS OF CRITICAL THINKING

While there is not a universally accepted definition of critical thinking, there is agreement that it is a complex process. The variety of definitions helps to provide insight into the myriad dimensions of critical thinking. Commonalities in definitions include an emphasis on knowledge, cognitive skills, beliefs, actions, problem identification, and consideration of alternative

TABLE 19–2 Definitions of Critical Thinking

Author	Definition
Watson and Glaser (1964)	Combination of abilities needed to define problems, recognize assumptions, formulate and select hypotheses, draw conclusions, and judge validity of inferences
Ennis (1989)	Reasonable reflective thinking focused on deciding what to believe or do
Paul (1992)	Process of self-disciplined, self-directed, rational thinking that verifies what we know and clarifies what we do not know
Delphi Report (1990); Facione, Facione, and Sanchez (1994)	Purposeful, self-regulatory judgments resulting in interpretation, analysis, inference, evaluation, and explanation
Alfaro-LeFevre (1999)	Purposeful and outcome-focused thinking
Bandman and Bandman (1995)	Rational examination of ideas, inferences, assumptions, principles, arguments, conclusions, issues, statements, beliefs, and actions

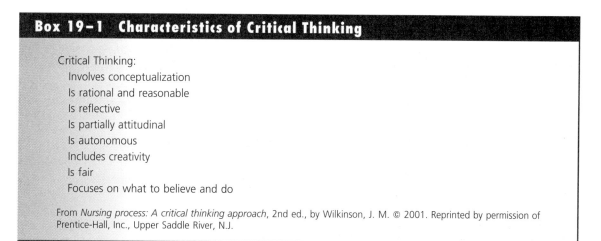

Box 19–1 Characteristics of Critical Thinking

Critical Thinking:

Involves conceptualization

Is rational and reasonable

Is reflective

Is partially attitudinal

Is autonomous

Includes creativity

Is fair

Focuses on what to believe and do

From *Nursing process: A critical thinking approach*, 2nd ed., by Wilkinson, J. M. © 2001. Reprinted by permission of Prentice-Hall, Inc., Upper Saddle River, N.J.

views and possibilities (Daly, 1998). The definitions presented earlier are summarized for comparison in Table 19–2, and characteristics of critical thinking are listed in Box 19–1.

The activities involved in the process of critical thinking include appraisal, problem solving, creativity, and decision making. The interrelationships between these concepts are illustrated in Figure 19–1. These activities are embedded

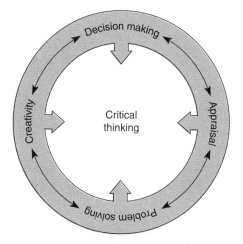

FIGURE 19–1 Critical thinking model. (Redrawn from *Role transition to patient care management* by M. K. Strader and P. J. Decker. © 1995. Reprinted by permission of Prentice-Hall, Inc., Upper Saddle River, N.J.)

in the critical thinking process in both nursing education and nursing practice.

Critical Thinking in Nursing

In nursing, critical thinking has often been portrayed as a rational linear process that is synonymous with problem solving and closely akin to the nursing process (Ford & Profetto-McGrath, 1994; Jones & Brown, 1993; Kintgen-Andrews, 1991). While the nursing process is one critical thinking competency that uses higher-order thinking to plan, provide, and evaluate nursing care, it is not all-encompassing. There is criticism that the nursing process constrains critical thinking because of its mechanistic approach (Conger & Mezza, 1996; Duchscher, 1999; Jones & Brown, 1993; Miller & Malcolm, 1990). Furthermore, equating critical thinking with problem solving implies that all critical thinking must be problem based. Models for critical thinking based on problem solving alone foster action according to predefined standards and objectives. The idea of predefinition is inconsistent with many of the tenets of critical thinking.

CRITICAL THINKING AND THE NURSING PROCESS

While critical thinking skills are important components of the nursing process and problem solving, they are not synonymous terms. The nursing process can serve as a tool for critical thinking, however. To effectively use the nursing process, the nurse must engage in critical thinking that is disciplined, logical, and reflective. Throughout the nursing process, the nurse uses a combination of abilities to sort and categorize data, identify patterns in the data, draw inferences, develop hypotheses that are stated in the form of outcomes, test these hypotheses as care is delivered, and make criterion-based judgments of effectiveness. Such critical thinking can distinguish between fact and fiction, thereby providing a rational basis for the delivery of nursing care. Although the components of the nursing process are described as separate and distinct steps, they become an integrated way of thinking as nurses gain more clinical experience. An overview of critical thinking throughout the nursing process is presented in Table 19–3.

Nursing literature about critical thinking addresses ways to teach critical thinking skills and to use critical thinking skills in clinical practice. "The use of critical thinking . . . with whatever theory or process selected, will enhance the validity, reliability, and worth of outcomes to clients, patients, and practitioners" (Bandman & Bandman, 1995, p. 99).

CURRICULUM INNOVATIONS FOR TEACHING CRITICAL THINKING

With a focus on critical thinking, nursing education is shifting from a purely problem-solving approach to one in which critical reflection mediates the relationship between knowledge and

TABLE 19–3 Overview of Critical Thinking Throughout the Nursing Process

Nursing Process	Critical Thinking
Assessment	Observing Distinguishing relevant from irrelevant data Distinguishing important from unimportant data Validating data Organizing data Categorizing data
Analysis/diagnosis	Finding patterns and relationships Making inferences Stating the problem Suspending judgment
Planning	Generalizing Transferring knowledge from one situation to another Developing evaluative criteria Hypothesizing
Implementation	Applying knowledge Testing hypotheses
Evaluation	Deciding whether hypotheses are correct Making criterion-based evaluations and judgments

Adapted from *Nursing process: A critical thinking approach*, 2nd ed., by Wilkinson, J. M. © 2001. Adapted by permission of Prentice-Hall, Inc., Upper Saddle River, N.J.

action. The ever-expanding rate of change in health care requires that students learn more, evaluate new knowledge, and monitor their own practice in light of the changes. In addition, the emphasis on critical thinking in education has been formalized in outcome measures for regional and specialized accreditation criteria. While there is general agreement that critical thinking skills should be supported and developed within educational programs, there is much less agreement on the methods of teaching these skills. Reviews of research in the literature reveal mixed findings, with no consistent evidence that nursing education contributes to an increase in critical thinking abilities in nursing students (Adams, 1999).

Incorporating and measuring critical thinking outcomes is a complex task leading to a variety of teaching methods. Keeping journals and using them to create action plans, using Socratic questioning, analyzing case studies from clinical practice, developing innovative clinical experiences, and modeling reflective problem solving are among the methods suggested for teaching critical thinking to students at all levels (Baker, 1996; Brock & Butts, 1998; Callister, 1996; Colucciello, 1999; Daley et al., 1999; Feingold & Perlich, 1999; Kelly, 1997; Mastrian & McGonigle, 1999; Paul & Heaslip, 1995; Perciful & Nester, 1996; Rossignol, 1997; Schumacher & Severson, 1996; Sedlak & Doheny, 1998; Wade, 1999). One carefully constructed framework for teaching and evaluating critical thinking was developed at the Indiana University School of Nursing (Dexter et al., 1997). Competencies were based on cognitive skills derived from *The Delphi Report*'s definition of critical thinking. These cognitive skills of interpretation, analysis, evaluation, inference, explanation, and self-regulation were operationalized and leveled for associate degree, baccalaureate, master's, and doctoral programs. Suggestions for faculty use in evaluating critical thinking accompany these definitions. Such frameworks provide useful guidance for teaching and measuring what is often seen as an elusive concept.

The University of Wyoming School of Nursing incorporates the analysis of newspaper articles in a course on professional issues (Beeken et al., 1997). At the University of Alabama in Huntsville College of Nursing, registered nurse students present paradigm cases of a clinical situation in refining their critical thinking abilities.

The goal of these strategies is to help students think critically and reflectively. The effective strategies support and encourage students in seeing new possibilities by going beneath the surface of a situation to examine underlying assumptions that constrain discourse and autonomous action. Critical reflection requires a disposition to listen; a tolerance for diversity, disagreement, and uncertainty; and an openness to new ideas. It includes critical examination of one's own practices. This self-examination enables an understanding of the personal perceptions and assumptions of a situation that guide one's practice. It also requires understanding a situation and the way the system works to maintain the status quo. This action involves risk taking, challenges the status quo, and requires a more active learning environment.

NURSING JUDGMENT MODEL

A critical thinking approach to clinical practice encourages nurses to challenge established theories and practices that are based on linear models of thinking. Clinical judgment, which makes use of reflective thinking, is strongly rooted in the critical thinking process (Duchscher, 1999). Kataoka-Yahiro and Saylor (1994) describe a model for nursing judgment and assert that the critical thinking process is "reflective and reasonable thinking about nursing problems without a single solution and is focused on deciding what to believe and do" (p. 352). This model identifies the outcome of critical thinking as discipline-specific clinical judgments.

Components of Critical Thinking. The critical thinking model for nursing judgment presents five components of critical thinking: specific knowledge, experience, competencies, attitudes, and standards of care.

KNOWLEDGE. Domain-specific knowledge is essential to successful clinical reasoning because knowledge provides the data for critical thinking processes. For example, one cannot identify appropriate actions for unexpected clinical symptoms without understanding the physiology involved. This example highlights the fact that for critical thinking to be productive, nurses must have a sound knowledge base.

EXPERIENCE. The lack of practical experience and opportunity to make decisions can limit the development of critical thinking. Understanding complex situations comes through experience in analyzing similar and contrasting situations. The importance of experiential knowledge as a nurse moves from novice to expert clinician has been emphasized by Benner (1984).

COMPETENCIES. The nursing judgment model features cognitive rather than psychomotor competencies. Cognitive competencies are of three types: general critical thinking competencies, specific critical thinking competencies in clinical situations, and specific critical thinking competencies in nursing. General critical thinking competencies are common to other disciplines and nonclinical situations and therefore are not unique to nursing. Examples include the scientific process, hypothesis generation, problem solving, and decision making. Specific critical thinking competencies in clinical situations are used by nurses and other health care providers and include diagnostic reasoning, clinical inferences, and clinical decision making.

ATTITUDES. *Attitudes* are "traits of the mind" and are central aspects of a critical thinker (Paul, 1992). According to Paul, critical thinking is impossible if one does not persevere at reasoning, does not fairly weigh evidence for an opposing viewpoint, or does not value curiosity or discipline. It is essential to cultivate independence, confidence, and responsibility, and to acknowledge the limits of one's personal knowledge or viewpoint. Thus, the critical thinking model for nursing judgment includes attitudes of confidence, independence, fairness, responsibility, risk taking, discipline, perseverance, creativity, curiosity, integrity, and humility.

STANDARDS. Both intellectual and professional standards are important to the nursing judgment model. Critical thinking must meet the universal intellectual standards identified by Paul (1992) and presented in Figure 19–2. Critical thinking also must be consistent with standards of professional nursing (e.g., the American Nurses Association's [ANA] *Code for Nurses* and *Standards of Professional Nursing Practice*). That is, nurses engage in critical thinking for the good of individuals or groups rather than to cause harm or to undermine a situation. Professional standards include criteria for ethical nursing judgment, evaluation, and professional responsibility.

Levels of Critical Thinking. In addition to the five components of critical thinking, three levels of thinking are included in the Kataoka-Yahiro and Saylor model. These levels are basic, complex, and commitment.

At the *basic* level, the nurse views answers as dichotomous and assumes that authorities have a correct answer for every problem. There is also acceptance that there is a diversity of opinions and values among authorities. Although the goal is to move to higher levels of thinking, movement can be restricted by lack of knowledge and experience as well as by inadequate competencies, inappropriate attitudes, and nonutilization of standards.

At the *complex* level, the nurse continues to recognize diversity in outlooks and perceptions and also has the ability to systematically detach, analyze and examine alternatives. Here the best answer to a problem might be "it depends." Alternative, perhaps conflicting solutions are recognized. An example of complex thinking is deciding to deviate from standard protocols or roles in a specific complex client situation.

At the *commitment* level, the nurse anticipates the necessity of making a personal choice

PERFECTION............VS.............IMPERFECTION OF THOUGHT

Clear............................vs.............Unclear

Precise........................vs.............Imprecise

Specific.......................vs.............Vague

Accurate......................vs.............Inaccurate

Relevant......................vs.............Irrelevant

Plausible......................vs.............Implausible

Consistent....................vs.............Inconsistent

Logical.........................vs.............Illogical

Deep............................vs.............Superficial

Broad...........................vs.............Narrow

Complete.....................vs.............Incomplete

Significant....................vs.............Trivial

Adequate for purpose...vs.............Inadequate

Fair...............................vs.............Biased or one-sided

FIGURE 19-2 Intellectual standards for thinking. (From Paul, R. (1992). *Critical thinking: What every person needs to know to survive in a rapidly changing world.* Santa Rosa, CA: Foundation for Critical Thinking.)

after the relative merits of alternatives have been examined. The nurse chooses an action or belief based on the alternatives identified at the previous level. If the chosen action is unsuccessful, alternative solutions are considered and used.

The three levels of thinking can be illustrated in a practice situation in which a nurse receives a physician's medication order. Nurses functioning at each level of thinking will handle the situation the following ways:

Basic: "Since Dr. Jones wrote it, it must be correct. However, last week we had a client with the same problem, and Dr. Smith ordered a different medication. There must be two ways to treat this problem."

Complex: "I wonder why we are treating identical clients in two different ways? I am going to explore this issue in more detail."

Commitment: "I have examined all the information I can find, and I think Dr. Jones made a mistake in the order. I am going to call and confer with her."

The requirement for critical thinking in nursing judgment is based on the complexity of sound clinical reasoning. Effective nursing care requires that the nurse avoid simplistic generalizations about procedures and routines in favor of rational individualized clinical judgment based on critical thinking. "Being able to make effective clinical judgments comes from a 'marriage' of theoretical and experiential knowledge" (Alfaro-LeFevre, 1999, p. 83).

CREATIVITY THINKING

Higher levels of thinking require a creative outlook. *Creativity thinking* is a process that leads to the development of ideas or products that are new and original. It is an essential component of critical thinking for health care providers, particularly as methods of health care delivery shift and demands for accountability increase. Creative thinkers are open to new ideas, provide alternatives, and are willing to dream and take risks. Challenging traditional ways of thinking and being open to new ways of thinking is the essence of creativity thinking. "As nurses we must reframe how we think about our jobs to be more creative, more open to a variety of possibilities, and more open to options that might work" (Grossman & Valiga, 2000, p. 100).

How does creativity thinking differ from critical thinking? A clear example of the difference is presented by Miller and Babcock (1996), who state that "creative thinking is the kind of thinking you use to construct a hypothesis and critical thinking is the kind of thinking you use when you test that hypothesis" (p. 116). The creative thinker projects an attitude of open-mindedness and flexibility, while the critical thinker is more tentative, cautious, and analytical. Creativity thinking is valued for its potential to facilitate change and enhance progress.

The environment in which students learn and nurses practice can either constrain or facilitate creativity thinking. An environment that impedes creative thinking is one that reinforces memorizing, retaining factual information, and following orders. An environment that is conducive to creative thinking is characterized by flexibility, openness, support for change, and risk taking. An environment that demands perfection and reinforces the status quo constrains both critical thinking and creativity thinking. Such an environment leads to the attitude, "If it is not going to be accepted, or even considered, why bother?"

Characteristics of Critical Thinkers

Eight interdependent traits of mind are essential to becoming a critical thinker (Paul & Elder 1999):

1. *Intellectual humility*—an awareness of the limits of one's knowledge and sensitivity to the possibility of self-deception.
2. *Intellectual courage*—involves willingness to listen and examine all ideas, including those to which there is a negative reaction.
3. *Intellectual empathy*—imagining oneself in the place of others in order to better understand them. It allows reasoning from the viewpoint of others.
4. *Intellectual integrity*—the application of rigorous and consistent standards of evidence and the admission of errors when they occur.
5. *Intellectual perseverance*—willingness to continually seek intellectual insights over a period of time and in the face of difficulties.
6. *Faith in reason*—reflects confidence in one's own ability to think rationally.
7. *Intellectual sense of justice*—holding to intellectual standards without seeking one's own advantage.
8. *Intellectual Autonomy*—having rational control of one's beliefs, values, and inferences.

Individuals who are critical thinkers have specific sets of characteristics. According to Alfaro-LeFevre (1999), active thinkers ask themselves such questions as "Am I seeing things correctly? "What does this really mean?" "Do I know why this is?" "How can I be more sure?" Other characteristics identified by Alfaro-LeFevre include being

- Knowledgeable about biases and beliefs
- Confident, patient, and willing to persevere
- A good communicator, who realizes that mutual exchange is essential to understanding the facts and finding the best solutions
- Open-minded, listening to other perspectives, and withholding judgments until all evidence is weighed
- Humble, realizing that no one has all the answers.

- Proactive, anticipating problems, and acting before they occur
- Organized and systematic in the approach to problem solving and decision making
- An active thinker with a questioning attitude
- Flexible, changing approaches as needed
- Cognizant of rules of logic, recognizing the role of intuition, but seeking evidence and weighing risks and benefits before acting
- Realistic, acknowledging that the best answers do not mean perfect answers
- Creative and committed to excellence, looking for ways to improve oneself and the way things get done

The Delphi Report's description of an ideal critical thinker also describes the attributes of a nurse with ideal clinical judgment:

The ideal critical thinker is habitually inquisitive, well-informed, trustful of reason, open-minded, flexible, fair-minded in evaluation, honest in facing personal biases, prudent in making judgments, willing to reconsider, clear about issues, orderly in complex matters, diligent in seeking relevant information, reasonable in the selection of criteria, focused in inquiry, and persistent in seeking results which are as precise as the subject and the circumstances of inquiry permit (American Philosophical Association, 1990, p. 3).

Disposition Toward Critical Thinking

Becoming a critical thinker involves more than developing a set of skills. It involves nurturing the disposition toward critical thinking to ensure the use of critical thinking skills outside of a structured setting, such as a classroom. Seven aspects of critical thinking disposition, based on the findings from *The Delphi Report*, are incorporated into the California Critical Thinking Disposition Inventory (CCTDI) (Facione et al., 1995). These dispositional subscales, designed

to be discipline neutral, have relevance for nursing practice:

- *Inquisitiveness* is intellectual curiosity and desire for learning even when there is not a readily apparent application for the knowledge. For nurses, a deficit here might signal a limited potential for developing expert knowledge and clinical practice ability. Nurses who routinely ask, "I wonder why—?" in the absence of a specific problem display inquisitiveness.
- *Systematicity* is the tendency toward organized, orderly, focused, and diligent inquiry. Asking questions such as "In what order did the client's symptoms occur?" and "Is there more information we should consider?" are examples of systematic inquiry. Organized approaches are essential for competent clinical practice.
- *Analyticity* is applying reasoning and the use of evidence to resolve problems, anticipating difficulties, and remaining alert to the need to intervene. An analytical nurse connects clinical observations with the theoretical knowledge base to anticipate clinical events.
- *Truth-seeking* is eagerness to seek the best knowledge in a given context, courage in asking questions, and objectivity and honesty, even if findings do not support self-interests or preconceived notions. Truth-seeking leads to continual reevaluation of new information. In nursing practice, the reason for why things are done a certain way is often given as "we have always done it that way." This response is contrary to truth-seeking behavior. Not being disposed to truth-seeking can lead to nursing practice that is based on habit rather than on tested theory and may therefore hamper the development of more effective practice.
- *Open-mindedness* is tolerance of divergent views and sensitivity to one's own biases. This disposition is central to the goal of culturally competent care. Absence of

open-mindedness might preclude provision of effective nursing care to populations that are different from the nurse.

- *Self-confidence* is trust in one's own reasoning processes. It permits trust in one's judgment and promotes leadership of others in resolving problems. The nurse who makes excellent assessments of client care situations but who is reluctant to bring these observations forward in interdisciplinary situations, especially if they differ from those made by the physician, shows a lack of self-confidence. Self-confidence to present the results of one's thinking is important in improving client care.

- *Maturity* is the disposition to be judicious in one's decision making. The critically thinking mature person approaches problems, inquiry, and decision making with the understanding that some problems are ill-structured, some situations have more than one plausible option, and many judgments must be made based on standards, contexts, and evidence for which the outcome is uncertain. This trait has important implications for ethical decision making in nursing.

A study to measure critical thinking dispositions in a sample of baccalaureate nursing students in their culminating clinical course was conducted by Colucciello (1999). Weaknesses in analyticity, self-confidence, inquisitiveness, and systematicity were found. Since the students were in their final clinical course, the lack of self-confidence or trust in their reasoning abilities was of particular concern. The group's maturity and truth-seeking abilities were relatively strong, however.

Strategies to Build Critical Thinking Skills

Critical thinking is enhanced in environments that are caring, nonthreatening, flexible, and re-spectful of diverse points of view. Nurses who are familiar with the nursing process, the scientific method, and research methods already know much about critical thinking because they are based on some of the same principles.

Strategies to enhance critical thinking include the following (Alfaro-LeFevre, 1999):

- Anticipate questions others might ask. This helps to identify a wider scope of questions that need to be answered to obtain relevant information. For example, "What will the client's family want to know?"
- Ask "what if" questions.
- Look for flaws in thinking for the purpose of evaluating assessments and solutions and making improvements. Ask "What is missing?" and "How could this be made better?"
- Ask others to look for flaws in thinking.
- Develop good habits of inquiry—habits that aid in the search for truth, such as keeping an open mind, clarifying information, and taking enough time.
- Use phrases such as "I need to find out" rather than "I don't know" or "I'm not sure."
- Turn errors into learning opportunities.

Persistent use of these strategies develops the skills and nurtures the disposition for critical thinking. Becoming a critical thinker is a life-long process; we can all be better than we are if we work at it.

Research and Measurement Issues Associated with Critical Thinking

While the concept of critical thinking is assuming a greater role in the design of instruction, the measurement of critical thinking remains difficult (Rane-Szostack & Robertson, 1996). There are few fully tested measures of critical thinking skills, and research with subjects other than students is quite limited.

CRITICAL THINKING MEASURES

One of the most widely used measures of critical thinking skills is the *Watson-Glaser Critical Thinking Appraisal* (WGCTA). The test is composed of a series of objective items designed to measure five aspects of critical thinking: inference, recognition of assumptions, deduction, interpretation, and evaluation of arguments. Scores on the five subtests are equally weighted to derive a total score.

The *Cornell Critical Thinking Test* (CCTT) is a multiple-choice test. It assesses deductive reasoning, identification of faulty reasoning, judgment of reliability of statements, evaluation of evidence, choice of useful hypothesis-testing predictions, and finding assumptions.

The *California Critical Thinking Skills Test* (CCTST) is based on *The Delphi Report*'s consensus definition of critical thinking. It provides an overall score on critical thinking skills and subscale scores on analysis, evaluation, inference, deductive reasoning, and inductive reasoning. The CCTST companion instrument, the California Critical Thinking Dispositions Inventory (CCTDI), is designed to measure dispositions toward critical thinking.

RESEARCH

Much of the research on critical thinking in nursing has been done with students rather than with practicing nurses. Thus, information relative to critical thinking in clinical practice is sparse. In an integrative review of 20 studies ranging from 1977 to 1995, Adams (1999) found varied and contradictory results about the relationship between critical thinking abilities and skills and nursing education. Some explanations for the inconsistency might be the design of the study (i.e., lack of randomization), an imprecise definition of critical thinking, lack of instruments to measure critical thinking in nurs-

ing (as opposed to general critical thinking abilities), and the failure to determine if teaching methods facilitated critical thinking.

The results of longitudinal studies that address the relationship between nursing education and critical thinking are mixed. Several studies that used the WGCTA found no significant difference in critical thinking between entry to and exit from upper-division nursing study (Bauwens & Gerhard, 1987; Maynard, 1996; Vaughan-Wrobel, O'Sullivan, & Smith, 1997). Sullivan (1987) also used the WGCTA and found no significant differences between entry and exit among RN students in a baccalaureate program. Similarly, Kintgen-Andrews (1988) found no significant gain over an academic year among practical nursing students, prehealth science freshmen, associate degree nursing students, and generic baccalaureate sophomore students. On the other hand, Frye, Alfred, and Campbell (1999), McCarthy et al. (1999), and Miller (1992) reported a positive relationship between education and critical thinking, with both associate degree and baccalaureate students scoring significantly higher as they moved through their program.

Cross-sectional studies also report mixed findings. Baccalaureate senior students scored higher on critical thinking than did second-year associate degree students (Frederickson & Mayer, 1977). Baccalaureate seniors also scored higher on the WGCTA than did associate degree and diploma nursing students (Scoloveno, 1981; Brooks & Shepherd, 1992). However, there were no significant differences between graduate and undergraduate students on the WGCTA (Matthews & Gaul, 1979).

Research relative to critical thinking in clinical practice is sparse. A study of critical thinking ability of practicing nurses was conducted by Pardue (1987). Baccalaureate- and master's-prepared nurses scored higher on the WGCTA than did those with diplomas or associate degrees, but there were no significant differences in self-reported difficulty in making decisions. Maynard (1996) explored the relationship between critical thinking and level of competence as defined by Benner's (1984) stages of skill acquisition and reported that the experiential component appears to have an influence on critical thinking development. May and colleagues (1999) also postulate that critical thinking might emerge as a factor associated with clinical competence as nurses become more experienced clinicians. Howenstein et al. (1996) studied 160 nurses practicing in two urban hospitals and found that age and years of experience were negatively correlated with critical thinking ability. Beeken (1997) interviewed and tested 100 staff nurses to determine relationships between critical thinking and self-concept. Comparison among nurses with varying levels of education showed higher levels of critical thinking ability in baccalaureate-prepared nurses.

None of these studies is definitive in its findings. The mixed findings in these studies also might be attributed to the fact that critical thinking is a complex process that is very difficult to measure, or to other factors in the research design.

Application of Critical Thinking in a Clinical Situation

All disciplines have a logic and nursing is no exception. . . . Nursing content is infused through, with, and continually shaped by nursing goals, nursing questions and problems, nursing ideas and concepts, nursing principles and theories, nursing evidence, data and reasons, nursing interpretations and claims, nursing inferences and lines of formulated thought, nursing implications and consequences, and a nursing point of view (Paul & Heaslip, 1995, p. 47).

Nursing information and data are transformed into knowledge, which then becomes the basis of sound and critically monitored nursing practice. The following example uses the elements of reasoning described by Paul (1993) and illustrated in Figure 19–3, which

work together to create a critical thinking environment.

SITUATION

Representatives of various agencies have come together to discuss the adequacy of health services for the elderly in their community. A registered nurse is selected as the leader of the group. Since the group is a loosely constructed one representing many different constituencies, the leader recognizes the potential for the lack of focus and the possibility of producing a product that does not meet the stated purpose or needs of the community. The nurse decides to consciously use the elements of critical thinking in leading the group through its task.

Identify the purpose. At the beginning of the first meeting, the leader states that their purpose is to analyze the adequacy of community health services for the elderly. During the course of subsequent meetings, the leader reiterates the purpose to keep the group focused. The major purpose often has to be distinguished from related purposes, such as expanding services for the elderly or assessing all health services in the community. Frequent reminders help in actually achieving the purpose and focusing thought and action.

Clearly and succinctly state the question being asked, the problem being solved, or the issue under discussion. In this situation the major question is, "Are there adequate health services for the elderly of the community?" This question can be further broken down into subquestions related to the type of services available, access to those services, the amount of use of the services, and unmet health needs of the elderly in the community. The questions should relate to the overall purpose and be answerable and relevant.

Recognize that all reasoning is done from some point of view. Because the group itself

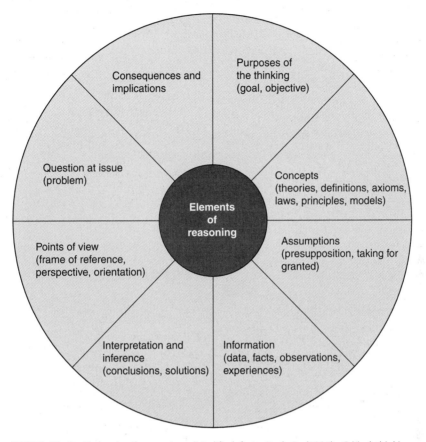

FIGURE 19–3 Elements of reasoning. (Modified from Paul, R. (1994). *Critical thinking: Transforming the quality of teaching, learning, and practice in the education of health professionals* [Workbook]. Santa Rosa, CA: Foundation for Critical Thinking.)

represents different constituencies, multiple points of view are expected to surface. In guiding the group, the challenge of the leader is to become aware of her own point of view and that of others, be fair in having all relevant points of view expressed, and allow evaluation of all perspectives while keeping the discussion focused on the purpose and relevant questions.

Understand that all reasoning is based on assumptions. Because assumptions are often embedded deeply in reasoning, it is sometimes difficult to identify them. However, not doing so places serious constraints on critical thinking and may distort the outcome. For example, the leader hears statements from one member of the group that health services for children are a greater problem than for the elderly. Another group member comments that because of their previous contributions to the community, health services for the elderly should have highest priority and no amount of service is adequate. The challenge to the nurse leader is to help the group to identify assumptions that influence the group's work, check the validity of the assumptions, and reexamine the questions being asked in light of the assumptions.

Clarify concepts and ideas that are necessary to explore the issue. The group should first define what is meant by "adequacy" and what is meant by "health services." These terms may have a wide range of meanings, depending on the points of view and assumptions of the group members. Clarifying these ideas may lead to further discussion and explication of assumptions stated earlier.

Examine the empirical data. At this point the group examines the available data. Examples of information that might be useful include the number and types of health services available in the community, whether or not there are elderly people who are unable to get access to those services, and the existence of health needs for which no services are provided. The challenge to the leader is to ensure that the data presented are complete and relevant to the question, to disregard information that is not relevant to the current issue, and to state the evidence clearly and fairly.

Draw inferences from the data. The leader must be sure that there is a link between the data and inferences, that they are reasonable given the data, and that they are consistent. In this situation, the group determined that institutional services were adequate for those elderly who could get to them. However, the lack of transportation services prevented many of the elderly from going to the settings where services were delivered. It was also determined that there was a lack of primary care and nutritional services.

Develop implications and consequences. At this stage the group must examine the conclusion of their reasoning and project the implications and consequences of that reasoning. Precise consequences for addressing or not addressing the issues must include both positive and negative consequences.

Comment

Today's health care environment requires nurses to solve complex problems, address complex questions, explore unique client situations, and evaluate the effectiveness of a wide range of interventions. Critical thinking is an integral part of effective nursing action. It is a complex process through which nurses can explore practice situations and search for effective outcomes. The conscious application of critical thinking principles can result in effective decision making and ultimately enhance the quality of care.

KEY POINTS

- Critical thinking is an evolving concept that is not easily defined.
- Critical thinking skills are important components of the nursing process and problem solving, but critical thinking, the nursing process, and problem solving are *not* synonymous terms.
- Clinical judgments are outcomes of critical thinking in nursing.
- Appraisal, problem solving, creativity, and decision making are interrelated concepts in critical thinking.
- Nurses with expert clinical judgment display characteristics of high-level critical thinking.
- To think critically, nurses must be able to see connections; use logic; differentiate between fact, inference, and assumptions; evaluate arguments; consider many sides of an issue; be creative; and believe in their ability to think and reason.
- Becoming a critical thinker involves not only acquiring a set of skills, but also developing a disposition toward critical thinking.
- Becoming a critical thinker is a lifelong process.
- More work needs to be done to enhance and examine critical thinking embedded in nursing practice. Two areas needing particular attention

are the development and refinement of instruments to measure critical thinking in practice and further exploration of the relationship between clinical judgment and critical thinking.

CRITICAL THINKING EXERCISES

1. Differentiate between critical thinking, problem solving, and decision making.

2. Think about a patient care situation that you have recently encountered. What questions are your colleagues likely to ask you when you present this situation to them?

3. Mr. Jones, age 82, is admitted to your hospital unit. In conducting his initial assessment, you notice that he is somewhat confused. His admitting notes indicate that he takes digoxin and Lasix. Describe the process that you will use to determine whether or not Mr. Jones is experiencing side effects from his medication. Focus on the questions you will ask yourself or others, not on the side effects themselves.

4. Describe the best and worst decision making you have seen by a nurse in a client care situation. Compare these two situations in terms of the thought process used, the underlying assumptions of the nurses, the accuracy of available information, the interpretation of information, and the soundness of the decision reached.

REFERENCES

Adams, B. L. (1999). Nursing education for critical thinking: An integrative review. *Journal of Nursing Education, 38,* 111–119.

Alfaro-LeFevre, R. (1999). *Critical thinking in nursing: A practical approach* (2nd ed.). Philadelphia: Saunders.

American Philosophical Association. (1990). *Critical thinking: A statement of expert consensus for purposes of educational assessment and instruction. The Delphi Report: Research findings and recommendations prepared for the Committee of Pre-college Philosophy.* (ERIC Document Reproduction Service No. ED 315-423)

Baker, C. R. (1996). Reflective learning: A teaching strategy for critical thinking. *Journal of Nursing Education, 35,* 19–22.

Bandman, E. L., & Bandman, B. (1995). *Critical thinking in nursing.* Norwalk, CT: Appleton & Lange.

Bauwens, E. E., & Gerhard, G. G. (1987). The use of the Watson-Glaser Critical Thinking Appraisal to predict success in a baccalaureate nursing program. *Journal of Nursing Education, 26,* 278–281.

Beeken, J. E. (1997). The relationship between critical thinking and self-concept in staff nurses and the influence of these characteristics on nursing practice. *Journal of Nursing Staff Development, 13,* 272–278.

Beeken, J. E., Dale, M. L., Enos, M. F., & Yarbrough, S. (1997). Teaching critical thinking skills to undergraduate nursing students. *Nurse Educator, 22*(3), 37–39.

Benner, P. (1984). *From novice to expert: Excellence and power in clinical nursing practice.* Menlo Park, CA: Addison-Wesley.

Brock, A. & Butts, J. B. (1998). On target: A model to teach baccalaureate nursing students to apply critical thinking. *Nursing Forum, 33*(3), 5–10.

Brooks, K., & Shepherd, J. (1992). Professionalism versus general critical thinking abilities of senior nursing students in four types of nursing curricula. *Journal of Professional Nursing, 8,* 87–95.

Callister, L. C. (1996). Maternal interviews: A teaching strategy fostering critical thinking. *Journal of Nursing Education, 35,* 29–30.

Catalano, J. (2000). *Nursing now: Today's issues, tomorrow's trends.* Philadelphia: Davis.

Colucciello, M. L. (1999). Relationships between critical thinking dispositions and learning styles. *Journal of Professional Nursing, 15,* 294–301.

Conger, M. M., & Mezza, I. (1996). Fostering critical thinking in nursing students in the clinical setting. *Nurse Educator, 21,* 11–15.

Daley, B. J., Shaw, C. R., Balistrieri, T., Glasenapp, K., & Piacentine, L. (1999). Concept maps: A strategy to teach and evaluate critical thinking. *Journal of Nursing Education, 38,* 42–47

Daly, W. M. (1998). Critical thinking as an outcome of nursing education. What is it? Why is it important to nursing practice? *Journal of Advanced Nursing, 28,* 323–331.

Dexter, P., Applegate, M., Backer, J., Claytor, K., Keffer, J., Norton, B., & Ross, B. (1997). A proposed framework for teaching and evaluating critical thinking in nursing. *Journal of Professional Nursing, 13,* 160–167.

Duchscher, J. E. B. (1999). Catching the wave: Understanding the concept of critical thinking. *Journal of Advanced Nursing, 29,* 577–583.

Ennis, R. H. (1987). Critical thinking and the curriculum. In M. Heiman & J. Slomianko (Eds.), *Thinking skills instruction: Concepts and techniques.* Washington, DC: National Education Association.

Ennis, R. H. (1989). Critical thinking and subject specificity: Clarification and needed research. *Educational
Researcher, 18,* 4–10.

Facione, P. A. (1990). Critical thinking: A statement of
expert consensus for purposes of educational assessment and instruction (executive summary). In *The
Delphi Report* (pp. 1–19) Millbrae, CA: California
Academic Press.

Facione, N. C., & Facione, P. A. (1996). Externalizing
the critical thinking in knowledge development and
clinical judgment. *Nursing Outlook, 44,* 129–136.

Facione, N. C., Facione, P. A., & Sanchez, C. A.
(1994). Critical thinking disposition as a measure of
competent clinical judgment: The development of the
California Critical Thinking Disposition Inventory.
Journal of Nursing Education, 33, 345–350.

Facione, P. A., Sanchez, C. A., Facione N. C., &
Gainen, J. (1995). The disposition toward critical
thinking. *The Journal of General Education, 44*(1),
1–25.

Feingold, C., & Perlich, L. J. (1999). Teaching critical
thinking through health-promotion contract. *Nurse
Educator, 24*(4), 42–44.

Ford, J. S., & Profetto-McGrath, J. (1994). A model for
critical thinking within the context of curriculum as
praxis. *Journal of Nursing Education, 33,* 341–344.

Frederickson, K., & Mayer, G. G. (1977). Problem solving skills: What effect does education have? *American
Journal of Nursing, 77,* 1167–1169.

Frye, B., Alfred, N. & Campbell, N. (1999). Use of the
Watson-Glaser Critical Thinking Appraisal with BSN
students. *Nursing and Health Care Perspectives, 20,*
253–255.

Grossman, S., & Valiga, T. M. (2000). *The new leadership challenge: Creating the future of nursing.* Philadelphia: Davis.

Howenstein, M. A., Bilodeau, K., Brogna, M. J., &
Good, G. (1996). Factors associated with critical
thinking among nurses. *Journal of Continuing Education in Nursing, 27*(3), 100–103.

Jones, S. A., & Brown, L. N. (1993). Alternative views
on defining critical thinking through the nursing process. *Holistic Nurse Practitioner 7,* 71–76.

Kataoka-Yahiro, M., & Saylor, C. (1994). A critical
thinking model for nursing judgment. *Journal of
Nursing Education, 33,* 351–356.

Kelly, E. (1997). Development of strategies to identify
the learning needs of baccalaureate students. *Journal
of Nursing Education, 36,* 156–162.

Kintgen-Andrews, J. (1988). Development of critical
thinking: Career ladder P.N. and A.D. nursing students, pre-health science freshmen, generic baccalaureate sophomore nursing students. *Resources in Education, 24*(1) (ERIC Document Reproduction Service
No. 297153)

Kintgen-Andrews, J. (1991). Critical thinking and nursing education: Perplexities and insights. *Journal of
Nursing Education, 30,* 152–157.

Mastrian, K. G., & McGonigle, D. (1999). Using technology assignments to promote critical thinking.
Nurse Educator, 24, 45–47.

Matthews, C. A., & Gaul, A. L. (1979). Nursing diagnosis from the perspective of concept attainment and
critical thinking. *Advances in Nursing Science, 2*(11),
17–26.

May, B. A., Edell, V., Butell, S., Doughty, J., & Lang-
ford, C. (1999). Critical thinking and clinical
competence: A study of their relationship in BSN
seniors. *Journal of Nursing Education, 38,* 100–
110.

Maynard, C. A. (1996). Relationship of critical thinking
ability to professional nursing competence. *Journal of
Nursing Education, 35,* 12–18.

McCarthy, P., Schuster, P., Zehr, P., & McDougal, D.
(1999). Research briefs: Evaluation of critical thinking in a baccalaureate program . . . are there differences between sophomore and senior students. *Journal of Nursing Education, 38,* 142–144.

McPeck, J. E. (1990). *Teaching critical thinking.* New
York: Routledge.

Meyers, C. (1991). *Teaching students to think critically.*
San Francisco: Jossey-Bass.

Miller, M., & Malcolm, N. (1990). Critical thinking in
the nursing curriculum. *Nursing and Health Care,
11*(2), 67–73.

Miller, M. A. (1992). Outcomes evaluation: Measuring
critical thinking. *Journal of Advanced Nursing, 17,*
1401–1407.

Miller, M. A., & Babcock, D. E. (1996). *Critical thinking applied to nursing.* St. Louis: Mosby.

Pardue, S. F. (1987). Decision-making skills and critical
thinking ability among associate degree, diploma,
baccalaureate, and master's prepared nurses. *Journal
of Nursing Education, 26,* 354–361.

Paul, R. (1992). *Critical thinking: What every person
needs to survive in a rapidly changing world.* Santa
Rosa, CA: Foundation for Critical Thinking.

Paul, R. (1993). The art of redesigning instruction. In J.
Willsen & A. J. A. Binker (Eds.), *Critical thinking:
How to prepare students for a rapidly changing world*
(p. 319). Santa Rosa, CA: Foundation for Critical
Thinking.

Paul, R. (1994). *Critical thinking: Transforming the
quality of teaching, learning, and practice in the education of health professionals* [Workbook]. Charleston,
SC: Medical University of South Carolina College of
Nursing.

Paul, R., & Heaslip, P. (1995). Critical thinking and
intuitive nursing practice. *Journal of Advanced Nursing, 22,* 40–47.

Paul, R., & Elder, L. (1999). *The miniature guide to critical thinking concepts and tools.* Dillon Beach, CA: Foundation for Critical Thinking.

Perciful, E. G., & Nester, P. A. (1996). The effect of an innovative clinical teaching method on nursing students' knowledge and critical thinking skills. *Journal of Nursing Education, 35*(1), 23–28.

Rane-Szostack, D., & Robertson, J. F. (1996). Issues in measuring critical thinking: Meeting the challenge. *Journal of Nursing Education, 35*(1), 5–11.

Rossignol, M. (1997). Relationship between selected discourse strategies and student critical thinking . . . the clinical post-conference. *Journal of Nursing Education, 36,* 467–475.

Schumacher, J., & Severson, A. (1996). Building bridges for future practice: An innovative approach to foster critical thinking. *Journal of Nursing Education, 35,* 31–33.

Scoloveno, M. (1981). Problem solving ability of senior nursing students in three program types. *Dissertation Abstracts International, 41,* 1396B.

Sedlak, C. A., & Doheny, M. O. (1998). Peer review through clinical rounds: A collaborative critical thinking strategy. *Nurse Educator, 23*(5), 42–45.

Strader, M. K., & Decker, P. J. (1995). *Role transition to patient care management.* Norwalk, CT: Appleton & Lange.

Sullivan, E. J. (1987). Critical thinking, creativity, clinical performance, and achievement in RN students. *Nurse Educator, 12*(2), 12–16.

U.S. Department of Education. (1995). *National assessment of college student learning: Identifying college graduates' essential skills in writing, speech and listening, and critical thinking.* Washington, DC: U.S. Government Printing Office.

Vaughan-Wrobel, B. C., O'Sullivan, P., & Smith, L. (1997). Evaluating critical thinking skills of baccalaureate nursing students. *Journal of Nursing Education, 36,* 485–488.

Wade, G. H. (1999). Using the case method to develop critical thinking skills for the care of high-risk families. *Journal of Family Nursing, 5*(1), 92–109.

Watson, G., & Glaser, E. M. (1964). *Critical thinking appraisal.* Orlando, FL: Harcourt Brace Jovanovich.

Wilkinson, J. M. (1996). *Nursing process: A critical thinking approach* (2nd ed.). Menlo Park, CA: Addison-Wesley Nursing.

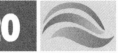
The Change Process

ANNE GRISWOLD PEIRCE, PhD, RN, AND NATHANIEL W. PEIRCE, EdD

OBJECTIVES

At the completion of this chapter, the reader will be able to:

- Discuss the various factors that influence change.
- Compare organizational development and transformation.
- Contrast the four models of planned change most commonly used in nursing.
- Apply the models of change to clinical situations.
- Discuss complexity in the change process.

PROFILE IN PRACTICE

Ola Burns Allen, RNC, DNS
Professor and Associate Dean for Academic Affairs
University of Mississippi Medical Center
School of Nursing
Jackson, Mississippi

In his Phi Beta Kappa address at Harvard in 1837, Ralph Waldo Emerson asserted, "each age must write its own books, the books of an older period will not fit." Certainly, in the world of nursing education, no truer words were ever spoken. J. B. Lon Hefferlin, in his 1969 article "Hauling Academic Trunks," notes that few institutions change spontaneously and suggests that the factors most influencing change are the conditions under which the institution operates and its ethos with respect to change. While the art of nursing has remained for the most part constant, the science of nursing undergoes constant change. Resistance to change in nursing faculty, just as in other disciplines and work settings, can be anticipated. Each institution and each department within the insti-

tution has its own historic orientation. Change in educational institutions with major resistance to change may take place at a time when older faculty retire or leave and are replaced with new and innovative faculty. The crucial challenge for administrators of nursing education programs, prior to implementing any educational innovation, is to identify faculty fears and then be sensitive to those fears when implementing strategies for change.

Change is everywhere in health care, making it a challenge for those who enjoy change and a major impediment for those who don't. Included among the many forces of change are the financial, clinical, technical, social, political, and even spiritual aspects of health care. Each of these forces separately, and all of them together, create a health care world that is very different from 5 years ago and one that will be even more changed in the future.

Nursing has traditionally embraced the mechanistic organizational model. In this model the analogy of the machine is used to describe the work of the organization. Machines, of course, are not composed of living organisms. Instead, machines operate in predictable ways based on energy input and production output. Organizations of people are far less predictable. Each individual can be counted on to act just a little differently than another, bearing little resemblance to cogs in a wheel. These individual differences result in a dynamic, ever-changing organization, again bearing little resemblance to a machine.

By using the tenets of complexity to model the workplace, nurses can be better prepared to deal with change that is inherent in health care. Complexity theory proposes that organizations are complex adaptive systems in which change is inherent and necessary. In this model change and

growth are necessary for survival. Without the ability to adapt to change, humanity would look very different.

The acknowledgment that change is good for the organization allows for several important changes in thinking, including that

- Changing organizations are innovative organizations.
- Adaptation can occur in a timely manner to changes in the environment.
- Unpredictable events can be just as positive a force as predictable events.
- Unchanging organizations are not viable in today's world.

Nurses who are interested in organizations that promote change should be alert to phrases such as "this is the way we do things here" or "everybody knows that this is the way it should happen." The underlying principle here is one of permanence rather than one of adaptation or change, which may create a very dissatisfying work environment.

"There is nothing permanent but change."
- *Heraclitus, 513 B.C.*

Change is the natural and inevitable process that transforms people, systems, organizations, cultures, and societies into new variations. Change is promoted in both public and private organizations as an indicator of progress, efficiency, and survival; paradoxically, it is also vilified as a threat to the individual and society. Likewise, the human response can be accepting and welcoming or avoidant and resistant.

The omnipresent nature of change compels all professions to analyze and understand its ramifications for individuals and organizations. Many of the current debates in health care have given the nursing profession the impetus to more closely examine what change means to the discipline. For example, the debate on health

care reform has already resulted in a multitude of changes, even if no legislative action ever occurs. In fact, Kobs (1999) asks in the title of her article, "Does the C in JCAHO Stand for Change?" Nursing's response will inevitably create further change in the profession and paradigms of care.

Nurses today need to have the courage and conviction to bring about change to improve the quality of care for patients. Although many changes in nursing practice and management are imposed by external forces, "nursing changes would be more efficient and effective if guided by internal as well as external change agents, because nursing experts have a greater understanding than outsiders of the manner in which various nursing system elements interact" (Gillies, 1994, p. 470). Lee and Alexander (1999a) note that while not all organizational change is equivalent, all change carries a price tag.

Planning for change and reacting to unplanned change is part of nursing. In fact these activities may be essential to nursing (Redmond et al., 1999). For these reasons it is necessary for nurses not only to become knowledgeable about planned change theory, but also to participate in the evolution of new change models and interventions. It is not enough just to use previously developed business models without considering how and why nursing is different.

Most models of change used by nursing are based on systems theory. *Systems theory* is a linear cause-and-effect model that uses the analogy of machines or computers to explain how people react to change. Recent work in many different fields has shown that dynamic, adaptive systems, such as people, cannot be examined in the same ways as linear, nondynamic systems. Dynamic systems have an emergent nature; they change and evolve in ways that cannot always be predicted. Rather than reflecting the machine world, dynamic systems more closely approximate biological models. Thus, it seems that change should be examined within a dynamic framework, for change is basically about people. This chapter presents information about chaos and complexity theories as an alternative framework that may be used to develop more realistic models of change for the nursing profession. Common frameworks currently used to examine change are also presented.

Defining Change

The dictionary defines change as both a noun and a verb. As a noun, *change* is defined as the act, process, or result of changing. It may also be defined as an alteration, transformation, or substitution. Other synonyms are mutation, permutation, variation, and vicissitude. As a verb, *change* means to make different in some partic-

ular way, to modify, to make radically different, to transform, or to give a different position, course, or direction. Other synonyms for the verb form of change include switch, exchange, modify, or undergo loss, transformation, transition, or substitution. From the dictionary definitions, then, change can be described as both a process and an outcome.

The nursing literature is replete with articles and books about change and the change process. Yet there are relatively few conceptual or operational definitions of change. The definitions that are offered are often simplistic or overreaching. For example, change is "a dynamic process by which an alteration is brought about that makes a distinct difference in something" (Grohar-Murray & DiCroce, 1992, p. 201) or "change is any alteration, regardless how slight or how major, or how large or how small" (Bernhard & Walsh, 1995, p. 162). Such succinct definitions do not take into account the complexity of change. Instead, Sheehan (1990) suggests that change is synonymous with conversion, innovation, novelty, metamorphosis, revolution, and transformation. Bruhn (1999) describes change as the alteration of an existing field of forces. It is clear that change is a complicated business, and can only be understood as such (Irvine & Phoenix, 1998).

Recent nursing literature includes whether transition should be the organizing construct rather than change, and Meleis and Trangenstein (1994) differentiate between the two. According to them, *transition* occurs over time and has a sense of movement and an internal orientation, in contrast to *change,* which implies a substitution and has a faster or more abrupt movement as well as a more external orientation.

It might appear that the use of *transition* would focus attention only on the human process during change. Transition instead may be embedded in all changes. If *change* is the movement from one state to the next, then *transition* may describe that movement. Transition may also be a richer term for describing the movement of an individual or organization through change.

In the business literature, change is often defined in terms of the type or magnitude of change produced. For example, *transactional change* is concerned with the change of everyday occurrences, such as the way in which nursing care is documented or a procedure is accomplished. *Transformational change* is that which fundamentally alters a behavior or attitude (Burke & Litwin, 1992). An example of transformational change would be the recent movement of nursing care out of the hospital and into the community.

Change is an integral part of each aspect of life, and thus it is not surprising that religious and philosophical views also influence its definition. The contrasting views of Eastern and Western philosophy and religion have been used to explicate change as a process (Eastern) and as an outcome (Western).

Although integral to life, it is easy to appreciate that change is also subjective. As such, the individual influences the view of change. Any individual who likes change will view it differently from one who does not accept or want change. In fact, the meaning that is attached to change is probably as individual as the person involved (Globerman, 1999).

Thus change is not easily defined. It is a process and an outcome, a movement and a state, expected and unexpected, gradual and rapid, good and bad, and all states in between. Change is altered by the reaction and perceptions of involved individuals and is illuminated through patterns of behavior. As we endeavor to understand change, it is important to remember that change is universal but may not always be understandable or predictable.

Elements of Change

The elements important to change are the change itself, the context, the time, and the individuals involved (Davis, 1991). Lack of awareness of these elements can be disastrous to those who want to promote change. Several crucial elements of change are considered in this chapter, including attitudinal, behavioral, language, metaphorical, informational, rate, volume, and cross-cultural factors of change. These elements are illustrated in Figure 20–1.

INDIVIDUAL-ATTITUDE CHANGE

Promoting change in people is difficult, since people are reluctant to give up old ways of thinking. Yet the promotion of organizational change, or any other type of change, is very dependent on a change in individual attitudes.

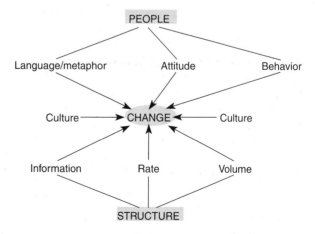

FIGURE 20-1 Elements of change.

For this reason, it is important to consider not only how to change structure when planning for change, but also how to change people.

Psychological theory can be used to guide the change process. Since much of change is about people, it is beneficial to have any knowledge that helps one deal more effectively with the people involved in innovation. One recommendation is that *Gestalt* theory be used in the plan for change (Stickland, 1992). *Gestalt theory* is based on the assumption that learning is a process of changing insights or thought patterns. An individual learns from using, perceiving, and receiving stimuli from the environment. Thought patterns change through a process of simultaneous, mutual interaction between the individual and the environment. For example, a nurse and client share the process and the experience of moving to optimal health. The interaction of their roles enables them to gain insights into each other, and this facilitates change. Another theory used to explicate change is Kubler-Ross's (1970) theory of loss. Gabel and Oster (1998) explain how loss can be an essential part of change and that the stages of loss can be reflected in those who must change.

A number of problems inherent in attitudinal change have been identified, and ways to effect attitudinal change have been proposed. The first step is to understand whether an attitude is changeable and to what degree. According to Beer and Walton (1987), there are three types of attitudinal change. *Alpha change* occurs when there is a real change in a measurement of the concept but no change in the way it is conceptualized. To illustrate, individuals may change the value they place on the use of alternative medicine, but they still consider these therapies an adjunct to real medicine. *Beta change* occurs when there is a real shift in expectations. For example, individuals might come to expect that *all* disease be treated with nutrition as part of an overall medical treatment regimen. *Gamma change* represents a complete and radical change, such as espousing the use of nutrition as the primary treatment for disease. Alpha

change is the easiest to promote and gamma the most difficult.

Bonalumi and Fisher (1999) say that among other factors to be considered is the resilience of the individuals involved. They employ the terminology used by Conner (1993) to describe resilient people; positive, focused, flexible, organized, and proactive. While not all individuals are resilient, they write that these characteristics can be taught and so should be considered when change is contemplated. No matter what strategy is used, change may fail if the individual's attitude is not considered. Salmond (1998) writes that understanding the human side of change is critical. She outlines a 12-step process to managing transition. Her process acknowledges that only about 15% of people welcome change; the rest are reluctant or resistant.

CHANGE IN BEHAVIOR

Whereas all three types of change—alpha, beta, and gamma—reflect changes in attitude, they do not ensure changes in behavior. When change can be viewed publicly, it is more likely to result in lasting behavioral change (Tice, 1992). Management should start a change process by requiring behavioral change of top executives. People believe in a change only when they see it work (Duck, 1993). Before that happens, it is just talk.

Involvement in the process of change can also facilitate behavioral change. How and what the individuals involved think about the change process affects their actions (Downey & Brief, 1986; Grossman & Valiga, 2000; Lowstedt, 1993; Potter et al., 1998). The more people are involved in the planning and implementation of the change process, the greater the chance of success (Armenakis, Harris, & Mossholder, 1993; Axelrod, 1992). For example, to improve the quality of working conditions on an obstetrical unit, a participation project to initiate needed change in scheduling practices was implemented. New models of the work schedule were developed with the staff, and the preferred schedule of the majority was implemented. After a trial basis, the new schedule was evaluated and adjustments were made by the staff. The overall satisfaction with the change was favorable, in part because of involvement in the process (Snell & Turner, 1991).

LANGUAGE AND METAPHOR OF CHANGE

The use of metaphor and language may also be important, since language is the vehicle used to discuss and conceptualize change. Gioia and Chittipeddi (1991) suggest that *sensemaker* and *sensegiver* be used as descriptive metaphors for the people involved in promoting change. These metaphors suggest a different involvement in the change process than does the term change agent, which is most frequently used in nursing. *Agent* suggests the external orientation of a manager, whereas *sensemaker* and *sensegiver* suggest the internal orientation of a guide to the change process.

Spitzer (1999) suggests that change has a fractal nature—that is, it is self-similar on many different levels. Her work suggests a more biologic model as she writes that the three phases of the change process are shedding light, restructuring, and growth. In yet another example of the use of metaphor and language, Kolorountis and Thorstenson (1999) use an ethics framework, with the terms such as caring, nurturing, and fairness to describe organizational change.

The appropriate uses of metaphor can also help provide needed reference points during the change process. Listening to the metaphors of speech can give important clues to understanding change in context (Marshak, 1993). For example, two metaphors that could be used to refer to change are "create a new vision" and "lay a good foundation." Each of these metaphors implies a different type of change. Their respective use by two persons to describe one change could signal a conflict in the rate and direction of change.

Changing the common vernacular, or metaphors, of an institution can even facilitate change as it occurs. For instance, the process of change in one psychiatric institution involved moving from a standard 28-day program for all patients to more fluid and individualized treatment plans. Simply changing the language from *treatment program* to *treatment process* helped the staff to better understand and accept the change of not rigidly adhering to 28 days of treatment (Hamm, 1992).

INFORMATION AND CHANGE

Information is a critical element in the change process. Although some argument can be made about the amount of information required, all planned change must include the transfer of information. Different types of information may be needed. Stickland (1992) suggests that both factual and sensory data are needed if change is to be successful. An alternative view is that the repetition of the message is important. When persons promoting change have talked about it so much they cannot bear to think about it any more, the message is just starting to get through (Duck, 1993).

Rational strategies for change depend heavily on information (Rogers, 1983). In fact, communication is the focus in these models. It is thought that if the individuals involved understand the need for change, their behavior will change, be rational, and be logical. The quality and amount of information exchanged is critical to the success of planned change, for only information will convince the individual of the need to change.

Normative strategies also rely on the transfer of information by educating those participating in the change process. Learning and change must be considered together, since one cannot learn without changing the brain's neural network, and one cannot change without learning (Kosko, 1993). Again, the quality and type of information exchanged is important. Even with power-coercive strategies, where change comes from those holding power or seeking control, there is some need to explain change in order to implement the innovation.

The change process usually involves the collection of information through an evaluation, needs assessment, or survey. Although other methods are available, survey methodology is recommended as the most comprehensive way to assess change factors (Armenakis, Harris, & Mossholder, 1993). For example, before implementing change on a nursing unit, nurse managers should survey the staff to determine the need for change, in addition to assessing other important and previously identified factors, such as resistance, language, attitude, and behavior.

The type of information collected is important to understanding both the need for change and the factors involved. Simpson (1999) writes that without computer-based information technology (IT) change is not going to be possible or probable in the future. Change factors such as information are termed the driving and restraining forces (Lewin, 1951). *Driving forces* are those that push the system toward the desired change, whereas *restraining forces* pull the system away. Only a very thorough analysis of the system can enable the person promoting change to understand those opposing forces. For example, driving forces for computerized documentation might include the perceived benefits of computerized charts being quicker and more accurate, whereas restraining forces could include lack of time, resources, and money to properly educate those involved.

Information is important to change, but correct information does not always ensure success, nor does more information always improve matters (Mawhinney, 1992). More information means more facts to consider and thus more variables to add to the equation. The problems encountered by adding more information are called *information-based complexity* (Traub & Wozniakowski, 1994). All information gathered in preparation for change contains a certain amount of inherent error. Thus, more information by definition means more error. While more information may indeed add to an understanding of change, the increased amount of error must also be considered. Newsworthy events illustrate this point. Even though journalists report much information, it is often inconsistent and sometimes incorrect. In reports of a natural disaster, for example, the number of people missing or dead varies among news sources and changes from day to day.

While not yet applied to change theory, it may be that *fuzzy logic,* which considers degrees of truth or correctness, can provide the best overall solution to a given problem of change (Kosko, 1993). Individuals and groups planning change could consider degrees of change in their evaluation of change rather than determining whether a situation is changed or unchanged. This way of thinking is more consistent with the real world, in which events are rarely black or white but rather shades of gray.

RATE AND VOLUME OF CHANGE

The rate at which change or changes occur also influences the response to change. Many life changes are both expected and gradual, such as the developmental changes of maturation. Even organizations have analogous developmental changes as they grow and mature. In many ways, these types of slow and gradual changes are easy to accept, and in some cases it may not even be obvious that a change has occurred. In part, this has to do with the predictability of the change.

However, other types of changes cannot and should not occur slowly. And while some change can be small in nature, many changes require large-scale alterations. Rapid change, large changes, or changes that are both rapid and large are not easily dealt with by most individuals (or organizations). There appears to be a natural preference for stability and/or control (Lewin, 1992). This resistance to change is influenced by habit; by selective attention to, and retention of, only confirming information; by fear of the unknown; and by fears related to the loss of security and income (Arnold, Capella, & Sumrall, 1987). That these real or perceived threats are directed to fundamental aspects of life may make the resistance to change more understandable (see Box 20–1).

Box 20–1 **Factors That Make It Harder to Change**

Rapid change
Large changes
Multiple changes
Unexpected changes

 ## Cross-Cultural Aspects of Change

Much of the theoretical work on change is deeply rooted within Western thought and thus may not be relevant to other cultures. In fact, planned change models that propose total system linearity and predictability may also not be realistic, even within some Western cultures. Marshak (1993) proposes that change theory based on Eastern thought, specifically Confucianism and Taoism, may present an alternative and important view.

In Eastern thought, life is cyclical, and therefore so is change. The change process does not have an end point but rather is ongoing and in constant need of refinement. Equilibrium and harmony are critical and must be maintained. Change is expected; it is not an aberration but rather an accepted part of life.

Planned Change

> "When you know a thing, to recognize that you know it, and when you do not know a thing, to recognize that you do not know it. That is knowledge."
>
> ● *Confucius*

The profession of nursing is undergoing massive change with the development of new practices, evolving health care policies, and the need to respond to organizational changes in the clinical setting. As a result, there has been extensive discussion in nursing on planned change theory and models. In a review of the literature, Tiffany and colleagues (1994) observed a "high frequency of citation of inappropriate or incomplete change theories combined with a low rate of evaluation of change theories." They concluded that practicing nurses need more understandable expositions and practical applications of planned change.

DEFINING PLANNED CHANGE

Three of the most cited definitions of planned change in the nursing literature are those proposed by Chin, Bennis and colleagues, and Zajc. Chin (1976) views *planned change* as the way in which a practitioner analyzes and works out situations of change. "These ways are embodied in the concept with which they apprehend the dynamics of the client system they are working with, their relationship to it, and their process of helping with its change" (p. 90). Bennis, Benne, and Chin (1985) view *planned change* as a purposeful, conscious implementation of one's understanding and acquired skills to manage the course of change. Finally, Zajc (1987) looks at *planned change* as a form of theory that describes how the change agent plans to proceed toward a desirable goal.

PLANNED CHANGE THEORIES AND MODELS

Much of the nursing discourse on planned change emerges from the business fields of organization development (OD) and, more recently, organization transformation (OT). Organization development is a term that has been used in the business literature to explicate change within an organization. Most OD theorists view organizations as open systems reacting to the environment. In an open system the manager has to have the expertise to understand and interpret the environmental changes in order to manage change. Thus, as a field, OD is concerned with the "theory and practice of managing the continual adaptation of internal organizational arrangements to changes in the external environment" (Beer & Walton, 1987, p. 340).

Although OD encompasses more than just change, all development requires change. According to Porras and Silvers (1991), the field of planned change is still evolving as a result of rapid change in the environment. This places a burden on organizations to adapt quickly in order to progress and survive. The model illustrated in Figure 20–2 summarizes the OT and OD models of change. The OD approach, the more traditional, has been synonymous with the term planned change. The OT approach is a

second-generation OD and represents an emerging field. At this point, the definition of OT is rapidly evolving.

Organization development is defined as "(1) a set of behavioral science theories, values, strategies, and techniques (2) aimed at the planned change of organizational settings (3) with the intention of generating alpha, beta, and/or gamma cognition change in individual organizational members, leading to behavioral change and thus (4) creating a better fit between the organization's capabilities and its current environmental demands, or (5) promoting changes that help the organization to better fit predicted future environments" (Porras & Silvers, 1991, p. 54).

Organization transformation is "(1) a set of behavioral science, theories, values, strategies, and techniques (2) aimed at the planned change of organization vision and work settings (3) with the intention of generating alpha, beta, gamma cognition change in individual organizational members, leading to behavioral change

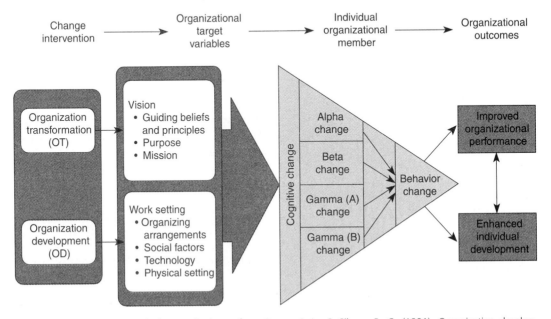

FIGURE 20–2 Organizational change. (Redrawn from Porras, J. L., & Silvers, R. C. (1991). Organization development and transformation. *Annual Review of Psychology, 42,* 51–78. Reproduced with permission by Annual Reviews, Inc.)

TABLE 20-1 Models of Planned Change

Model	Anticipated Resistance to Change	Amount of Force Behind Change Approach	Major Approach of Model
Rational	Low	Low	Education and communication
Normative	Moderate	Moderate	Persuasion and participation
Paradoxical	Moderate	Moderate	Rethinking
Power-coercive	High	High	Force

From Tappen, R. M. (1989). *Nursing leadership and management* (2nd ed.). Philadelphia: Davis.

and thus (4) promoting paradigmatic change that helps the organization better fit or create desirable future environments" (Porras & Silvers, 1991, p. 54).

Thus OT is distinguished from OD as being an approach to create a new vision for the organization. OD, on the other hand, is designed to help an organization adapt to a changing environment or improve its alignment with expected environments (Porras & Silver, 1991). OT draws from more recent developments in psychology, systems theory, and transpersonal psychology.

There are those that contend that the development of a third-generation theory would be more beneficial than either OD or OT (Beer & Walton, 1987; Duck, 1993; Mawhinney, 1992). This third-generation theory could include all types of interventions as well as applications to the myriad of circumstances faced by organizations. Complexity theory, described later in the chapter, may provide the framework needed for the newest approach to change theory.

In examining planned change, there are several theories and models that have been cited by nurses for application in the clinical setting. Four types of models are commonly discussed:

rational, normative, paradoxical, and power-coercive. Table 20–1 lists characteristics of the four models and their relationship to persuasion and power as the forces for change.

Rational Model. Rational models are proposed to be effective in a system that is universally ready for change (Armenakis, Harris, & Mossholder, 1993; Backstrom, 1999; Tappen, 1995). The premise of *rational models* is that, with good information, most people will make the logical choice to change. The rational models are least dependent on power, as illustrated in Figure 20–3. They assume that people behave rationally and that there is little need to force action. The models propose that communication is the key to the process.

STEPS IN THE CHANGE PROCESS. The rational models generally present the following three steps as necessary to the change process: development of the change, communication about the change, and consequences (acceptance or rejection) of the change.

Step 1. *Development.* In rational models of change, there is a critical need to fully develop the proposed change before its presentation to those involved. For instance, a nurse who wanted to develop a change in an institution's

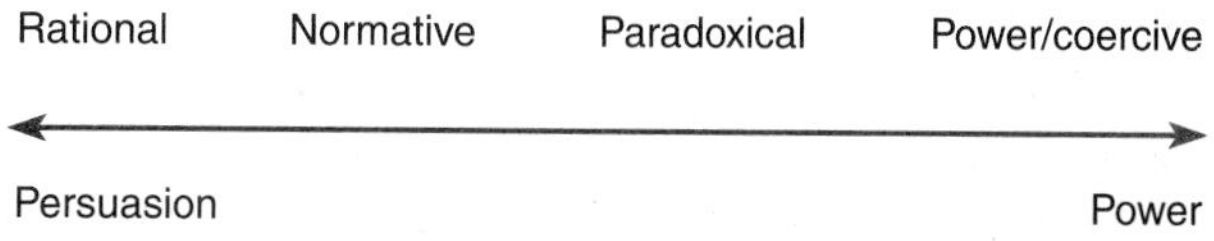

FIGURE 20-3 Power-persuasion continuum of planned change.

Rational   Normative   Paradoxical   Power/coercive

Persuasion ←————————————————→ Power

method of documentation would collect information about the existing methods of documentation. The nurse would evaluate this information and would choose the best documentation method to present to those involved in decision making.

Step 2. *Communication.* The method chosen for communication is critical to the success of the process. All individuals concerned must receive the information, understand it, and accept the reasoning that led to its choice. The person responsible for the proposed change must understand the characteristics of those who will experience the change and the characteristics of the change itself before deciding on the most appropriate method of dissemination. Various methods of communication might include booklets, memos, one-on-one discussion, and group discussions. Communication is most persuasive when it comes from a variety of different sources (Armenakis, Harris, & Mossholder, 1993).

In the rational model, a trial period or pilot study is often attempted before widespread implementation of the change. The trial period allows problems to be identified and worked out before full-scale implementation. Also, human nature is such that a partial commitment may be viewed more favorably by those involved in the change than forcing a full commitment. And, most important, a trial period allows for more communication.

Step 3. *Consequences.* Once the change is instituted, the expectation is that it will be accepted because it was the rational choice. Steps included in the model for development and communications are thought to ensure subsequent adoption of the change.

EXAMPLE OF A RATIONAL MODEL. One of the best-known rational models is Rogers' (1983) diffusion of innovation process. This is a five-stage model and is summarized in Box 20–2.

In this model, the first stage is knowledge, in which the individual becomes aware of the innovation and its function. The leader prepares for the proposed change by gathering all pertinent information related to the innovation. In the second stage, persuasion, the individual forms a favorable or unfavorable attitude toward the innovation. In the third stage, the individual decides to accept or reject the innovation. The fourth stage of implementation occurs when the individual puts the innovation into action. In the final stage, the individual considers the consequences of the change. In this stage, the change is either adopted or rejected.

The adoption of a change has three phases: trial, installation, and institutionalization. The trial phase is a pilot study of the change. If the pilot is successful, then in the second phase, the change becomes fully integrated into the system as a regular routine. Finally, in the third phase of adoption, the change becomes deeply rooted in the behavior pattern.

Introducing an innovation in an organization rests in the linkage of the change agent with the change agency and client (Rogers, 1983), as illustrated in Figure 20–4. Seven roles can be identified for the change agent who is introducing a single innovation (see Box 20–3). The goal of the change agent is to develop self-renewing behavior and "shift the client from a position of reliance on the change agent to self-reliance" (Rogers, 1983, p. 317).

Box 20–2 Rogers' Diffusion of Innovation Process

Stage 1   Knowledge
Stage 2   Persuasion
Stage 3   Acceptance or rejection
Stage 4   Implementation
Stage 5   Consequences

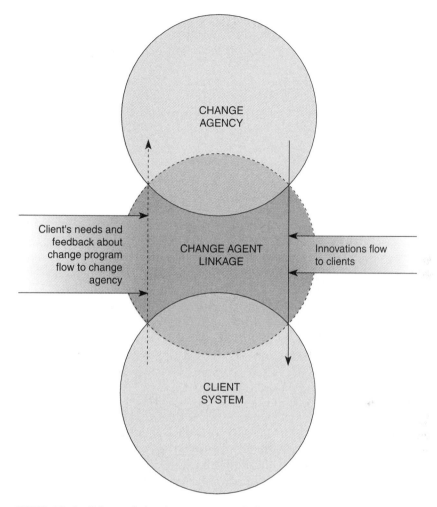

FIGURE 20–4 Linkage of the change agent with the change agency and client. (Reprinted with the permission of The Free Press, a Division of Simon & Schuster, Inc., from *Diffusion Innovations,* Third Edition, by Everett M. Rogers. Copyright © 1962, 1971, 1983 by The Free Press.)

Box 20–3 The Change Agent's Seven Roles

1. Develops a need for change
2. Establishes an informational-exchange relationship with client
3. Diagnoses client's problem
4. Creates intent to change the client
5. Translates intent into action
6. Stabilizes adoption of innovation and presents discontinuances
7. Moves client to a self-reliant position

CRITIQUE OF THE RATIONAL MODEL. Rational models are based on the assumption that if individuals know that the change is the rational choice, they will accept it. Rational models further assume that individuals know what each choice means and understand all the implications for each choice. Recent work by Langer (1989) has shown that much of human decision making is far from rational. Furthermore, even if it is the most rational choice, it may not always be the correct choice in a given situation. All decision making must consider numerous variables, and each variable has some uncertainty attached to it. It may be unrealistic to think that there is always one best solution or that the consequences of any decision can be predicted with certainty (Kosko, 1993).

Normative Model. When the resistance to change is more pronounced, it is suggested that change agents consider a normative model. *Normative models* focus on the norms of individuals targeted for change and on the actions of the leader. The norms thought to be important to change are attitudes, needs, values, and feelings. One major assumption of this model is that if both the leader and the target group actively participate in the change process, resistance will be mitigated. Three major theorists have developed normative-type models.

Lewin's model (1951) consists of three stages labeled *unfreezing, changing,* and *refreezing.* In the first stage (unfreezing), there is a careful assessment of the forces driving and restraining change. The leader conducts a detailed analysis of the environment, the characteristics of the change, and the potential responses to the change. After a careful analysis, the status quo is "unfrozen" by a deliberate introduction of disequilibria to move the organization to a desired state. Once there is movement toward change, the leader can begin to implement the planned change process by introducing new information, encouraging new behavior, providing opportunities for feedback, clarifying goals, and maintaining open communication. In the final stage (refreezing), the goal is to stabilize and integrate the change so that it becomes internalized in the system.

Havelock's (1973) and Lippitt's (1973) models center on the action of the leader rather than the environment, as in Lewin's normative change model. Their models use a participatory and democratic style of leadership for the planning and implementation of change. The models place the leader in the role of change agent and require the participation of those involved at the beginning of the planning phase.

The action of the leader follows five steps (Box 20–4). First, the leader builds a relationship with those involved that is based on trust and respect. It is critical during this phase that the leader listens well, communicates clearly, and is very open. In the second step, the target group is very involved in diagnosing the problem and establishing the need for change. The leader guides the process. Generally, consensus for change is developed through collaboration between the leader and the group. In the third step, the resources (time, skills, money, commitment) that are needed for the planned change are assessed. After the assessment is completed, specific and attainable goals are set by the group (fourth step). In the last step,

---

Box 20–4 Steps of Normative Change

Step 1   Build relationship.
Step 2   Establish need for change.
Step 3   Assess resources.
Step 4   Set goals.
Step 5   Support change process.

which is similar to Lewin's refreezing and Rogers' institutionalization, the leader continues to provide support for the change, feedback on progress, and maintenance of the actions needed to continue the change. A similar process was described by Cameron and Wren (1999) for changing organizational values in a continuing care program.

CRITIQUE OF THE NORMATIVE MODEL. Normative models are proposed to work when there is low to moderate resistance to change and a consensus can be built. Even when conditions are appropriate, change is not that easily accomplished. In part, change is not easy because any attempt to isolate the relevant factors denies the real and complex nature of most problems. That is, any attempt to isolate causation for change or reactions to change is futile because most change events are multicausal (Duck, 1993).

The normative models do not consider the history or underlying culture of the organization. Schein (1985) and others have stressed the importance of organizational culture to the change process. Organizational culture tends to vary with an organization's life cycle. Therefore leaders and managers will be more successful in implementing change if "change problems, strategy, and tactics are tied to a life-cycle framework" (Beer & Walton, 1987, p. 47) rather than a strict adherence to a normative model. Thus change attempted on a newly constructed nursing unit where change is expected may be easier to accomplish than change on a unit that is more mature and "set in its ways."

The normative models consider such norms as trust and individual feelings important to the change process, since change is thought to occur more easily when it focuses on feelings and when there is trust. Trust in the change process is based on the predictability of the events and the perceived capability of those involved (Duck, 1993). During change, individuals want to know the intentions of those promoting the change and the ground rules. People also want to understand who is responsible for the specific activities and what steps will need to be accomplished to bring about the change. Although trust and capability are the basis for the normative models, they are not easily obtained and should not be assumed. Instead, it should be remembered that the process of change by its very nature reduces predictability and, sometimes, capability.

Paradoxical Model. The paradoxical model is rooted in psychotherapy and focuses on the manner in which problems are viewed and solved (Westenholz, 1993). It has been noted in psychotherapy that an illogical plan or way of looking at a problem may succeed in changing a system or organization that cannot be changed by logic. *Paradoxical thinking* helps others think in new ways about old problems. Sometimes only a very illogical plan is capable of forcing a new way of thinking (Westenholz, 1993). Remember, it may be human nature to work against the change in order to maintain a consistent frame of reference.

Much of this work comes from the observations of Watzlawick, Weakland, and Fisch (1974). In the paradoxical model there are two levels of change: first- and second-order changes. In a *first-order change,* the patterns of behavior and the nature of relationships remain the same despite attempts at change (Watzlawick, Weakland, & Fisch, 1974). The change paradoxically serves to reinforce the status quo. For example, following decentralization of a hospital, the managers were having difficulty relating to each other as peers. The communication pattern had been top-down, or superior to subordinate in nature. Following the change, when one manager approached another as an equal and attempted to change the pattern of communication, the other manager retreated further into the previous mode of communicating only with the hospital president. Thus, even though an attempt was made to change the pattern, no real change occurred. In fact, the patterns of behavior that needed to change became more entrenched.

Second-order change may be needed to alter

the former patterns of behavior. A second-order change requires reframing the problem from a new perspective. Watzlawick and colleagues (1974) suggest four steps:

- Clearly define the problem.
- List all solutions tried.
- Clearly define parameters of realistic change.
- Create a paradoxical, second-order change strategy.

In the final step, the selection of a new second-order strategy is usually in direct opposition to former attempts to bring about planned change. As such, in attempting to change communication patterns in the example given above, the leader may try the paradoxical move of not allowing managers to communicate during a selected meeting. This move might force managers to talk to one another outside of the meeting, thus setting up a new pattern of peer communication.

CRITIQUE OF THE PARADOXICAL MODEL. As with the other models, there are drawbacks to this change model as well. First, the leader who promotes paradoxical thinking has to be highly motivated and be willing to carry out what appears to be strategies that are at odds with the normal ways of doing things. Second, the strategy means taking a risk that can backfire. A leader who presents a paradoxical way of thinking can become so associated with that view that he or she is unable to talk to others about the original problem and solution and so loses credibility with those involved. Finally, reframing the problem requires imagination and creativity. It is not easy to look at a problem from a new point of view, and few individuals are able to think paradoxically.

Power-Coercive Model. The power-coercive model is promoted as a way to deal with both strong resistance to change and inability to reach consensus. In *power-coercive* models, direct force moves the target system toward change. "When using power-based strategies,

people's needs, feelings, attitudes and values may be recognized but they are not necessarily respected" (Tappen, 2001, p. 442).

In the power-coercive model, six phases of the change process are initiated by the change agents (Tappen, 2001):

- Define the issue and identify the opponent.
- Organize a following.
- Build a power base.
- Begin action phase.
- Keep the pressure on.
- Use stronger tactics to overcome the resistance (the final struggle).

The person or group involved in the change (not necessarily the leader) assumes the risks of this strategy. These steps can be followed by people who are the "have-nots" in a system and who want to use various forms of power (money, position, legal system, control of access to resources, public support, etc.) to bring about change (Alinsky, 1972; Haley, 1969).

CRITIQUE OF THE POWER-COERCIVE MODEL. The power-coercive model uses power to force change. There are times, of course, when this method may be necessary. However, most change situations probably do not require force. Forcing others to change against their will can lead to unforeseen consequences in an organization. When this method is employed, those involved must be prepared to deal with the resistance. With forced change, the unforeseen will occur. In fact, Lee and Alexander (1999b) cite the importance of peripheral change in managing organizations in turbulent times.

Unplanned Change

> "Chaos is the law of nature; order is the dream of man."
> ● *Henry Adams*

Change is not always planned. External events and crises may cause more changes than does planned change. Suffice it to say, events happen, people change, and life evolves in ways that cannot be known. Even planned changes can unfold in ways that are unpredictable.

The models of planned change are based on the assumption that organizations are predictable, linear systems. Yet many systems are far from that, especially systems that encompass human beings. *Complexity theory* is the study of nonlinear, dynamic systems, such as people and organizations. Within this theory, both order and disorder coexist as natural parts of the system. Among the tenets of complexity theory are that (1) systems exhibit behavior that is more than the sum of their parts, (2) much behavior is nonlinear and irreversible, (3) uncertainty is a part of every system, and (4) systems can generate random, nonpredictable behavior. Rather than the world envisioned by Plato, where disorder is error and order is the norm, complexity theorists envision the world as Heraclitus did, in a perpetual state of flux where disorder is expected.

Chaos and Complexity

Underlying most work in the social sciences are implicit assumptions about cause and effect and the predictability of events. Recent research in fields such as physics, anthropology, economics, biology, and even mathematics has revealed that absolute predictability and control may not be a realistic goal. It appears that dynamic systems, even simple ones, can generate random, unpredictable behavior. Consider, for example, the weather. Despite access to large-scale computers with which to calculate a vast knowledge base of weather predictors in combination with timely satellite pictures, weather forecasts are still not 100% accurate. Weather just does not represent a predictable linear model. Furthermore, if weather cannot be modeled as a linear system, human behavior, of which we know even less, certainly cannot.

One reason for the apparent inability to predict such phenomena as weather, disease progression, and response to change is the notion of sensitivity to initial conditions. In changing and evolving systems, small chance events or differences in conditions have the ability to lead to very different outcomes. As an example, any small shift in temperature, wind direction, or barometric pressure is enough to cause major differences in the weather. In part, this is due to the iterative effects of positive feedback; in other words, the small change becomes magnified as the system grows. Small errors do not always stay small (Kellert, 1993).

Unfortunately, chaos can appear in any stable system when the system is given the right push (Pool, 1989). *Chaos* has been defined as the unpredictable behavior that can arise from systems (Lipsitz & Goldberger, 1992). It appears that most systems have points where they are the most sensitive to disturbance. Rather than absorbing the effects of the disturbance, the system begins to respond in unpredictable ways. For example, electrical stimulation given at the right point in the cardiac cycle can cause the heart rhythm to show bifurcations and other abnormal rhythms. The point where a system exhibits change is known by many names, depending on the discipline. Periods of change are called "crisis points" by developmental psychologists, "hinge points" by archaeologists, "punctuations" by biologists, and "phase transitions" by physicists.

Familiarity with an organization or a person may reveal obvious points of weakness or concern. These points should be thought of as places where the person or system is vulnerable or even unstable. For example, a change of administration is probably not well thought out if it is scheduled to occur during a major holiday time.

Dynamic systems are remarkably resilient and show an ability to maintain order despite the surrounding disorder. The type of disturbance, the magnitude of the disturbance, the susceptibility of the system, and happenstance can all influence how a system responds (Cambel,

1993). *Complexity theory* tells us that it may not be possible to know all the points of vulnerability within a system despite careful analysis and planning. All plans regarding change should include discussions of how to recognize and deal with critical points. When unexpected change occurs, the system should be supported in order to avoid chaos.

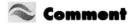 **Comment**

"Change can provide opportunities for growth, survival, extinction, or retrenchment" (Lancaster, 1999, p. 150). As external forces continue to drive the financing and delivery of health care, nurses need to have the knowledge, courage, and conviction to bring about change to improve the quality of care for patients. Understanding the process of change is essential for effective nursing practice in today's changing health care environment and for the continued advancement of the nursing profession.

KEY POINTS

- Change is a natural and unavoidable aspect of life.
- Change affects everything, including people, organizations, societies, and nations.
- While some change can be planned, much of change is unplanned, and even planned change does not always unfold as designed.
- Change has been viewed as a hypothetical linear system where each part of the system was thought to be understandable and controllable.
- The rational model of planned change is based on the assumption that with good information, most people will make the logical choice to change.
- The normative model of change is based on the assumption that if both the leader and the target group participate in the change process, resistance to change will be reduced.
- The paradoxical model of change is based on the

notion that an illogical plan or way of looking at a problem may succeed in changing a system where logic failed.
- The power-coercive model is useful when dealing with both strong resistance to change and inability to reach consensus.
- While all the models have valid aspects, none of the models has been shown to be effective in all situations.
- Recent work in many different disciplines has shown that more information or more structure does not always ensure smooth change.
- Systems under stress, such as those experiencing change, can act in a variety of strange and unpredictable ways called chaos.
- Complexity theory has shown that the behavior of a part of a system cannot be used to predict the behavior of the whole system.
- New models of change should take into account the dynamic nature of change, specifically patterns of behavior during change, areas of vulnerability during the change process, and the roles involvement and information play.
- The change process should be considered complex and not a process that can be reduced to a few rules or clichés.

CRITICAL THINKING EXERCISES

1. Look at a recent change in your clinical area. Explain or evaluate the process of change according to one of the change theories discussed in this chapter. Who were the supporters and resistors? What obstacles needed to be overcome? How was the change implemented, and what was the outcome?

2. If you were going to institute a major change in a home health agency, what would be your first step? How would this differ if you wanted to make a change in a hospital? Which model of planned change would be most effective in each situation, and why?

3. Describe a situation in which an unexpected event occurred during the implementation of a change. Why do you believe the unexpected event occurred? How could this have been avoided? Was the outcome a positive or negative one?

REFERENCES

Alinsky, S. D. (1972). *Rules for radicals: A practical primer for realistic radicals.* New York: Vintage Books.

Armenakis, A. A., Harris, S. G., & Mossholder, K. W. (1993). Creating readiness for organizational change. *Human Relations, 46,* 681–703.

Arnold, D. R., Capella, L. M., & Sumrall, D. A. (1987). Hospital challenge: Using change theory and processes to adopt and implement the marketing concept. *Journal of Health Care Marketing, 7*(2), 15–24.

Axelrod, D. (1992). Getting everyone involved: How one organization involved its employees, supervisors, and managers in redesigning the organization. *Journal of Applied Behavioral Science, 28,* 499–509.

Backstrom, T. (1999). Intra-organization work for change: A model and two tools. *American Journal of Industrial Medicine, Supplement 1,* 61–63.

Beer, M., & Walton, A. E. (1987). Organization change and development. *Annual Review of Psychology, 38,* 339–367.

Bennis, W. G., Benne, K. D., & Chin, R. (Eds.). (1985). *The planning of change* (4th ed.). New York: Holt, Rinehart & Winston.

Bernhard, L. A., & Walsh, M. (1995). *Leadership: The key to the professionalism of nursing* (3rd ed.). St. Louis: Mosby.

Bonalumi, N., & Fisher, K. (1999). Health care change: Challenge for nurse administrators. *Nursing Administration Quarterly, 23*(2), 69–73.

Bruhn, J. G. (1999). Energizing yourself for change. In K. Lancaster (Ed.), *Nursing issues in leading and managing change* (pp. 609–625). St. Louis: Mosby.

Burke, W. W., & Litwin, G. H. (1992). A causal model of organizational performance and change. *Journal of Management, 18,* 523–545.

Cambel, A.B. (1993). *Applied chaos theory: A paradigm for complexity.* San Diego, CA: Academic Press.

Cameron, G., & Wren, A. M. (1999). Reconstructing organizational culture: A process using multiple perspectives. *Public Health Nursing, 16*(2), 96–101.

Chin, R. (1976). The utility of systems models and developmental models for practitioners. In W. G. Bennis, K. D. Benne, R. Chin, & K. Corey (Eds.), *The planning of change* (3rd ed.). New York: Holt, Rinehart & Winston.

Conner, D. R. (1993). *Managing at the speed of change.* New York: Villard Books.

Davis, P. S. (1991). The meaning of change to individuals within a college of nurse education. *Journal of Advanced Nursing, 16,* 108–115.

Downey, K., & Brief, A. (1986). How cognitive structures affect organizational design. In H. Sims & D. Gioia (Eds.), *The thinking organization.* San Francisco: Jossey-Bass.

Duck, J. D. (1993, November-December). Managing change: The art of balancing. *Harvard Business Review, 71*(6), 109–118.

Gabel, S., & Oster, G. D. Mental health providers confronting organizational change: Process, problems, and strategies. *Psychiatry, 61,* 302–316.

Gillies, D.A. (1994). *Nursing management* (3rd ed.). Philadelphia: Saunders.

Gioia, D. A., & Chittipeddi, K. (1991). Using sensemaking and sensegiving in strategic change initiatives. *Strategic Management Journal, 12,* 433–448.

Globerman, J. (1999). Hospital restructuring: Positioning social work to manage change. *Social Work in Health Care, 28*(4), 13–30.

Grohar-Murray, M. E., & DiCroce, H. R. (1992). *Leadership and management in nursing.* Norwalk, CT: Appleton & Lange.

Grossman, S., & Valiga, T. M. (2000). *The new leadership challenge: Creating the future of nursing.* Philadelphia: Davis.

Haley, J. (1969). *The power tactics of Jesus Christ and other essays.* New York: Avon Books.

Hamm, F. B. (1992). Organizational change required for paradigmatic shift in addiction treatment. *Journal of Substance Abuse Treatment, 9,* 257–260.

Havelock, R. G. (1973). *The change agent's guide to innovation in education.* Englewood Cliffs, NJ: Educational Technology Publications.

Irvine, Y., & Phoenix, E. (1998). The new change process: Always a work in progress. *Perspectives, 22*(4), 2–5.

Kellert, S. H. (1993). *In the wake of chaos.* Chicago: University of Chicago Press.

Kobs, A. E. J. (1999). Does the C in JCAHO stand for change? *Nursing Administration Quarterly, 23*(2), 83–85.

Koloroutis, M., & Thorstenson, T. (1999). An ethics framework for organizational change. *Nursing Administration Quarterly, 23*(2), 9–18.

Kosko, B. (1993). *Fuzzy thinking: The new science of fuzzy logic.* New York: Hyperion.

Kubler-Ross, E. (1970). *On death and dying.* London: Tavistock.

Lancaster. K. (1999). *Nursing issues in leading and managing change.* St. Louis: Mosby.

Langer, E. (1989). *Mindfulness.* Redwood City, CA: Addison-Wesley.

Lee, S. Y., & Alexander, J.A. (1999a). Consequences of organizational change in U.S. hospitals. *Medical Care Research and Review, 56,* 227–276.

Lee, S. Y., & Alexander, J. A. (1999b). Managing hospitals in turbulent times: Do organizational changes improve hospital survival? *Health Services Research, 34,* 923–946.

Lewin, K. (1951). *Field theory in social science: Selected theoretical papers*. New York: Harper & Row.

Lewin, R. (1992). *Complexity: Life at the edge of chaos*. New York: Macmillan.

Lippitt, G. L. (1973). *Visualizing change: Model building and the change process*. La Jolla, CA: University Associates.

Lipsitz, L. A., & Goldberger, A. L. (1992). Loss of complexity and aging: Potential applications of fractals and chaos theory to senescence. *JAMA, 267,* 1806–1809.

Lowstedt, J. (1993). Organizing frameworks in emerging organizations: A cognitive approach to the analysis of change. *Human Relations, 46,* 501–526.

Marshak, R. J. (1993). Lewin meets Confucius: A review of the OD model of change. *Journal of Applied Behavioral Science, 29,* 393–415.

Mawhinney, T. C. (1992). Evolution of organizational cultures as selection by consequences: The Gaia hypothesis, metacontingencies, and organizational ecology. *Journal of Organizational Behavior Management, 12*(2), 1–26.

Meleis, A. I., & Trangenstein, P. A. (1994). Facilitating transitions: Redefinition of a nursing mission. *Nursing Outlook, 42*(6), 255–259.

Pool, R. (1989). Is it chaos, or is it just noise? *Science, 242*(4887), 25–28.

Porras, J. I., & Silvers, R. C. (1991). Organization development and transformation. *Annual Review of Psychology, 45,* 51–78.

Potter, M. L., Dawson, A. M., Barton, N. M., & Nitz, R.E. (1998). Change . . . ouch. *Nursing Management, 29*(11), 27–29.

Redmond, G., Riggleman, J., Sorrel, J. M., & Zerull, L. (1999). Creative winds of change: Nurses collaborating for quality outcomes. *Nursing Administration Quarterly, 23*(2), 55–64.

Rogers, E. M. (1983). *Diffusion of innovation* (3rd ed.). New York: Free Press.

Salmond, S. W. (1998). Managing the human side of change. *Orthopaedic Nursing, 17*(5), 38–51.

Schein, E. (1985). *Organizational culture and leadership*. San Francisco: Jossey-Bass.

Sheehan, J. (1990). Investigating change in a nursing context. *Journal of Advanced Nursing, 15,* 819–824.

Simpson, R.L. (1999). Changing world, changing systems: Why managed care health care demands information technology. *Nursing Administration Quarterly, 23*(2), 86–88.

Snell, L., & Turner, D. (1991, May-June). A new master rotation on a labor and delivery unit. *Canadian Journal of Nursing Administration, 4*(2), 19.

Spitzer, A. (1999). Steering an academic department through a paradigm shift: The case of a new paradigm for nursing. *Journal of Nursing Education, 38,* 312–318.

Stickland, G. (1992). Positioning training and development departments for organizational change. *Management Education and Development, 23,* 307–316.

Tappen, R. M. (1989). *Nursing leadership and management* (2nd ed.). Philadelphia: Davis.

Tappen, R. M. (2001). *Nursing leadership and management: Concepts and practice* (4th ed.). Philadelphia: Davis.

Tice, D. M. (1992). Self-concept and self-presentation: The looking glass self is also a magnifying glass. *Journal of Personality and Social Psychology, 63,* 435–451.

Tiffany, C.R., Cheatham, A.B., Doornbos, D., Loudermelt, L., & Momadi, G. G. (1994). Planned change theory: Survey of nursing periodical literature. *Nursing Management, 25*(7), 54–59.

Traub, J. F., & Wozniakowski, H. (1994). Breaking intractability. *Scientific American, 266*(1), 102–107.

Watzlawick, P., Weakland, J. H., & Fisch, R. (1974). *Change: Principles of problem formation and problem resolution*. New York: Norton.

Westenholz, A. (1993). Paradoxical thinking and change in the frames of reference. *Organization Studies, 14*(1), 37–58.

Zajc, L. S. (1987). *Models of planned educational change: Their ideational and ideological contexts and evolution since the late 1950s*. Unpublished manuscript, available from University Microfilms International, Ann Arbor, MI.

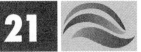

21

Nursing Research

AUDREY G. GIFT, PhD, RN, FAAN

OBJECTIVES

At the completion of this chapter, the reader will be able to:

- Define nursing research and describe how it has evolved over the past 40 years.
- Describe the process by which research can be implemented in practice.
- Compare and contrast the different approaches to nursing research and how they can be used to answer different nursing questions.
- Describe the research process and the parts of the research report.
- Describe the ethical considerations in conducting a nursing research study, such as protecting human subjects in a study and maintaining the integrity of the research.
- List several sources for funding a research study.

PROFILE IN PRACTICE

Celia Wills, PhD, RN, FAAN
Assistant Professor
College of Nursing
Michigan State University
East Lansing, Michigan

Scientific inquiry has been a lifelong interest of mine. This interest was fostered by my parents, who were both scientists and academicians in chemistry and chemical engineering. I have always been intensely analytic and curious about how things work in terms of cause-and-effect relationships. As an undergraduate student at the University of Virginia School of Nursing, certain faculty members noted my potential for graduate level work and encouraged me to think about applying to graduate school.

As a registered nurse in the psychiatric/mental health nursing specialty area, I became strongly impressed by the need for improved mental health services for people coping with depressive disorders. I recognized that treatment was often inadequate, and that decisions of both health care providers and patients played important roles in the outcomes of depression treatment. Health care providers had to rely on the decision making of patients to implement depression treatment, yet little was known about how patients made such decisions about their treatment. This gap in knowledge became the focus of my research program when I entered graduate school.

During my graduate studies at the University of Wisconsin–Madison I had two outstanding mentors. I worked with Carolyn Dawson, PhD, RN, who introduced me to theoretical foundations of nursing research and clinical nursing research methods. I also worked with Colleen F. Moore, PhD, a cognitive-developmental psychologist, who helped me to further develop my skills in research methods and statistics.

As a graduate student, I conducted a series of survey research studies to model basic processes of patient judgment and decision making about medication acceptance (Wills, 1997; Wills & Moore, 1994a, 1994b, 1996). These early studies showed that decision making about medication involves a highly complex process of weighing and combining multiple considerations. These studies allowed me to begin to model the complex process of how people make decisions about medications and to understand both the general and situation-specific circumstances under which a medication is likely to be accepted or declined.

Although I continue my line of basic research on health-related judgment and decision-making processes (see Holzworth & Wills, 1999, and Wills, 1999, for recent examples), as a faculty member at Michigan State University, I have extended my earlier research to more applied contexts which included clinical samples. I was able to work with an interdisciplinary health-related decision-making research team at Michigan State University, testing an educational intervention as decision support for menopausal women (Rothert et al., 1997). I also completed a study with 97 depressed primary care patients, exploring relationships between decision making and patterns of antidepressant medication use (Wills & Holmes-Rovner, 1998). This study allowed an assessment of the psychometric properties of several recently developed standardized measures of decision making for a depressed primary care patient population.

This study served as a pilot study for a grant sponsored by the National Institute of Mental Health, which includes two projects: (1) a longitudinal study of relationships between depressed primary care patient decision making, medication use, health status, and cost and utilization of health services outcomes; and (2) preliminary testing of a patient decision support intervention for primary care depression treatment. These projects will extend my prior research in two ways: (1) linking individual-level patient decision making to macro-level health services outcome, and (2) extending descriptive-level research to studies testing a decision support intervention.

The biggest challenges I have faced as a researcher have been resource limitations, which constitute barriers to research in almost any setting: for example, access to research participants, obtaining adequate research funding, and having sufficient release time to devote to research and writing. In some senses, the more daunting challenges to a successful career as a researcher are personal, such as self-doubts about the value of my own ideas and scholarship. Other challenges include managing the general pressures of an academic career as well as resolving or managing decisional conflict about how I should be spending my time and energy—that is, what amount of effort should be devoted to research versus my other academic roles in teaching and service. The best part of being a researcher is having a job where I can spend time pursuing a heartfelt interest, as well as the intellectual challenge and stimulation of doing research and writing.

Inadequately treated depression is a serious public health problem because of its high prevalence in the general population and its substantial adverse impact on morbidity, mortality, and quality of life. Effective treatments such as antidepressant medication are available for the treatment of major depression, but most primary care patients who are prescribed antidepressant medication either refuse or discontinue the medication soon after starting it, before the benefits of the medication can be realized. Health care providers must rely on patients to make decisions on implementing treatment for depression, but to date, there has been little research into how patients make treatment decisions, or how one can support them in effective decision making. I look forward to examining the macro-level outcomes affected by individual-level patient decision making. This research will allow me to better understand patient decision-making processes and will facilitate the development of improved patient decision support interventions that may be implemented by nurses to make positive depression treatment outcomes in primary care more likely.

Nursing research is directed toward gaining an understanding of nursing care of individuals and groups. Its purpose is to develop a knowledge base that will guide practice. The National Institute of Nursing Research (NINR) indicates in its mission statement that it supports clinical and basic research to establish a scientific basis for the care of individuals across the life span, from the management of patients during illness and recovery to the reduction of risks for disease and disability. Promoting healthy lifestyles, promoting quality of life in those with chronic illness, and care for individuals at the end of life are particular areas of emphasis for the institute (NINR, 1999). The institute "seeks to understand and ease the symptoms of acute and chronic illness, to prevent or delay the onset of disease or disability or slow its progression, to find effective approaches to achieving and sustaining good health, and to improve the clinical settings in which care is provided." Nursing research involves clinical care in a variety of settings, including the community and home, in addition to more traditional health care sites. The NINR's research extends to problems encountered by patients, families, and caregivers. It also emphasizes the special needs of at-risk and underserved populations. These efforts are crucial in the creation of scientific advances and their translation into cost-effective health care that does not compromise quality" (NINR, 1999, p. 7). The intent of nursing research is to ensure that nursing care is scientifically based rather than based on tradition. For this to happen, however, nurses must be aware of research and use it in practice.

To fully cover nursing's role in research, this chapter is divided into the following sections: the history of nursing research, reading and using research in practice, conducting a research study, ethics in research, and funding for research.

History of Nursing Research

Nursing research has often been described as beginning with the detailed observations made by Florence Nightingale during the Crimean War. She observed and recorded details about the environment (ventilation, temperature, cleanliness, purity of water, and diet) and linked these observations to patient outcomes. She realized that providing a clean environment reduced mortality in soldiers. However, few who followed her engaged in these systematic recordings.

Studies of the effectiveness of public health teaching date back to before World War I. Then, in the 1920s, case studies of patients first began to appear in the *American Journal of Nursing*. During the 1940s and 1950s the focus was on nursing services research, which includes the organization and delivery of nursing services. Time and motion studies were done, and statewide surveys of personnel were conducted.

The 1950s saw increased activity supporting nursing research. In 1952 *Nursing Research*, the first journal devoted exclusively to nursing research, was published. In 1953 the Institute for Research and Service in Nursing Education was established at Teachers College, Columbia University, and provided learning experiences in research for doctoral students. The focus of this program, however, was on nursing education (Burns & Grove, 1997).

In 1955 federal funding first became available for grants in nursing through the Division of Nursing within the Bureau of Health Professions in the Health Resources and Services Administration of the U.S. Public Health Service. The aim was to provide resources for faculty development, including nursing research. Funding was minimal and nonrecurring, thus requiring an allocation annually. This continued until the 1980s.

Also in 1955 the American Nurses' Foundation was chartered as the research and education subsidiary of the American Nurses Association (ANA). One of its main goals has been to raise funds and distribute grants to support beginning nurse scientists. Since 1955 more than 500 nurse researchers have benefited from more than $2 million in grants Recently it was decided that the amount of some basic research grants would be increased to $5,000 where possible, with two awards available at $10,000.

The first research institution to emphasize clinical nursing research was established in 1957 as the Department of Nursing Research in the Walter Reed Army Institute of Research (Stevenson, 1986). At this time also, specialty organizations began to appear, and the need for nursing research to provide the basis for nursing practice standards became evident.

Regional research organizations, such as the Southern Regional Education Board (SREB) and the Western Interstate Commission on Higher Education (WICHEN), were formed. Their goals were to provide opportunities for nurse researchers to meet and disseminate nursing research findings and techniques. These regional research societies have changed names or geographic boundaries, but they remain an important factor in nursing research today.

Nursing research in the 1960s included studies focusing on nursing education, nursing delivery systems, and clinical practice. The 1970s saw the development of models, conceptual frameworks, and theories to guide nursing practice. Nurses began to use models from a variety of sources to provide direction for clinical nursing research. By the late 1970s three additional research journals appeared in nursing: *Advances in Nursing Science,* which publishes nursing research that focuses on nursing theories, and *Research in Nursing and Health* and the *Western Journal of Nursing Research,* both of which publish nursing research studies. This expanded the forum for communication of nursing research findings. More recently, research-focused specialty journals have begun to appear for the communication of research findings.

The beginning doctoral programs in nursing focused on nursing education, with many of the graduates taking administrative positions in higher education. Few nurses established careers in nursing research. In the 1980s, however, there was a dramatic increase in the number of doctoral programs in nursing. In 2000 there were 71 doctoral programs in nursing. This is in contrast to 1979, when there were only 22 doctoral programs in nursing. The percentage of graduates pursuing a research career is continuing to rise, with most being employed in educational institutions, but an increasing number taking positions in clinical settings. With the advent of managed care, however, nurse researchers in a clinical setting have experienced changes from a focus on improving patient care for individuals to documentation of effective outcomes for groups of patients.

NATIONAL INSTITUTE OF NURSING RESEARCH

In 1986 the National Center for Nursing Research was established within the National Institutes of Health (NIH). The name was changed to the National Institute of Nursing Research (NINR) in 1993. Dr. Ada Sue Hinshaw was the first director, serving from 1986 to 1994, followed by Dr. Patricia Grady, who has served from 1995 to the present.

The NINR accomplishes its mission by allocating supporting grants to universities and other research organizations with most of its budget. A smaller percentage of its budget is used to conduct research intramurally at laboratories in Bethesda, Maryland. There are currently two intramural laboratories, a Wound Healing Laboratory and a Health Promotion Laboratory. A laboratory on symptom management is also planned for the intramural program. The rest of the budget is used for comprehensive research training, career development, and core centers in specialized areas of research inquiry to prepare individuals with requisite skills to conduct research in an interdisciplinary setting. Extramural programs provide funding to researchers in universities, hospitals, and other research centers across the country and are presently organized into seven areas:

1. Research in chronic illness and long-term care, including health issues of individuals with arthritis, diabetes, and urinary incontinence. This area also encompasses family caregiving and long-term care.
2. Research in health promotion and risk behaviors, including studies of women's health; developmental transitions, such as adolescence and menopause; environmental health; and health behavior research, such as studies of exercise, nutrition, and smoking cessation.
3. Research in cardiopulmonary health and critical care, including prevention and the care of individuals with cardiac or respiratory conditions. This area also includes research in critical care, trauma, wound healing, and organ transplantation.
4. Research in neurofunction and sensory conditions, including pain management, sleep disorders, and symptom management, in persons with cognitive impairment or chronic neurological conditions. This area also includes research on patient care in acute care settings.

5. Research in immune responses and oncology, including symptoms primarily associated with cancer and AIDS, such as fatigue, nausea and vomiting, and cachexia. Prevention research on specific risk factors is also included.
6. Research in reproductive and infant health, including premature labor and low birth weight, reduction of health risk factors during pregnancy, labor and delivery, and the postpartum period, and issues related to prenatal care, neonates, infant growth and development, and fertility.
7. Research in end-of-life and palliative care, including clinical management of physical and psychological symptoms, communication, ethics and clinical decision-making, caregiver support, and care delivery issues (NINR, 1999).

One activity of the NINR is the setting of the National Nursing Research Agenda. The purpose of this is to provide structure, depth, and direction for nursing research. A subcommittee of the National Advisory Council for Nursing Research provides oversight for this activity. The first priorities were for 1989 to 1994, and the following seven areas were selected:

1. Low birth weight—mothers and infants
2. HIV infection—prevention and care
3. Long-term care for older adults
4. Symptom management—pain
5. Nursing informatics—support for patient care
6. Health promotion for children and adolescents
7. Technology dependency across the life span (NINR, 1993)

The second conference identified the next priorities for 1995 to 1999. These were:

1. Community-based nursing models
2. Health-promoting behaviors and HIV/AIDS
3. Remediation of cognitive impairment

4. Living with chronic illness
5. Biobehavioral factors related to immuno-competence

The NINR recently underwent strategic planning and set the following scientific goals and objectives for the 5-year period of 2000–2004 (NINR, 1999):

Goal 1: Identify and support research opportunities that will achieve scientific distinction and produce significant contributions to health. The leadership areas identified include end-of-life/palliative care research, chronic illness experiences, quality of life and quality of care, health promotion and disease prevention research, symptom management, telehealth interventions and monitoring, implications of genetic advances, cultural and ethnic considerations.

Goal 2: Identify and support future areas of opportunity to advance research on high-quality, cost-effective care and to contribute to the scientific base for nursing practice.

Goal 3: Communicate and disseminate research findings resulting from NINR-funded research.

Goal 4: Enhance the development of nurse researchers through training and career development opportunities.

Federal funding for nursing research has increased over the years. For instance, there was a rise in obligated dollars from $16.2 million in 1986 to $44.9 million in 1992 (NINR, 1993) and exceeding $77 million in 1999 (NINR, 1999). However, the NINR remains the smallest institute within the NIH, with the lowest percentage of approved proposals receiving funding of any NIH institute. There is presently a national effort on the part of nursing deans and associate deans for research to educate Congress about the accomplishments and needs of the NINR and to request support for a designated percentage increase in appropriation specific for this institute. More information about the NINR is available on its web site (http://www.nih.gov/ninr/).

Using Research in Practice

It is vital that nursing base its practice on nursing research rather than tradition. Many practices are ingrained in nursing and have been allowed to continue because nurses have not questioned the rationale for the practice. The first step is to question routines by examining the research base. This requires nurses to read nursing research and include the findings in their practice. This is not easily done but appears to be becoming more common as nurses are increasingly being given more autonomy for their practice (Coyle & Sokop, 1990).

An important step in research utilization is learning about the research findings (Box 21–1). Common nursing problems such as pressure ulcer care and pain management are the problems with the largest nursing research base and therefore those most used to guide practice (Buss et.al., 1999). Nurses report that they learn about research by reading the professional nursing literature, attending conferences and inservices, and observing the practice of others (Coyle & Sokop, 1990). When these activities are encouraged by administration, utilization of research increases. The culture of the organizations in which nurses work and the resources available are vital in supporting the use of research in practice (Omery & Williams, 1999). One way in which nurses can share research findings is in nursing practice committees to update policies and procedures. The role models displayed in these committees can be a valuable asset for research utilization in nursing.

Another way to learn about research findings is through the use of standards and practice guidelines available from national agencies and organizations, such as the Agency for Healthcare Research and Quality (AHRQ). Research on selected topics, such as the management of

Box 21-1 Ways to Incorporate Research into Practice

RESEARCH IN CLINICAL NURSING JOURNALS

Several clinical journals now have sections in which they summarize and evaluate recent research studies. They then have a section in which the implications of the research for nursing practice are included. An example of such a journal is *Heart and Lung*. Other journals, such as *Applied Nursing Research,* focus on research designed specifically for the clinical setting.

NURSING PRACTICE COMMITTEE

Practice committees are charged with writing and reviewing nursing policies and procedures for a hospital. It is important to consider the current relevant research when writing or revising policies and procedures. The committee can be asked to share reviews of the current research when the policy is presented. Also, there may be a list of references used in establishing the policy that are printed at the end.

JOURNAL CLUB

Many practice settings have journal clubs that meet to discuss recent research related to the patient population under their care. If your institution does not have a journal club, you might want to consider establishing one. This will attract nurses interested in reading, evaluating, and discussing research. Each person could be assigned a journal to read and report about each month. This saves each nurse from trying to read all journals each month.

NURSING RESEARCH COMMITTEE

Nursing research committees have been established in many hospitals to educate nursing staff about research and to inform potential investigators of institutional requirements for conducting nursing research. The objective is to facilitate nursing research while maintaining high-quality patient care (Vessey & Campos, 1992).

acute pain, urinary incontinence, or pressure ulcers, is reviewed and recommendations are made for clinical practice. The goal is for all health professionals to implement the recommendations in practice. These guidelines are available at the web site www.guideline.gov.

One of the most significant changes that will enhance the retrieval and dissemination of research findings and make them more available is the use of electronic publishing. For a list of electronic journals and other electronic nursing sources, see the article by Susan Sparks (1999). Electronic publishing makes information more accessible. There is a fear that it will also limit the peer review, but others suggest that the critique could be made more public by including it along with the electronic publication and thus increase the intellectual exchange (Sparks, 1999). To support this notion the NIH is establishing a web-based repository for barrier-free access to primary reports in the life sciences. This repository will be called PubMed Central and will evolve by having the existing PubMed biomedical literature database extend its coverage to include plant and agriculture research while continuing its linkage to external on-line journals. The plan is to have PubMed Central archive, organize, and distribute peer-reviewed reports from journals, as well as reports that have not been peer-reviewed. The PubMed web site is accessed at http://www.ncbi.nlm.nih.gov/PubMed/. What this means for the practicing nurse is that the need for electronic connection to the Internet is becoming more and more essential to having a research-based practice.

In addition to electronic sources, there are other resources being developed for the evaluation of nursing research studies and communication of the findings. An example is the Council for the Advancement of Nursing Science, which was recently developed within the American Academy of Nursing to support the development, conduct, and utilization of nursing science. Facilitating nursing scientists and sharing research findings with nurses and the community at large are also goals. Further details on the council are available on their web site, http://www.nursingworld.org/aan/webad.htm. Another example is the Sarah Cole Hirsh Institute for Best Nursing Practices Based on Evidence at the Frances Payne Bolton School of Nursing at Case Western Reserve University, School of Nursing, which is a clearinghouse for nursing practice guidelines (Youngblut & Brooten, 2000). A source of research synthesis, not specific to nursing but which does include nursing research is the Cochrane Library, ongoing meta-analysis of evidence documenting effective health care practices. This is a global enterprise with centers around the world and reviews available on the web for those who register (Estabrooks, 1998).

A number of models have been proposed to describe the application of research findings to clinical practice. Most, such as the Stetler/Marram model (Stetler, 1994), are based on the premise that nurses desire knowledge, and the model explains how and why it is sought out. Titler and colleagues (1994), however, have developed the Iowa model, which depicts a different type of model for research utilization (Fig. 21–1). They describe what they call problem-focused triggers to research utilization. This occurs when a clinical problem is repeatedly encountered in practice, risk management, or quality improvement programs and leads to the use of research in practice. They give the example of learning that 50% of critical care patients

reported a mean pain intensity of 7.5 on a 10-point scale, which led to the implementation of a research-based pain management protocol (Titler et al., 1994). Quality improvement data are a rich source of ideas for nursing research.

The decision to use research to enhance practice requires an evaluation of the available research on the topic. The quality, quantity, and applicability of the research to the practice setting are considered. If the research is absent or insufficient, conducting a research study should be considered. This is discussed in the next section. However, if there is a sufficient research base to suggest appropriate changes for practice, these would have to be tested in the practice setting before being adopted.

When a change in practice is to be implemented, Titler and colleagues (1994) recommend first setting criteria and selecting outcome measures for evaluating the effects of the change. Documentation of the current situation is necessary so that it can be used as a comparison with an assessment made using the same outcome measures after the change is implemented. The nature of the practice change determines whether the intervention is developed from a multidisciplinary or independent nursing perspective. For example, a change in pain management would most likely require the cooperation of physicians, nurses, and perhaps anesthesiologists for a successful program to be implemented. There are, however, other activities that fall solely within the domain of nursing.

Pilot testing the change on one or two units before implementing the change throughout the institution is advisable. This will allow potential problems to be corrected ahead of time. If the staff nurses on the pilot units are educated about the research base and evaluate the change as desirable, they can assist in orienting others and discussing the positive outcomes of the change (Titler et al., 1994).

Outcomes to be included in the evaluation of a practice change should include not only patient outcomes but the financial implications of the change as well. A change in practice re-

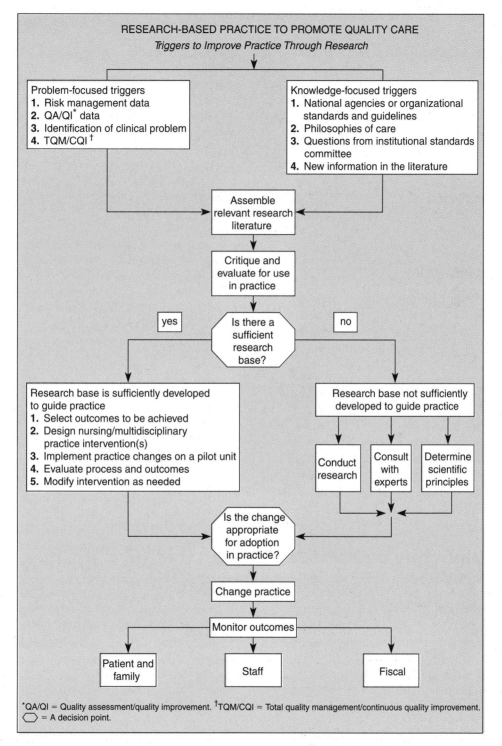

FIGURE 21–1 Iowa model of problem-focused triggers to research utilization. (Copyright University of Iowa Hospital and Clinics. Redrawn from Titler, M. C., et al. (1994). Infusing research into practice to promote quality care. *Nursing Research, 43,* 307–313.)

quires the orientation of staff, changing of forms, changes in other areas of practice. This can be costly to the institution. Such changes are warranted, however, if they result in significantly better patient outcomes. Other outcomes to evaluate would be the satisfaction of the staff with the practice change. Increased staff satisfaction will contribute to staff retention and a reduction in the cost of orienting new staff. Using research as a basis for practice has as its goal improvement in the patient, staff, and financial outcomes for the institution.

PRACTICE GUIDELINES

By definition, clinical practice guidelines are based on research. They are a summary and evaluation of the current research with recommendations made for clinical practice. Guidelines are put forward by specialty nursing organizations as well as by the AHRQ (http://www.guideline.gov). The ANA has published a booklet describing how to evaluate and use guidelines (Ferrell et al., 1994). It has also published a manual to be used by specialty organizations indicating how to develop guidelines (Marek, 1994). Of particular note in this manual are the scoring sheets used by the various guideline panels in evaluating research studies.

Conducting a Research Study

Although reading, evaluating, and using research in practice is every nurse's responsibility, involvement in conducting research varies with the nurse's level of education. Those with a baccalaureate degree are critical to the identification of problems for research. They are the nurses who are in the best position to identify the gaps in nursing knowledge. Baccalaureate degree nurses may also be asked to assist nurse researchers in identifying subjects meeting the inclusion criteria for a study and in gaining ac-cess to clinical sites. They may also assist with data collection (ANA, 1993).

In the present cost-containment environment, nurses' time has become even more valuable than before. When a nurse is hired to care for patients, that must remain the primary focus for the nurse. However, there are rewards that can be gained from involvement in nursing research. One of the most exciting can be learning the answer to the question being explored. This is particularly exciting when it results in an improvement in practice. Another reward is the contribution to the knowledge base of nursing and the advancement of the profession. Involvement in research is often a requirement for career advancement, but in some cases it may also provide other rewards. Rewards may be personal, such as increased knowledge, satisfaction with one's performance, or seeing one's name in print.

These rewards for involvement in research are negotiated with the researcher on the basis of the time that will be required. For instance, if all that is required is the identification of subjects admitted with a certain diagnosis or the recording of routine data on a separate sheet, the reward may be simply the sharing of research findings. If, on the other hand, what is required is increased monitoring or the recording of more complex patient data, these activities would put more of a burden on the nursing staff and the reward would be expected to be more extensive. Nurses may be paid to collect research data or may negotiate shared authorship if they make a significant contribution to the research study.

Nurses at all levels of practice are involved in nursing research. Nurses with a master's degree might be involved by collaborating with other investigators, facilitating data collection, and providing expert clinical consultation. The design and coordination of research studies is a role most commonly reserved for the doctorally prepared nurse (ANA, 1993). Guidance on how to obtain assistance in designing and conducting a nursing research study is described in Box 21–2.

Box 21–2 How to Obtain Assistance in Conducting a Research Study

NURSE RESEARCHERS IN AN ACADEMIC SETTING

Faculty in most universities are expected to conduct research. Nursing faculty are no exception to this expectation. Those prepared at the doctoral level have had the advantage of courses in research design and statistics. If they have had experience conducting clinical studies, they can be a valuable asset in deigning a research study. In addition, many institutions have personnel who can assist with data entry or other aspects of statistical analysis. If the school has a nursing research center, this would be a good place to locate such personnel.

NURSE RESEARCHERS IN A HOSPITAL SETTING

Many hospitals employ nurses to conduct independent research studies. The objective is to generate the data needed to maintain or improve high-quality patient care. Many are responsible for quality improvement within the institution. Such offices may have personnel available to assist the nursing research enterprise.

CONTACTING RESEARCHERS FROM PUBLISHED STUDIES

If researchers have used a particular measurement instrument or an analytical technique that you are interested in, contact them to learn of their experiences. Published studies indicate the institution where the researcher is employed, making it possible to contact them by phone, letter or email. Ask them to share any problems they may have had in using the instrument or technique. They may also be helpful in directing you to other recent literature on the topic.

PROFESSIONAL ORGANIZATIONS

Specific research organizations previously described have Research Interest Groups. (RIGs). These provide a useful forum for beginning and advanced researchers to meet.

THE RESEARCH PROCESS AND THE RESEARCH PROPOSAL

The research process involves planning the research, conducting the research, and then communicating the findings. Research begins with the question that is to be answered. This is often motivated by the nurse's desire to answer a clinical question or to find a better way to perform a nursing intervention, or by an interest in a particular phenomenon. When a research question is being formulated, the previous research done in the area is reviewed so that the study can be developed in a manner that will add to the body of knowledge. While reviewing, critiquing, and synthesizing the research literature, one should also note the details of the research. For instance, noting how variables are defined and measured in the studies will aid in writing the research proposal.

The research proposal is the plan for the research and is written to communicate what is to be done in the study. It will undergo many revisions as the plan evolves and becomes stronger. The research proposal begins with the significance section, which uses data to indicate why the research is important. This is a short section that ends by indicating the purpose of the study and the research questions or hypotheses that are to be examined in the study. The significance section is usually developed along with the review of the literature.

The focus of the literature review section is to place the present study in the context of previous research. Research studies are described by indicating the focus of the study, the design, the number and type of subjects used, what and how variables were measured, and the findings. Strengths and weaknesses of studies are also included. The goal of this synthesis is to set the stage conceptually for the study. The conceptual framework used to guide the study is presented and indicates how the variables of the study are expected to be related to one another. As the literature is being reviewed, the details of the published studies are noted and plans for the methods to be used in the present study are developed.

The methods section of the proposal consists of several subdivisions that are usually planned at the same time but written in a standard order. It begins with the research design. The type of study to be conducted depends on the question being asked and what is already known about the particular phenomenon. The practical aspects of implementing the study in the clinical setting also need to be considered. A design should be chosen to best answer the question and have the least impact on the clinical setting so that patient care is not compromised.

The next section describes the sample to be included in the study and the site of the study. The measurement subsection follows and describes the measures to be used in the study. The measurement section includes a description of each instrument's reliability and validity and the method by which it was established. In addition, measures need to be evaluated for their appropriateness to the study population, their appropriateness to the variable definition, and the feasibility of using them in the clinical setting, although this may not appear in the written report. Scoring techniques for the instrument are described and indicate the level of measurement for the instrument. For clinical or physiological measures, it is important to identify the exact instrument to be used to measure the variable, including its accuracy and preci-

sion. If the study involves the testing of different treatments, a section in which they are described must be included.

The procedures that will be followed for the study need to be decided. For instance, how will potential subjects be identified? The procedures section of the proposal states exactly what is to be done to the subjects in the study, including the times that all measures are to be taken and treatments given. A plan is then developed and indicated in the proposal for the analysis that will be used to answer each research question.

It is usually after the research question and design have been developed that the title is chosen, even though it appears on the first page of the proposal. The ideal title indicates the topic, the study design, variables of interest, and the population to be studied. The abstract, which is usually the last part of the study to be written, even though it becomes the first section of the proposal, is a brief but comprehensive summary of the research proposal.

The reference section goes at the end and lists all the journal articles or other sources of information cited in the text. The appendix is the section in which all supporting documents, such as data collection tools and letters of support, are contained.

Once the planning is completed and the proposal written, the forms required for human subjects' review or any other review (discussed later in the chapter) need to be written, submitted, and approved. Data collection can then begin. This is usually the most time-consuming phase of the research process and tends to take longer than expected. The data can be entered into a computer program as they are collected. This will allow analysis to proceed according to the research plan. Analysis, however, is not the final step in the research process. The study is not completed until the findings are communicated to the health care community. This can be by verbal presentation, a poster session, or, most important, by publishing the findings.

Classification of Nursing Research Studies

There are several ways to classify nursing research studies. One way is to refer to the topics explored. Most commonly that involves characterizing studies that focus on nursing care, such as clinical nursing studies, and those focusing on the delivery of nursing services, such as nursing services research or health systems research. Another way to describe nursing research is according to how the knowledge that is generated will be used. This is most commonly referred to as basic research and applied research. Basic research involves the generation of knowledge for knowledge's sake. Findings from these studies are not always directly useful in practice. Basic research is often considered synonymous with research conducted in a biological laboratory, sometimes using human tissues, blood, cells, and so forth, or animal models, but is not required to be only research done in that setting. An example of a basic research study might be to examine the response of tissue to pressure. Applied research, on the other hand, is conducted to answer a clinical question or solve a nursing practice problem more directly. It often uses the knowledge generated in basic research. An example would be the use of patients to evaluate the effectiveness of pressure-relieving devices in preventing skin breakdown.

A third way to define nursing research is in terms of the types of questions asked in a particular study. These are considered to be hierarchical, with research at the lower or beginning levels being required before the higher or more advanced levels of research can be undertaken. It is essential to understand a phenomenon before attempting to change it. The first level of research is a study that focuses on describing a phenomenon of interest to nursing and is called a descriptive study. An example would be describing the informational needs of surgical patients following discharge (Jacobs, 2000). Exploratory studies are those that describe relationships, such as the relationship between smoking behavior and socioeconomic status. Explanatory studies are those that test a theory. A theory is an abstract conceptualization about interrelationships among phenomena. An explanatory study provides a richer understanding of relationships than does an exploratory study (Polit & Hungler, 1999). It will usually follow an exploratory study. An example is the use of the health belief model to predict factors associated with participation by Mexican migrant farmworkers in a tuberculosis screening program (Poss, 2000). The fourth level of research is that of prescription. The goal is to identify the results of actions, such as testing the effectiveness of nursing interventions. This labeling of nursing studies can be in addition to other ways of describing a particular study.

QUANTITATIVE AND QUALITATIVE APPROACHES TO RESEARCH

There are two major scientific approaches to nursing research, both of which are essential to nursing science. The most familiar category is the quantitative approach. This method requires that something be known ahead of time about the phenomenon of interest. A theory is chosen or formulated to explain relationships. The research methodology then involves a systematic, controlled collection and analysis of data. The goal is to offer support for the theory as an explanatory device for the phenomenon of interest.

Qualitative research is the other major approach to research. This involves the collection of data that are more holistic, contextual, and subjective, usually in the form of interviews and observations in a natural setting. The goal of this research is to understand the human experience. It results in the generation of theory rather than the testing of theory. The appropriate research methodology is determined by the question being asked and the extent of the knowledge already established in relation to the phenomenon of interest.

RESEARCH METHODS

Both research approaches are essential for the advancement of nursing knowledge. Some researchers combine the two approaches when studying a particular phenomenon and believe that this is the best way to gain a comprehensive understanding of complex nursing phenomena.

Quantitative Research. Within each of these major approaches to research there are specific methodologies that can be used. Within the quantitative approach to research, the goal is most often to establish cause. Thus an approach is used that eliminates as many extraneous variables as possible, allowing the causal relationship between two or more variables to be examined. Three criteria are necessary to establish cause:

1. If an event is believed to cause an outcome, then the event must precede the outcome in time.
2. Whenever the outcome occurs, the event must always have been present before it.
3. There must be a theory or other explanation for the relationship between the event and the outcome.

In this research design, the cause, or the event, is called the independent variable and the effect, or the outcome, is called the dependent variable.

EXPERIMENTAL RESEARCH. The quantitative research design that is considered the best for establishing cause is the experimental design. The three criteria that are necessary for a design to be considered experimental are (1) more than one group is used, (2) subjects participating in the study are randomly assigned to groups, and (3) the researcher has control over the independent variable (Cook & Campbell, 1979). The independent variable (commonly a treatment) is routinely administered to one group, with outcomes compared with those of a control group that does not receive the treatment or that receives another type of treatment. This design is sometimes referred to as a ran-domized controlled trial. The goal is to remove all other possible explanations for the effect on the dependent variable except that contributed by the independent variable. An example of an experimental study is one that tested the effectiveness of personalized decision exercise in assisting women to make and act on informed decisions that are consistent with their values in respect to menopause and hormone replacement therapy. Women were randomly assigned to one of three intervention formats—written material only, guided discussion, or the personalized decision exercise. The investigators found that women were able to learn information regarding treatment options and were able to adhere to their own plans. They were surprised, however, to learn that the guided discussion was the most effective intervention (Rothert et al., 1997). Box 21–3 provides an example of an experimental study on an inpatient unit.

QUASI-EXPERIMENTAL RESEARCH. When the research design includes having an independent variable that is manipulated but subjects are not randomly assigned to groups, the study is called a quasi-experimental study (Cook & Campbell, 1979; Polit & Hungler, 1999). An example of a quasi-experimental design would be the testing of an educational program in an acute care setting. To randomly assign patients to receive or not receive the teaching would mean that patients who did receive the teaching and patients who did not might be located in beds next to one another. They would be likely to talk, and the person not receiving the teaching might benefit from the information shared. There might also be resentment from those who were excluded from the teaching. To prevent this, the researcher would have to separate the treatment groups and experimental groups geographically or by time. The challenge to the researcher would be to separate the effect due to the teaching from the effect due to the initial noncomparability between groups. The ability to make causal claims is therefore more limited when a quasi-experimental design is used than when an experimental design is used.

Box 21-3 Example of an Experimental Design

APPLICATION

Research can and should be used to guide nursing practice. Although a change of practice should not be based on only one study, some studies have direct applicability to practice and, because of their implications for the comfort of the patient, indicate a need to change and evaluate present practice. An example of one such study is the testing of the effectiveness of bed rest after cardiac catheterization (Keeling et al., 1994). Although practice requires that patients remain in bed for 12 hours, this research study did not document benefit from placing such a requirement on patients. Since there was no research supporting the requirement for 12 hours of bed rest after cardiac catheterization, the research- ers decided to randomly assign patients to 6 or 12 hours of bed rest and to monitor outcomes in both groups to determine if there was more bleeding in those with fewer hours of bed rest. After observing 109 patients, they did not detect differences in the incidence of bleeding between the two groups. Patients kept in bed for a shorter time did not have an increased incidence in bleeding from the catheter insertion site. The bleeding that did occur was initiated long after the standard 12 hour bed rest period, and it occurred in patients receiving IV heparin after the procedure. The researchers could not implicate early ambulation as a cause of bleeding but rather suspected that the prolonged clotting times, dressing removal, cough, or activity the day after the procedure were more likely explanations. A shorter period of required bed rest would be more comfortable for the patients and might result in a reduction in narcotic analgesics. There is also less risk from any of the ventilatory or circulatory complications of immobility. A shortened time in bed might also reduce hospital costs by reducing nursing care requirements and perhaps resulting in a shorter length of stay.

NONEXPERIMENTAL RESEARCH. Nonexperimental designs include those in which the independent variable is not manipulated. Nonexperimental research designs are less expensive to implement and may be used for that reason. These designs need to be used when it is unethical or impossi- ble to manipulate the independent variable, such as when studying the effects of smoking or widowhood. The ex post facto or case-control design is a type of nonexperimental design. Subjects are selected because of differences in the dependent variable, such as those with a particular condition and those without the con- dition, and their past history is examined in an attempt to determine differences that might have contributed to the condition. An example is a study by Skoner, Thompson, and Caron (1994) in which they selected women with stress urinary incontinence and those without it and found that the factors contributing to in-continence were a history of delivering a baby vaginally, having an episiotomy or tear during delivery, and having a mother with stress uri- nary incontinence. High parity (four or more pregnancies) was not associated with increased risk. Another situation in which an ex post facto research design is frequently used is with re- search examining the factors contributing to nosocomial infections.

Surveys are nonexperimental research studies that obtain information from respondents using a self-report methodology. They usually ask people about their behaviors or what they plan to do. They tend to be broad in scope but superficial in nature because they are limited by the extent to which respondents are willing to report on the topic. Surveys can include a mailed questionnaire, telephone interview, or the like. A recent example of a clinical survey design research study is the comparison of symptom experiences of lung transplant recipients analyzed by comparing across sex, pretransplant diagnosis and type of transplant (Lanuza et al., 1999).

Other nonexperimental designs are descriptive studies in which the focus is to determine frequencies of occurrence of certain phenomena or to describe relationships among variables. No attempt is made to establish causal claims. Nonexperimental research can be used to describe the current state of practice and used as an incentive to change practice. After the change is implemented, it can be evaluated using research methods, such as an experimental design (Box 21–4).

Qualitative Research. Qualitative research also includes different research designs, depending on the phenomenon being studied. The three types of qualitative research designs used most commonly in nursing are phenomenology, ethnography, and grounded theory research.

Box 21–4 Use of a Descriptive Study to Improve Practice

Many advances have been made in surgery in the past 10 years. The use of fiberoptic technology and microsurgery has changed the detail work that can be accomplished in surgery, and this increased precision has resulted in the patient being on the operating room table for a much longer time than in the past. My colleagues and I began to notice that more patients who came in for elective surgery were experiencing skin breakdown a few days after surgery. Since these patients were healthy, we decided that the loss of skin integrity was likely to be preventable. However, we were not able to elicit support for a practice change. It was believed that before we could correct the problem, we needed to be more certain about the extent of the problem and the factors related to it. Was skin breakdown related to the length of time on the operating table, the positioning devices used, the type of surgery or the surgeon, the patient's age, the patient's individual risk of skin breakdown, or other factors?

To examine this problem more fully, a descriptive study was undertaken (Grous, Reilly, & Gift, 1997). The purposes of the study were to determine the incidence of skin breakdown in those undergoing prolonged surgery and to determine factors related to pressure ulcer formation. A proposal was written, and approval was obtained from the Institutional Review Board to conduct the study.

Subjects consisted of 33 adult patients undergoing operative procedures of 10 hours or longer. Fifteen (45%) were found to develop state I or II pressure ulcers within 48 hours of surgery. No significant differences were found between those who did and those who did not develop pressure ulcers in relation to age, gender, preoperative Braden Scale score, position on the operating room table, or type or length of surgery. A significant difference was found in relation to the type of device placed on the operating room table under patients. A warming blanket was used more often on those who developed pressure ulcers (75%) than on those who did not. It was recommended that warming blankets be used in the operating room only when essential.

The results of the study were shared with the staff and other personnel in the operating room. There was then widespread support for a practice change. Criteria were developed to define situations where it would be essential to use a warming blanket. Otherwise, alternative warming devices were to be used. This change was simple to implement, since it had the support of the operating room personnel. We are presently involved in evaluating the effectiveness of the change by repeating the descriptive study. The incidence of pressure ulcer formation before and after the practice change will be compared.

PHENOMENOLOGY. Phenomenology is used when the goal is to describe particular phenomena or experiences (Streubert & Carpenter, 1995). The focus is on the meaning ascribed to the phenomenon by the person. Therefore the primary method of data collection is to listen to the voices of the people experiencing the phenomenon. This usually takes the form of interviews.

An example of a phenomenological study is one in which hermeneutical phenomenological techniques were used to explore the lived experiences of ten African-American and Latino grandmothers who were the primary caregivers for their HIV-positive grandchildren. Four themes—upholding the primacy of family, living in the child-centered present, being strong as mature women, and living with a constricting environment—were identified. The Latino and African-American women were found to be more alike than different (Caliandro & Hughes, 1998).

Another example of a phenomenological study is one in which a deeper understanding of the meaning of living with violence was gained from the descriptions offered by women who were living among and inseparable from violence, abuse, and maltreatment (Draucker & Madsen, 1999). The researchers found that violence left the women alienated, unsettled, unprotected, and distrustful. They went to great lengths to protect others and create a safe place for themselves.

ETHNOGRAPHY. Ethnography focuses on describing culture (Streubert & Carpenter, 1995). The basic question is, What is the nature of the group? That which is implicit in a culture is made explicit. This requires an intimacy with the participants beyond simply talking to them. The researcher becomes a participant observer in the culture. This is accomplished by going to the location of the culture, observing their behaviors, and having them describe the meaning for the behaviors. This methodology is especially helpful in understanding complex cultures, such as a health care system, and is used extensively in anthropology.

An example of ethnography is a study by Wolf (1988), in which the author describes the therapeutic and occupational rituals of nurses. Therapeutic rituals are those that improve the condition of patients, whereas occupational rituals are symbolic actions that facilitate the transition of professional neophytes into their professional role. These rituals enable nurses to carry out their caring activities for ill or dying patients. They also help to reaffirm the values and beliefs of nurses.

GROUNDED THEORY. The third commonly used qualitative methodology in nursing is grounded theory research, which is the exploration of the processes of human interaction (Streubert & Carpenter, 1995). It explores the richness and diversity of human experience. A constant comparative analysis technique is used to generate themes or categories of the phenomenon of interest. Grounded theory research will often contribute to the development of middle-range theories.

An example of a grounded theory study that led to a mid-range theory of self-care is the study by Leenerts and Magilvy (2000). For the 12 women in the study, self-care practices developed over time and were categorized into four categories: focusing on self, fitting resources, feeling emotions, and finding meaning. The categories were linked through the core category, investing in self-care, and carried the explanatory power for developing mid-range theory.

Ethics in Research

In addition to selecting a research methodology, the researcher must be concerned with ethical issues. There are two main areas of ethical concern in nursing research: the use of humans as subjects and maintaining the integrity of the nursing research process.

PROTECTING THE RIGHTS OF SUBJECTS

Research involving human subjects raises complex ethical issues. First, in planning a research study involving humans, one must consider the ethical principles of beneficence versus nonmaleficence. Researchers are obligated to consider the risks and benefits of their work—both the risks and benefits to the individual participating in the study and the risks and benefits to society as a whole. Research differs from the provision of therapy in that participation in research often will not be directly beneficial to the individual. The researcher often benefits more than the individual. However, even studies that pose little or no risk to the individual participating must show some benefit, or the researcher will not be permitted to conduct the study (Weijer, Dickens, & Meslin, 1997).

Justice is the ethical principle considered when subjects are chosen for participation in a study. Those people who are unable to speak for themselves (such as children and those who are mentally deficient or otherwise incapacitated) are considered vulnerable. Such subjects should not be included in a research study simply because they are available. They should be included only if the researcher is interested in a study dealing specifically with that population. For instance, if one were studying nursing care of children, then children would be expected to be included as subjects.

It is essential that researchers also consider the diversity of research participants and protect against negative differentiation toward individuals or groups on the basis of their diversity (Silva, 1995). There has been much consideration given lately to the inclusion of women and minorities in research studies. Researchers, such as those testing new drugs, are required to design studies and include samples that will establish the effectiveness of such therapies in women and minorities, not only Caucasian men (Moreno et al., 1998). The nurse researcher is directed to be sensitive to women as well as men, to those of different cultures or ethnic backgrounds, and to choose appropriate frameworks to guide research, measurement instruments, and methodologies for data collection. Subjects from different cultures interpret and communicate health information in a different fashion (Padonu et al., 1996), which will influence the findings of a research study if not considered in the design. Analysis should examine the findings by comparing across genders, cultures, ethnic groups, and the like.

The ethical principle of autonomy is most important when humans are asked to participate in a research study. Each individual is valued in our society, and each is therefore given the right to make decisions about his or her own life. The process by which individuals are provided with truthful information about a research study and invited to participate without coercion must be identified for each study. The researcher is expected to maintain the participants' confidentiality. Individuals also have the right to withdraw from a study at any time if they so desire. By the same token it must be remembered that those from different ethnic groups make decisions differently. If potential subjects wish to include other family members in their decision making, they should be allowed to do so. Researchers are required to have certain elements such as the purpose of the study, reason for them being invited to participate, what the study will entail, potential benefits and risks, alternative therapies, their rights as research subjects, contact information, and the like, in the written consent. For a web-based training module regarding research involving human subjects, see the web site, http://helix.nih.gov:8001/ohsr/newcbt/.

MAINTAINING THE INTEGRITY OF THE STUDY

The second major area of ethical concern in research is maintaining the integrity of the research study. This involves avoiding scientific misconduct in the design, conduct, or reporting of the research and is governed by the current regulations at 45 CFR 689 (NSF) and 42 CFR

50 (NIH). Basically, principal investigators, those responsible for directing the study, are responsible for seeing that the study is well designed, addresses a question of sufficient value to justify the risk posed to participants, is conducted honestly following the stated protocol, and is reported accurately and promptly. There are three terms that are used to describe research improprieties: fabrication, falsification, and plagiarism. Although these terms are not defined in the current regulation, they are made more explicit in the proposed regulation ("Proposed federal policy," 1999).

Fabrication is the making up of data for the purpose of deception, whereas *falsification* is manipulating research materials, equipment, or processes, or changing or omitting data or results such that the research is not accurately represented in the research record. These improprieties are generally agreed to include the reporting of data that were not obtained according to the research protocol, the selective reporting of findings, and the omission of conflicting data. *Plagiarism* is the appropriation of another person's ideas, processes, results, or words without giving appropriate credit, including those obtained through confidential review of others' research proposals and manuscripts. Basically it is the presenting of another person's work as one's own (Korenman et al., 1998). Improprieties of authorship are often included under plagiarism.

It is the responsibility of the principal investigator to monitor not only his or her own behavior but also that of others involved in the project. Ignorance is not an acceptable excuse for academic misconduct. Those involved in a research project must be taught proper techniques for carrying out the research in a timely, cost-effective, and ethical manner. The principal investigator needs also to monitor the activities of research assistants as the research is being conducted. This may involve scheduled meetings of the entire research team, having research assistants demonstrate the research protocol during announced and unannounced visits to

the site, having another person verify data entry, and performing ongoing evaluation of all research staff (Gift, Creasia, & Parker, 1991). Federally funded research studies are subject to an audit of all aspects of the research study, from the selection of subjects to the analysis of data (Rudy & Kerr, 2000).

The Office of Research Integrity (ORI) has recently been moved from the NIH to within the U.S. Department of Health and Human Services. This separated ORI from those conducting the research, enhancing their oversight capability. The ORI is charged with the development and promulgation of policies, procedures, rules, and regulations aimed at preventing, monitoring, and imposing administrative actions concerning misconduct of research. For more information about this government office see their web site, http://ori.dhhs.gov. They publish improprieties of researchers and attempt to avoid improprieties by promoting scientific integrity through a variety of educational programs and activities.

Although most nursing research involves humans, it is also understood that researchers involved in animal research will conduct their work with the least possible harm or suffering to the animal. Animals are selected for a research study only if they are the most appropriate species for the needs of the research (Silva, 1995). All studies involving animals must be preapproved by an Institutional Animal Review Board before the research can be conducted.

Review of a Research Proposal

There are several reasons why a research proposal is reviewed before a study is begun. It is reviewed for its scientific merit—to determine whether the research question will make a contribution to science and whether the proposed research design, sampling techniques, measurement, and analysis will answer the question in the best manner possible. This form of review is conducted in a variety of situations. One is in an academic setting when professors review a study to decide if a student researcher should proceed with the study. The goal is to have the student design the best study possible.

Researchers serving on review panels for funding agencies engage in scientific review of studies to decide which studies should receive funding. Often the results of this scientific review are then integrated into a decision about which studies are in line with the mission of the funding organization. Those with the most scientific merit and most in line with the mission of the agency receive the funding.

Another form of review is that done to gain access to subjects. This is usually necessary when the research is to be conducted in a setting where potential subjects are cared for by others. Those responsible for caring for the potential subjects will usually have a mission other than research, such as providing health care. The institution will want to be sure that a research study will not interfere with their primary mission or disturb their patients unnecessarily.

The only form of research review that is mandated by law is that which is done for the protection of human subjects or animals. The National Research Act of 1974, Title 45, Part 46, Code of Federal Regulations, and other related laws and regulations mandate the review of research involving humans. A review by an institutional review board (IRB) ensures that risks to subjects are minimal and reasonable in relation to the benefits of the investigation. It mandates that selection of subjects and informed consent be equitable and appropriate to the research.

Every research study involving humans must be reviewed by an IRB before data collection begins. If the proposal is written for the IRB, the researcher indicates the level and type of risk involved for subjects who participate in the study. How the subjects' confidentiality will be maintained, as well as how other federal guidelines for human subjects will be followed in the study, must be indicated. If consent is required,

the consent form should be included in the appendix.

The level of review by the IRB, however, depends on the nature of the study and the potential risks to the subject. The levels of review include exempt review, expedited review, and full committee review. Exempt review is for those studies that are conducted in an educational setting and that involve normal educational practices or educational tests. Studies involving the collection or study of existing data, documents, records, or specimens would also receive an exempt review. Demonstration programs evaluating public benefit of service programs, as well as studies evaluating food taste, food quality, or consumer acceptance, would also receive an exempt review.

The category of expedited review is for those studies involving no more than minimal risk to subjects. These include studies involving the collection of hair, nails, or teeth, secretions, excreta, or other materials that would normally be removed from the body. Research involving the recording of data from noninvasive procedures routinely employed in clinical practice, as well as research focusing on drugs or devices that are not classified as experimental, would receive an expedited review by the IRB. Minor invasive procedures, such as the venipuncture removal of small amounts of blood or the collection of plaque and calculus, as well as voice recordings, moderate exercise of healthy volunteers, and research concerned with individual or group behaviors or characteristics, would receive an expedited review. All other research would require a full committee review.

All studies requiring a full committee review and most studies requiring an expedited review will involve the use of a written informed consent. A consent form is a succinct statement written in clear, understandable language. It gives information about the reason why the person was chosen to be included in the study as well as the purpose, procedures, benefits, risks, and duration of the study. The name and telephone number of the responsible researcher and a 24-hour emergency number are provided. The consent form must indicate that the subject has the right to refuse to participate in the study or to withdraw from the study after it has begun without any penalty. Each adult subject or legal guardian who signs a consent form must receive a written copy of the document. In some special situations permission is given to enroll subjects in a study using an oral informed consent. The exact wording of the consent information is written and submitted to the IRB for approval along with the research proposal before the study can begin.

The government agency that oversees human subjects research is the Office for the Protection from Research Risks. More information about informed consent procedures is available on their web site, http://grants.nih.gov/grants/oprr/oprr.html. This agency has recently been moved from its former location within NIH, where it reported to the Office of the Director, NIH, to its present location in the Office of Public Health and Science within the Office of the Secretary of the U.S. Department of Health and Human Services. This was done to elevate its stature and effectiveness in ensuring the safely and welfare of people who participate in research, as well as the humane care and use of animals in research (http://www.hhs.gov/news/press/1999pres/991104c.html).

Quality Improvement Versus Research

Often in a clinical setting it is difficult to decide where a quality improvement project ends and a research study begins. When quality assurance advanced to quality improvement, it became common to alter the practice environment and measure the benefits of that alteration. These activities often resemble research. One distinction, however, is mandated by law: a research study must be approved by the IRB before data collection can begin. Therefore, if a project begins as a quality improvement project, it cannot be turned into a research study afterward. An-

other factor dividing the two is the intended use of the project. If the findings were to be used only at a specific institution, it would be classified as a quality improvement project, whereas a project to be published in a research journal and shared with others would be classified as a research project. However, there are quality assurance journals in which quality assurance projects are published. To decide on the difference between the two, the relationship of the practice or product being studied to the routine standard of care needs to be examined. Quality improvement projects would involve only routine practices. The design of the project also influences the distinction, with the use of a randomized clinical trial most likely being a research project. The difference between research and quality improvement needs to be examined before data are collected for the project. That decision will affect how the results of the project can be used after it is completed.

Seeking Funding for a Research Study

In seeking funding for a research study, the first consideration is the match between the researcher's idea and the funding mission of the agency. Funding for research can come from a variety of sources.

FUNDING AGENCIES

Nursing Organizations. Nursing organizations such as Sigma Theta Tau, the American Association of Critical Care Nurses, and the Oncology Nursing Society have research programs that allow them to fund small research projects. Information packets that contain guidelines indicating the focus of their particular research interests, what to include in a proposal, submission deadlines, and funding amounts can be obtained from the organization.

Businesses and Corporations. If a research proposal involves the testing of a particular piece of equipment or a commercially available product, it is possible that the company producing the product will fund the research. The dollar amounts of research awards from these sources are often small, but many companies will also supply their products for the study.

Nonprofit Agencies. These agencies, which include organizations such as the American Heart Association, American Cancer Society, and American Lung Association, have a focus for their research effort that is usually obvious from the title of the organization. Funding success is determined by how well the project and experience of the researcher meet their guidelines.

Foundations. A foundation is a nongovernmental, nonprofit organization with its own funds. Often these are from an individual, family, or corporation. A foundation usually has programs established to maintain or aid charitable, religious, educational, social, or other activities serving the common good. Those that have funded nursing research include the Robert Wood Johnson Foundation, the American Nurses' Foundation, and the W.K. Kellogg Foundation. Directories listing these funding opportunities are available.

Federal Research Agencies. In 2000 the U.S. Public Health Service published *Healthy People 2010,* which launched its national health promotion and disease prevention initiative to increase health care quality and years of healthy life and to eliminate health disparities. These goals provide a guideline for research funding priorities for most federal funding agencies. The NIH is the agency within the U.S. Public Health Service that funds biomedical research. Nurse researchers are eligible for funding from any institute within the NIH; however, their research interests make them more likely to seek funding from the NINR and such institutes as the National Institute on Aging, the National Institute of Mental Health, and the National Institute of Child Health and Human Development. AHRQ is another government agency that supports research. This agency is the lead agency charged with supporting research designed to improve the quality of health care, reduce its cost, and broaden access to essential services. All federal funding for research is highly competitive and designed to support the experienced researcher.

FORMS TO BE SUBMITTED

Funding agencies usually require a copy of the research proposal as well as additional information. The funding agency requests these extra sections to evaluate the match between the proposed research and their funding mission, as well as to evaluate the competence of the researcher and the resources available to carry out the research.

A funding institution usually requires a budget and budget justification section. A budget consists of a listing of the money required to carry out the research proposal, and the justification section is an indication of how that money will be used. This is done to allow the funding agency to decide if the project is worth the expense.

Biographical sketches of key personnel, other sources of support, and a description of the resources and environment for research are sections that are required in most funding proposals. If a section indicating previous work of the principal investigator is required, it is usually called preliminary studies and is presented after the background of the study. It is essential that the researcher use these sections to indicate how the research study being proposed meets the funding objectives of the agency.

KEY POINTS

- Nursing research has high-quality patient care as its ultimate objective.
- Research is a recent development in nursing.
- The National Institute of Nursing Research, an institute of the National Institutes of Health, provides federal funding for nursing research.

- Using research to improve the quality of patient care is the responsibility of all nurses.
- Nursing research methods are commonly divided into quantitative and qualitative approaches.
- The principal investigator in a nursing research study must protect the rights of the humans who are subjects in the study.
- The integrity of the research study protocol, data analysis, and publication is vital to conducting research studies.
- All research that involves humans must be approved by a federally mandated institutional review board before data collection can begin.
- Funding for nursing research can come from nursing organizations, businesses, nonprofit agencies, foundations, or federal research agencies.

CRITICAL THINKING EXERCISES

1. If you were to learn that a clinical procedure is not being performed in your institution according to the latest nursing research findings, what process would you recommend for changing that practice? Who would be the supporters of this change, and who would need to be convinced of its merit?

2. Think of a clinical problem you are currently encountering. How would you design a research study to solve the problem? What questions would you need to answer before you began the study? What type of ethical issues would need to be resolved? What are the major barriers that would prevent you from conducting this study?

3. Describe the review procedures you would go through if you were to conduct a nursing research study in the clinical setting most familiar to you.

4. What would you do if you were asked to collect data for a research study on a patient who did not know he or she was part of the study? Would this ever be acceptable? Under what conditions?

REFERENCES

American Nurses Association. (1993). Position paper: Education for participation in nursing research. Washington, DC: Author.

Burns, N., & Grove, S.K. (1997). *The practice of nursing research: Conduct, critique and utilization* (3rd ed.). Philadelphia: Saunders.

Buss, I. C., Halfens, R.J.G., Abu-Saad, H.H., & Kok, G. (1999). Evidence-based nursing practice: Both state of the art in general and specific to pressure sores. *Journal of Professional Nursing, 15*(2), 73–83.

Caliandro, G., & Hughes, C. (1998). The experience of being a grandmother who is the primary caregiver for her HIV-positive grandchild. *Nursing Research, 47,* 107–113.

Cook, T. D., & Campbell, D. T. (1979). *Quasi-experimentation: Design and analysis issues for field studies.* Chicago: Rand McNally.

Coyle, L. A., & Sokop, A. G. (1990). Innovation adoption behavior among nurses. *Nursing Research, 39,* 176–180.

Draucker, C. B. & Madsen, C. (1999). Women dwelling with violence. *Image: Journal of Nursing Scholarship, 31,* 327–332.

Estabrooks, C. A. (1998). Will evidence-based nursing practice make practice perfect? *Canadian Journal of Nursing Research, 30*(1), 15–36.

Ferrell, M. J., DiCarlo, B., Anderson, J., Baker, C., Bell, D., Brunt, B., & Kelly, K. C. (1994). *Utilization of agency for health care policy and research guidelines.* Washington, DC: American Nurses Association.

Gift, A. G., Creasia, J., & Parker, B. (1991). Utilizing research assistants and maintaining research integrity. *Research in Nursing & Health, 14,* 229–233.

Grous, C., Reilly, N. & Gift, A. (1997) Skin integrity in patients undergoing prolonged operations. *Journal of Wound, Ostomy & Continence Nursing, 24*(2), 86–91.

Holzworth, R. J., & Wills, C. E. (1999). Nurses' judgments regarding seclusion and restraint of psychiatric patients: A social judgment analysis. *Research in Nursing and Health, 22*(3), 89–201.

Jacobs, V. (2000). Informational needs of surgical patients following discharge. *Applied Nursing Research, 13*(1). 12–18.

Keeling, A. W., Knight, E., Taylor, V., & Nordt, L. A. (1994). Postcardiac catheterization time-in-bed study: Enhancing patient comfort through nursing research. *Applied Nursing Research, 7*(1), 14–17.

Korenman, S. G., Berk, R., Wenger N. S., & Lew, V. (1998). Evaluation of the research norms of scientists and administrators responsible for academic research integrity. *Journal of the American Medical Assoication, 279,* 41–47.

Lanuza, D. M., McCabe, M., Norton-Rosko, M., Corliss, J. W., & Garrity, E. (1999). Symptom experiences of lung transplant recipients: Comparisons across gender, pretransplantation diagnosis, and type of transplantation. *Heart and Lung, 28,* 429–437.

Leenerts, M. H., & Magilvy, J. K. (2000). Investing in self-care: A midrange theory of self-care grounded in the lived experience of low-income HIV-positive white women. *Advances in Nursing Science, 22*(3), 58–75.

Marek, K. D. (1994). *Manual to develop guidelines.* Washington, DC: American Nurses Association.

Moreno, J., Caplan, A. L., Wolpe, P. R., & Members of the Project on Informed Consent, Human Research Ethics Group. (1998). Updating protections for human subjects involved in research. *Journal of the American Medical Association, 280,* 1951–1958.

National Institute of Nursing Research. (1993). *Nursing research at the National Institutes of Health, fiscal years 1989–1992.* Washington, DC: U.S. Department of Health and Human Services, U.S. Public Health Service.

National Institute of Nursing Research. (1999). *Strategic planning for the 21st century* "on-line". Available: http://www.nih.gov/ninr/strategic plan.htm

National Institutes of Health. (1994). Responsibilities of NIH and awardee institutions for the responsible conduct of research. In *NIH guide* (pp. 23, 42). Washington, DC: U.S. Department of Health and Human Services, U.S. Public Health Service.

Omery, A., & Williams, R. P. (1999). *An appraisal of research utilization across the United States.* Pasadena, CA: Divisional Nursing Services, Kaiser Permanente.

Padonu, G., Holmes-Rovner, M., Rothert, M., Schmitt, N., Kroll, J., Rovner, D., Talarczyk, G., Breer, L., Ransom, S., & Gladney, E. (1996). African-American women's perception of menopause. *American Journal of Health Behavior, 20,* 242–251.

Polit, D. F., & Hungler, B. P. (1999). *Nursing research: Principles and methods* (6th ed.). Philadelphia: Lippincott.

Poss, J. E. (2000). Factors associated with participation by Mexican migrant farmworkers in a tuberculosis screening program. *Nursing Research, 49,* 20–28.

Proposed federal policy on research misconduct to protect the integrity of the research record. Office of Science and Technology Policy. (1999, October 14). *Federal Register, 64* (198), 55722–55725.

Rothert, M. L., Holmes-Rovner, M., Rovner, D., Kroll, J., Breer, L., Talarczyk, G., Schmitt, N., Padonu, G., & Wills, C. (1997). An educational intervention as decision support for menopausal women. *Research in Nursing and Health, 20,* 377–387.

Rudy, E. B., & Kerr, M. E. (2000). Auditing research studies. *Nursing Research, 49,* 117–120.

Silva, M. C. (1995). *Ethical guidelines in the conduct, dissemination, and implementation of nursing re-search.* Washington, DC: American Nurses Association.

Skoner, M. M., Thompson, W. D., & Caron, V. A. (1994). Factors associated with risk of stress urinary incontinence in women. *Nursing Research, 43,* 301–306.

Sparks, S. (1999). Electronic publishing and nursing research. *Nursing Research, 48,* 50–54.

Stetler, C.B. (1994). Refinement of the Stetler/Marram model for application of research findings to practice. *Nursing Outlook, 42,* 15–25.

Stevenson, J.S. (1986). Forging a research discipline. *Nursing Research, 36,* 60–64.

Streubert, H. J., & Carpenter, D.R. (1995). *Qualitative research in nursing: Advancing the humanistic imperative.* Philadelphia: Lippincott.

Titler, M. G., Kleiber, C., Steelman, V., Goode, C., Rakel, B., Barry-Walker, J., Small, S., & Buckwalter, K. (1994). Infusing research into practice to promote quality care. *Nursing Research, 43,* 307–313.

Vessey, J. A., & Campos, R. G. (1992). The role of nursing research committees. *Nursing Research, 41,* 247–249.

Weijer, C., Dickens, B., & Meslin, E.M. (1997). Bioethics for clinicians: Research ethics. *Canadian Medical Association Journal, 156,* 1153–1157.

Wills, C. E. (1997). Young adult medication decision making: Similarities and differences among mental versus physical health treatment contexts. *The Journal of Nursing Science, 2*(3/4), 59–72.

Wills, C. E. (1999). On the role of framing effects in assessment of health-related utilities [invited editorial]. *Medical Decision Making, 19,* 505–506.

Wills, C. E., & Holmes-Rovner, M. (1998). Preliminary validation of the satisfaction with decision scale with depressed primary care patients [abstract]. *Medical Decision Making, 18,* 464.

Wills, C. E., & Moore, C. F. (1994a). A controversy in scaling of subjective states: Magnitude estimation versus category rating methods. *Research in Nursing and Health, 17,* 231–237.

Wills, C. E., & Moore, C. F. (1994b). Judgment processes for medication acceptance: Self-reports and configural information use. *Medical Decision Making, 14,* 137–145.

Wills, C. E., & Moore, C. F. (1996). Perspective taking judgments of medication acceptance: Inferences from relative importance about the impact and combination of information. *Organizational Behavior and Human Decision Processes, 66,* 251–267.

Wolf, Z. R. (1988). *Nurses work: The sacred and profane.* Philadelphia: University of Pennsylvania Press.

Youngblut, J. M., & Brooten, D. (2000). Moving research into practice: A new partner. *Nursing Outlook, 48*(2), 55–56.

22

Health Care Informatics

TERESA L. PANNIERS, PhD, RN, AND SUSAN K. JACOBS, MLS, RN

OBJECTIVES

At the completion of this chapter, the reader will be able to:

- Discuss the implications of health care informatics for nursing practice.
- Outline, with examples, the use of advanced health care technologies used to support patient care.
- Compare and contrast the various nursing taxonomies used to document nursing's contribution to patient care.
- Discuss the evolution of the specialty of nursing informatics.
- Recognize that information literacy requires unique cognitive knowledge of how information is structured and accessed.
- Understand that scholarly information is gathered and arranged in standard formats and accessed using print or electronic indexes.
- Recognize that the Internet contains both scholarly and nonscholarly information and that critical evaluation is crucial.

PROFILE IN PRACTICE

Barbara M. Tully, MSN, MS, RN, CS, CNOR
Program Director
Age Center of the Worcester Area, Inc.
Worcester, Massachusetts

Just as for many nurses who came before me and those who will come after me, the path I followed started in childhood. The first step on the path is the question, "What do you want to be when you grow up?" The journey then develops into the challenge of finding professionals to be mentors, to observe their chosen professions and imagine ourselves doing what they do. Another source of influence is books that provide the accounts of famous people. I knew when I was quite young what I would be doing, not from reading books but from looking at family pictures. In those photographs were pictures of a young student nurse, my mother. Through observation of her, teaching by her, and being a recipient of her ministrations, there was no doubt in my mind: I was going to be a registered nurse.

My career started literally at my mother's knee and continued on through my completing a certificate as an adult nurse practitioner and a master of science in nursing degree. In this master's program I was introduced to computers, software, and the potential of this technology. As Florence Nightingale stated in *Notes on Nursing*, an extremely important aspect of nursing, when providing care to patients is observation, which in turn produces "momentous minutiae." Today's health care environment is even more prolific with regard to data, which needs to be collected, manipulated, and communicated. I therefore recognized the need for nurses to define and articulate the place for "informatics" as it relates to the provision of nursing care. To this end I continued my education and completed a master of science in nursing informatics.

When reading Nightingale's tome the reader becomes aware that the fundamentals of caring for people remain basically the same. It is also obvious there have been many changes and advances in the hundred-plus years since she wrote her book. Nursing passes on from one generation to the next, keeping the basics and adding to its body of knowledge. So, too, there have been generations of computers, and it is up to nursing to be part of this and to blend technology to the fullest with the end result—the provision of the highest quality care to the individual patient and community.

Health Care Informatics: A Driving Force for Nursing Practice

Mandel (1993) describes *health care informatics* as an umbrella term used to encompass the rapidly evolving discipline of using computing, networking, and communications—methodology and technology—to support the health related fields, such as medicine, nursing, pharmacy, and dentistry. Health care informatics has evolved dramatically since the inception of computerization of data in the early 1960s. For example, hospital information systems were the mainstay of systems used in the 1970s. These systems were developed in response to a concern for reimbursement of the costs incurred by hospitalized individuals. Financial, charge-capture, and communication activities were carried out using mainframe computers that processed information in a centralized manner. In the 1980s, with the advent of personal computers, information was able to be processed in a decentralized manner. Nurses found that data related to critical elements of care could be captured and that the information gleaned could be used to improve nursing practice. There was

a greater emphasis placed on nursing information systems that defined and supported nursing care delivered at the bedside. Systems for care plans, documentation, and quality assurance were developed to support nursing practice. During the 1980s, systems also became more comprehensive, and attempts were made to integrate nursing data with data from other departmental systems.

The 1990s heralded the era of telecommunications, with the trend being one of open systems and communication over wide-area networks. The term *open systems* refers to the ability of different types of computers to communicate with one another. *Wide-area networks* refers to the linkage of computers located in different buildings in the same geographic area or, more broadly, across the country and around the world. As we enter the 21st century, ownership of information about health care options is increasingly being taken by consumers. In fact, Lynch (1999) describes a cultural revolution wherein the technologies of networked information will provide the enabling tools to allow consumers not only to have access to public information, but access to most of the same information resources used by health care professionals. Increasingly, consumers will continue to demand such information and will use it to make better informed choices about their health care options.

THE SPECIALTY OF NURSING INFORMATICS

In the field of health care informatics, nursing has developed the specialty of nursing informatics to delineate the contribution made by nurses in an environment of interdisciplinary teams and patient-centered care. *Nursing informatics* has been defined as a combination of computer science, information science, and nursing science designed to assist in the management and processing of nursing data, information, and knowledge to support the practice of nursing and the delivery of nursing care (Graves & Corcoran, 1989). As a specialty, nursing informatics develops applications, tools, processes, and structures that assist nurses in managing data in taking care of clients or in supporting the practice of nursing. Nursing informatics supports client care, either directly or indirectly, by supporting nursing education, research, and administration (American Nurses Association [ANA], 1994).

Nursing informatics is taught as a specialty in many graduate programs (*Peterson's Guide*, 1999/2000). Nursing informatics is also part of the core curriculum in many nursing baccalaureate programs (Vanderbeek et al., 1994). In addition to the educational focus on nursing informatics, the American Nurses' Credentialing Center (ANCC) (1995) certifies nurses in the specialty of nursing informatics. This certification declares a level of excellence in practice for nurses who practice in the field of nursing informatics.

Health Care Informatics Applications and Nursing

As nurses interact with consumers and other health care providers, they use a vast array of information technologies to support and enhance the care provided to clients. Consider the following case study:

Mr. Lazarus has been undergoing cancer chemotherapy for treatment of a lymphoma in an outpatient oncology center. In the past 24 hours, he has developed fever, chills, and pleuritic chest pain and is experiencing a productive cough. He has been admitted to the hospital for suspected pneumonia. On admission, the history of Mr. Lazarus's condition and the treatment regimen at the outpatient center are transferred electronically to establish an electronic client record.

On initial examination in the medical unit, the previous history and physical data are available to the resident physician, Dr. Cassidy, allowing him to update the client record with the information required to care for Mr. Lazarus during this acute episode of his illness. Following the initial workup, a chest x-ray is obtained and blood is drawn. While Mr. Lazarus is being evaluated by Nurse Matthews, the radiologist is reading the x-ray film and subsequently enters the results directly using a point-of-care application that is part of a larger point-to-point integrated clinical information system. At the same time, the technician in the clinical laboratory is entering the results of the culture and sensitivity testing of the sputum sample directly into the integrated system.

Nurse Matthews and Dr. Cassidy are able to retrieve these results at the client's bedside using the point-of-care system at the patient's bedside. Dr. Cassidy confirms the diagnosis and prescribes the appropriate antibiotic by entering it directly into the point-of-care system. The order is transmitted to the pharmacy, where it is immediately filled and transported to the unit, allowing Nurse Matthews to begin the antibiotic treatment. Nurse Matthews has been entering Mr. Lazarus's vital signs using a handheld computer throughout the shift and is able to access a graphical depiction of the temperature, blood pressure, pulse, and respirations. She notes that his temperature is slowly returning to normal and his respirations are less rapid. In providing comprehensive care, Nurse Matthews logs into the database and queries the Nursing Interventions Classification related to care for patients receiving chemotherapy and receives information about nursing activities appropriate to this clinical condition.

Mr. Lazarus has recovered enough to return home. Since he lives alone, he will be followed at home mainly through a telehealth application and, when needed, be visited in person by a community health nurse for follow-up care. The visiting nurse communicates with the medical center using the telehealth technology to conduct a clinical consultation with specialists at the medical center. In addition, the nurse documents Mr. Lazarus's care using a point-of-care device. When Mr. Lazarus no longer requires the personal services of the community health nurse, he continues to receive care and advice through a videophone that connects him directly to the medical center. Mr. Lazarus continues to be treated directly at the medical center when needed, but his visits to the center are less frequent since he has gained access to the center via videophone.

The case study shows the seamless depiction, transmittal and storage of data that are needed to provide the sophisticated level of care for Mr. Lazarus. Let's take a closer look at some of the many health care informatics applications integral to nursing that support this level of care.

POINT-OF-CARE COMPUTING

Point-of-care computing allows the health care practitioner to process patient care data at the point where the service is being provided. In Mr. Lazarus's case, the point-of-care computing took place in a variety of settings, including his bedside, the pharmacy, and the radiology department. Using point-of-care computing increases the accuracy of data capture, affords rapid processing, and decreases redundancy in record keeping. Point-of-care applications can vary in type from hand-held pen computers that are carried by nurses to record patient care activities to high-end integrated personal computers (PCs) that are attached to a medical cart and used by a multidisciplinary team during clinical rounds (Schutzman, 1999). All point-of

care technologies rely on the concept of networking. *Networking* means that communications equipment is used to connect two or more computers and their resources (Capron, 1998). Networks can be classified as local-area networks (LANs) or wide-area networks (WANs). A *local-area network* is a computer network in a hospital, a clinic, or an office. A *wide-area network* is a network that provides communication services to more than one hospital, clinic, or office. The latest type of networking, one that allows mobile computing, is that of wireless local area networks (WLANs). *Wireless local area networks* are data communication systems that provide peer (PC-to-PC) and point-to-point (LAN-to-LAN) connectivity within a building or among buildings on a campus (Schutzman, 1999). Wireless networks make use of radio signals to transmit data signals through the air without any physical connection (Simpson, 1996). It is important to note that WLANs augment the more traditional hard-wired LANs and are used where wiring is difficult, costly, or inconvenient to employ.

Using networking technology, nurses are able to share client data as well as computer applications software among computers. For example, in Mr. Lazarus's case, while he is being treated in the hospital, Nurse Matthews can access his clinical record using a wireless laptop computer. At the same time she can use other point-of-care technologies such as a pulse oximeter and a point-of-care blood analyzing system to ascertain physiological measures that can assist in her assessment of his health status. These technologies can be integrated in such a way that all data are automatically uploaded into Mr. Lazarus's clinical record, which is maintained in a central location accessible through a hard-wired network. Ultimately, the use of point-of-care computing enables more prompt patient assessment and treatment and can result in an increase in the quality of the care provided to patients such as Mr. Lazarus.

TELEHEALTH

Telehealth is an innovation resulting from the integration of information and communications technologies that is used to support the delivery of clinical services directly to the patient in the location where he or she works or lives (Brennan, 1999). Telehealth allows the transmission of health care information over distance and time (Kazman & Westerheim, 1999). Two primary modes of telehealth transmission are available: interactive live video and the store-and-forward method. The cost of the live method is much greater than the cost of the store-and-forward method and is a consideration in any telehealth application. Equipment required for telehealth includes a *computer platform,* which is the hardware and software combination that makes up the basic functionality of a computer; a *network protocol,* which is a set of rules for the exchange of data between two or more computers, and a local area network (LAN) and/or a wide area network (WAN) that allows practitioners to share data and resources among several computers over a local or wide geographical area (Capron, 1997). Patients such as Mr. Lazarus can benefit from the efficient comprehensive communications between health care providers, and the ability to synthesize patient data, including diagnoses, procedures, lab results, specialist referrals, and even prescriptions (Kazman & Westerheim, 1999).

There are many examples of successful telehealth applications that have been developed by health care practitioners. For example, Nakamura, Takano, & Akao (1999) conducted a study in Japan in which they evaluated the effectiveness of teleheath through the use of a videophone system using an integrated systems digital network (ISDN) installed in individual homes of clients and health care providers. Two groups of elderly patients were studied: one group was provided with videophones and one group received care in the usual manner. Functional independence was measured in both groups before the installation of the video-

phones and 3 months after the home health care was started, with and without videophones. The use of videophones led to demonstrated improvements in the activities of daily living, communication, and social cognition independence in the group of patients using the videophones. The researchers concluded that the use of videophones in home health care improved the quality of service to clients.

A physician (Flowers, 1999) found that, in an economically disadvantaged South Central Los Angeles location, people were going blind needlessly. There were only seven ophthalmologists to care for the 1.4 million people living in the area being served. A solution to this problem was the development of teleophthalmology. Here, the use of teleophthalmology was successful because it was a natural extension of the routine practice of ophthalmology and much of the equipment currently used already captured and stored images of ocular structures in compressed digital format, allowing them to be transported over existing telecommunications transmission media. The result of using this telehealth application was that the average consultation time was cut from half an hour to less than 5 minutes. During the system's first year of operation, approximately 30% of the patients who would never have been seen by an ophthalmologist were diagnosed with sight-threatening conditions that required follow-up care or additional tests.

In another important demonstration, two universities in Texas have joined forces to establish a cutting-edge telehealth clinic to provide comprehensive health care and rehabilitative services to children (Green et al., 2000). Through the use of telehealth technology, children who routinely commuted as much as 2 to 3 hours to receive care are now able to receive the services of a specialized interdisciplinary health care team. One of the main benefits resulting from development of the telehealth clinic was that children could be assessed by the whole team in one telehealth visit as compared to the children visiting each specialist separately. This effort resulted in greater efficacy and efficiency in treating children with specialized needs.

As can be seen in the case study, Mr. Lazarus continues to obtain high-quality care including interactions with specialists by means of telecommunications and the efficient receipt and transfer of data to support the nursing care he is receiving at home. Also, Mr. Lazarus can receive support by communicating with a cancer support group using technologies such as an electronic chat room wherein cancer patients share information and advice with each other.

DECISION SUPPORT SYSTEMS

A *decision support system* (DSS) is another health care informatics application that assists nurses in providing quality patient care. A DSS increases the nurse's decision-making effectiveness when he or she is faced with a complex clinical situation that has one or more plausible choices of treatment and a certain amount of risk associated with each of the treatment choices. An example of a decision support system that is used by nurses and physicians is a system called *Iliad* (Warner et al., 1988) that teaches diagnostic reasoning. Iliad is composed of an inference engine and a knowledge base (Lange et al., 1997). The *inference engine* is simply a set of rules that are applied in decision making, and the *knowledge base* is a comprehensive data set specific to a content domain. Iliad generates a differential diagnosis based on individual patient data and recommendations for further treatment. Iliad offers consultation, simulation, and reference. The most recent version of this DSS has a knowledge base built on actual clinical findings in over 500,000 documented patient encounters (http://www.cmea.com/catalog/670.html).

In a study of nurse practitioner (NP) students (Lange et al., 1997), Iliad was used to determine the effects of this DSS on the NP students' diagnostic skill performance. The study found that the use of Iliad improved NP students' diagnostic reasoning. In another study

with physicians, Friedman et al. (1999) found that using Iliad as a "hands-on" diagnostic DSS improved the diagnostic reasoning of physicians. In both studies, the authors viewed Iliad as a useful tool to assist practitioners in making clinical diagnoses. With regard to Mr. Lazarus's case, suppose the patient continues to experience fever, chills, and pleuritic chest pain despite the treatment for pneumonia that has been instituted. Nurse Matthews could use Iliad to relate these specific clinical findings to the condition of lymphoma. In essence, Nurse Matthews would have available the combined knowledge of many experts in the field and would be able to get immediate, specific feedback to augment her own intuitive skills. Iliad would provide Nurse Matthews with evidence-based, objective data to assist her in understanding how a differential diagnosis is made related to these new symptoms exhibited by Mr. Lazarus.

NURSING LANGUAGES

When considering applications such as point-of-care computing and telehealth, it is imperative that nurses be able to record patient data using a standard language. Although the data, information, and knowledge required to provide client care may be derived from a number of sources, nursing leaders have begun to distinguish those elements that describe the unique contributions of nursing to the promotion of health of individuals, families, and communities. The Nursing Minimum Data Set and established nursing taxonomies are examples of the progress made toward defining the diagnoses, interventions, and outcomes that are directly attributable to nursing and provide input to health care informatics databases.

The Nursing Minimum Data Set. The Nursing Minimum Data Set (NMDS), developed at the University of Wisconsin, Milwaukee, was generated to acknowledge the contribution of nursing to client outcomes. As the importance of nationwide health databases increases, it is important that a minimum number of essential nursing elements be included in those databases. The *Nursing Minimum Data Set* is defined as "a minimum set of items of information with uniform definitions and categories concerning the specific dimension of professional nursing, which meet the information needs of multiple data users in the health care system" (Werley, 1988). The NMDS comprises a nursing diagnosis, nursing intervention, nursing outcome, intensity of nursing care measure, and health record number. The system also includes a unique identifier for the nurse provider and data elements in common with the Uniform Hospital Discharge Data Set (UHDDS). Because this system is compatible with the UHDDS, there is great potential for documenting nursing's contributions to health care to insurers, hospital decision makers, nurse administrators, chief information officers, chief nursing officers, and informatics nurse specialists. A major purpose of the NMDS is to establish a comparison of client-centered data that can be used to evaluate the effectiveness of nursing care across practice settings and geographic boundaries. The NMDS recognizes personnel delivering care, the type of nursing care provided, the impact of that care on client outcomes, and the costs of nursing care. This system can enhance greatly the ability of nursing to conduct research and to create health policy.

Nursing Taxonomies. Nursing taxonomies are languages that provide data that can complete the NMDS framework. In other words, the NMDS provides the structure for what data are needed to describe nursing practice, and the nursing taxonomies provide the specific data, which fall into large categories such as nursing diagnosis, interventions, and outcomes. Some of the taxonomies developed include the North American Nursing Diagnosis Association (NANDA) taxonomy, the Nursing Interventions Classification (NIC), the Nursing Outcomes Classification (NOC), the Omaha Problem Classification, the Home Health Care Classification (HHCC), the Ozbolt Patient Care Dataset, and the Perioperative Nursing Data Set.

The *NANDA classification system* was developed to standardize nomenclature for nursing diagnoses. The work began initially in 1973 when a group of nurses met at the first national conference, and in 1982, following several conferences, the North American Nursing Diagnosis Association was formalized. In its most recent version (NANDA, 1999), the terms that were originally based on human response patterns are being refined and simplified (Clark, 1999).

The Iowa Intervention Project has produced a taxonomy of nursing interventions called the *Nursing Interventions Classification* (NIC). The project is the outgrowth of years of collaborative work by scholars and clinicians headed by McCloskey and Bulechek at the University of Iowa College of Nursing. The taxonomy consists of three levels that classify nursing interventions initially as abstract domains, then as related sets of interventions, and finally as a very concrete set of 433 intervention labels. Examples include abuse protection, bathing, emergency care, and learning facilitation. This system is dynamic, with new labels added as nurse researchers continue to study the phenomena of nursing (McCloskey & Bulechek, 1996; McCloskey, Bulechek, & Donohue, 1998). An example of an intervention from the NIC that would assist Nurse Matthews in providing care to Mr. Lazarus related to chemotherapy management is provided in Box 22–1.

The *Nursing Outcomes Classification* (NOC) is a classification system that provides a standard vocabulary and measures for patient outcomes that are influenced by nursing interventions (Johnson & Maas, 1998). The NOC contains over 2,000 outcomes organized in six domains and 24 classes. An *outcome* is described as "a variable concept" representing a patient or family caregiver state, behavior, or perception that is measured along a continuum and responsive to nursing interventions. As in the NIC, each

---

Box 22-1 Example of a Nursing Intervention Using the Nursing Interventions Classification (NIC)

Nursing Intervention: Chemotherapy management

Definition: Assisting the patient and family to understand the action and minimize the side effects of antineoplastic agents

Activities*:

Monitor for side effects and toxic effects of chemotherapeutic agents

Provide information to patient and family on how antineoplastic agents work on cancer cells

Instruct patient and family on ways to prevent infection, such as avoiding crowds and using good hygiene and hand-washing techniques

Instruct patient and family to promptly report fevers, chills, nosebleeds, excessive bruising, and tarry stools

Institute neutropenic and bleeding precautions

Administer antiemetic drugs for nausea and vomiting

Ensure adequate fluid intake to prevent dehydration and electrolyte imbalance

Provide nutritious, appetizing foods of patient's choice

* These activities are an abbreviated list; see the NIC manual for the complete list.

From McCloskey, J. C., & Bulechek, G. M. (Eds.). (2000). *Iowa Intervention Project: Nursing Interventions Classification* (NIC) (3rd ed., pp. 210-211.) St. Louis: Mosby.

NOC outcome has a definition, a list of indicators, a measurement scale, and a short list of references used in the development of the outcome. For example, Johnson & Maas (1998) describe the outcome Self-Esteem that is defined as "personal judgment of self-worth." Nurses can identify the outcome and, using a Likert-type scale, can assess the patient on several concrete indicators of self-esteem. What does this add to the NIC? It adds a concrete way of measuring the actual effectiveness of a nursing intervention. Using such a classification system can now link the actual intervention to the outcome achieved. It also holds the potential to determine the cost/benefit of nursing interventions and can demonstrate nursing's accountability for patient care.

The *Omaha Problem Classification,* commonly referred to as the Omaha System, is a classification scheme used with clients treated in a community health setting. It consists of three components: the Problem Classification Scheme, the Intervention Scheme, and the Problem Rating Scale for Outcomes. Insofar as nurses provide the majority of community health care, this system has a direct impact on the provision of that care (Martin & Norris, 1996; Martin & Scheet, 1992).

Saba (1994) developed a *Home Health Care Classification* (HHCC) of nursing diagnoses and interventions. The HHCC uses a framework of 20 home health care components to classify and code nursing diagnoses and interventions specific to home health. Its major purpose is to classify clients, predict resource requirements, and measure outcomes. This system allows data to be computerized and uses the format of the ICD-10 classification scheme whereby the home health care component, the nursing service category, the subcategory, and actions are defined and coded.

The *Ozbolt Patient Care Dataset* is a set of standard terms and codes that are compatible with an existing patient-level database. Standard terms have been developed for 209 nursing diagnoses/patient care problems, 122 expected patient outcomes, and 545 interventions/patient care activities (Ozbolt, 1996).

The *Perioperative Nursing Data Set* is an automated language that describes the specialty practice of perioperative nursing. Four domains—safety, physiologic response to surgery, patient and family behavioral response to surgery, and the health system—compose the data set. Each domain has defined outcomes, nursing interventions, and nursing diagnoses that relate to perioperative nursing (Kleinbeck, 1999).

These classification systems are important in providing the data necessary to proclaim nursing's contribution to the health and well-being of individuals who receive health care, and clinical systems should be evaluated for inclusion of these standard nursing languages. To this end, the ANA has formed the group Nursing Information Data Set Evaluation Committee (NIDSEC) (Simpson, 1998) to create standards specifically related to nursing that must be included in clinical information systems that are marketed to health care agencies. In order for a clinical information system to be NIDSEC certified, the system must meet the standards developed by NIDSEC for inclusion of pertinent nursing documentation. The goal of the NIDSEC is to certify vendors' clinical information systems as being compliant with standard nursing documentation. Certification of a clinical information system means that nurses can be confident that the system includes standard nursing language and other necessary components of nursing documentation processes.

In summary, Nurse Matthews now has several nursing taxonomies that can be used to support her practice. Clark (1999) states that nurses need standardized language to identify and measure the outcomes of nursing practice. Using such systems affords visibility, accountability, and recognition for nurses as they provide care to their patients.

～ Health Sciences Library Information Resources to Support Nursing Practice

In addition to the previously mentioned informatics technologies, Nurse Matthews has a world of information resources available to support her practice, accessible via health sciences library gateways. Resources that were traditionally housed in the hospital library are now accessible from remote sites, on the patient unit or from a home computer. The literature search is enhanced and expedited by the use of information technology. On-line catalogues are widely accessible to explore the holdings of a library. Electronic databases, mostly accessed via subscription, are powerful tools for searching the journal literature by subject. A wide variety of documents, data, graphics, sound, and video are now available on the Internet.

When Nurse Matthews leaves Mr. Lazarus's bedside she has the option of exploring these sources to retrieve information relevant to his nursing care. A literature search may be conducted to find research-based journal articles. Her institution may allow her to retrieve the full text of some of these electronically. She may already subscribe to electronic mailing lists or table of contents services and participate in on-line chat rooms or support groups for oncologic nurses. She may access an Internet web portal (also known as a start-up page) that integrates access to her e-mail, information retrieval from both free and fee-based databases, and assists her in organizing information. She may use the Internet to take advantage of distance learning opportunities to earn continuing education credits. The following sections will explain more about using technology to retrieve and organize information.

INFORMATION LITERACY

Any discussion of electronic retrieval must begin with *information literacy:* understanding the basic architecture of information and the need to do critical evaluation. Although nurses may be comfortable with computer applications for word processing, e-mail, presentation software, spreadsheets, and other applications, the conceptual skills needed for effectively using electronic search tools are unique.

Primary sources (e.g., research articles, books, dissertations, other documents) are those that contain original information, not previously published, and include the peer-reviewed journal literature. *Secondary sources* provide a synthesis of information published elsewhere (e.g., textbooks, newspaper articles, comments, letters, review articles). Print indexes (e.g., the *Cumulative Index to Nursing and Allied Health Literature* and *Index Medicus*) and their electronic counterparts, the *bibliographic databases,* index the primary and secondary sources.

USING LIBRARY ON-LINE CATALOGUES

Library holdings are generally accessed using on-line public access catalogues (OPACs). In addition to titles of books owned, users may also ascertain what newspaper and journal titles a library subscribes to; often on-line catalogues may be freely accessed from remote sites. Information in published books is often several years old and should be considered for background information in health topics. For the most up-to-date information, users should consult the journal literature.

SELECTING AND ACCESSING A BIBLIOGRAPHIC DATABASE

A *database* is defined as "a collection of information organized in such a way that a computer program can quickly select desired pieces of data. You can think of a database as an electronic filing system" (Webopedia, 1996).

Access to bibliographic databases varies from one institution to another. Databases are costly to produce and maintain, and they are generally accessed via institutional license agreements.

The print index *Cumulative Index to Nursing and Allied Health Literature* had its beginnings in the 1940s, and it has been available in electronic form since 1982 as the CINAHL database (produced by Cinahl Information Systems, Inc., http://www.cinahl.com).

Access to CINAHL is available from several commercial vendors; although the content is the same, different search interfaces have varied functionality. CINAHL currently provides access to more than 1,220 active journals in nursing, allied health disciplines, and alternative/complementary therapy journals from 1982 to the present; selected journals are also indexed in the areas of consumer health and biomedicine, many with abstracts (Cinahl Information Systems, 2000b). Full text is included for selected state nursing journals and some newsletters, standards of practice, practice acts, government publications, research instruments, and patient education material. A sample search will be detailed later in this chapter.

MEDLINE (MEDlars onLINE), the premier biomedical database (produced by the U.S. National Library of Medicine), indexes over 4,300 journals in medicine, nursing, dentistry, veterinary medicine, the health care system, and the preclinical sciences. MEDLINE is the electronic version of the print *Index Medicus.* Containing more than 10 million records, dating back to 1966, MEDLINE is available from a number of commercial vendors and is also free on the web as PubMed (http://www.ncbi.nlm.nih.gov/entrez/query.fcgi/). MEDLINE includes the journals in the *International Nursing Index* and is needed for comprehensive searching of the nursing literature.

When selecting any database, searchers should consider the time period covered and how often a database is updated, as well as the type of literature indexed. For example, in addition to journal articles, CINAHL indexes book chapters, research instruments, audiovisuals, and web sites. A database like Information Access Company's Health Reference Center—Academic indexes both professional and consumer-oriented literature. EMBASE (Elsevier Science) covers over 4,000 journals from approximately 70 countries, including comprehensive coverage of drug research and pharmacology, which may not be indexed elsewhere (Elsevier Science, 2000). Some other specialized databases useful to nurses include those presented in Table 22–1. A biennial list, "Essential Nursing References," can assist nurses in keeping up to date and locating related databases (Interagency Council of Information Resources for Nursing [ICIRN], 1998).

The interdisciplinary nature of nursing topics dictates that related information may be found in other specialized databases. For example, information about a topic in palliative care might be related to ethical, legal, theological, economic, or historical literature. Librarians can help you identify these databases.

Database Records. The building block of a database is the citation or record (Box 22–2) which has separate searchable fields. The citation includes enough information for the searcher to locate the full article; specialized features of databases index selected additional information. The subject heading field displays the assigned descriptors or subject headings. These controlled vocabulary terms are assigned by professional indexers who review the articles. A controlled vocabulary of terms ensures consistency and increases the likelihood that similar items will be grouped together. MEDLINE is based on the hierarchical MeSH vocabulary (the National Library of Medicine's Medical Subject Headings, which contains more than 19,000 main headings) (U.S. National Library of Medicine [NLM], 1999). CINAHL uses MeSH as the model for its thesaurus. Approximately 70% of the headings searched using CINAHL are MeSH headings. However, CINAHL also incorporates into its database more than 2,500 unique headings for concepts in nursing and allied health, including nursing specialties, NANDA nursing diagnoses, the Iowa Nursing Interventions Classification (NIC), major nurs-

ing models, terms for all recognized nursing specialties, and access to research designs, data analysis techniques, and data collection methods (Levy, 1996).

MeSH terms are added to and modified on a yearly basis by the National Library of Medicine as new concepts appear in the literature (Lowe & Barnett, 1994). For example, "Acquired Immunodeficiency Syndrome" was added to MeSH in 1983. The CINAHL thesaurus is also revised yearly (Levy, 1996). Thesauri embedded in database programs are used to help searchers translate or "map" language to the preferred term. For example, a searcher who enters the term "Lou Gehrig's Disease" or "ALS" is directed to the controlled vocabulary term "Amyotrophic Lateral Sclerosis." MeSH indexing is "a form of intelligent preprocessing that should be taken advantage of whenever possible" (Lowe & Barnett, 1994).

MeSH terms are arranged hierarchically in a thesaurus. These "tree structures" may also be browsed electronically (http://www.ncbi.nlm.nih.gov/htbin-post/Entrez/meshbrowser?) or in a print version, *Medical Subject Headings—Tree Structures* (U.S. NLM, 2000) and users have the option of selecting broader terms or including narrower terms ("exploding" the search). Similarly, the CINAHL subject headings may be explored using the online thesaurus or a print version, *CINAHL Subject Headings* (Cinahl Information Systems, 2000a). Scope notes (definitions of terms) are also available electronically. Subject headings may be assigned as "major," those that capture the main focus of the article indexed and are identified in the record shown with an asterisk.

In addition to the assigned MeSH or CINAHL terms, subheadings are often attached. In the CINAHL example shown in Box 22–2, the subheading "ae [adverse effects]" has been appended to the subject heading "chemotherapy, cancer." Indexers assign the most specific headings and subheadings possible, and searchers should use the subject heading/

TABLE 22–1 Bibliographic Databases

Database (Years Covered)/Producer	Description
AIDSLINE (AIDS information onLINE) (1980–present) U.S. National Library of Medicine http://www.nlm.nih.gov	References to the published literature on HIV infections and AIDS, covering research, clinical aspects, and health policy issues. The citations are derived from the MEDLINE, HealthSTAR, and BIOETHICSLINE files, and the meeting abstracts from the International Conferences on AIDS and other AIDS-related meetings, conferences, and symposia.
BIOETHICSLINE (BIOETHICS onLINE) (1973–present) Produced jointly by the Kennedy Institute of Ethics and the U.S. National Library of Medicine http://www.nlm.nih.gov	Indexes English-language materials on bioethics. Documents are selected from the disciplines of medicine, nursing, biology, philosophy, religion, law, and the behavioral sciences. Selections from popular literature are also included.
CANCERLIT (1983–present) National Cancer Institute http://cnetdb.nci.nih.gov/cancerlit.shtml	This index deals with the physiology of cancer and agents stimulating cell division. Also covered are the related topics of therapy, causative agents and carcinogenic mechanisms, biochemistry, and immunology.
CINAHL (Cumulative Index to Nursing & Allied Health Literature) (1982–present) Cinahl Information Systems, Inc. http://www.cinahl.com/	Citations to articles in more than 1,220 active journals in nursing, allied health disciplines, and alternative/complementary therapy journals, along with the publications of the American Nurses Association and the National League for Nursing.
Cochrane Database of Systematic Reviews Cochrane Collaboration http://cochrane.co.uk/	Regularly updated systematic reviews prepared and maintained by collaborative review groups. Also included are protocols for reviews currently being prepared (background, objectives, and methods of reviews in preparation).
Embase (1974–present) Elsevier Science http://www.elsevier.com/	Includes citations and abstracts of the biomedical literature from more than 4,000 international journals from 70 countries. Comprehensive coverage of drug research, pharmacology, pharmacy, pharmacoeconomics, pharmaceutics and toxicology, human medicine (clinical and experimental), basic biological research, health policy and management, public, occupational and environmental health, substance dependence and abuse, psychiatry, forensic science, biomedical engineering and instrumentation. Selective coverage of nursing, allied health, dentistry, veterinary medicine, psychology, and alternative medicine.
ERIC (1966–present) U.S. Department of Education's Educational Resources Information Center	Citations to literature covering all aspects of the field of education. These include articles appearing in more than 700 journals and hundreds of significant research reports (federal, state, and local).
Health Reference Center—Academic (Last 4 years + current year) Information Access Company http://library.iacnet.com	Index with selected full-text links to nursing, allied health, and medical journals; consumer health magazines; newsletters; pamphlets; newspaper articles; topical overviews; reference books; includes selective indexing for articles in approximately 1,500 additional general interest titles.
HealthSTAR (Health Services, Technology, Administration, and Research) (1975–present) Produced cooperatively by the National Library of Medicine (NLM) and the American Hospital Association (AHA) http://www.nlm.nih.gov	Citations and abstracts to articles, including both the clinical and the nonclinical aspects of health care and delivery. Includes all of the management-related citations from MEDLINE.

TABLE 22-1 **Bibliographic Databases** *Continued*	
Database (Years Covered)/Producer	**Description**
MEDLINE (MEDlars onLINE) (1966–present) Produced by the National Library of Medicine http://www.nlm.nih.gov	Provides citations (and some abstracts) to articles on all health-related topics from over 4,000 biomedical journals. (Holdings also include journals indexed in the *International Nursing Index.*)
PsycINFO (1887–present) American Psychological Association http://www.apa.org/psycinfo/	Covers the professional and academic literature in psychology and related disciplines. Includes records from the printed *Psychological Abstracts,* plus material from *Dissertation Abstracts International* and other sources.
RNdex (1992–present) Information Resources Group, Inc. http://www.rndex.com/rndex.htm	Index and abstracts to articles in more than 150 of the leading English-language nursing, case management, and managed care journals.
Social Science Citation Index (SSCI) (1988–present) Institute for Scientific Information http://www.isinet.com/	International multidisciplinary index to the literature of the social, behavioral, and related sciences, including nursing. Features the ability to search cited references.
Sigma Theta Tau International Registry of Nursing Research Virginia Henderson International Nursing Library http://www.stti.iupui.edu/library/	Bibliographic database and abstracts for over 11,000 English-language studies contributed by nurse researchers internationally.

From Health Sciences Library, University of Maryland, Baltimore, Maryland.

subheading combination when possible to increase precision, rather than combining two subject headings (Lowe & Barnett, 1994).

Other access points such as author, words in the title or abstract, journal title, institution, and so forth may be used for retrieval. For example, in the 1997 record shown, "supportive therapies" is searchable as a key word in the title and abstract fields. When selecting title words as well as terminology used in the abstract and text of an article, nurse authors should consult database thesauri and consider how searchers will find their article (Allen, 1998).

Search Strategies. *Boolean operators* (connectors) serve as powerful tools to shape retrieval. A search command using the term "AND" dictates that *both* terms must be in the retrieved record. Use of the "OR" connector retrieves records that contain *either* term, and is often used with synonyms to expand the search results (for example, "palliative care OR supportive therapies OR end-of life care"). *Truncation* is another technique for expanding search results; a truncation symbol (e.g., $, #, *, etc.) is used after the root of a word in a search command to retrieve all terms that begin with the root (e.g., the command therap$ would retrieve records containing "therapy," "therapist," "therapeutic," etc.). A database help screen helps the user identify the truncation symbol used in a database.

Search strategies for limiting retrieval in databases like MEDLINE and CINAHL include using the focus feature (an asterisk in front of the term) to retrieve articles that have been determined to have the subject heading as a major focus of the article. A retrieved set of articles may be further limited by year of publication or type of publication (e.g., a case study versus a

Box 22-2 Sample Record from CINAHL

Authors
Houston D.

Institution
Coordinator, Clinical Systems, The University of Texas, M.D. Anderson Cancer Center, Patient Care Information Systems, 1515 Holcombe Blvd., Houston, Texas 77030

Title
Supportive therapies for cancer chemotherapy patients and the role of the oncology nurse

Source
Cancer Nursing. 20(6):409–13, 1997 Dec. (23 ref)

Abbreviated Source
CANCER NURS. 20(6):409–13, 1997 Dec. (23 ref)

Document Delivery
NLM Serial Identifier: C05740000

Journal Subset
Core Nursing Journals
Nursing Journals
Peer Reviewed Journals
USA Journals.

Special Interest Category
Oncologic Care

CINAHL Subject Headings
Bone Marrow / de [Drug Effects]
Cancer Patients
*Chemotherapy, Cancer / ae [Adverse Effects]
Mouth Care
Nausea and Vomiting / pc [Prevention and Control]
Nutrition Disorders / pc [Prevention and Control]
*Oncologic Nursing
*Quality of Life

Abstract
Cancer chemotherapy often causes severe side effects, such as neutropenia, nausea and vomiting, and oral complications, which adversely affect patients' quality of life and may interfere with treatment success. A number of supportive therapies, such as colony stimulating-growth factors and antiemetics, have been developed to ameliorate these side effects, however, but often are underutilized. Oncology nurses, who serve as liaisons between oncologists and patients, can have a positive effect on patients' quality of life by educating them about potential side effects and the availability of supportive therapies, and by bringing patients' quality of life concerns and priorities to the attention of physicians. This article reviews the side effects of chemotherapy and the supportive therapies currently available to treat them and explores the role of oncology nurses as advocates for improved quality of life for chemotherapy patients. (23 ref)

Box 22–2 **Sample Record from CINAHL** *Continued*

ISSN
0162-220X
Publication Type
Journal Article
Language
English
Entry Month
199803

A search command "Oncologic Nursing AND Quality of Life" would retrieve this citation because both terms are present as CINAHL subject headings. A key word search command "supportive therapies" would also retrieve this citation because the phrase is found in the title as well as in the abstract.

clinical trial). Publication type can be a powerful indicator of the usefulness of the information retrieved, as will be discussed subsequently in the section on evidence-based health care. Geographic terms and age groups are other attributes that may be applied by the indexers and used as limits by searchers. Journal subsets provide another way to limit. For example, a search in MEDLINE may be limited to the "nursing" subset of journals; a CINAHL search may be limited to "core nursing journals."

A good search strategy is to find an article that is highly relevant and notice the other subject headings assigned to generate ideas for a new search. When viewing records retrieved for a search on adverse effects of chemotherapy, the searcher might notice the associated term "nutrition disorders" and use that to search for related articles. The MEDLINE PubMed interface has a "related articles" function to do this electronically. *The Social Science Citation Index* database has a similar feature.

Another basic tenet of bibliographic searching is knowing whether the search interface used defaults to "phrase" or "key word" searching. For example, when the software default is phrase searching, the term "high blood pressure" is searched as a connected phrase (or translated to the controlled vocabulary term

"hypertension") and the records retrieved will be relevant. If the software program understands the terms as key words, records retrieved will have the terms "high," and "blood," and "pressure" somewhere in each citation retrieved, not necessarily connected, and may include many irrelevant articles. Particularly in MEDLINE, the search result may be tremendous and unmanageable, and may *not* necessarily include all of the articles assigned the term "hypertension"! Often the less one knows of the complexity of a database, the greater the initial sense of success when retrieving information (R. Faraino, personal communication, February 11, 2000). It is very easy to retrieve a large number of articles from a database; developing the skills to focus on retrieving relevant articles to support clinical practice ("filtering") takes experience and cognitive understanding of how the database is structured. A sample search on supportive therapies for oncology patients' nausea related to chemotherapy is presented in Table 22–2.

Free versus Fee-Based Options for MEDLINE.
Searchers have choices of free and fee-based interfaces to MEDLINE. Free PubMed from the National Library of Medicine, Biomednet (http://www.biomednet.com/), and others

offer varied functionality, and their features are compared in print and web sources. Searchers and institutions may prefer the enhancements of fee-based services, particularly for help translating natural language into subject headings (mapping) or for context-sensitive help screens (Anagnostelis & Cooke, 1997; Brown & Rankow, 1999). When evaluating a MEDLINE interface, the user should determine whether the full MEDLINE database is included, how often it is updated, whether key words are translated to MeSH terms (mapped), what the search default mode is, whether searches can be saved, and so forth (R. Faraino, personal communica-

tion, February 11, 2000). CINAHL is available only via commercial vendors (the full CINAHL database is not available free on the web), and each of the vendor interfaces has unique characteristics and features.

Users should consult the online help screens to determine the default mode. Consult a health sciences librarian. "Web-based versions of MEDLINE, with their graphic interfaces and language mapping, are easier to use than their predecessors, but beneath the many user-friendly interfaces that clothe MEDLINE is a search engine of complex and powerful design. Using MEDLINE is a bit like driving a power-

TABLE 22-2 Sample Search in CINAHL

Search Strategy	Search Set No.	Search Command	No. of Articles Retrieved
Plan your search by deciding on one or more main concepts: *Find research on supportive therapies for oncology patients' nausea related to chemotherapy*			
	1	chemotherapy, cancer/	845
	2	nausea/	162
Consider synonyms to expand each search set using the OR operator	3	(antineoplastic agents/ OR chemotherapy, cancer/)	1,987
	4	nausea/ OR "nausea and vomiting"/	629
Combine concepts using AND	5	set 3 AND set 4	206
Limit the set to articles that have been designated with the publication type, "Research"	6	Limit set 5 to *Research* articles	69
Evaluate results; consider alternate search strategies			
View the subject headings in relevant records to generate ideas for related searching		*Related subjects for further searching:* nursing interventions/ oncologic care/ oncologic nursing/ antiemetics/ [therapeutic use] relaxation techniques/ nutrition disorders/	

ful racing car that has been modified for street use. It can transport you with astonishing speed to places you don't want to go" (Katcher, 1999, p. 11). Promotion of PubMed as a source for consumers has been misleading. MEDLINE is not the optimal database for consumers in search of health information. Naive searchers are not known to be comprehensive; consumers in search of health information are often in need of reassurance ("good news") and are not likely to differentiate a case study from a clinical trial. The National Library of Medicine's site MEDLINEPlus (http://www.nlm.nih.gov/medlineplus/) provides a mediated interface to selected topics in MEDLINE, and consumers should be directed to this site rather than to MEDLINE.

Specialized Databases for Nursing and Biomedical Information.

Evidence-based health care, which is defined as "the conscientious, explicit and judicious use of current best evidence in making decisions about the care of individual patients" (Sackett et al., 1996, p. 71), provides a formal approach to accessing the best information by applying quality filters to database searches. McKibbon describes the hierarchical nature of biomedical literature as a "wedge," with "idea" papers, editorials, and opinions at the wide end of the wedge and clinical trials at the narrow point of the wedge (McKibbon, et al. 1999). It is estimated that only one idea in 5,000 eventually becomes available for clinical application; the majority of published articles should not be used to "inform practice" (Greenhalgh, 1997). The term *evidence-based nursing* is often used to mean "research-based practice," but its strict definition is to describe practices that have been critically appraised using defined criteria and are "ready for clinical application" (McKibbon & Marks, 1998b). Evaluated abstracts of these studies (as well as "systematic reviews," which synthesize the findings of many studies) are published in many nursing journals such as *Evidence Based Nursing*

and the *Online Journal of Knowledge Synthesis for Nursing.* These articles are indexed in CINAHL and are examples of a "distilled" information source; the studies meet rigorous criteria based on research methodology and are presented with evaluated abstracts by expert clinicians (McKibbon & Marks, 1998a).

There are also specialized databases that contain "consolidated" information sources, which synthesize the findings of many studies (e.g., systematic reviews) and then statistically combine them (a meta-analysis) (McKibbon & Marks, 1998a). *The Cochrane Database of Systematic Reviews* includes many nursing topics, the result of an international collaboration. A fuller discussion of evidence-based practice is beyond the purview of this text, but sources for further reading are listed in the bibliography.

The *Sigma Theta Tau Registry of Nursing Research* is a unique resource that contains abstracts of studies that may be unpublished or ongoing, submitted by nurse researchers. Available to members or by institutional subscription via the Virginia Henderson International Nursing Library, over 11,000 English-language studies have been indexed by variables or phenomenon of study, as well as by author, title, or key words provided by the researchers (http://www.stti.iupui.edu/library/). Studies are not peer reviewed for quality. It is up to the individual registrant to provide enough information about his or her work to allow users to evaluate relevance and quality.

Links to Full Text.

Whether free on the World Wide Web or fee-based, bibliographic databases may include selected links to the full text of journal articles. MEDLINE, via PubMed, links to the full text of recent editions of several hundred of the 4,300 journals it indexes (U.S. NLM, 1999). The user should consult a librarian to explore access to full text links, full-text electronic journals and archives, as well as options for interlibrary loan and document delivery at the user's institution.

THE INTERNET

The global information network known as the *Internet* allows information to be shared among any users with a personal computer and connectivity. The Internet is a source of vast amounts of information and has sophisticated capabilities for searching and locating data, files, databases, digitized library collections, software, graphics, sound, and video.

Originally called the ARPAnet, the network was an experimental project developed in 1969 by the Advanced Research Projects Agency in the U.S. Department of Defense. ARPAnet was designed so that research could be shared between military and university sources and, more important, so that such communication could be sustained in the event of a nuclear attack. Not long after ARPAnet was designed, the Defense Department developed a standard protocol called Transmission Control Protocol/Internet Protocol (TCP/IP), a data communications standard that determines how two computers will exchange information. By using TCP/IP, other networks could also establish a gateway to the Internet. A *gateway* is a computer system that transfers data between normally incompatible computer networks. With these technologies, the Internet has become available for everyone's use.

In addition to e-mail, which allows individuals to communicate, and electronic mailing lists, which allow users with shared interests to post and distribute information to those subscribed to a list, there are Internet protocols for *Telnet* (allows remote logins to other computer systems), *FTP* (file transfer protocol software, which enables electronic files to be transferred from one site to another), *newsgroups* ("global bulletin boards," which enable users to post and exchange information), and *gopher* (an early web tool that allows browsing linear menus; most gopher documents are now readable as web documents). More comprehensive discussions of each of these features of the Internet are found in many specialized guides such as

Computers in Nursing's Nurses' Guide to the Internet, 2nd ed. (Nicoll, 1998), and new Internet users will find tutorials and guides on the Internet itself, such as

- "Learn the Net," at http://www. learnthenet.com/english/index.html
- "Finding Information on the Internet: A Tutorial," at http://www.lib.berkeley.edu/TeachingLib/Guides/Internet/FindInfo.html

The most common and most popular use of the Internet since the mid-1990s is via the World Wide Web.

The World Wide Web. The emergence of the World Wide Web is the result of the development of graphical user interfaces (GUIs), which enable the use of user-friendly point-and-click browsing hypertext links (replacing the command-driven text-based systems that were previously mediated by information professionals). Using a browser (a software program such as Netscape Navigator or Microsoft Explorer) enables the user to view both text and graphics displayed on the screen. Behind the scenes, *hypertext markup language* (html) enables the information to be displayed. *Hypertext transfer protocol* (http) is used by the end user (client) to locate a unique address, a URL (uniform resource locator), and request a document from a host or "server" that delivers web documents to the end user. This client-server architecture is the framework that supports the World Wide Web.

Dispelling Misperceptions. The World Wide Web provides a forum for freely accessing any print or graphical material that anyone with a computer may *post* and anyone with a computer may *access.* The web has the capability of providing more up-to-date information than any other medium. And the web contains and has the potential to disseminate valuable data that may profoundly affect lives. At the same time, information may be outdated, incorrect, or harmful.

Many users share the widespread misperception that *everything* is available on the Internet and that everything is *free*. Users frequently use the terms "on the Internet," "on line," and "available electronically" interchangeably, but the discussion of bibliographic databases earlier in this chapter illustrates that users won't find most of the databases of the peer-reviewed scholarly literature freely available. Although the Internet may be its mode of transmission, scholarly, peer-reviewed literature is expensive to produce and organize, and most bibliographic databases and full-text electronic journals are only obtained by license arrangements as institutional subscriptions. A survey of 221 key nursing journals found that while 111 (50%) are available on-line in full text (either free on the web, by publisher subscription, included in an aggregated full-text database, or via fee-based access to individual articles), only seven (3.3%) of these 221 journals are completely free on the web, and most of these have published just a few articles (Allen, 1999, 2000). The fee-based links to electronic journals usually archive recent years only, perhaps back 5 years. Although many journals offer free on-line versions of their continuing education articles, or partial access to current or archived titles, comprehensive searchers cannot rely on this small fraction of the literature.

Yet the current publishing scheme is evolving, profoundly impacted by new technology. It has been noted that health care and research facilities will continue to grow increasingly networked (Lynch, 1999), databases that are beginning to license full-text links to articles will increase, and a "cultural revolution" is occurring with regard to the scholarly process and preprints (Lynch, 1999). Former National Institutes of Health Director Harold Varmus has proposed PubMed Central, an electronic server for "all biomedical research reports, both reviewed and unreviewed, with a sophisticated search engine and free access for anyone in the world." (Burke, 2000). As plans for the PubMed Central site evolve, the site's mission is to include reports that have been "screened but not formally peer-reviewed" (National Institutes of Health, 1999). Another site, Netprints (http://clinmed.netprints.org/), an electronic archive of articles posted prior to peer review, was launched in December 1999 by the *British Medical Journal* and the Highwire Press (Delamothe et al., 1999).

In addition to the plethora of Internet resources and uses for health care professionals, nurses in their role as health educators find themselves confronted with consumers who have become more proactive about retrieving their own information and are more involved about their own care. Nurses are "physically present in more settings than any other health care worker" and need to respond to more informed consumers (National League for Nursing, 1997). Patients may be motivated by "a distrust of managed care, insurance companies, and [the] medical establishment," and are enabled by access to much of the same information that was once only accessible to either health or information professionals (Lynch, 1999). Consumers with "a little knowledge" may challenge health professionals with the results of their own research gathered on the web (Jeffrey, 1998). Yet the quality of the information consumers retrieve, even when it comes from sources such as teaching centers, news services, and health departments, has been deemed variable (McClung et al., 1998).

Consumers as well as professionals are faced with a daily barrage of media attention focused on the Internet. There are ever-present "how-to" articles in popular magazines and newspapers (as well as in the scholarly literature) that list both web sites and tips for users and also provide warnings. The issues are vast and complex.

Navigating the Web. Unlike library catalogues and other databases, the World Wide Web is not organized according to any one scheme (although the information contained at any individual site may be an organized database). No one organization owns, monitors, or controls the Internet. There is no controlled vocabulary. As a result, finding information can be challenging and requires combining strategies.

One way to locate information on the web is to know the site one is looking for (typing in a URL). Newspapers and periodicals, along with broadcasting and advertising media, abound with lists of discipline-specific sites, for example "Web Sites for Midwives" (Anderson, 1999) or "Internet Technology: Resources for Perinatal Nurses," (Drake, 1999). A published list of selected sites "Essential Nursing References," compiled biennially by ICIRN (ICIRN, 1998) is another place to start. From these suggested sites, users may use hypertext links to browse or "surf" the web for related information. But, because the web is arranged in a nonlinear way, this is not an efficient strategy for locating specific information.

Search tools are commonly used to search the World Wide Web. Three types of tools are Directories, Search Engines, and Metasearch tools (Thede, 1999). *Directories* (or web guides such as Yahoo at http://www.yahoo.com or Britannica Web's Best at http://www.britannica.com) are tools compiled by human indexers who assign subject headings to the contents of web sites. For example, by browsing the categories arranged hierarchically in Yahoo, one can locate a site by category:

Health
  Nursing
    History
      Florence Nightingale
        Florence Nightingale: Rural Hygiene (essay)

Several sites devoted to Florence Nightingale are identified, including the full text document "Florence Nightingale: Rural Hygiene," an essay written by Nightingale on the subject of hygiene, which is part of the Internet Modern History Sourcebook (Internet Modern History Sourcebook, 1997) Searching a web directory is similar to browsing the table of contents of a book or a telephone yellow pages directory. One tries to decide how someone else might have classified information by browsing categories.

Search engines, the second type of tool, employ software "spiders" or "robots" that crawl electronically to collect web sites (e.g., Google at http://google.com) and then add them to their catalogue. Using a search engine is similar to searching the index of a book. The searcher enters a word and the engine retrieves records with key words matching the term entered. Although valuable for obscure information, key word searching may result in large, unwieldy lists, and terms are retrieved out of context. For example, a search using the word "nursing" may retrieve sites related to nursing as a discipline as well as sites including graphics of lactating sheep! Each search engine has its own rules for determining how sites are indexed and how the results are ranked according to relevance. Some give a higher ranking to terms based on its frequency of occurrence in the retrieved document; others may consider whether the term is found in titles or headings (Sparks & Rizzolo, 1998). Search engines have different rules for entering a search string, using Boolean connectors, use of quotation marks for phrases, truncation symbols, and so forth. Some search engines also include a subject directory of the included sites. The user should look for a "help" link on the search engine's home page to determine how to enter a search. Searchers should always consider using several search tools because no one search engine covers the entire contents of the web. Sites that describe how search engines work and compare the features of search engines can provide helpful information (e.g., Search Engine Watch at http://www.searchenginewatch.com/).

Metasearch tools, a third type, search several selected search engines simultaneously and are able to eliminate duplicates (Sparks & Rizzolo, 1998). For example, entering a term in MetaCrawler (http://www.metacrawler.com/) prompts the metasearch tool to simultaneously search multiple search engines. Metasearch tools are useful when the search request is a simple key word. Because the search engines have different rules for entering search strings, the words should not be linked with Boolean connectors; phrase searching may not be supported. The disadvantage of a metasearch tool is that it cannot take advantage of the individual features of each search engine to customize searches (Sparks & Rizzolo, 1998). As no metasearch tool covers the entire web, searchers should consider a combined strategy and explore using more than one metasearch tool. See "Finding Information on the Internet: A Tutorial" at http://www.lib.berkeley.edu/TeachingLib/Guides/Internet/FindInfo.html for comparisons of recommended metasearch tools.

Evaluating the Web. Critical evaluation is a crucial step in any search for information on the World Wide Web. Unlike the scholarly peer-reviewed literature, organized into journals and cited in standard records by the bibliographic databases, the web contains documents in many nonstandard formats, contributed by non-screened sources and unevaluated for quality. Anyone can publish on the Internet, which has been called "the world's largest vanity press" (Silberg, Lundberg, & Musacchio, 1997).

One strategy for searching the World Wide Web is to find places where respected searchers have preevaluated web sites. Selected meta-sites for nursing information (such as the Hardin Meta Directory of Nursing Internet Sites, http://www.lib.uiowa.edu/hardin/md/nurs.html, or Healthweb Nursing at the University of Michigan, at http://healthweb.org/browse.cfm?subject=60) provide evaluated, annotated links.

As the World Wide Web evolves, steps are being taken to ensure consistency and establish standards. The Health on the Net (HON) Foundation, a not-for-profit, international collaboration, has published a code of conduct that suggests standards for producers of health information web sites (http://www.hon.ch/HONcode/Conduct.html).

There are basic, agreed-upon criteria for evaluating web sites. As health professionals interacting with patients, nurses need to be alert to the context in which information is presented. Patients reading information intended for professionals may misinterpret information; the information may not be false, but it may still do harm (Eysenbach & Diepgen, 1998). Although the date a web site was modified may be recent, this does not ensure that the information is up to date. Nurses should approach all information critically and use the criteria in Table 22–3 to evaluate web sites.

≈ Strategies for Managing Information

Electronic access to information, for both professionals and consumers, provides a rich resource for up-to-date access as well as the challenge of managing information overload. A good strategy for nurses is to begin by subscribing to several relevant electronic mailing lists in a specialty (for example, ONCO-NURSE is a discussion list for oncology nurses). As patient advocates, nurses can use Internet directories to locate support groups for patients, including on-line support groups for home-bound patients. Free e-mail accounts are available via several web services (supported by advertising). Journal table of contents services (receiving a journal table of contents via e-mail) may be available from individual web sites or by subscription. News groups are another type of electronic discussion group where one may post and read messages. Explore what electronic databases are available via your institution and inquire about library orientation and database training that may be offered at a health sciences library. Locate help guides and local web resources at your library.

As nurses explore the content of what is available on the web, both free and fee-based, bookmarking (or selecting "favorite") web sites

TABLE 22–3 Criteria for Evaluating Health Information on the Internet	
Content	What is the scope of the site? What does it purport to cover? If it's a database, what years are covered?
Audience	Who is the intended audience? Health professionals? Health consumers? What is the context?
Authority	Who is the creator? What are their credentials? Is the site based at or affiliated with an institution?
Accuracy	Is the author qualified to write this document? Are references cited? Can the same information be verified elsewhere?
Purpose/Objective	Is the site an opinion? For profit? For education? For self-promotion? For advertising? What is the bias?
Structure/ Organization	What does the site look like? Is it readable and well organized? Can users get to linked information in three or fewer clicks?
Currency	When was the site last updated? When was the content updated? Are the links active and up to date?

Data from Goldsborough (1999); Hodson-Carlton & Dorner (1999); Kapoun (1998); Silberg, Lundberg, & Musacchio (1997); Walther & Speisser (1997).

is a good way to begin to customize your information gateway. Options for customizing a web portal are available at many institutions or search engine sites. Portals provide users with multiple services (e-mail, chat rooms, journals and databases, stock quotes, news links, and so forth) to attract users to these advertiser- or institution-supported pages. Selected web sites available for nursing information are presented in Table 22–4.

Bibliographic management software (e.g., Pro Cite or Reference Manager) can assist nurses in building a personal database of articles and information retrieved. The web offers resources for learning simple html (e.g., "A beginner's guide to HTML," at http://www.ncsa.uiuc.edu/General/Internet/WWW/HTMLPrimer.html) and building one's own web site as another way to connect with health professionals with similar interests and to disseminate information.

Comment

In this age of high-technology client care, nursing practice requires vast amounts of information to formulate plans of care and uses sophisticated technologies to provide care. Nurses must synthesize information efficiently to support and enhance their practice. To strengthen their practice, nurses must evaluate technologies within the framework of health care informatics to discern the effects of these technologies in producing high-quality outcomes for patients. Nurses must be educated consumers of information resources and active participants in developing practice innovations resulting from the use of information technology. Information technology has dramatically changed the environment of information retrieval, and will no doubt continue to evolve. Nurses need a foundation in the principles of information literacy to continue to apply new technologies and to build on for lifelong learning. By undertaking these actions, nurses will be assured of having leadership positions in the provision of client care in the information age.

TABLE 22–4 Representative Examples of the Types of Web Sites Available for Nursing Information

Name of Site and URL	Type of Site	Description of Contents
Britannica www.britannica.com	Web directory, free encyclopedia, free full-text articles. Selected, annotated, and ranked by humans.	Supported by advertising, this site aggregates a free encyclopedia (*Britannica*); links to selected full-text periodical articles; and a web directory of "expertly reviewed" sites.
Cable News Network http://www.cnn.com/HEALTH	News.	Up-to-date links to health related national and international news articles.
CHID http://chid.nih.gov/	Free bibliographic database.	Index of health promotion and health education materials contributed by health-related federal agencies.
Finding Information on the Internet: A Tutorial http://www.lib.berkeley.edu/ TeachingLib/Guides/Internet/ FindInfo.html	A free Internet tutorial.	Hypertext linked Internet tutorial, for beginners to advanced searchers.
Google http://google.com	A general search engine.	Indexes 90–100 million web sites, ranking by popularity.
Hardin Meta Directory of Nursing Internet Sites http://www.lib.uiowa.edu/hardin/md/ nurs.html	A metadirectory of nursing information.	"Best of the best"—list of sites related to nursing.
Health Web—nursing communication—electronic discussion groups http://www.healthweb.org/ browse.cfm?categoryid=1723	A list of links in one category.	Links to subscribing information for electronic discussion groups in selected nursing specialties.
HSTAT http://text.nlm.nih.gov/ National Library of Medicine	A free database.	Electronic resource that provides access to the full text of documents useful in health care decision making. Includes clinical practice guidelines.
Lippincott's Nursing Center http://www.nursingcenter.com/	A site provided by a publisher of nursing texts and journals.	Selected full-text access to journals (may require free registration); opportunities to earn on-line CE credit; career and association links; forum discussions.
MetaCrawler http://www.metacrawler.com/	A meta-search engine.	Simultaneously searches nine search engines and consolidates results in a ranked list.
National Academy Press http://www.nap.edu/	Full-text books in electronic form.	Full-text, searchable hypertext versions of books published by NAP.
National Library of Medicine http://www.nlm.nih.gov/databases/ databases.html	Free databases.	MEDLINE, Bioethicsline, Cancerlit, Visible Human Project, and others.
NOAH: New York Online Access to Health http://www.noah-health.org	Consumer-oriented health information, full text.	Bilingual (English and Spanish) links to information, web sites, fact sheets, glossaries, clinical trials. Searchable by topic.
Online Journal of Issues in Nursing http://www.ana.org/ojin	Free electronic nursing journal.	A full-text electronic journal available free on the Internet.
Resources for Nurses and Families http://pegasus.cc.ucf.edu/~wink/	Searchable metasite.	Nursing and teaching resources, searchable and organized by category, maintained by Dr. Diane Wink, University of Central Florida.

KEY POINTS

- Health care informatics will be used to support and enhance nursing practice in the 21st century.

- Nurses will use advanced technologies such as point-of-care systems, teleheath, and decision support systems to provide comprehensive care to clients.

- Consumers will use networking technologies to gain access to information that will enable them to make informed choices about their health care options.

- Nursing will experience rapid developments in information technology and integrate these developments into practice.

- Nursing will continue to be challenged to develop its nursing language, as in the Nursing Minimum Data Set, the North American Nursing Diagnosis Association Taxonomy, the Nursing Interventions Classification, the Nursing Outcomes Classification, the Perioperative Classification System, the Ozbolt Patient Care Data Set, the Omaha Problem Classification, and the Home Health Care Classification of Nursing Diagnoses and Interventions.

- Information systems are used to support nurses' clinical decision making and critical thinking.

- Integrated management systems are used to support the effective administration of nursing practice in a variety of settings.

- Nurses will continue to communicate globally using the Internet to enhance education, practice, and research.

- A revolution is taking place in the world of access to scholarly information. Information technology has made information available more directly and there are movements to circumvent the traditional peer review process.

- Information on the World Wide Web requires evaluation. There is no formal peer review process to regulate the quality or accuracy of what is posted.

- Online information is both free and fee-based. Most of the full-text scholarly literature is available by institutional subscription or for a fee.

CRITICAL THINKING EXERCISES

1. Consider how you would use a point-of-care system to access, process, retrieve, and store patient care data in your agency. How would using such a system contrast with the present processes used for patient care documentation?

2. Review the nursing taxonomies in this chapter. Which of these taxonomies best fits with your own practice? Why?

3. Use an Internet search engine (e.g., http://google.com) to search for a phrase. Evaluate several of the retrieved sites based on the evaluation criteria given in Table 22–3.

4. Browse links from a nursing metasite (e.g., the Hardin Meta Directory of Nursing Sites, at http://www.lib.uiowa.edu/hardin/md/nurs.html). Evaluate the usefulness of these evaluated, annotated links and compare to what you find on your own using a search engine.

5. Compare the information found at a web site to that found in a journal article. How is it organized, cited, and arranged?

REFERENCES

Anagnostelis, B., & Cooke, A. (1997, December 9–11). Evaluation criteria for different versions of the same database: A comparison of Medline services. Paper presented at Online Information 97: The 21st International Online Information Meeting, London.

Allen, M. (1998, Winter). Selecting keywords: Helping others find your article. *Nurse Author and Editor, 8*(1), 4.

Allen, M. (1999). *Key nursing journals: Characteristics and database coverage,* [on-line]. Available: http://www.library.kent.edu/nahrs/resource/reports/specrpts.htm

Allen, M. (2000). Nursing journals: No, they're not all online for free. *NAHRS Newsletter, 20*(1), 7–9.

American Nurses Association. (1994). *The scope of practice for nursing informatics.* Washington, DC: Author.

American Nurses' Credentialing Center. (1995). *Informatics nurse certification catalog.* Washington, DC: Author.

Anderson, D. A. (1999). Web sites for midwives. *Medical Reference Services Quarterly 18*(3), 39–56. Available: http://omni.ac.uk/agec/iolim97/

Brennan, P. F. (1999). Telehealth: Bringing health care to the point of living. *Medical Care, 37,* 115–116.

Brown, H. A., & Rankow, V. G. (1999). MEDLINE on the Internet. In M. S. Wood (Ed.), *Health care resources on the Internet: A guide for librarians and health care consumers.* New York: Haworth Information Press.

Burke, M. (2000). PubMed Central: Be careful what you ask for. *College and Research Libraries News, 61*(1), 21–23.

Capron, H. L. (1998). *Computers: Tools for an information age* (5th ed.) Reading, MA: Addision-Wesley Longman.

Cinahl Information Systems. (2000a), *Cumulative Index to Nursing and Allied Health Literature Cinahl Subject Headings.* Glendale, CA: Author.

Cinahl Information Systems. (2000b). *Cinahl Information Systems products and services.* Available: http://www.cinahl.com/prodsvcs/prodsvcs.htm

Clark, J. (1999). A language for nursing. *Nursing Standard, 21*(31), 42–47.

Delamothe, T., Smith, R. Keller, M. A., Sack, J., & Witscher, B. (1999). Netprints: The next phase in the evolution of biomedical publishing. *British Medical Journal, 319,* 1515–1516

Drake, E. (1999). Internet technology: Resources for perinatal nurses. *JOGNN: Journal of Obstetric, Gynecologic, and Neonatal Nursing, 28*(1), 15–21.

Elsevier Science. (2000). *EMBASE: The Excerpta Medica database.* Available: http://www.elsevier.com/inca/publications/store/5/2/3/3/2/8/index.htt

Eysenbach, G., & Diepgen, T. L. (1998). Towards quality management of medical information on the Internet: Evaluation, labeling, and filtering of information. *British Medical Journal, 317,* 1496–1500.

Flowers, C. W. (1999). Caring for the inner city: Telemedicine's newest niche. *Health Management Technology, 20*(9), 12–14.

Friedman, C. P., Elstein, A. S., Wolf, F. M., Murphy, G. C., Franz, T. M., Heckerling, P. S., Fine, P. L., Miller, T. M., & Abraham, V. (1999). Enhancement of clinicians' diagnostic reasoning by computer-based consultation. *Journal of the American Medical Association, 282,* 1851–1856.

Goldsborough, R. (1999). Information on the net often needs checking. *RN, 62*(5), 22–24.

Grassian, E. (1997). *Thinking critically about World Wide Web resources.* Los Angeles: UCLA College Library. Available: http://www.library.ucla.edu/libraries/college/instruct/web/critical.htm

Graves, J., & Corcoran, S. (1989). The study of nursing informatics. *Image: Journal of Nursing Scholarship, 21,* 227–231.

Green, A., Esperat, C., Seale, D., Chalambaga, M., Smith, S., Walker, G., Ellison, P., Berg, B., & Robinson, S. (2000). The evolution of a distance education initiative into a major telehealth project. *Nursing and Health Care Perspectives. 21*(2), 66–70.

Greenhalgh, T. (1997). *How to read a paper: The basics of evidence-based medicine.* London: British Medical Journal.

Hodson-Carlton, K., & Dorner, J. L. (1999). An electronic approach to evaluating web resources. *Nurse Educator 24*(5), 21–26.

Interagency Council of Information Resources for Nursing. (1998). *Essential nursing references* [On-line] New York: Author. Available: http://icirn.org/essrefs.htm

Internet Modern History Sourcebook. (1997). *Florence Nightingale: Rural hygiene* [On-line]. Available: http://www.fordham.edu/halsall/mod/nightingale-rural.html

Jeffrey, N. A. (1998, October 19). Doctors and patients—a little knowledge—doctors are suddenly swamped with patients who think they know a lot more than they actually do. *Wall Street Journal,* R8.

Johnson, M., & Maas, M. (1998). The Nursing Outcomes Classification. *Journal of Nursing Care Quality, 12*(5), 9–20.

Kapoun, J. (1998). Teaching undergrads web evaluation: A guide for library instruction. *College and Research Libraries News, 59,* 522–523.

Katcher, B. (1999). *Medline: A guide to effective searching.* San Francisco: Ashbury Press.

Kazman, W., & Westerheim, A. (1999). Telemedicine leverages the power of clinical information. *Health Management Technology, 20*(9), 8–11.

Kleinbeck, S. V. M. (1999). Development of the Perioperative Nursing Data Set. *Association of Operating Room Nurses Journal, 70*(1), 15–27.

Lange, L. L., Haak, S. W., Lincoln, M. J., Thompson, C. B., Turner, C. W., Weir, C., Foerster, V., Nilasens, D., & Reeves, R. (1997). Use of Iliad to improve diagnostic performance of nurse practitioner students. *Journal of Nursing Education, 36*(10), 36–45.

Levy, J. R. (1996). *Mastering the database search: Self-study and class guide to the use and understanding of the CINAHL database* (2nd ed.). Glendale, CA: Cinahl Information Systems.

Lowe, H. J., & Barnett, G. O. (1994). Understanding and using the medical subject headings (MeSH) vocabulary to perform literature searches. *JAMA, 271,* 1103–1108.

Lynch, C. (1999). Medical libraries, bioinformatics, and networked information: A coming convergence? *Bulletin of the Medical Library Association, 87,* 408–414.

Mandel, S. H. (1993). A global perspective of informatics in health in developing countries. In S. H. Mandel, M. Korpela, D. Forster, K. Moidi, & P. Byass

(Eds.), *Health informatics in Africa—HELINA 93* (pp. 3–8). Amsterdam: Excerpta Medica.

Martin, K. S., & Norris, J. (1996). The Omaha System: A model for describing practice. *Holistic Nursing Practice, 11*(1), 75–83.

Martin, K. S., & Scheet, N. J. (1992). *The Omaha system: Applications for community health nursing*. Philadelphia: Saunders.

McCloskey, J., & Bulechek, G. M. (Eds.). (1996). *Iowa Intervention Project: Nursing Interventions Classification (NIC)* (2nd ed.). St. Louis: Mosby.

McCloskey, J. C., & Bulechek, G. M. (Eds.). (2000). *Iowa Intervention Project: Nursing Interventions Classification (NIC)* (3rd ed.) St. Louis: Mosby.

McCloskey, J. C., Bulechek, G. M., & Donohue, W. (1998). Nursing interventions core to specialty practice. *Nursing Outlook, 46*(2), 67–76.

McClung, H. J., Murray, R. D., & Heitlinger, L.A. (1998). The internet as a source for current patient information. *Pediatrics 101*(6), E2.

McKibbon, A., with Eady, A., & Marks, S. (1999). *Evidence-based principles and practice*. Hamilton, Ontario: Decker.

McKibbon, K. A. (1998). Evidence-based practice. *Bulletin of the Medical Library Association 86*, 396–401.

McKibbon K., & Marks S. (1998a). EBN notebook: Searching for the best evidence. Part 1. Where to look. *Evidence-Based Nursing, 1*(3), 68–70.

McKibbon K., & Marks S. (1998b). EBN notebook: Searching for the best evidence. Part 2. Searching CINAHL and MEDLINE. *Evidence-Based Nursing, 1*(4), 105–107.

Nakamura, K., Takano, T., & Akao, C. (1999). The effectiveness of videophones in home healthcare for the elderly. *Medical Care, 37*, 117–125.

National Institutes of Health. (1999, August 30). PubMed Central: An NIH-operated site for electronic distribution of life sciences research reports [on-line]. Available: http://www.nih.gov/welcome/director/pubmedcentral/pubmedcentral.htm

National League for Nursing. (1997, April). *Final report: Commission on a Workforce for a Restructured Health Care System* [On-line]. New York: National League for Nursing. Available: http://www.nln.org/infrest1.htm

Nicoll, L. H. (1998). *Computers in nursing's Nurses' Guide to the Internet* (2nd ed.). Philadelphia: Lippincott.

North American Nursing Diagnosis Association. (1999). *Nursing diagnoses: Definition and classification 1999–2000*. Philadelphia: Author.

Ozbolt, J. G. (1996). From minimum data to maximum impact: Using data to strengthen patient care. *Advanced Practice Nursing Quarterly, 1*(4), 62–69.

Peterson's guide to nursing programs 1999/2000 (5th ed.). (1999). Princeton: Peterson's Guides.

Saba, V. K. (1994). *Home health care classification (HHCC) of nursing diagnoses and interventions*. Washington, DC: Georgetown University.

Sackett, D. L., Rosenberg, W. W., Gray, T. A., Haynes, R. B., & Richardson, W. S. (1996). Evidence based medicine: What it is and what it isn't. *British Medical Journal, 312*, 71–72.

Schutzman, A. (1999). Easy steps to point-of-care computing. *Health Management Technology, 20*(6), 20–24.

Silberg, W. M., Lundberg, G. D., & Musacchio, R. A. (1997). Assessing, controlling, and assuring the quality of medical information on the internet: Caveat lector et viewor—let the reader and the viewer beware. *Journal of the American Medical Association, 277*, 1244–1245.

Simpson, R. L. (1996). Wireless communications: A new frontier in technology. *Nursing Management, 27*(11), 20–21.

Simpson, R. L. (1998). Setting the informatics standard: An overview of NIDSEC's information systems evaluation criteria. *Nursing Economics, 16*, 279–281.

Sparks S. (1999). Electronic publishing and nursing research. *Nursing Research, 48*, 50–54.

Sparks, S. M., & Rizzolo, M. A. (1998) World Wide Web search tools. *Image: The Journal of Nursing Scholarship, 30*, 167–171.

Thede, L. Q. (Ed.).(1999). *Computers in nursing: Bridges to the future*. Philadelphia: Lippincott.

U.S. National Library of Medicine. (1999). NLM's web site gets a new look. *NLM Newsline, 54*(2–3), 1–4.

U.S. National Library of Medicine. (2000). *Medical subject headings* [Factsheet] [On-line]. Available: http://www.nlm.nih.gov/pubs/factsheets/mesh.html

U.S. National Library of Medicine (2000). *Medical subject headings, tree structures 2000*. Bethesda: Author.

Vanderbeek, J., Ulrich, D., Jaworski, L.W., Hergert, D., Beery, T., & Baas, L. (1994). Bringing nursing informatics into the undergraduate classroom. *Computers in Nursing, 12*, 227–231.

Walther, J. H., & Speisser, N. (1997, Fall). Developing and delivering medical reference source instruction in a special library [On-line]. *Issues in Science and Technology Librarianship, 16*. Available:http://www.library.ucsb.edu/istl/97-fall/article2.html

Warner, H. R., Haug, P., Bouhaddou, O., Lincoln, M., Warner, H., Jr., Sorensen, D., Williamson, J. W., & Fam, C. (1988). Iliad as an expert consultant to teach differential diagnosis. In *Proceedings of the Twelfth Annual Symposium on Computer Applications in Medical Care* (pp. 371–376). Washington, DC: IEEE Computer Society Press.

Webopedia. (1996, September 1). *Webopedia definition and links* [On-line]. Available: http://www.pcwebopaedia.com/TERM/d/database.html

Werley, H. H. (1988). *Identification of the nursing minimum data set*. New York: Springer.

Index

Note: Page numbers in *italics* refer to illustrations; page numbers followed by t refer to tables.

A

Accommodation, in management, 172
Accountability, 52, 54–55, 278
Accreditation, educational, 37
Adaptation, in systems theory, 104
Adaptation model, of Sister Callista Roy, 127–128, 134t
Adaptive model of health, 331t, 332
Administrative law, 257–261, *260*
Administrative model, of professional governance, 65
Administrative Procedure Act, 260
Adult learner, 56–57
Advance directive, 281
Advanced practice nurse, 90–91
 as physician substitute, 237–238, 247
 history of, 20–22
 standards for, 222
 vs. physician, 259
Advocacy, client, 84–85, 276–278, 288
Aesthetic knowledge, 389, 390t
African-American nurses, history of, 16–18, *16*
Age, of nursing workforce, 193
Agenda for Health Care Reform, 22
AIDSLINE, 476t
Almshouses, 5
Alpha change, 426
Alternative therapies. See *Complementary and alternative practices and products.*
Altruism, 49, 52
American Association of Colleges of Nursing, 67–68, 217
American Nurses Association, 7, 65–66
American Nurses' Credentialing Center, 218
American Nurses' Foundation, 444
American Red Cross, volunteer nurse's aides program of, 15
American Society of Superintendents of Training Schools for Nurses of the United States and Canada, 7
Americans With Disabilities Act, 220t, 221, 261
Anaclitic depression, 318
Analyticity, critical thinking and, 413
Andragogy, 56–57, 390–391, 390t, 391t. See also *Patient teaching.*
Anger management, 340–341
Apitherapy, 367
Army Nurse Corps, 14
Ascorbic acid, 357t
Assault, 267–268
Assertiveness, in management, 171
Associate degree programs, 19–20, 30, 34t–35t, 40
Assumptions, 120

Attitudes, change of, 425–426, *425*
 in critical thinking, 410
Audiovisual materials, for patient teaching, 396, 397t
Authorization bills, 210
Autonomy, of nurse, 48t, 50, 55, 64
 of patient, 281
 of research subject, 458
Avoidance, in management, 172

B

Baccalaureate programs, 28–29, 34t–35t, 39–40
Balanced Budget Act, 186, 210–211, 220t
Battery, 267–268
Bee venom therapy, 367
Behavior, unpredictable, 437–438
Behavioral change, *425*, 426–427
Behavioral system model, of Dorothy Johnson, 132–133, 135t
Behavioral theories, of learning, 386–387, 387t
Beneficence, 280
Benner, P. A., novice-to-expert model of, 60–62, 61t–62t
Bergstrom, Nancy, 216, 224
Beta change, 426
Beta-carotene, 357t
Betts, Virginia Trotter, 216
Bias, cultural diversity and, 302–303
Bibliographic databases, 474–481, 476t–477t
 for evidence-based nursing, 481
 full-text links of, 481
 management of, 485–486
 MeSH terms for, 475, 477
 on Internet, 482–485
 records of, 475, 477
 search strategies for, 477–479
Biculturalism, 58
Bioelectromagnetic modalities, 368–369
BIOETHICSLINE, 476t
Biofield therapy, 363–364, 365t–366t
Blanchard and Hersey, situational leadership theory of, 163t, 166
Blue Cross, history of, 12
Board certification, 37–38
Board of nursing practice, 260–261, *260*
Bolton, Frances Payne, 14
Boolean operators, for database search, 477
Boundary, in systems theory, 97, 98
Breach of confidentiality, 269